Dimitrios Linos (Editor)
Jon A. van Heerden (Editor)

Adrenal Glands

Dimitrios Linos (Editor)
Jon A. van Heerden (Editor)

Adrenal Glands

Diagnostic Aspects and Surgical Therapy

With 187 Figures
in 251 Separate Illustrations, Mostly in Color
and 52 Tables

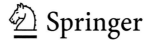 Springer

Professor Dr. Dimitrios Linos
Director 1st Surgical Clinic, Hygeia Hospital
227 Kifissias Avenue, 14561 Kifissia, Greece

Professor Dr. Jon A. van Heerden
Department of Surgery, Mayo Clinic
First Street SW 200, Rochester, MN 55905, USA

ISBN 3-540-41099-6 Springer-Verlag Berlin Heidelberg New York

Library of Congress Control Number: 2004104845

Springer is a part of Springer Science+Business Media
springeronline.com

© Springer-Verlag Berlin Heidelberg 2005
Printed in Germany

Editor: Gabriele Schröder, Heidelberg, Germany
Desk editor: Stephanie Benko, Heidelberg, Germany
Production editor: Ingrid Haas, Heidelberg, Germany

Cover-Design: Frido Steinen-Broo, Pau, Spain
Illustrations: Rüdiger Himmelhan, Heidelberg, Germany
Typesetting: Fotosatz-Service Köhler GmbH, Würzburg, Germany
Printing and bookbinding: Stürtz AG, Würzburg, Germany

Printed on acid-free paper.   24/3150 ih - 5 4 3 2 1 0

Preface

ως δ' εκείνον μεν ζων, δια τούτον δέ καλώς ζων.

(Πλούταρχος 75 π. Χ)

Plutarch wrote that Alexander the Great once said that he owed his life to his father but he owed learning how to live well to his teacher, Aristotle.

This book is a tribute to my teacher in surgery Jon van Heerden. "Jon," for his many friends, yet always "Dr. van Heerden" for me (who never managed to overcome the anxiety I felt, as a chief resident, when interrupting a golf game to discuss patient problems) has inspired many surgeons worldwide.

It is not accidental that in this book most of the renowned participants have been directly or indirectly students, and/or friends, of Jon van Heerden. The remaining contributors who are not surgeons have known, respected and admired him for his contribution to the field of adrenal surgery.

The magic of JvH, as he is affectionately known in the surgical community, is his keen insight into a complicated subject and his ability to transform complexity into simplicity. And thus even the complexities of some esoteric adrenal diseases are today readily understood by both generalists and specialists. One of his favorite quotes is in fact: "If it is not awfully simple, it is usually simply awful."

Skills can be sharpened, knowledge acquired, but what is even more important is the fact that some people transfer their knowledge to others. It could be argued that greatness in the intellect of a person is only surpassed by the ability to inspire greatness in others; this then is the essence of JvH, who once stated "The greatest satisfaction in surgery lies in the achievements which others are inspired to perform."

JvH was a Consultant at the Mayo Clinic for 31 years and has influenced and stimulated innumerable trainees to perform the Art of Surgery with integrity and humility. Many, many more surgeons have benefited from his devotion to teaching, educating, knowledge sharing, and technical pearls at meetings locally, nationally, and internationally.

As impeccable as he was in his lectures, he was even more meticulous in the operating room. His operating rooms at Mayo were models of decorum, punctuality, expert teamwork, attention to minutiae, the abhorrence of blood loss, and ultimate respect not only for tissues, but most importantly for the patient. He truly believed in the aphorism: "The most important person in the operating room is the patient – not the surgeon." Jon van Heerden was just and understanding but he was not lenient or flexible with members of the operating team and there was no margin for error.

In this book, integrity, skill, validity and reliability are among the qualities the authors have aspired to as they tackle the captivating "mysteries" that shroud the adrenal glands. Precision and concision were strived for in all chapters, which are both up to date and informative. With concrete data on the different aspects of adrenal anatomy, physiology and pathology, and the practical and appropriate application of the surgical treatment, the reader can expect to be challenged and enlightened, surprised as well as comforted, and foremost – educated.

I cannot stress adequately how indebted I feel to the gracious contributions from the world-renowned physicians and surgeons who rose to the challenge of producing this ambitious project with enthusiasm. Without their contribution this would have never been a possibility, since neither the editors nor the publishers would accept anything less than the very best available. A note of special thanks is due to Ms. Stephanie Benko, from Springer-Verlag, and to my assistant Mary Kostopoulou, who were both enthusiastic and tireless in their organizational skills.

Dimitrios A. Linos, MD, FACS

Preface

You, our readers, are justified to ask "Why is there a need for yet another textbook on a rare aspect of endocrine surgery?" We, your editors, albeit biased, feel that the answer is an affirmative one and is based on a number of closely interrelated factors.

Much has changed in the understanding, elucidation, and identification and management of almost all aspects of diseases that affect the adrenal glands. We have, indeed, come a long way since Thomas Addison in 1855 succinctly stated "It will hardly be disputed that at the present moment, the function of the suprarenal capsules, and the influence they exercise in the general economy are almost or altogether unknown."

Similarly, the surgical approach to these retroperitoneal glands has undergone an amazing revolution in the most recent decade. We wonder if Hugh-Young, famous for developing and popularizing the posterior open approach to the adrenal glands, could have, in his wildest dreams, ever imagined outpatient laparoscopic adrenalectomy. We think not!

Today, and in the future, the emphasis is going to be on teamwork with close cooperation and communication between many disciplines when caring for patients with adrenal pathology. Surgeons, in particular, will need to change their daily vocabulary from *I* to *we*. This is an essential factor which this textbook hopefully clearly emphasizes and exemplifies, and the various disciplines are indeed well represented by our contributors.

The medical/surgical world is shrinking due to improved and rapid communications and ease of travel. The contributors to this volume represent many different countries, which is most gratifying. We believe that this international flavor will only increase in the future and that this increase is good for all concerned, patients in particular.

We are deeply indebted to all of the contributors to this publication, be they physicians, surgeons, radiologists, anesthesiologists, artists, or publishers. They have unselfishly given us and you not only their expertise but their most precious possession – their time.

Lastly, both of us stand on the shoulders of our teachers and our role models, who have enabled us to see a little further than perhaps they did. Humbly, we thus thank Jim Priestley, Bill Remine, Dick Welbourne, Sheldon Sheps, and Bill Young. You, our revered teachers, collectively exemplify to us the thoughts eloquently expressed by Halsted.

It is our sincere wish that you, who have honored us by reading this introduction and what follows, will derive a modicum of pleasure as you peruse *Adrenal Glands: Diagnostic Aspects and Surgical Therapy*. If you per chance read something that may benefit patient care, this educational endeavor will have been well worth the effort and our wishes shall have been granted and fulfilled.

Jon van Heerden

Table of Contents

List of Contributors

Åkerström, Göran, MD
Professor, Department of Surgery
Akademiska Sjukhuset, Uppsala Universitet
75185 Uppsala, Sweden
Email: goran.akerstrom@kirurgi.uu.se

Armstrong, Jonathan, MD, MB BS, FRACS
Priory Thatch, Priory Green
Dunster, Somerset, TA 24 6RY, United Kingdom
Email: zoedog68@hotmail.com

Ayala, Alejandro, MD
Pediatric and Reproductive Endocrinology Branch
National Institutes of Health
Building 10, Room 9D-42, 10 Center Drive
Bethesda, MD 20892, USA
Email: ayalaa@nih.gov

Beuschlein, Felix, MD
Abteilung Innere Medizin II
Schwerpunkt Endokrinologie & Diabetologie
Medizinische Klinik und Poliklinik
Universitätsklinikum Freiburg
Hugstetter Strasse 55
79106 Freiburg, Germany
Email: beuschlein@medizin.ukl.uni-freiburg.de

Boger, Michael Sean, MD, PharmD
Department of Internal Medicine
Wake Forest University Baptist Medical Center
Medical Center Boulevard
Winston-Salem, NC 27157, USA
Email: mboger@wfubmc.edu

Brauckhoff, Michael, MD
Klinik für Allgemein-, Viszeral- und Gefäßchirurgie
Martin Luther Universität Halle/Wittenberg
Ernst-Grube-Strasse 40
06097 Halle/Saale, Germany
Email: michael.brauckhoff@medizin.uni-halle.de

Charmandari, Evangelia, MD
Pediatric and Reproductive Endocrinology Branch
National Institute of Child Health
and Human Development (NICHD)
National Institutes of Health
31 Center Drive, Building 10, Room 9D42
Bethesda, MD 20892-1583, USA
Email: charmane@mail.nih.gov

Chrousos, George, MD
Chairman, Department of Pediatrics
Agia Sophia University Hospital
125-127 Kifissias Avenue
11524 Ampelokipoi, Athens, Greece
Email: chrousog@exchange.nih.gov

Doherty, Gerard M., MD
Professor, Section Head, General Surgery
A. Alfred Taubman Health Care Center
University of Michigan
Room, 2920, 1500 East Medical Center Drive
Ann Arbor, MI 48109, USA
Email: gerardd@umich.edu

Dralle, Henning, MD
Professor, Klinik für Allgemein-, Viszeral-
und Gefäßchirurgie
Martin Luther Universität Halle/Wittenberg
Ernst-Grube-Strasse 40
06097 Halle/Saale, Germany
Email: henning.dralle@medizin.uni-halle.de

Duh, Quan-Yang, MD
Professor of Surgery, Surgical Service
Veterans Affairs Medical Center
University of California
4150 Clement Street
San Francisco, CA 94121, USA
Email: quan-yang.duh@med.va.gov

España, Nayví, MD
Surgical Resident, Department of Surgery
Instituto Nacional de Ciencias Médicas
y Nutrición Salvador Zubirán
Vasco de Quiroga 15
Tlalpan 14000, Mexico City, MEXICO
Email: nayvi@hotmail.com

Farley, David. R., MD
Professor, Department of Surgery, Mayo Clinic
200 First Street, SW
Rochester, MN 55905, USA
Email: farley.david@mayo.edu

Gimm, Oliver, MD
Abteilung für Allgemein-, Viszeral-
und vaskuläre Chirurgie
Martin Luther Universität Halle/Wittenberg
Ernst-Grube-Strasse 40
06097 Halle/Saale, Germany

Gordon, Richard D., MD
Professor, Department of Medicine
Greenslopes Hospital
4120 Brisbane, Australia
Email: med.greenslopes@ug.edu.au

Hamberger, Bertil, MD, PhD, FRCS
Professor of Surgery
Department of Surgical Sciences
Section of Surgery, Karolinska Hospital
17176 Stockholm, Sweden
Email: bertil.hamberger@kirurgi.ki.se

Harris, Dean A., MB, ChB, MRCS
Clinical Research Fellow, Institute of Nephrology
College of Medicine, University of Wales
Heath Park
Cardiff, Wales CF14 4XN, United Kingdom

Heinz-Peer, Gertraud, MD
Assistant Professor of Radiology
Department of Radiology
Division of Surgical Radiology
Medical University of Vienna
Währinger Gürtel 18-20
1090 Wien, Austria
email: gertraud.heinz@meduniwien.ac.at

Hellman, Per, MD
Department of Surgical Sciences
Universiy Hospital
75185 Uppsala, Sweden
Email: per.hellman@kirurgi.uu.se

Herrera, Miguel F., MD, PhD
Professor, Department of Surgery
Instituto Nacional de Ciencias Médicas
y Nutrición Salvador Zubirán
Vasco de Quiroga 15
Tlalpan 1400, Mexico D.F. Mexico
Email: herreram@quetzal.innsz.mx

Hodin, Richard Aaron, MD
Professor, Chief of Endocrine Surgery
Department of Surgery
Massachusetts General Hospital
Gray 504, 55 Fruit Street
Boston, MA 02114-2696, USA
Email: rhodin@partners.org

Iacconi, Pietro, MD
Dipartimento di Chirurgia
Facoltà di Medicina e Chirurgia, Università di Pisa
Via Roma 67
56126 Pisa, Italy

Kaczirek, Klaus, MD
Department of Surgery
Section of Endocrine Surgery
Division of General Surgery
Medical University of Vienna
Währinger Gürtel 18-20
1090 Wien, Austria
email: klaus.kaczirek@meduniwien.ac.at

Kanaka-Gantenbein, Christina, MD
Pediatric Endocrinologist
Unit of Endocrinology, Diabetes and Metabolism
First Department of Pediatrics
Agia Sophia Children's Hospital,
University of Athens
Thivon 3 & Mikras Asias Street
11527 Goudi, Athens, Greece

Kurtaran, Amir, MD
Associate Professor of Nuclear Medicine
Department of Nuclear Medicine
Medical University of Vienna
Währinger Gürtel 18-20
1090 Wien, Austria
email: amir.kurtaran@meduniwien.ac.at

Kyrou, Ioannis, MD
16 Agias Aikaterinis Str.
17352 Agios Dimitrios
Athens, Greece
e-mail: kyrouj@otenet.gr

Lamb, M. Nicole, MD
Surgical Resident, Morehouse School of Medicine
720 Westview Drive SW
Atlanta, GA 30310-1495, USA

Linos, Dimitrios A., MD, Professor
Director of 1st Surgical Clinic, Hygeia Hospital
Consultant in Surgey, Massachusetts General Hospital
Boston, MA, USA
227 Kifissias Avenue
14561 Kifissia, Athens, Greece
Email: dlinos@hol.gr
Email: dlinos@hms.harvard.edu

Marescaux, Jacques, MD, FRCS
Chirurgie A, Hôpital Civil, IRCAD-EITS Institute
1 Place de l'Hôpital, BP 426
67091 Strasbourg Cedex, France
Email: Jacques.Marescaux@ircad.u-strasbg.fr

Mastorakos, Georgios, MD
3 Neofytou Vamva Str.
10674 Athens, Greece
Email: mastorak@mail.kapatel.gr

Merke, Deborah P.
Chief of Pediatric Services
Clinical Center of the National Institute of Child
Health & Human Development (NICHD)
9000 Rockville Pike
Bethesda MD 20892, USA
E-mail: merked@mail.nih.gov

Memtsoudis, Stavros G., MD
Department of Anaesthesiology
Preoperative and Pain Medicine
Brigham and Women's Hospital
75 Francis Street
Boston MA 02115, USA
Email: smemtsoudis@comcast.net

Miccoli, Paolo, MD
Professor, Dipartimento di Chirurgia
Facoltà di Medicina e Chirurgia, Università di Pisa
Via Roma 67
56126 Pisa, Italy
Email: p.miccoli@dc.med.unipi.it

Niederle, Bruno, MD, Professor
Professor of Surgery, Department of Surgery
Section of Endocrine Surgery
Division of General Surgery
Medical University of Vienna
Währinger Gürtel 18-20
1090 Wien, Austria
email: bruno.niederle@meduniwien.ac.at

Nuchtern, Jed G., MD
Associate Professor of Surgery and Pediatrics
Baylor College of Medicine
Texas Children's Cancer Center
6621 Fannin, CC650.00
Houston, TX 77030, USA
Email: nuchtern@bcm.tmc.edu

Pantoja, Juan Pablo, MD
Staff Surgeon, Department of Surgery
Instituto Nacional de Ciencias Médicas
y Nutrición Salvador Zubirán
Vasco de Quiroga 15
Tlalpan 14000, Mexico City, Mexico
Email: pantoja@quetzal.innsz.mx

Pattou, Francois N., MD
Assistant Professor of Surgery
General Surgical and Endocrine Unit
Hospital Huriez
Rue Michel Polonovski
59037 Lille Cedex, France
Email: fpattou@univ-lille2.fr

Perrier, Nancy Dugal, MD, FACS
Associate Professor of Surgery
Department of Surgical Oncology
University of Texas, MD Anderson Cancer Center
1400 Holcombe Boulevard
Houston, TX 77230-1402, USA
Email: nperrier@mdanderson.org

Proye, Charles A.G., MD, Prof.
Service de Chirurgie Générale Endocrinienne
Clinique Chirurgicale Est, Hôpital Claude Huriez
University de Lille
Rue Michel Polonovski
59037 Lille Cedex, France

Psoma, Maria, MD
Anesthesiologist, Hygeia Hospital
Consultant in Anesthesia, Mayo Clinic
Rochester, MN, USA
Kifissias Avenue & 4 Erythrou Stavrou Street
151 23 Marousi
Athens, Greece
Email: psoma.maria@mayo.edu

Reincke, Martin, MD
Professor, Abteilung Innere Medizin II
Medizinische Klinik, Universitätsklinikum Freiburg
Hugstetter Strasse 55
79106 Freiburg, Germany
Email: reincke@med1.ukl.uni-freiburg.de

Richards, Melanie L., MD
Associate Professor, Department of Surgery
University of Texas Health Science Center
Room 213E, 7703 Floyed Curl Drive
San Antonio, TX 78229-3900, USA
Email: richardsm@uthscsa.edu

Roman, Sanziana, MD, FACS
Assistant Professor of Surgery
Chief of Endocrine Surgery, Department of Surgery
Yale University, School of Medicine
333 Cedar Street
New Haven, CT 06520, USA
Email: sanziana.roman@yale.edu

Rubino, Francesco, MD
IRCAD-EITS Institute
1 Place de l'Hôpital, BO 426
67091 Strasbourg, France
Email: F.rubino@lycos.com

Russell, Heidi V., MD
Assistant Professor of Pediatrics
Baylor College of Medicine
Texas Children's Cancer Center
6621 Fannin
Houston, TX 77030, USA
Email: hvrussell@txccc.org

Shohet, Jason M., MD, PhD
Assistant Professor of Pediatrics
Baylor College of Medicine
Texas Children's Cancer Center
6621 Fannin
Houston, TX 77030, USA
Email: jshohetbcm.tmc.edu

Soler, Luc, PhD
IRCAD-EITS Institute
1 Place de l'Hôpital, BP 426
67091 Strasbourg, France
email: luc.soler@ircad.u-strasb.fr

Souvatzoglou, Athanasios, MD
92 Vassilis Sofias Avenue
11528 Athens, Greece
email: dkpim@ath.forthnet.gr

Stephen, Antonia E.
Division of Surgical Oncology
Massachusetts General Hospital
55 Fruit Street
Boston, MA 02114, USA
Email: astephen@partners.org

Stowasser, Michael, PhD, FRACP
Associate Professor, Hypertension Unit
Princess Alexandra Hospital
Wooloongabba
4120 Brisbane, Australia
Email: mstowasser@ug.edu.au

Sturgeon, Cord, MD
Department of Surgery
Veterans Affairs Medical Center
University of California
4150 Clement Street
San Francisco, CA 94121, USA

Swamidoss, Cephas, MD
Department of Anesthesiology
New York-Presbyterian Hospital
Weill-Cornell Medical College
525 East 68th Street, Floor G3
New York, NY 10021, USA

Thalassinos, Nikolas, MD
Professor
24 Ravine Street
11521 Athens, Greece
Email: endo.evangel@acisgroup.gr

Thompson, Geoffrey B., MD
Professor, Department of Surgery
Mayo Clinic and Mayo Foundation
200 First Street SW
Rochester, MN 55905, USA
Email: thompson.geoffrey@mayo.edu

Tsagarakis, S., MD
Department of Endocrinology
Diabetes and Metabolism, Evangelismos Hospital
45-47 Ipsilantou Street
10676 Kolonaki
Athens, Greece

Tsakayannis, Dimitrios E., MD
16 Karneadou Street
10675 Athens, Greece
Email: dtsak@ath.forthnet.gr

Tsigos, Constantine, MD
Professor, Hellenic National Center for Research,
Prevention and Treatment of Diabetes Mellitus
and Its Complications
3, Ploutarchou Street
10675 Athens, Greece
Email: ctsigos@hndc.gr

Udelsman, Robert, MD, MBA
Professor, Chairman, Department of Surgery
Yale-New Haven Hospital
330 Cedar Street, FMB 102
New Haven, CT 06520, USA
Email: robert.udelsman@yale.edu

Vassiliadi, D., MD
Department of Endocrinology
Diabetes and Metabolism, Evangelismos Hospital
45-47 Ipsilantou Str.
10676 Kolonaki
Athens, Greece

Walz, Martin K., MD
Professor, Abteilung für Chirurgie
Zentrum für Minimalinvasive Chirurgie
Kliniken Essen-Mitte
Henricistrasse 92
45136 Essen, Germany
Email: martin.walz@uni-essen.de
Email: mkwalz@kliniken-essen-mitte.de

Wheeler, Malcom H., MD
Professor, Department of Endocrine Surgery
University Hospital of Wales
Heath Park
Cardiff CF4 4XW, United Kingdom
Email: M.H.Wheeler@btinternet.com

Young, Abbie L., MS
Professor, Genetic Counselor
Minnesota Department of Health
717 Delaware Street SE
Minneapolis, MN 55440, USA
email: Abbie.Young@health.state.mn.us

Young, William F., Jr. MD, MSc, FACP, FRCP (Edin)
Professor of Medicine, Division of Endocrinology
and Metabolism and Nutrition, Mayo Clinic
200 First Street S.W.
Rochester, MN 55905, USA
email: Young.William@Mayo.edu

1 History of Adrenal Surgery

Dean A. Harris, Malcolm H. Wheeler

1.1 Introduction

The adrenal glands were first depicted by Bartholomaeus Eustachius in 1552. They were drawn onto copper plates, Eustachius being the first anatomist to use this method, and reproduced in print in 1563 [1]. The early anatomists such as da Vinci, Galen and Vesalius had overlooked the glands, first named "glandulae renibus incumbents" (glands lying on the kidneys) by Eustachius. Successive names include "glandulae renales", coined by Thomas Wharton, physician to St. Thomas' Hospital, London, in 1656 [2], and "capsulae suprarenales", used by Jean Riolan of Paris in 1629 [3]. The terms cortex and medulla, to describe the two component parts of the adrenal, were first used by Emil Huschke, anatomist and embryologist at Jena, in 1845.

The function of the adrenals was the subject of much speculation in the 19th century with the suggestion that they might release "a peculiar matter into the blood," or conversely "absorb humid exudates from the large vessels nearby". The fundamental, but controversial, proposal that the adrenal glands produced 'internal secretions' ('secretion interne') was made by the Parisian physiologist Claude Bernard in 1855 [4].

Remarkably, in the same year, Thomas Addison described 11 patients showing clinical features attributable to adrenal insufficiency, namely anemia, debility, feebleness of the heart, irritability of the stomach, and a change in skin color. The autopsy findings were adrenal destruction by unilateral or bilateral tuberculosis, metastatic carcinoma, or simple atrophy. These observations were presented to the South London Medical Society in 1849, focusing on the anemia component of the syndrome, but the classical description of Addison's disease (the eponym being ascribed by Armand Trousseau [5]) was published 6 years later as a monograph, *On the Constitutional and Local Effects of Disease of the Suprarenal Capsules* [6]. Although the publication stimulated much interest, some controversy, and important experimental work, the syndrome of Addison's disease was not universally accepted for many years.

Charles Édouard Brown-Séquard concluded that the adrenals were essential for life (*essentials à la vie*) after carrying out a series of experiments on dogs, cats, hares and guinea pigs in which bilateral adrenalectomy always resulted in death in a few hours and even unilateral adrenalectomy was often fatal [7].

William Osler was the first to attempt treatment of adrenal insufficiency in 1896, using an extract of pig's adrenal [8]. The isolation of epinephrine by Abel in 1897 [9], following Oliver and Schäefer's work with adrenal extract in 1894 [10], had attracted great interest, and the absence of this chemical was thought to be responsible for the weakness and low blood pressure of Addison's disease and the fatal consequences of adrenalectomy. Epinephrine was used at the Mayo Clinic in 1920 to treat a patient with symptoms of Addison's disease following nephrectomy [11]. Although administration of epinephrine resulted in temporary relief of the patient's weakness, he later succumbed. Others reported the lack of efficacy of this medullary hormone, and it soon became clear that Addison's disease affected the adrenal cortex only.

In 1926, cortical extracts were used successfully in adrenalectomized animals, but it was not until the 1940s that cortisone was isolated and synthesized, work led by Edward Kendall of the Mayo Clinic[12], and Tadeus Reichstein of Basle [13], later to be awarded the Nobel Prize for their remarkable achievements. It was realized that the adrenal cortex produced several steroids, with deoxycorticosterone being the first to be synthesized. Aldosterone, initially called electrocortin, was discovered later by James Tait and Sylvia Simpson in London [14], and was found to exert influence over electrolyte fluxes.

Development of techniques to measure urinary and plasma steroids subsequently facilitated the assessment of adrenal gland function and paved the way for the precise identification and investigation of a whole range of pathological conditions of the adrenals, including Cushing's syndrome, Addison's disease and Conn's syndrome.

In common with the investigation of most disorders of the endocrine glands, once the hormonal dysfunction has been confirmed it became necessary to localize the site of the pathological lesion. With regards to the adrenals there was an initial dependence upon the insensitive method of plain abdominal radiography. The first attempt of specific adrenal imaging was by retroperitoneal gas insufflation [15]. This technique was not reliable and many preferred pyelography. Caval venous sampling, first performed in 1955 to assay catecholamines, was a significant breakthrough [16]. The refinement of selective adrenal venous sampling subsequently aided localization of adrenal pathology, and indeed remains a most valuable diagnostic tool today [17]. Phlebography, whilst being a sensitive technique, was associated with complications such as adrenal rupture or gland infarction [18], and never really gained favor. Scintigraphy, developed by Beierwaltes and colleagues at Ann Arbor, Michigan [19], employed radiolabeled cholesterol and was useful to diagnose hyperplasia and functioning tumors of the adrenal cortex.

Cross-sectional imaging with computed tomography (CT) was first used in 1975 [20], and along with magnetic resonance imaging (MRI) [21] remains the mainstay of localization investigation today.

1.2   Milestones in the Surgical Treatment of Adrenal Disease

Despite a growing understanding of adrenal anatomy and physiology and several reports of surgical removal of pathologically enlarged adrenal glands it is believed that no adrenal tumor was precisely diagnosed preoperatively before 1905 [22].

Knowsley Thornton is thought to have performed the first successful adrenalectomy for suprarenal tumor in London in 1889, reported in 1890 [23]. The patient, a 36-year-old woman with hirsutism secondary to the tumor, survived 2 years, until the disease recurred. The tumor weighed in excess of 20 lbs, necessitating concomitant nephrectomy.

Although Harvey Cushing (Fig. 1) had defined the fundamental role of the pituitary basophil cell in Cushing's disease [24], others soon recognized that the development of Cushing's syndrome required the presence of the adrenal cortex [25]. Therefore exploration of the therapeutic avenue of surgical adrenalectomy for this disorder was the next logical step.

Results of ten adrenalectomies for Cushing's syndrome, performed by Walters and Priestley, were published in 1934 [26]. They found four carcinomas, one adenoma, three cases of hyperplasia, and two normal glands. Even when subtotal adrenalectomy was performed there was 30% mortality [27]. The outlook for patients undergoing adrenalectomy for Cushing's syndrome was dramatically transformed once cortisone became available for therapeutic replacement. The first recorded perioperative use of cortisone in adrenalectomy for Cushing's syndrome was in 1949 at the Mayo Clinic and the mortality rate fell to zero for the subsequent 18 reported cases [27]. Replacement cortisone therapy was then continued postoperatively, a procedure which of course today is routine practice. This development had a major impact on endocrine surgery, not only making adrenalectomy a safe procedure but also facilitating the operation of total hypophysectomy.

Two years after the discovery of aldosterone the syndrome of primary aldosteronism, characterized by hypertension and hypokalemia, was reported by Jerome Conn in 1955 [28] (Fig. 2). His patient was a 34-year-old woman suffering from tetany, periodic paralysis, paresthesia, polyuria, polydipsia and hypertension. She was thought to have bilateral adrenal hyperplasia, but at exploration of the right adrenal, a 4-cm cortical adenoma was discovered, removal of which cured the patient of her hypertension and metabolic abnormalities. Conn subsequently published details of 108 collected patients with aldosterone producing adenomas [29]. Seventy-nine of these underwent surgery, and hypertension was cured in 66%, improved in 20% but remained unchanged in 14%.

With the initial enthusiasm for diagnosing Conn's syndrome it was thought that the condition might account for a significant proportion of hypertensives, but by 1980 it was apparent that less than 1% of the hypertensive population suffered from this surgically treatable disorder.

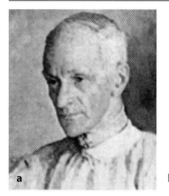
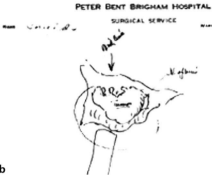
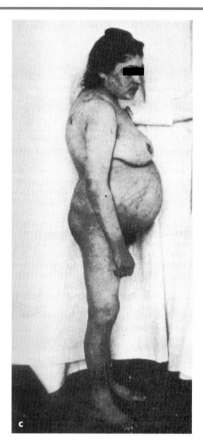

Fig. 1. a Henry Cushing as depicted in a portrait at the Peter Bent Brigham Hospital. **b** Cushing's surgical notes on a patient with the syndrome that bears his name, pituitary tumor. Taken from *Endocrine Surgery* (Linos 1984). **c** Minnie G., the first patient seen by Dr. Cushing, with the obvious signs of the disease that carries his name

Adrenaline was the first adrenal hormone to be discovered, but its crucial role in the clinical syndrome caused by pheochromocytoma was not defined until many years later when the hormone was extracted from adrenal tumors [30]. Fränkel provided the first report of a patient with a probable pheochromocytoma, an 18-year-old female suffering from intermittent palpitations, tachycardia and anxiety attacks [31]. She died after a severe episode of chest pain and dys-

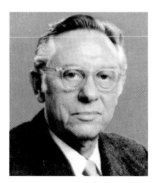

Fig. 2. Dr. Jerome Conn, Professor of Medicine at the University of Michigan. (From *Endocrine Surgery*, Linos 1984)

pnea, and at autopsy was noted to have highly vascular bilateral adrenal tumors. The term pheochromocytoma was coined by Pick [32] in 1912 and the first successful removal of a pheochromocytoma was by Cesar Roux in Lausanne in 1926 [33] followed by Dr. Charles Mayo in Rochester, Minnesota, the following year [34].

It soon became apparent that surgery for this condition was extremely hazardous with a high mortality related to the uncontrolled preoperative hypertension, severe hypertensive surges during intraoperative tumor manipulation and postoperative hypotension. With improving anesthetic techniques and a greater understanding of the pathophysiology of the disease, allied to the use of agents such as phentolamine and noradrenaline to control blood pressure, Priestley was able by 1956 to report a remarkable series of 51 patients undergoing surgery without any mortality [35].

Further advances in diagnosis with HPLC (high pressure liquid chromatography) methods for catecholamine assay, localization with CT, MRI or MIBG ($[^{131}I]$meta-iodobenzylguanidine), improved pharmacological control of blood pressure, evolving surgical methods and a multidisciplinary approach have now rendered the surgical treatment of pheochromocytoma a relatively safe event with a low morbidity and virtually zero mortality.

In the 1960s it had become apparent that pheochromocytoma could also occur in association with other endocrine tumors, including medullary thyroid carcinoma, within a familial setting as part of the MEN IIa and IIb syndromes [36, 37, 38]. The search for the underlying genetic defect coincided with spectacular advances in molecular biology and culminated in the identification of the RET proto-oncogene mutations on chromosome 10 [39]. These dramatic developments paved the way for genetic screening of family members predisposed to the hereditary forms of the disease.

The increasing application of abdominal cross-sectional imaging with CT and MRI resulted in adrenal lesions being discovered when investigations were performed for unrelated reasons. The vast majority of these so-called incidentalomas are non-secreting adrenocortical adenomas. The precise management of these lesions still remains somewhat controversial, but it is agreed that the key issues to be considered before making a decision to perform surgery are biochemical evaluation of possible hormonal secretory excess and assessment of malignant potential [40]. The advent of minimally invasive techniques for adrenalectomy, with their attendant minimal morbidity and mortality, has introduced the risk of changing the indications for performing adrenalectomy in these circumstances.

1.3   The Development of the Surgical Technique of Adrenalectomy

The first adrenalectomy was performed through a T-shaped subcostal incision similar to that previously described in 1882 by Carl von Langenbüch for cholecystectomy [41]. Most of these early operations on the adrenal were for the removal of large tumors, but because the incisions employed, whether anterior transperitoneal, lateral or retroperitoneal, were essentially similar to those used for renal surgery it was found that these approaches were frequently too low to permit adequate access. Therefore surgeons began to site their incisions at a progressively higher level usually resecting the 11th or 12th ribs. In 1932 Lennox Broster of London devised an operation which provided almost ultimate access to the adrenal, utilizing a transpleural, trans-diaphragmatic approach through a long, posterior intercostal incision [42]. In 1927, Charles Mayo used a flank incision when performing the first adrenalectomy in the United States for pheochromo-

cytoma [34]. Various anterior, lateral and retroperitoneal incisions became established each with their own merits and problems.

Anterior incisions, roof-top (bilateral subcostal) or midline permitted a full exploration of the abdominal cavity, especially important when operating for lesions such as pheochromocytoma which might be multiple or ectopic, before the development of accurate localization studies. The anterior approach still has special utility when operating for large tumors such as adrenocortical carcinoma. It is possible to gain excellent access by subcostal extension and on rare occasions even converting to a thoraco-abdominal exposure.

Lateral incisions with 11th rib removal gave excellent access, but bilateral pathology such as Cushing's syndrome due to hyperplasia required the patient to be turned to allow access to the contralateral side.

Hugh Young designed a posterior approach, removing the 12th rib, which would also permit bilateral simultaneous exposure of both adrenals [43]. Although an excellent method for removal of smaller tumors such as Conn's adenomas, access could often be difficult and totally inadequate for dealing with larger lesions over 5 cm in diameter.

Open removal of the adrenal was unchallenged until 1992, when Gagner [44] described a transperitoneal laparoscopic approach to the gland. This exciting new method was enthusiastically embraced by the endocrine surgical community and others described a posterior retroperitoneal endoscopic approach [45]. These methods have a wide range of application especially for Conn's tumors, Cushing's syndrome and pheochromocytoma, offering the patient very real benefits with respect to postoperative pain, speed of recovery and ultimately cosmesis. Laparoscopic techniques, however, are not generally appropriate for the removal of larger tumors >8 cm in diameter, malignant and potentially malignant tumors. However, it must be appreciated that this question of size and malignancy remains something of a gray area with divided opinion. The international body of evidence in favor of minimally invasive adrenalectomy for small, benign, functioning adrenal lesions suggests that this method is now the new surgical 'gold standard'.

References

1. Eustachii B (1975) Opuscula Anatomica. Quoted by Harrison TS, Gann DS, Edis AJ, Egdahl RH. Surgical disorders of the adrenal gland. Grune and Stratton, New York, pp 1–2

2. Wharton T (1659) Adenographia: sive Glandularum totius corporis descriptio, 2nd edn. (Coll: London: Socio) Amstelaedami, p 139

3. Medvei VC (1982) A history of endocrinology. MTP Press, Lancaster, England, p 125

4. Bernard C (1855–1856) Leçons de physiologie expérimentale appliquée à la médicine, 2 vols. JB Ballière, Paris

5. Trousseau, A. Bronze (1856) Addison's disease. Arch Gén Méd 8:478

6. Addison T (1855) On the constitutional and local effects of disease of the suprarenal capsules. S. Highley, London

7. Brown-Séquard E (1856) Recherches éxperimentales sur la physiologie et la pathologie des capsules surrénales. Arch Gén Méd (Paris) 8:385–401

8. Osler W (1896) Six cases of Addison's disease. Int Med Mag 5:3–11

9. Abel JJ, Crawford AC (1897) On the blood-pressure raising constituent of the suprarenal capsule. Johns Hopkins Hosp Bull 8:151–157

10. Oliver G, Schäefer EA (1894) On the physiological action of extract of the suprarenal capsules. J Physiol 16: 1–4

11. Rolleston HD (1936) The endocrine organs in health and disease, with a historical review. Oxford University Press, London, p 355

12. Kendall EC, Mason HL, Myers CS, Allers WD (1936) A physiologic and chemical investigation of the suprarenal cortex. J Biol Chem 114:57–58

13. Reichstein T (1936) Constituents of the adrenal cortex. Helv Chim Acta 19:402–412

14. Simpson SA, Tait JF, Bush JE (1952) Secretion of a salt retaining hormone by the mammalian adrenal cortex. Lancet ii:226–232

15. Cahill GF (1935) Air injections to demonstrate the adrenals by x-ray. J Urol 34:238–243

16. Melby JC, Spark FF, Dale SL, Egdahl RH, Khan PC (1967) Diagnosis and localisation of aldosterone producing adenomas by adrenal vein catheterization. N Engl J Med 277:1050–1056

17. Doppmann JL, Gill JR (1996) Hyperaldosteronism: sampling the adrenal veins. Radiology 198:309–312

18. Adamson U, Efendic S, Granberg PO, Lindvall N, Lins PE, Low H (1980) Preoperative localization of aldosterone-producing adenomas. An analysis of the efficiency of different diagnostic procedures made from 11 cases and from a review of the literature. Acta Med Scand 208:101–109

19. Thrall JH, Freitas JE, Beierwaltes WH (1978) Adrenal scintigraphy. Semin Nucl Med 8:23–41

20. Sheedy PF, Stephens DH, Hattery RR, Muhm JR, Hartman GW (1976) Computed tomography of the body: initial clinical trial with the EMI prototype. Am J Roentgenol 127:23–51

21. Sohaib SA, Peppercorn PD, Allan C, Monson JP, Grossman AB, Besser GM, Reznek RH (2000) Primary hyperaldosteronism (Conn syndrome): MR imaging findings. Radiology 214:527–531

22. Richards O (1905) Growths of the kidneys and adrenals. Guy's Hosp Rep 59:217–332

23. Thornton JK (1890) Abdominal nephrectomy for large sarcoma of the left suprarenal capsule: recovery. Trans Clin Soc Lond 23:150–153

24. Cushing H (1932) The basophil adenomas of the pituitary body and their clinical manifestations (pituitary basophilism). Johns Hopkins Hosp Bull 50:137–195

25. Kepler EJ (1949) Cushing's disease: a primary disorder of the adrenal cortices? Ann NY Acad Sci 50:657–678

26. Walters W, Wilder RM, Kepler EJ (1934) The suprarenal cortical syndrome. Ann Surg 100:670–688

27. Priestley JT, Sprague RG, Walters W, Salassa RM (1951) Subtotal adrenalectomy for Cushing's syndrome. Ann Surg 134:464–475

28. Conn JW (1955) Primary aldosteronism, a new syndrome. J Lab Clin Med 45:3–17

29. Conn JW (1961) Aldosteronism and hypertension. Arch Intern Med 107:813–828

30. Kelly HM, Piper MC, Wilder RM, Walters W (1936) Case of paroxysmal hypertension with paraganglioma. Proc Mayo Clin 11:65–70

31. Fränkel F (1886) Ein Fall von doppelseitigem, völlig latent verlaufenen Nebennierentumor und gleichzeitiger Nephritis. Virchows Arch Pathol Anat Klin Med 103: 244–263

32. Pick L (1912) Das Ganglioma embryonale sympathicum. Berl Klin Wochenschr 49:16–22

33. Mühl von der R (1928) Contribution à l'étude des paragangliomes. Thesis, L'Université de Lausanne, Lausanne, p 32

34. Mayo CH (1927) Paroxysmal hypertension with tumour of retroperitoneal nerve. JAMA 89:1047–1050

35. Kvale WF, Roth GM, Manger WM, Priestley JT (1956) Pheochromocytoma. Circulation 14:622–630

36. Sipple JH (1961) The association of phaeochromocytoma with carcinoma of the thyroid gland. Am J Med 31:163–166

37. Steiner AL, Goodman AD, Powers SR (1968) Study of a kindred with phaeochromocytoma, medullary thyroid carcinoma, hyperparathyroidism and Cushing's disease: Multiple endocrine neoplasia type 2. Medicine 47:371–409

38. Williams ED. A review of 17 cases of carcinoma of the thyroid and phaeochromocytoma. J Clin Pathol 18:288–292

39. Mulligan L, Kwok J, Healy C, Elsdon MJ, Eng C, Gardner E, Love DR, Mole SE, Moore JK, Papi L, et al. (1993) Germ-line mutations of the RET proto-oncogene in multiple endocrine neoplasia type 2A (MEN2A). Nature 363:458–460

40. Brunt ML, Moley JF (2001) Adrenal incidentaloma. World J Surg 25:905–913

41. von Langenbüch C (1882) Ein Fall von Exstirpation der Gallenblase. Berlin Klin Wochenschr 19:725–727. Quoted

by Welbourn RB in The history of endocrine surgery. Praeger, London, p 151

42. Broster LR, Hill HG, Greenfield JG (1932) Adreno-genital syndrome and unilateral adrenalectomy. Br J Surg 19: 557–570

43. Young HH (1936) Technique for simultaneous exposure and operation on the adrenals. Surg Gynaecol Obstet 63:179–188

44. Gagner M, Lacroix A, Bolte E (1992) Laparoscopic adrenalectomy in Cushing's syndrome and phaeochromocytoma. N Engl J Med 327:1033

45. Mercan S, Seven R, Ozarmagan S, Tezelman S (1995) Endoscopic retroperitoneal adrenalectomy. Surgery 118:1071–1075

46. Linos D (1984) Endocrine Surgery. BHTA Publications, Athens

2   Surgical Anatomy

Nancy Dugal Perrier, Michael Sean Boger

2.1   Introduction

The small paired adrenal glands have a grand history. Eustachius published the first anatomical drawings of the adrenal glands in the mid-sixteenth century [17]. In 1586, Piccolomineus and Baunin named them the suprarenal glands. Nearly two-and-a-half centuries later, Cuvier described the anatomical division of each gland into the cortex and medulla. Addison would describe the classical symptoms of the condition still bearing his name in 1855, igniting intense interest in the gland [1]. The next year, Brown-Séquard proved the vital necessity of the glands by performing adrenalectomies in animals [3]. Harvey Cushing described hypercortisolism in 1912, and Conn detailed primary hyperaldosteronism in 1955 [4, 6]. The first successful resections for pheochromocytoma were performed in 1926 by Charles Mayo in America and Roux in Switzerland [5]. Because of the relative frequency of adrenal disorders, endocrine surgeons must have a sound knowledge regarding appropriate management [11]. A solid understanding of adrenal anatomy lays the groundwork for future chapters in this textbook.

2.2   Morphology

The paired retroperitoneal adrenal glands are found in the middle of the abdominal cavity, residing on the superior medial aspect of the upper pole of each kidney (Fig. 1). However, this location may vary depending on the depth of adipose tissue. By means of pararenal fat and perirenal fascia, the adrenals contact the superior portion of the abdominal wall. These structures separate the adrenals from the pleural reflection, ribs, and the subcostal, sacrospinalis, and latissimus dorsi muscles [2]. Posteriorly, the glands lie near the diaphragmatic crus and arcuate ligament [10]. Laterally, the right adrenal resides in front of the 12th rib and the left gland is in front of the 11th and 12th ribs [2]. Each adrenal gland weighs approximately

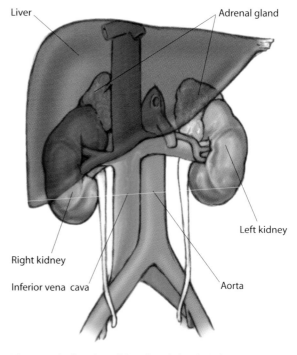

Fig. 1. In situ location of the adrenal glands. (After [10, p. 152])

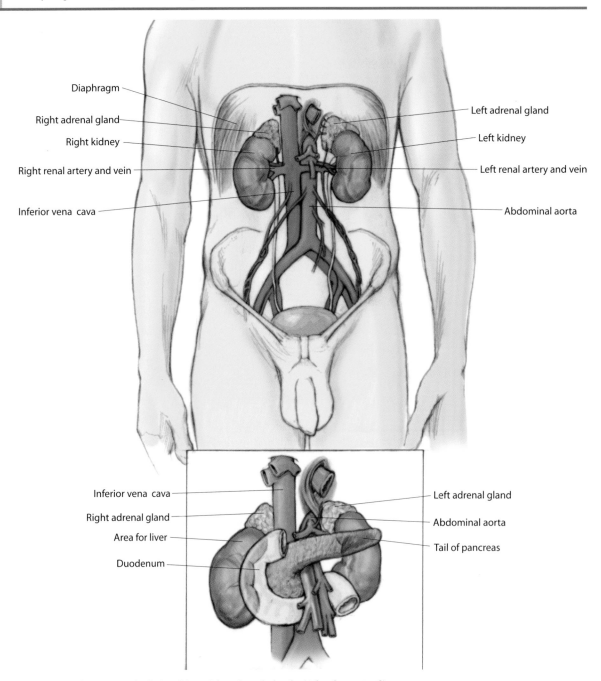

Fig. 2. Normal anatomical relationships of the adrenal glands. (After [12, p. 274])

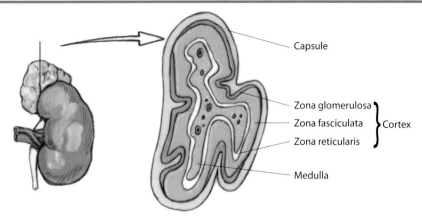

Fig. 3. Microscopic anatomy of the adrenal gland. (After [9, p. 1904])

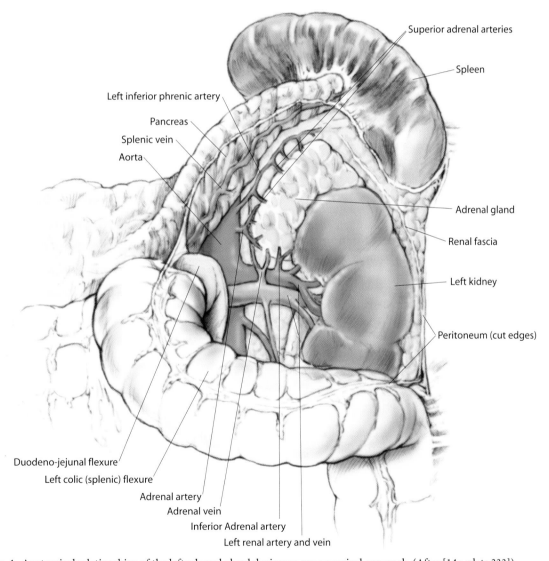

Fig. 4. Anatomical relationships of the left adrenal gland during an open surgical approach. (After [14a, plate 333])

3–6 g and measures roughly 5×2.5×0.5 cm [10]. Adrenal weight may increase by nearly 50% during periods of stress and pregnancy and pathologic glands may reach 700 g [12, 16].

The pyramid-shaped right adrenal gland (Fig. 2), sometimes called the "witch's hat," lies posterior and lateral to the inferior vena cava; it often touches the right diaphragmatic crus and bare area of the liver. The semilunar left adrenal gland (Fig. 2) is larger and flatter. It is located just lateral to the aorta, immediately posterior to the superior border of the pancreas, and medial to the superior pole of the kidney [8]. A thick, collagenous capsule sends deep trabeculae into the cortex and contains an arterial plexus supplying branches to the adrenal gland [9].

The adrenal cortex is a characteristic bright chrome yellow with a finely granular surface and firm consistency, allowing it to be readily differentiated from surrounding adipose tissue [2, 5]. The cortex is divided into three zones (Fig. 3) [9]. The *zona glomerulosa* secretes the mineralocorticoid aldosterone, which regulates salt and water homeostasis. The *zona fasciculata* secretes the glucocorticoid cortisol, which regulates carbohydrate metabolism. It comprises 75% of the cortical region [15]. The *zona reticularis* secretes sex steroids (progesterone, estrogen precursors, and androgens). The adrenal cortex is derived from the urogenital portion of the coelomic mesoderm [10]. The central medulla is dark red or pearly gray, depending on the blood content, and is rather friable. It secretes catecholamines which modulate the fight-or-flight response to stress [2, 5, 9, 14]. It originates from neural crest ectoderm and accounts for approximately one-tenth of the gland [9, 10]. It is completely enclosed by the adrenal cortex, except at the hilum [9].

True accessory adrenal glands contain both cortical and medullary tissue – these are very rare. However, nodules of adrenal cortical tissue are not uncommonly located in periadrenal fat, and ectopic cortical tissue may be found in the spleen, below the kidneys, or with the testes or ovaries [10]. Three percent of the general population has macroscopic adrenal nodules [12].

2.3 Relationship of the Adrenal Glands to the Kidneys

The adrenal glands are enclosed with their corresponding kidney via Gerota's (perirenal) fascia and are embedded in perirenal fat (Fig. 4) [10]. A transverse lamella separates the adrenals from the kidneys, enabling separate removal of either organ. The glands are attached to the diaphragm via ventral and dorsal layers of renal fascia, allowing them to move with the diaphragm, occasionally causing difficult hemostasis [2].

2.4 Blood Supply, Innervation, and Lymphatics

2.4.1 Arterial

The arterial supply of the adrenal gland is contributed by 12 small arteries from the aorta, inferior phrenic, renal and intercostal arteries. These tributaries branch to form a subcapsular arteriolar plexus from which capillaries enter the cortex in a radiating, spoke-like fashion (Fig. 5) [7, 10]. The adrenal arteries are also referred to as suprarenal arteries in many textbooks. The *superior adrenal artery* is a branch of the inferior phrenic artery and is located along the superior medial margin of the gland. The *middle adrenal artery* originates from the abdominal aorta. The *inferior adrenal artery* arises from the renal artery and is found along the inferior-medial margin of the gland [8, 16]. These arteries anastomose over the surface of the gland, and small unbranched arteries descend through the capsule. The right adrenal is mainly supplied by the superior and inferior adrenal arteries, whereas the left adrenal is mostly supplied via the middle and inferior adrenal arteries. Arterial and venous capillaries within the gland integrate the function of the cortex and medulla. Cortisol-rich effluent flows from the cortex to the medulla, where it stimulates the synthesis and activity of phenylethanolamine-*N*-methyl transferase, leading to the conversion of norepinephrine to epinephrine. Extra-adrenal chromaffin tissues lack this mechanism, thereby secreting mostly norepinephrine [16].

2.4.2 Venous

In contrast to the intricate arterial network, there is a single central vein exiting at the hilum of the adrenal glands (Fig. 5) [18]. Blood percolates within the gland from the medulla to the central medullary system, forming the large *adrenal vein*. Many accessory adrenal veins follow the course of the arteries and empty into the inferior phrenic vein, renal vein, or a venous arc in connection with the azygous system and posterior gastric veins. These collaterals form a caval or portal shunt and can enlarge with significant tumors [2].

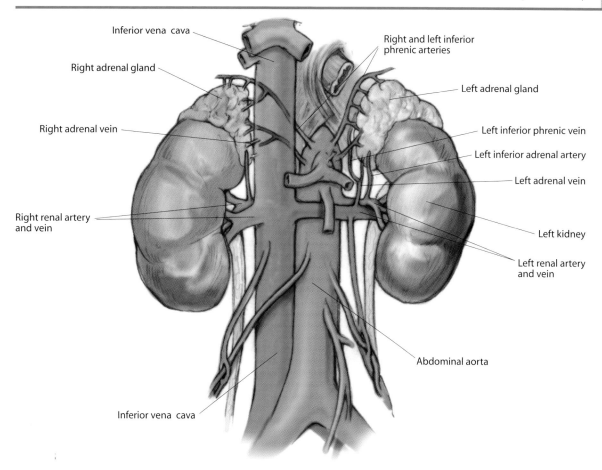

Fig. 5. Arterial supply and venous drainage of the adrenal glands. (After [12, p. 275])

2.4.3 Innervation

Innervation of the adrenal glands is via visceral affer- ent fibers arising from the *celiac, aorticorenal,* and *renal ganglia.* These fibers connect with the posterior *vagus nerve, phrenic nerve,* and greater and lesser *splanchnic nerves* (Fig. 6). They provide sensory or indirect vasomotor innervation as they pass through the cortex. They terminate in the medulla as pregan- glionic sympathetic fibers. It should be remembered that the adrenal medulla is a postsynaptic sympathetic nerve, belonging to the nervous system as such [2].

2.4.4 Lymphatic

The lymphatic drainage of the adrenal glands arises from a plexus deep in the adrenal capsule and a plexus in the adrenal medulla, emptying into the renal lymph nodes (Fig. 7). They follow the large vessels in three main pathways. On the right, a pathway terminates in the right lateral *lumbar (aortic) nodes* in front of the right diaphragmatic crus, proximal to the celiac trunk. A second pathway ends in the right lateral aortic nodes proximal to the junction between the left renal vein and vena cava. A third pathway ends in the *thoracic duct* or in the *posterior mediastinal nodes* after pierc- ing the crura of the diaphragm. This is an important route for metastatic spread of adrenal cortical tumors. Of note, lymphatic vessels drain only the cortex, not the medulla [2].

2.5 Left Adrenal Gland Relationships

The left adrenal gland is related to the left hemi- diaphragm, tail of the pancreas, splenic artery, and left renal vein (Fig. 8A, B). The visible relationships of the left adrenal gland during a laparoscopic approach contrast with those during an open surgical approach (Figs. 4, 9). This gland is crescentric, being convex medially and concave laterally. The superior border is

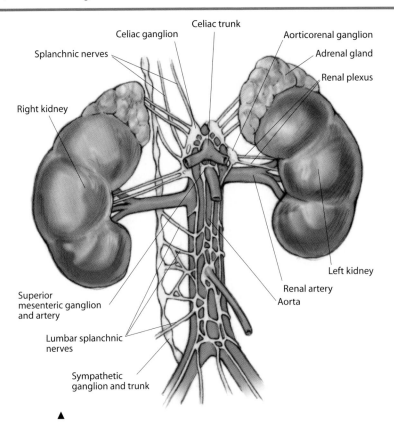

Fig. 6. Innervation of the adrenal glands. (After [1a, p. 157])

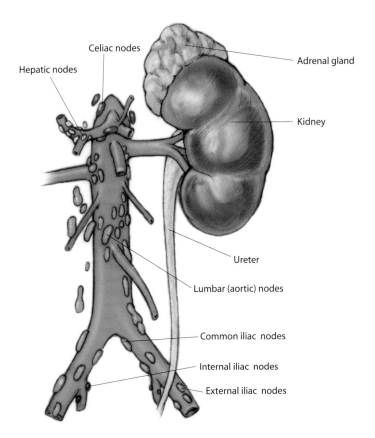

Fig. 7. Lymphatics of the adrenal glands. (After [14, p. 290])

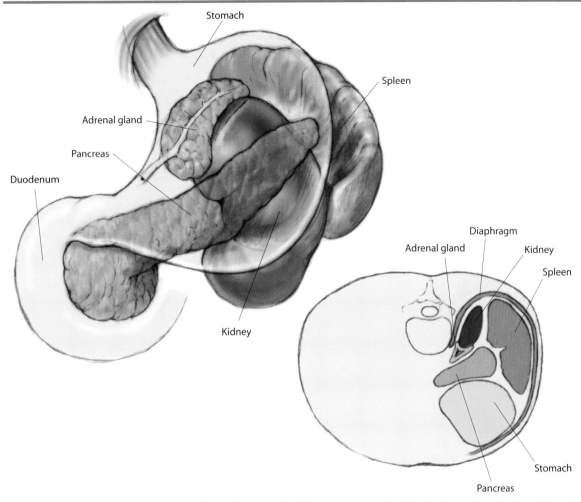

Fig. 8. Anterior anatomical relationships of the left adrenal gland. Posterior anatomical relationships of the left adrenal gland. (After [9, p. 1902])

sharp and the inferior border is rounded. In contrast to the right adrenal gland, the superior half of the *anterior surface* of the left adrenal gland is covered anteriorly via peritoneum of the lesser sac (Fig. 10) [18]. This separates the gland from the cardia of the stomach and the posterior pole of the spleen. Inferiorly, where the gland contacts the pancreas and splenic artery, there is no peritoneum [9, 18]. The left adrenal vein emerges at the hilum of the gland. A ridge divides the *posterior surface* into a lateral area adjoining the kidney and a smaller medial region contacting the left crus of the diaphragm. The *medial border* is convex and related to the inferomedial left celiac ganglion and to the left inferior phrenic and left gastric arteries, which ascend on the left diaphragmatic crus [9].

The ventral aspect of the left adrenal gland is attached to the dorsal viscera of the stomach and to the medial border of the spleen and the body of the pancreas. Both the splenic vein and the splenic artery are inferior to the left adrenal gland. The avascular segment of the gastrocolic ligament is commonly divided during surgery on the left adrenal gland. The transverse mesocolon attaches along the inferior border of the pancreas; it is retracted inferiorly and medially for operative exposure [2].

The left adrenal gland is located in front of the origin of the celiac trunk but it is separated from the aorta by a space of several millimeters [2]. The left adrenal vein is approximately 2–3 cm long, passing inferiorly from the lower pole of the gland, receiving the inferior phrenic vein, then taking an oblique downward course to enter the left renal vein (Fig. 5) [2, 8]. Occasionally, the vein empties into the left inferior phrenic vein (which then enters into the left renal vein)

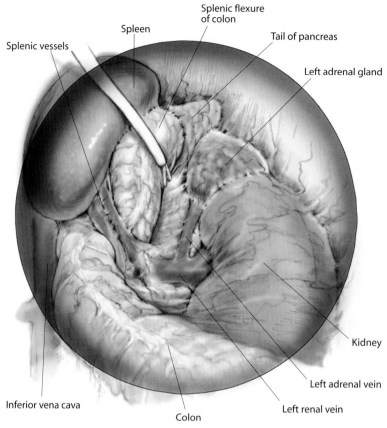

Fig. 9. Anatomical relationships of the left adrenal gland during a laparoscopic approach. (After [18, pp. 172, 173])

or crosses over the aorta to enter directly into the inferior vena cava [10]. The length of the left adrenal vein allows for ready vascular control during left adrenalectomy [2].

2.6   Right Adrenal Gland Relationships

The right adrenal gland is posterior to the inferior vena cava and right hepatic lobe and anterior to the diaphragm and superior pole of the right kidney (Fig. 11A, B) [9]. The anatomical relationships of the right adrenal gland appear quite different in a laparoscopic versus an open surgical approach (Figs. 12, 13). The *anterior surface*, which faces slightly laterally, has a narrow vertical medial area devoid of peritoneum which is posterior to the inferior vena cava. The anterior surface is nearly totally covered by the bare area of the liver (Fig. 10) [10, 18]. The upper portion of the lateral triangular area is also devoid of peritoneum and contacts the inferomedial angle of the bare area of the liver. The inferior portion of the lateral part may be

covered by peritoneum reflected from the inferior layer of the coronary ligament; the duodenum may overlap this region as well. Below the apex, near the anterior border of the gland, is the short hilum where the right adrenal vein emerges to join the inferior vena cava [9].

The ventral-lateral region of the right adrenal gland is overlapped by the peritoneum between the liver, kidney, and hepatic flexure of the colon [18]. The ventral-medial area is behind the inferior vena cava, separating the gland from the epiploic foramen anteriorly and the third portion of the duodenum and pancreatic head posteriorly. The body of the pancreas separates the adrenal gland from the lesser sac (omental

Fig. 10 (above). Peritoneal attachments of the adrenal glands. ▶ (After [18, p. 169])

Fig. 11 (below). A Anterior anatomical relationships of the right adrenal gland. **B** Posterior anatomical relationships of the right adrenal gland. (After [9, p. 1902])

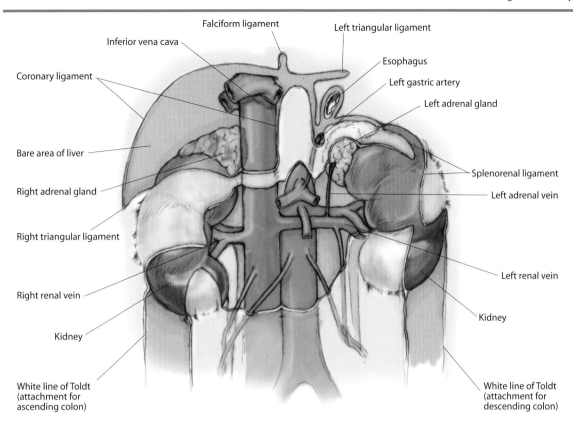

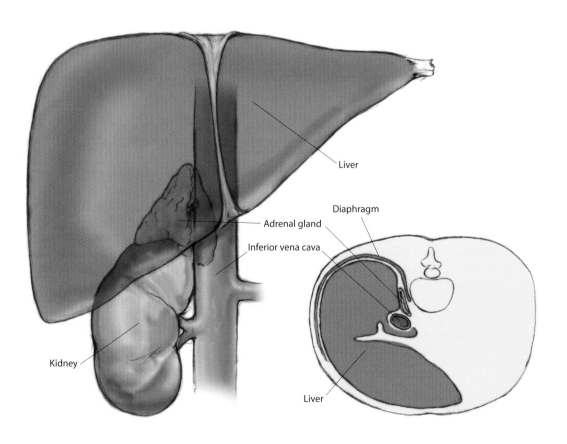

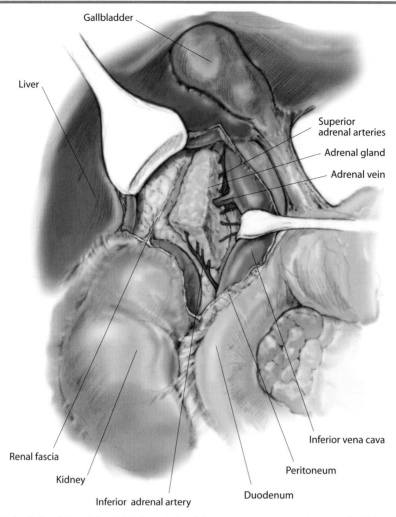

Fig. 12. Anatomical relationships of the right adrenal gland during an open surgical approach. (After [14a, plate 333])

bursa) and stomach [2]. The *posterior surface* is divided into upper and lower areas via a curved transverse ridge: its upper area, slightly convex, rests on the diaphragm, while the lower concave area contacts the superior pole and adjacent anterior surface of the right kidney. The thin *medial border* is related to the right celiac ganglion and the right inferior phrenic artery [9]. The medial border contacts, and may extend posteriorly towards, the inferior vena cava and is sometimes tucked behind it [10, 18]. If the inferior layer of the right coronary ligament is high, the right adrenal gland may partially reside in the right paracolic gutter (Morrison's pouch) where it contacts the peritoneum [18].

The right adrenal vein exits the hilum on the anteromedial surface of the gland (Fig. 5) [18]. It emerges for a mere 1 cm and takes a short, almost transverse route, at a 45° angle, to empty into the posterior segment of the inferior vena cava [8, 18]. The right adrenal vein cannot be exposed until the adrenal gland is mobilized [18]. The origin of this vein may be obscured by an enlarged gland. This is extremely important since accidental nicking of the inferior vena cava during adrenalectomy may cause fatal hemorrhage [2, 13]. Therefore, expert care is necessary when dissecting the right adrenal vein [12]. The right inferior phrenic vein is usually very small and is a direct tributary of the inferior vena cava [18]. Additional smaller veins are found in 5–10% of right adrenal glands. Rarely, aberrant veins may drain into the right hepatic vein or right renal vein. Knowledge of such anomalies is essential to avoid accidental ligation of the renal vein [12].

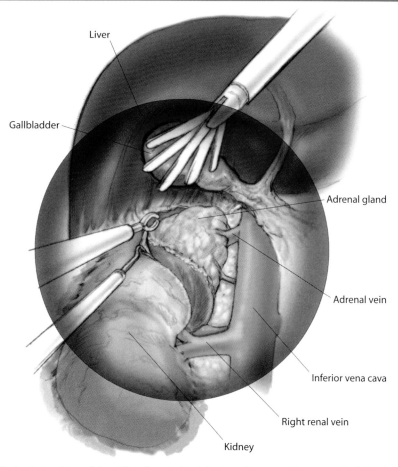

Liver

Gallbladder

Adrenal gland

Adrenal vein

Inferior vena cava

Right renal vein

Kidney

Fig. 13. Anatomical relationships of the right adrenal gland during a laparoscopic approach. (After [18, pp. 170, 171])

2.7   Summary

The adrenal gland represents two endocrine systems – the cortex and the medulla. Although these regions are small in comparison to many organs, they can lead to significant pathology from either primary or metastatic hyperfunctioning neoplasia or hyperplasia. The details of various adrenal disorders will be discussed in subsequent chapters. From the miraculous work of renowned surgeons like Mayo, Thorton and Young, adrenalectomy became a safe and effective therapy for adrenal disorders [12]. Because adrenal surgery is often the primary treatment modality for a multitude of adrenal conditions, a strong working knowledge of adrenal anatomy is essential.

References

1. Addison T (1855) On the constitutional and local effects of disease of the supra-renal capsules. Highley, London
1a. Agur AM, Lee MJ (eds) (1999) Grant's atlas of anatomy. Lippincott, Philadelphia, pp 273–288
2. Avisse C, Marcus C, Patey M, Ladam-Marcus V, et al (2000) Surgical anatomy and embryology of the adrenal glands. Surg Clin North Am 80:403–415
3. Brown-Séquard CE (1856) Recherches experimentales sur la physiologie et la pathologie des capsules adrenals. Arch Gen Med 5:385–401
4. Conn JW (1955) Primary aldosteronism, a new clinical entity. J Lab Clin Med 45:3–17
5. Couldwell WT, Simard MF, Weiss MH, Norton JA (1999) Pituitary and adrenal. In: Schwartz SI, Shires GT, Spencer FC, Daly JM, et al (eds) Principles of surgery. McGraw-Hill, New York, pp 1613–1661
6. Cushing H (1932) The basophil adenomas of the pituitary body and their clinical manifestations (pituitary basophilism). Bull Johns Hopkins Hosp 50:137–195

7. Dobbie JW, Symington T (1966) The human adrenal gland with special reference to the vasculature. J Endocrinol 34:479–489

8. Duh QY, Lui C, Tyrrell JB, Biglieri EG (2003) Adrenals. In: Way LW, Doherty GM (eds) Current surgical diagnosis and treatment. Lange, New York, pp 797–813

9. Dyson M (1995) Endocrine system. In: Bannister LH, Berry MM, Collins P, Dyson M, et al (eds) Gray's anatomy. Churchill Livingstone, New York, pp 1882–1907

10. Edis AJ, Grant CS, Egdahl RH (1984) Surgery of the adrenals. In: Edis AJ, Grant CS, Egdahl RH (eds) Manual of endocrine surgery. Springer-Verlag, New York, pp 151–242

11. Jossart GH, Burpee SE, Gagner M (2000) Surgery of the adrenal glands. Endocrinol Metab Clin North Am 29:57–68

12. Kebebew E, Duh QY (2001) Operative strategies for adrenalectomy. In: Doherty GM, Skogsed B (eds) Surgical endocrinology. Lippincott, Philadelphia, pp 273–288

13. Libertino JA (1988) Surgery of adrenal disorders. Surg Clin North Am 68:1027–1056

14. Moore KL, Dalley AF (1999) Abdomen. In: Moore KL, Dalley AF (eds) Clinically oriented anatomy. Lippincott, Philadelphia, pp 174–330

14a. Netter FH (2003) Atlas of human anatomy. Icon Learning Systems, Teterboro

15. Neville AM, O'Hare MJ (1985) Histopathology of the human adrenal cortex. Clin Endocrinol Metab 14:791–820

16. Newsome HH (2001) Adrenal glands. In: Greenfield LJ, Mulloholland MW, Oldham KT, Zelenock GB, et al (eds) Surgery: scientific principles and practice. Lippincott, Philadelphia, pp 1307–1323

17. Norton JA (1999) Adrenal. In: Schwartz SI, Shires GT, Spencer FC, Daly JM, et al (eds) Principles of surgery. McGraw-Hill, New York, pp 1630–1655

18. Paterson EJ (2002) Laparascopic adrenal anatomy. In: Gagner M, Inabnet WB (eds) Minimally invasive endocrine surgery. Lippincott, Philadelphia, pp 167–173

3 Hypothalamic-Pituitary-Adrenal Axis

Ioannis Kyrou, Constantine Tsigos

CONTENTS

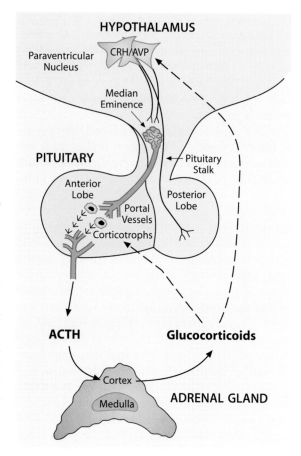

Fig. 1. A schematic representation of the components of the hypothalamic-pituitary-adrenal axis and their hormonal interactions. Stimulatory effects are represented by *solid lines* and inhibitory effects by *dashed lines* (*CRH*, corticotropin-releasing hormone; *AVP*, arginine vasopressin)

3.1   Introduction

The hypothalamic-pituitary-adrenal (HPA) axis outlines the tight hormonal coupling of the hypothalamus, the anterior pituitary and the adrenal cortex (Fig. 1). A linear progression characterizes the downstream activation of the axis while reciprocal feedback loops exist at each level to fine-tune the potency of the response and ensure optimal hormone secretions. The HPA axis is a vital component of the stress system and mediates a variety of adaptive responses to stressors that threaten body homeostasis. Basal and stress-related homeostasis depend on the integrity of the HPA axis, which additionally exerts profound regulatory effects on other systems (immune, endocrine and metabolic) in order to orchestrate a response that will allow endurance against any imposed challenge and preserve the internal milieu. Dysfunction at any level of the HPA axis can cause either prolonged or inadequate activation and leads to syndromal states that consistently share various degrees of impaired response to stress.

3.2   HPA Axis: A Multilevel Endocrine System

3.2.1   Hypothalamus: Corticotropin-Releasing Hormone and Arginine Vasopressin

The hypothesis that pituitary corticotropin (ACTH) secretion is controlled by a hypothalamic factor was first suggested in the late 1940s. A decade later, in vitro studies supported the existence of such a hypothalamic corticotropin-releasing factor by demonstrating that hypothalamic extracts could stimulate pituitary corticotroph cells to secrete ACTH. In 1981, Vale and his colleagues announced the sequence of a 41-amino-acid peptide from ovine hypothalami, designated corticotropin-releasing hormone (CRH), which showed greater ACTH-releasing potency in vitro and in vivo than any other previously identified endogenous or synthetic peptide.

Following the isolation of CRH, data from anatomic, pharmacologic, and behavioral studies made evident that CRH not only triggers the hormonal cascade of the HPA axis but also plays a complex role in the response to stressors. The wide distribution of CRH receptors in many extrahypothalamic sites of the brain, including parts of the limbic system and the central arousal-sympathetic systems in the brain stem and spinal cord, suggests the implication of CRH in a broader spectrum of neural circuits that control the stress response. In addition, experimental studies proved that central administration of CRH sets into motion a coordinated series of physiologic and behavioral responses, which apart from the activation of the pituitary-adrenal axis and the sympathetic nervous system, also include enhanced arousal, suppression of appetite and sexual behaviors, hypothalamic hypogonadism, and changes in motor activity, all characteristic of stress behaviors [95, 105, 110]. Conversely, central administration of CRH peptide antagonists suppresses many aspects of the stress response. Finally, CRH type 1 receptor knockout mice are characterized by a striking failure to properly answer to induced stress [108].

An intricate neuronal network regulates the secretion of hypothalamic CRH from parvicellular neurons of the paraventricular nucleus (PVN) (Fig. 2). These neurons have axons that terminate in the median eminence and secrete CRH into the hypophyseal portal system and axons that terminate in the locus ceruleus (LC)/norepinephrine (NE) sympathetic system neurons in the brainstem [28, 101]. Neurons of the latter systems send projections, mostly noradrenergic, to the PVN [30]. Thus, a reverberatory neural circuit is formed between the CRH neurons and those of the LC/NE sympathetic systems, with CRH and norepinephrine stimulating each other (Fig. 2) [16, 125]. Furthermore, CRH activates an ultra-short negative feedback loop on the CRH neurons [18], while a similar loop exists in the LC/NE-sympathetic system neurons, with norepinephrine inhibiting its own secretion via collateral branches and inhibitory α_2-noradrenergic receptors [1, 41]. In addition, neurotransmitters from parallel neuronal systems, like serotonin, acetylcholine, catecholamines (α_1-receptors) and neuropeptide Y, stimulate CRH secretion [18, 44], whereas the GABA/benzodiazepine system and endogenous opioids exert inhibitory effects [17, 82]. Regulatory opioid peptides are also produced by arcuate nucleus proopiomelanocortin (POMC) neurons that produce ACTH, α-MSH, and β-endorphin, all of which are inhibitory to CRH secretion [17, 82], and by CRH and arginine vasopressin (AVP) neurons which co-secrete dynorphin along with CRH and AVP [97]. A significant long negative feedback loop is also mediated by the glucocorticoids released from the adrenal cortex in response to ACTH in order to inhibit the prolongation of pituitary ACTH secretion and the activation of the hypothalamic CRH neurons and the LC/NE sympathetic systems [18, 71]. It is obvious that CRH secretion is tightly interweaved in the neurocircuitry of stress, which utilizes a complex network of interacting pathways in order to initiate and orchestrate an effective response to stressors.

In the hormonal cascade of the HPA axis activation, CRH exerts its effect on pituitary ACTH secretion via high-affinity transmembrane CRH receptors on the corticotrophs that couple to guanine nucleotide-binding proteins and stimulate the release of ACTH by a cAMP-dependent mechanism [2]. In addition to enhancing ACTH secretion, CRH also stimulates the de novo biosynthesis of POMC, the ACTH precursor, in corticotrophs resulting in a biphasic release of ACTH [71]. Two distinct CRH receptor subtypes (CRH-R1 and CRH-R2) have been characterized, encoded by distinct genes that are differentially expressed [21, 121]. CRH-R1 is the most abundant subtype found in anterior pituitary and is also widely distributed in the brain. The CRH-R2 subtype is expressed mainly in the peripheral vasculature and the heart, as well as in subcortical structures of the brain [132]. It is notable that CRH availability is also regulated by specific binding of the peptide to CRH binding protein [83], with which it partially colocalizes in various tissues [84].

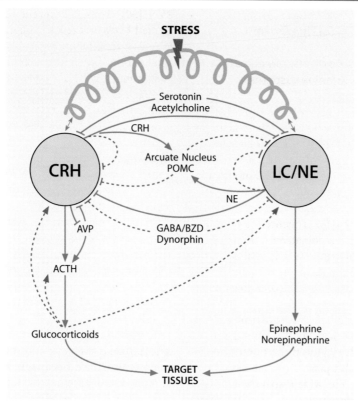

Fig. 2. A simplified, schematic representation of the intricate neuronal network that regulates the secretion of hypothalamic corticotropin-releasing hormone (*CRH*) from parvicellular neurons of the paraventricular nucleus (*PVN*). The HPA axis is tightly integrated with the main central nervous systems involved in the stress response. Activation is represented by *solid lines* and inhibition by *dashed lines* (*CRH*, corticotropin-releasing hormone; *ACTH*, corticotropin; *POMC*, pro-opiomelanocortin; *LC/NE*, locus ceruleus/norepinephrine-sympathetic system; *AVP*, arginine vasopressin; *GABA*, γ-aminobutyric acid; *BZD*, benzodiazepine)

At the level of the anterior pituitary, CRH is the most potent but not the sole regulator of the corticotroph ACTH secretion. AVP, a nonapeptide also produced by parvicellular neurons of the PVN and secreted into the hypophyseal portal system, is considered the second most important modulator of pituitary ACTH secretion [9]. Whereas CRH appears to directly stimulate the ACTH secretion, AVP and other factors, such as angiotensin II, have synergistic or additive effects [45, 94, 124]. AVP shows synergy with CRH in vivo, when the peptides are coadministered in humans [67]. Furthermore, physiologic elevations of plasma AVP in response to hyperosmolality, apparently produced by magnocellular neurons of the PVN, have additive rather than synergistic effects with CRH on stimulating ACTH secretion [91]. AVP interacts with a V1-type receptor (V1β, also referred as V3) and exerts its effects through calcium/phospholipid-dependent mechanisms [8]. In nonstressful situations, both CRH and AVP are secreted in the portal system in a pulsatile fashion, with approximately 80% concordance of the pulses [7, 40]. It has been shown that during stress, the amplitude of the pulsations increases, whereas, if the magnocellular AVP-secreting neurons are involved, continuous elevations of plasma AVP concentrations are seen. The aforementioned data support a reciprocal positive interaction between hypothalamic CRH and AVP at the corticotrophs. It is noteworthy that oxytocin, a nonapeptide produced by parvicellular neurons of the PVN like AVP, has no significant ACTH-releasing action in humans in vivo, while in the rat it appears to be an important coregulator of ACTH secretion [92]. Finally, it should be mentioned that catecholamines stimulate CRH secretion but have no direct effects on human pituitary ACTH secretion, while ghrelin, a novel GH secretagogue factor, appears to stimulate predominantly the AVP secretion [6, 64].

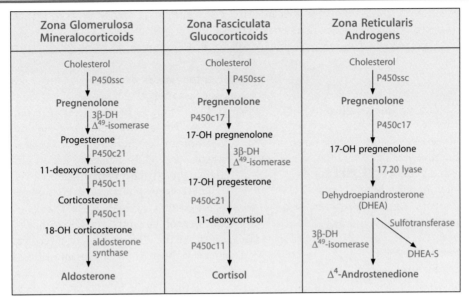

Zona Glomerulosa Mineralocorticoids	Zona Fasciculata Glucocorticoids	Zona Reticularis Androgens

Fig. 3. The pathway of steroidogenesis in the three zones of the adrenal cortex

3.2.2 Anterior Pituitary: Adrenocorticotropin

The signal of the initial HPA axis activation is transferred to the systemic circulation by adrenocorticotropin (ACTH). ACTH is a 39-amino-acid peptide secreted from the basophilic corticotrophic cells of the anterior pituitary which are distributed in the median wedge, anteriorly and laterally, and posteriorly adjacent to the pars nervosa. ACTH is a proteolytic product of a 266-amino-acid precursor, pro-opiomelanocortin (POMC) [38]. In the human anterior pituitary, POMC is processed into ACTH and two large polypeptides, N-terminal peptide and β-lipotropin, cosecreted in the circulation in approximately equimolar amounts [65, 79]. Subsequently, normal or abnormal regulation of ACTH secretion could be inferred by changes in the secretion of co-secreted products. Small, variable amounts of β-endorphin may also be produced and secreted by the human pituitary, but further processing of ACTH to smaller fragments, such as α-MSH and corticotropin-like intermediate lobe peptide (CLIP), does not occur in humans [65, 106]. It is of interest that the POMC precursor peptide is secreted in detectable amounts [115].

The regulatory influence of CRH on pituitary ACTH secretion varies diurnally and changes during stress [66]. The plasma ACTH concentration peaks at 6 A.M. to 8 A.M., and the lowest concentrations are found at about midnight. Episodic bursts of secretion appear throughout the day [58, 128]. The central mechanisms responsible for the circadian release of CRH/AVP/

ACTH in their characteristic pulsatile manner are not completely defined, but appear to be controlled by one or more central pacemakers [37]. Plasma cortisol concentrations generally follow those of ACTH, but owing to differences in bioavailability and pharmacokinetics between the two hormones, the correlation between their plasma concentrations is not perfect [54, 130]. The diurnal variation of ACTH and cortisol secretion is disrupted when a stressor is imposed or by changes in zeitgebers, e.g. lighting and activity.

The adrenal cortex is the principal target organ for ACTH, which acts as the major regulator of cortisol and adrenal androgen production by the *zonae fasciculata* (central zone) and *reticularis* (inner zone), respectively. ACTH is also essential for aldosterone biosynthesis from the *zona glomerulosa* (outer zone), although aldosterone secretion is primarily under the control of the renin-angiotensin axis [4, 111]. The biologic activity of ACTH resides in the N-terminal portion, with the first 24 amino acids necessary for maximal activity. ACTH interacts with specific high affinity cell membrane receptors (melanocortin receptor 2, MC2), expressed in all three cortical zones that couple to G-proteins to stimulate adenylyl cyclase and generate cAMP [76]. The latter activates a cAMP-dependent protein kinase, which stimulates cholesterol ester hydrolase, the key enzyme in the adrenocortical response of steroidogenesis to ACTH [51]. In addition, ACTH increases the uptake of cholesterol from plasma lipoproteins, enhances later steps in the steroidogenesis and has a trophic effect on the adrenal cortices (Fig. 3) [58]. It should be noted that ACTH when hypersecreted stimulates the melanocytes via the skin α-MSH receptor (MC1) [76], causing skin hyperpigmentation.

3.2.3 Adrenal Cortex: Glucocorticoids

At the level of the adrenal cortex, glucocorticoids synthesized in the *zona fasciculata* are the final effectors of the HPA axis and direct the stress response toward the goal of maintaining homeostasis. Cortisol, the main endogenous glucocorticoid in humans, is secreted by the adrenals into the circulation to reach the peripheral target tissues, where it exerts its effects via specific cytoplasmic receptors. In the unbound/inactive state, the glucocorticoid receptors are found as hetero-oligomers with heat shock protein (hsp) 90 and other proteins, which include hsp 70 and immunophillin [100, 107]. The ligand-bound receptors dissociate from the hetero-oligomer, homodimerize, and translocate into the nucleus, where they interact with glucocorticoid responsive elements (GREs) of the DNA to transactivate appropriate hormone-responsive genes [85]. The activated glucocorticoid receptors also interact at the protein level with the c-jun component of the activator protein-1 (AP-1) transcription factor, preventing this factor from exerting its effect on AP-1-responsive genes [57, 133].

Glucocorticoids play a key regulatory role on the basal control of HPA axis activity and on the termination of the stress response by acting at suprahypothalamic centers, the hypothalamus, and the pituitary gland [31, 42, 63]. The presence of a direct glucocorticoid negative feedback is crucial for the attenuation of the ACTH secretory response, in order to conserve the capacity of the HPA axis to respond to subsequent stressors. In addition, this negative feedback loop limits the duration of the total tissue exposure to glucocorticoids, thus minimizing the catabolic, antireproductive, and immunosuppressive effects of these hormones. Interestingly, a dual receptor system exists for glucocorticoids in the central nervous system, including the glucocorticoid receptor type I, or mineralocorticoid receptor, which responds to low levels of glucocorticoids and is primarily activational, and the classic glucocorticoid receptor (type II), which responds to higher levels of glucocorticoids and is dampening in some systems and activational in others [31].

3.3 HPA Axis: Other System Interactions

3.3.1 HPA Axis: Immune System

Over the last few decades compiling evidence has revealed a variety of interactions between the HPA axis and the immune system, suggesting an alliance of these systems against immune challenges. In states of inflammatory or immune stress, the overall adaptive mobilization of the organism can be described as a combination of the immune system activation and the typical stress response. Cytokines and other humoral mediators of inflammation have been proven as potent activators of the central stress response and can be regarded as the afferent limb of a feedback loop that mediates the immune system and HPA axis crosstalk (Fig. 4).

The three main inflammatory cytokines, tumor necrosis factor-alpha (TNF-α), interleukin-1, and interleukin-6, are secreted in inflammatory sites in a cascade-like fashion, with TNF-α appearing first followed by IL-1 and IL-6 in tandem [5]. Although TNF-α and IL-1α are primarily auto/paracrine regulators of inflammation, both can be found in the general circulation along with IL-1β and IL-6, the main

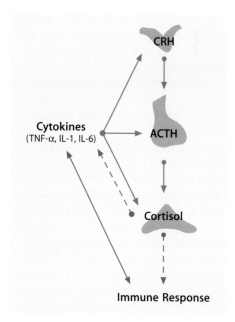

Fig. 4. A simplified, schematic representation of the interactions between the hypothalamic-pituitary-adrenal axis and the immune system. Stimulatory effects are represented by *solid lines* and inhibitory effects by *dashed lines* (*CRH*, corticotropin-releasing hormone; *ACTH*, corticotropin; *IL-1*, interleukin-1; *IL-6*, interleukin-6; *TNF-α*, tumor necrosis factor-α)

endocrine inflammatory cytokines [88]. All three inflammatory cytokines are able to directly and indirectly enhance the synthesis and secretion of CRH and AVP at the level of the hypothalamus and their effects are synergistic [13, 78, 102]. In addition, several eicosanoids and other inflammatory mediators such as platelet-activating factor (PAF), bradykinin, and serotonin show strong CRH-releasing properties [12, 44, 26]. Most striking has been the ability of interleukin-6 to acutely and chronically activate the HPA axis in humans [117]. The acute ACTH response to a single subcutaneous dose of IL-6 has been the highest ever seen in response to any stimulus, while antibodies to IL-6 almost completely block the stimulatory effect of bacterial lipopolysaccharide on the HPA axis [75, 14]. IL-6 seems to be the critical cytokine regulator in the immune stimulation of the HPA axis in chronic inflammatory stress. It is not clear, however, which of the above effects are endocrine and which are paracrine. Presence of cytokinergic neural pathways and local involvement of eicosanoids and PAF in CRH secretion are certain. Direct effects, albeit delayed, of most of these cytokines and mediators of inflammation on pituitary ACTH secretion also have been shown [43], and direct effects of these substances on adrenal glucocorticoid secretion also appear to be present [99, 131]. Finally, indirect activation of the HPA axis is also mediated through cytokine induced stimulation of the central noradrenergic stress system.

Conversely, activation of the HPA axis has profound inhibitory effects on the inflammatory immune response, because virtually all the components of the immune response are inhibited by cortisol (Fig. 4). Glucocorticoids act as potent anti-inflammatory and immunosuppressive factors by influencing the traffic of circulating leukocytes and inhibiting vital functions of the immune cells. Furthermore, they decrease the production of cytokines and other mediators of inflammation (e.g. platelet-activating factor, nitric oxide, prostanoids), induce cytokine resistance and inhibit the expression of adhesion molecules and their receptors on the surface of immune cells [77, 26]. It is interesting that glucocorticoids and catecholamines secreted during stress exert an immunomodulative effect by suppressing the T-helper 1 (Th1) response and causing a Th2 shift, thus protecting the tissues from the potentially destructive actions of type 1 proinflammatory cytokines and other products of activated macrophages [39].

An interesting aspect of the immune response is that CRH is also secreted peripherally at inflammatory sites (peripheral or immune CRH) by postganglionic sympathetic neurons and by cells of the immune system (e.g. macrophages, tissue fibroblasts) [61]. The secretion of immune CRH has been examined both in experimental animal models of inflammation [61] and in patients with rheumatoid arthritis [29] and Hashimoto's thyroiditis [112]. Immune CRH secretion is suppressed by glucocorticoids and somatostatin [61]. Mast cells are considered as the primary target of immune CRH where, along with substance P, it acts via CRH type 1 receptors causing degranulation. Subsequently, histamine is released, causing vasodilation, increased vascular permeability and other manifestations of local inflammation. Thus, locally secreted CRH has proinflammatory properties, whereas central CRH alleviates the immune response [26, 39].

3.3.2   HPA Axis: Other Endocrine Axes

The HPA axis is closely linked to the endocrine axes that control reproduction and growth. The survival of the individual and the species in general requires adequate nourishment, growth and reproduction, which are achieved through biologically costly pathways that threaten the stability of the internal milieu. Under conditions of serious danger to survival, the stress-dependent HPA axis activation intervenes to exert multilevel inhibitory effects on the gonadal and growth axes, until the imposed challenge is counteracted.

3.3.2.1 Gonadal Axis

The reproductive axis is inhibited at all levels by various components of the HPA axis (Fig. 5) [72, 86, 95]. At the hypothalamic level, CRH suppresses the gonadotropin hormone releasing hormone (GnRH) neurons of the arcuate nucleus. CRH-induced β-endorphin secretion by the arcuate POMC neurons mediates this suppression, but direct inhibitory action of CRH is also suggested [25]. In addition, glucocorticoids exert inhibitory effects on the hypothalamic GnRH neuron, the pituitary gonadotroph, and the gonads themselves and render target tissues of sex steroids resistant to their actions [86]. Hypothalamic functional amenorrhea is a typical example of stress induced inhibition of the female reproductive axis, while suppression of the gonadal function by chronic HPA axis activation has been also demonstrated in highly trained athletes of both sexes and in individuals with anorexia nervosa or sustaining starvation [52,

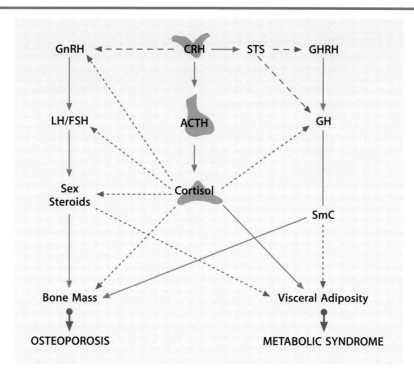

Fig. 5. A schematic representation of the regulatory effects of the hypothalamic-pituitary adrenal (*HPA*) axis on the reproductive axis, the growth axis and the metabolism. Dysfunction of the HPA axis may lead to osteoporosis and manifestations of the metabolic syndrome. Stimulatory effects are represented by *solid lines* and inhibitory effects by *dashed lines* (*CRH*, corticotropin-releasing hormone; *ACTH*, corticotropin; *GnRH*, gonadotropin-releasing hormone; *LH*, luteinizing hormone; *FSH*, follicle-stimulating hormone; *STS*, somatostatin; *GHRH*, growth hormone-releasing hormone; *GH*, growth hormone; *SmC*, somatomedin C)

68, 62]. It is interesting that during inflammation, circulating cytokines suppress the reproductive functions by activating the hypothalamic secretion of CRH and POMC-derived peptides, by enhancing the adrenocortical secretion of glucocorticoids and by inhibiting steroidogenesis at both ovaries and testes [93, 119].

Finally, a reciprocal interaction between CRH and the sex hormones is suggested by the presence of estrogen responsive elements in the promoter area of the CRH gene and by the direct stimulatory effects that estrogen exerts on CRH gene expression [126]. This finding implicates the CRH gene and consequently the HPA axis as a potentially important target of ovarian steroids and a potential mediator of gender related differences in the stress response and HPA axis activity.

3.3.2.2 Growth Axis

Growth is also sacrificed in order to preserve homeostasis under stressful conditions through a variety of inhibitory effects mediated by the HPA axis (Fig. 5)

[34, 96]. Prolonged activation of the HPA axis results in increased circulating levels of glucocorticoids which suppress the secretion of growth hormone (GH) and inhibit the action of somatomedin C and other growth factors on their target tissues [15, 122, 57]. However, it should be noted that at the onset of the stress response or after acute administration of glucocorticoids an acute elevation of growth hormone concentration in plasma may occur, presumably as a result of GH gene stimulation by glucocorticoids through glucocorticoid-responsive elements in its promoter region [19]. At the level of the hypothalamus, CRH stimulates the secretion of somatostatin, which is the most potent inhibitor of the growth hormone secretion by the somatotroph cells of the anterior pituitary, providing a centrally acting mechanism of growth suppression by the HPA axis.

The anabolic function of the thyroid gland is also interrupted by the activated HPA axis in order to conserve energy during stress. Increased circulating levels of glucocorticoids suppress the pituitary production of thyroid-stimulating hormone (TSH) and inhibit the conversion of the relatively inactive thyroxine to the more biologically active triiodothyronine in peripheral tissues (the "euthyroid sick" syndrome) [11, 36]. Inhibition of TRH and TSH secretion by CRH-stimulated increases in somatostatin might also participate in the central component of thyroid axis suppression during stress. Especially in the case of inflammatory stress, inhibition of TSH secretion is attributed in part to the direct action of cytokines on the hypothalamus and the pituitary [112, 117].

3.3.2.3 Metabolism

Glucocorticoids, the hormonal end-product of the HPA axis, exert primarily catabolic effects as part of a generalized effort to utilize every available energy resource against the challenge posed by intrinsic or extrinsic stressors. Thus, glucocorticoids increase hepatic gluconeogenesis and plasma glucose concentration, induce lipolysis (although they favor abdominal and dorsocervical fat accumulation) and cause protein degradation at multiple tissues (e.g. muscle, bone, skin) to provide amino acids that would be used as an additional substrate at oxidative pathways. In addition to their direct catabolic actions, glucocorticoids also antagonize the beneficial anabolic actions of GH, insulin and sex steroids on their target tissues [27]. This shift of the metabolism toward a catabolic state under the control of the activated HPA axis normally reverses upon retraction of the enforced stressor. Indeed, chronic activation of HPA axis would be damaging as it is expected to increase visceral adiposity, decrease lean body (muscle and bone) mass, suppress osteoblastic activity and cause insulin resistance (Fig. 5). Interestingly, the phenotype of Cushing's syndrome, characterized by abdominal and trunk fat accumulation and decreased lean body mass, in combination with manifestations of the metabolic syndrome (visceral adiposity, insulin resistance, dyslipidemia, hypertension), is present in a variety of pathophysiologic conditions, collectively described as pseudo-Cushing's states. The pseudo-Cushing's states are presumably attributed to HPA-induced mild hypercortisolism or to adipose tissue-specific hypersensitivity to glucocorticoids [27, 118].

The balance of metabolic homeostasis is also centrally affected by the neuroendocrine integration of the HPA axis to the CNS centers that control energy expenditure and intake. Indeed, CRH stimulates the POMC neurons of the arcuate nucleus which, via α-MSH release, elicit antiorexigenic signals and increase thermogenesis [89]. Conversely, glucocorticoids at the hypothalamic level enhance the intake of carbohydrates and fat and inhibit energy expenditure by stimulating the secretion of neuropeptide Y, which is the most potent appetite stimulator [20].

3.4   HPA Axis: Pathophysiology

Generally, the activation of the HPA axis is tightly regulated and is intended to be acute or at least of a limited duration. The time-limited nature of this process renders the induced adaptive antireproductive, antigrowth, catabolic and immunosuppressive effects temporarily beneficial rather than damaging and prevents significant adverse consequences [114]. In contrast, prolongation of the HPA axis activation, as documented in chronic stressful conditions, would lead to the stress syndromal state that Selye described in 1936 characterized by anorexia, loss of weight, depression, hypogonadism, peptic ulcers, immunosuppression, adrenal enlargement and involution of the thymus and lymph nodes [104]. Because CRH coordinates behavioral, neuroendocrine and autonomic adaptation during stressful situations, increased and prolonged production of CRH could explain the pathogenesis of the syndrome [120].

The prototypic example of prolonged dysregulation leading to hyperactivation of the HPA axis is manifested in melancholic depression with dysphoric hyperarousal and relative immunosuppression [46]. Indeed, cortisol excretion is increased and plasma ACTH response to exogenous CRH decreased. Hypersecretion of CRH has been shown in depression and suggests that CRH may participate in the initiation or perpetuation of a vicious cycle. Thus, owing to chronically hyperactive CRH neurons, patients with melancholic depression may sustain several severe somatic sequelae, such as osteoporosis, features of the metabolic syndrome, varying degrees of atherosclerosis, innate and Th-1-directed immunosuppression and certain infectious and neoplastic diseases [26]. If untreated, these patients have a compromised life expectancy curtailed by 15–20 years after excluding suicides.

In addition to melancholic depression, a spectrum of other conditions may be associated with increased and prolonged activation of the HPA axis (Table 1) including anorexia nervosa [47], obsessive-compulsive disorder [56], panic anxiety [24], excessive exercising [70], malnutrition [73], chronic active alcoholism [129], alcohol and narcotic withdrawal [10, 90], diabetes mellitus [120], hyperthyroidism [59] and pre-

Table 1. Pathophysiology of the hypothalamic-pituitary-adrenal axis (HPA) axis

	HPA axis activity		
	Increased	Decreased	Disrupted
Severe chronic disease	+		
Melancholic depression	+		
Anorexia nervosa	+		
Obsessive-compulsive disorder	+		
Panic disorder	+		
Chronic excessive exercise	+		
Malnutrition	+		
Diabetes mellitus	+		
Chronic alcoholism	+		
Hyperthyroidism	+		
Central obesity	+		
Pregnancy	+		
Atypical depression		+	
Seasonal depression		+	
Chronic fatigue syndrome		+	
Fibromyalgia		+	
Hypothyroidism		+	
Post glucocorticoid therapy		+	
Post stress		+	
Postpartum		+	
Rheumatoid arthritis		+	
Cushing's syndrome			+
Glucocorticoid deficiency			+
Glucocorticoid resistance			+
Congenital adrenal hyperplasia			+
ACTH resistance			+

menstrual tension syndrome [87]. Notably, patients with central (upper body) obesity exhibit higher levels of circulating inflammatory cytokines [116] while a subpopulation of these patients were also found to have mild hypercortisolism [81, 27].

Pregnancy is another condition characterized by hypercortisolism of a degree similar to that observed in mild Cushing's syndrome, severe depression and anorexia nervosa. Gestation is the only known physiologic state in humans in which CRH circulates in plasma at levels high enough to cause activation of the HPA axis [103]. Although circulating CRH, which is of placental origin, is bound with high affinity to CRH-binding protein [69, 83], it appears that the circulating free fraction is sufficient to explain the observed hypercortisolism. Hypercortisolism of pregnancy is associated with suppression of hypothalamic secretion of CRH, persisting in the postpartum [49].

On the other side of the spectrum of HPA axis dysregulation, another group of states is characterized by hypoactivation, rather than sustained activation, in which chronically reduced secretion of CRH may result in pathologic hypoarousal (Table 1). Patients with seasonal depression and the chronic fatigue syndrome fall into this category [32, 127]. Similarly, patients with fibromyalgia have decreased urinary free cortisol excretion and frequently complain of fatigue [50]. Hypothyroid patients also have clear evidence of CRH hyposecretion and often present depression of the "atypical" type [60]. It is interesting that in Cushing's syndrome, the clinical manifestations of hyperphagia, weight gain, fatigue, and anergia are consistent with the suppression of the hypothalamic CRH neurons by the associated hypercortisolism [48].

It is believed that an excessive HPA axis response to inflammatory stimuli would mimic the stress or hypercortisolemic state and would lead to increased susceptibility of the individual to a host of infectious agents or tumors as a result of Th-1 suppression, but enhanced resistance to autoimmune/inflammatory disease [39]. In contrast, a defective HPA axis response to such stimuli would reproduce the glucocorticoid-deficient state and would lead to relative resistance to infections and neoplastic disease, but increased susceptibility to autoimmune/inflammatory disease, such as Hashimoto's thyroiditis or rheumatoid arthritis [26]. Thus, an increasing body of evidence suggests that patients with rheumatoid arthritis have a mild form of central hypocortisolism [22]. Dysfunction of the HPA axis may actually play a role in the development or perpetuation of autoimmune disease, rather than being an epiphenomenon [109]. The same rationale may explain the high incidence of autoimmune disease in the period after cure of hypercortisolism, as well as in glucocorticoid underreplaced adrenal insufficiency [74].

Disruption of the HPA axis may present as a result of destructive processes involving the hypothalamus, pituitary, or adrenal glands, leading eventually to adrenal insufficiency (Table 1). On the other hand, eutopic or ectopic autonomous production of CRH, ACTH, or cortisol results in the development of Cushing's syndrome and suppression of the hypothalamic CRH neuron and normal pituitary corticotroph. It is interesting that the HPA axis of patients cured from Cushing's syndrome or after discontinuation of chronic glucocorticoid therapy requires a period of 6 months to 2 years to normalize [35]. It appears that the locus of such chronic glucocorticoid-induced adrenal suppression is primarily suprapituitary involving the CRH neuron [49].

Finally, genetic defects can cause disruption of the HPA axis. These include the various types of congenital adrenal hyperplasia due to enzymatic defects at different steps of steroidogenesis and the rare syndromes of ACTH and glucocorticoid resistance, whereby the defect lies in the ACTH and glucocorticoid receptor gene, respectively [55, 113]. All these hereditary abnormalities lead to attenuation or complete loss of the glucocorticoid negative feedback, resulting in compensatory increases of CRH and ACTH secretion [23].

References

1. Aghajanian GK, Van der Maelen CP (1982) α₂-Adrenoreceptor-mediated hyperpolarization of locus ceruleus neurons: Intracellular studies in vivo. Science 215:1394–1396
2. Aguilera G, Flores M, Carvallo P, et al (1990) Receptors for corticotropin-releasing factor. In: DeSouza EB, Nemeroff CB (eds) Corticotropin-releasing factor: Basic and clinical studies of a neuropeptide. CRC Press, Boca Raton, FL, pp 154–159
3. Aguilera G, Millan MA, Hauger RL, et al (1987) Corticotropin-releasing factor receptors: Distribution and regulation in brain, pituitary, and peripheral tissues. Ann NY Acad Sci 512:48–66
4. Aguilera G (1993) Factors controlling steroid biosynthesis in the zona glomerulosa of the adrenal. J Steroid Biochem Mol Biol 45:147–151
5. Akira S, Hirano T, Taga T, et al (1990) Biology of multifunctional cytokines: IL-6 and related molecules (IL-1 and TNF). FASEB J 4:2860–2867
6. Al-Damluji S, Cunnah D, Grossman A, et al (1987) Effect of adrenaline on basal and ovine corticotropin-releasing factor-stimulated ACTH secretion in man. J Endocrinol 112:145–150
7. Alzein J, Jeandel L, Lutz-Bucher B, et al (1984) Evidence that CRF stimulates vasopressin secretion from isolated neurointermediate pituitary [letter]. Neuroendocrinology 6:151
8. Antoni FA (1987) Receptors mediating the CRH effects of vasopressin and oxytocin. Ann NY Acad Sci 512:195–204
9. Antoni FA (1993) Vasopressinergic control of pituitary adrenocorticotropin secretion comes of age. Front Neuroendocrinol 14:76–122
10. Bardeleben U, Heuser I, Holsboer F (1989) Human CRH stimulation response during acute withdrawal and after medium-term abstention from alcohol abuse. Psychoneuroendocrinology 14:441–449
11. Benker G, Raida M, Olbricht T, et al (1990) TSH secretion in Cushing's syndrome: Relation to glucocorticoid excess, diabetes, goiter, and the "the sick euthyroid syndrome." Clin Endocrinol 133:779–786
12. Bernardini R, Chiarenza A, Calogero AE, et al (1989) Arachidonic acid metabolites modulate rat hypothalamic corticotropin releasing hormone in vitro. Neuroendocrinology 50:708–715
13. Bernardini R, Kamilaris TC, Calogero AE, et al (1990) Interactions between tumor necrosis factor-alpha, hypothalamic corticotropin-releasing hormone, and adrenocorticotropin secretion in the rat. Endocrinology 126:2876–2881
14. Besedovsky HO, del Rey A (1992) Immune-neuroendocrine circuits: Integrative role of cytokines. Frontiers Neuroendocrinol 13:61–94
15. Burguera B, Muruais C, Penalva A, et al (1990) Dual and selective actions of glucocorticoids upon basal and stimulated growth hormone release in man. Neuroendocrinology 51:51–58
16. Calogero AE, Gallucci WT, Chrousos GP, et al (1988) Effect of the catecholamines upon rat hypothalamic corticotropin releasing hormone secretion in vitro. J Clin Invest 82:839–846
17. Calogero AE, Gallucci WT, Chrousos GP, et al (1988) Interaction between GABAergic neurotransmission and rat hypothalamic CRH in vitro. Brain Res 463:28–36
18. Calogero AE, Gallucci WT, Gold PW, et al (1988) Multiple regulatory feedback loops on hypothalamic CRH secretion. Potential clinical implications. J Clin Invest 82:767–774

19. Casanueva FF, Burguera B, Muruais C, et al (1990) Acute administration of corticosteroids: A new and peculiar stimulus of growth hormone secretion in man. J Clin Endocrinol Metab 70:234–237

20. Cavagnini F, Croci M, Putignano P, Petroni ML, Invitti C (2000) Glucocorticoids and neuroendocrine function. Int J Obesity 24 Suppl 2:S77–S79

21. Chen R, Lewis KA, Perrin MH, et al (1993) Expression cloning of a human corticotropin releasing factor receptor. Proc Natl Acad Sci USA 90:8967–8971

22. Chikanza IC, Petrou Ñ, Chrousos GP, Kingsley Ï, Panayi G (1992) Defective hypothalamic response to immune/inflammatory stimuli in patients with rheumatoid arthritis. Arthr Rheumatol 35:1281–1288

23. Chrousos GP, Detera-Wadleigh S, Karl M (1993) NIH Conference. Syndromes of glucocorticoid resistance. Ann Intern Med 119:1113–1124

24. Chrousos GP, Gold PW (1992) The concepts of stress system disorders: Overview of behavioral and physical homeostasis. JAMA 267:1244–1252

25. Chrousos GP, Torpy DJ, Gold PW (1998) Interactions between the hypothalamic pituitary adrenal axis and the female reproductive system: Clinical implications. Ann Intern Med. 129:229–240

26. Chrousos GP (1995) The hypothalamic-pituitary-adrenal axis and immune-mediated inflammation. N Engl J Med. 332:1351–1362

27. Chrousos GP (2000) The role of stress and the hypothalamic-pituitary-adrenal axis in the pathogenesis of the metabolic syndrome: Neuro-endocrine and target tissue-related causes. Int J Obes Relat Metab Disord 24 Suppl 2:S50–55

28. Chrousos GP (1992) Regulation and dysregulation of the hypothalamic-pituitary-adrenal axis: The corticotropin-releasing hormone perspective. Endocrinol Metab Clin N Am 21:833–858

29. Crofford LJ, Sano H, Karalis K, et al (1993) Corticotropin-releasing hormone in synovial fluids and tissues of patients with rheumatoid arthritis and osteoarthritis. J Immunol 151:1587–1596

30. Cunningham ET Jr, Bohn MC, Sawchenko PE (1990) The organization of adrenergic inputs to the paraventricular and supraoptic nuclei of the rat hypothalamus. J Comp Neurol 292:651–667

31. de Kloet ER, Vreugdenhil E, Oitzl MS, Joels M (1998) Brain corticosteroid receptor balance in health and disease. Endocr Rev 19:269–301

32. Demitrack M, Dale J, Straus S, et al (1991) Evidence of impaired activation of the hypothalamic-pituitary-adrenal axis in patients with chronic fatigue syndrome. J Clin Endocrinol Metab 73:1224–1234

33. DeSouza EB, Insel TR, Perrin MH, et al (1985) Corticotropin-releasing factor receptors are widely distributed within the rat central nervous system. J Neurosci 5:3189–3203

34. Dieguez C, Page MD, Scanlon MF (1988) Growth hormone neuroregulation and its alterations in disease states. Clin Endocrinol (Oxf) 28:109–143

35. Doherty GM, Nieman LK, Cutler GB Jr, et al (1990) Time to recovery of the hypothalamic pituitary adrenal axis following curative resection of adrenal tumors in patients with Cushing's syndrome. Surgery 108:1085–1090

36. Duick DS, Wahner HW (1979) Thyroid axis in patients with Cushing's syndrome. Arch Intern Med 139:767–772

37. Dunlap JC (1999) Molecular bases for circadian clocks. Cell 96:271–290

38. Eipper BA, Mains RE (1980) Structure and biosynthesis of proadrenocorticotropin/endorphin and related peptides. Endocr Rev 1:1–27

39. Elenkov IJ, Webster EL, Torpy DJ, Chrousos GP (1999) Stress, corticotropin-releasing hormone, glucocorticoids, and the immune/inflammatory response: Acute and chronic effects. Ann N Y Acad Sci 876:1–11; discussion 11–13

40. Engler D, Pham T, Fullerton MJ, et al (1989) Studies on the secretion of corticotropin releasing factor and arginine vasopressin into hypophyseal portal circulation of the conscious sheep. Neuroendocrinology 49:367–381

41. Foote SL, Bloom FE, Aston-Jones G (1983) Nucleus locus ceruleus: New evidence for anatomical and physiological specificity. Physiol Rev 63:844–914

42. Frim DM, Robinson BG, Pasieka KB, et al (1990) Differential regulation of corticotropin releasing hormone mRNA in rat brain. Am J Physiol 258:E686–692

43. Fukata J, Usui T, Naitoh Y, et al (1988) Effects of recombinant human interleukin-1α, IL-1β, IL-2 and IL-6 on ACTH synthesis and release in the mouse pituitary tumor cell line AtT-20. J Endocrinol 122:33–39

44. Fuller RW (1992) The involvement of serotonin in regulation of pituitary-adrenocortical function. Front Neuroendocrinol 13:250–270

45. Gillies GE, Linton EA, Lowry PJ (1982) Corticotropin-releasing activity of the new CRF is potentiated several times by vasopressin. Nature 299:355–357

46. Gold PW, Chrousos GP (1999) The endocrinology of melancholic and atypical depression: Relation to neurocircuitry and somatic consequences. Proc Assoc Am Physicians 111:22–34

47. Gold PW, Gwirtsman H, Avgerinos P, et al (1986) Abnormal hypothalamic-pituitary-adrenal function in anorexia nervosa: Pathophysiologic mechanisms in underweight and weight-corrected patients. N Engl J Med 314:1335–1342

48. Gold PW, Loriaux DL, Roy A, et al (1986) Responses to the corticotropin-releasing hormone in the hypercortisolism of depression and Cushing's disease: Pathophysiologic and diagnostic implications. N Engl J Med 314:1329–1335

49. Gomez MT, Magiakou MA, Mastorakos G, Chrousos GP (1993) The pituitary corticotroph is not the rate-limiting step in the postoperative recovery of the hypothalamic pituitary adrenal axis in patients with Cushing's syndrome. J Clin Endocrinol Metab 77:173–177

50. Griep EN, Boersma JW, de Kloet ER (1993) Altered reactivity of the hypothalamic pituitary adrenal axis in the primary fibromyalgia syndrome. J Rheumatol 20:469–474

51. Gwynne JT, Strauss JF 3rd (1982) The role of lipoproteins in steroidogenesis and cholesterol metabolism in steroidogenic glands. Endocr Rev 3:299–329

52. Hackney AC (2001) Endurance exercise training and reproductive endocrine dysfunction in men: Alterations in the hypothalamic-pituitary-testicular axis. Curr Pharm Des 7:261–273

53. Harris (1948) Neural control of the pituitary gland. Physiol Rev 28:139

54. Horrocks PM, Jones AF, Ratcliffe WA, et al (1990) Patterns of ACTH and cortisol pulsatility over 24 hours in normal males and females. Clin Endocrinol (Oxf) 32:127–134

55. Hurley DM, Accili D, Stratakis C, et al (1991) Mutation of the glucocorticoid receptor gene in familial glucocorticoid resistance. J Clin Invest 87:680–686

56. Insel TR, Kalin NH, Guttmacher LB, et al (1982) The dexamethasone suppression test in obsessive-compulsive disorder. Psychiatry Res 6:153–160

57. Jonat C, Rahmsdorf HJ, Park KK, et al (1990) Antitumor promotion and anti-inflammation: Down modulation of AP-1 (fos/jun) activity by glucocorticoid hormone. Cell 62:1189–1204

58. Kahri AI, Huhtaniemi I, Salmenpera M (1976) Steroid formation and differentiation of cortical cells in tissue culture of human fetal adrenals in the presence and absence of ACTH. Endocrinology 98:33–41

59. Kamilaris TC, Calogero AE, Johnson EO, et al (1989) Effects of hypothyroidism and hyperthyroidism on the basal activity of the hypothalamic-pituitary-adrenal axis (abstract). Clin Res 37:360A

60. Kamilaris TC, DeBold CR, Pavlou SN, et al (1987) Effect of altered thyroid hormone levels on hypothalamic-pituitary-adrenal function. J Clin Endocrinol Metab 65:994–999

61. Karalis K, Sano H, Redwine J, et al (1991) Autocrine or paracrine inflammatory actions of corticotropin-releasing hormone in vivo. Science 254:421–423

62. Kazis K, Iglesias E (2003) The female athlete triad. Adolesc Med 14:87–95

63. Keller-Wood ME, Dallman MF (1984) Corticosteroid inhibition of ACTH secretion. Endocr Rev 5:1–24

64. Korbonits M, Kaltsas G, Perry LA, et al (1999) The growth hormone secretagogue hexarelin stimulates the hypothalamo-pituitary-adrenal axis via arginine vasopressin. J Clin Endocrinol Metab 84:2489–2495

65. Krieger DT, Liotta AS, Brownstein MS, et al (1980) ACTH, β-lipotropin, and related peptides in brain, pituitary and blood. Recent Prog Horm Res 36:277–344

66. Krieger DT (1975) Rhythms of ACTH and corticosteroid secretion in health and disease and their experimental modification. J Steroid Biochem 6:785–791

67. Lamberts SW, Verleun T, Oosterom R, et al (1984) Corticotropin-releasing factor and vasopressin exert a synergistic effect on adrenocorticotropin release in man. J Clin Endocrinol Metab 58:298–303

68. Laue L, Gold PW, Richmond A, Chrousos GP (1991) The hypothalamic-pituitary-adrenal axis in anorexia nervosa and bulimia nervosa: Pathophysiologic implications. Adv Pediatr 38:287–316

69. Linton EA, Wolfe CD, Behan DP, et al (1988) A specific carrier substance for human corticotropin releasing factor in late gestational maternal plasma which could mask the ACTH releasing activity. Clin Endocrinol (Oxf) 28:315–324

70. Luger A, Deuster P, Kyle SB, et al (1987) Acute hypothalamic-pituitary-adrenal responses to the stress of treadmill exercise: Physiologic adaptations to physical training. N Engl J Med 316:1309–1315

71. Lundblad JR, Roberts JL (1988) Regulation of proopiomelanocortin gene expression in pituitary. Endocr Rev 9:135–158

72. MacAdams MR, White RH, Chipps BE (1986) Reduction in serum testosterone levels during chronic glucocorticoid therapy. Ann Intern Med 140:648–651

73. Malozowski S, Muzzo S, Burrows R, et al (1990) The hypothalamic-pituitary-adrenal axis in infantile malnutrition. Clin Endocrinol (Oxf) 32:461–465

74. Masi AT, Chatterton RT, Aldag JC, Malamet RL (2002) Perspectives on the relationship of adrenal steroids to rheumatoid arthritis. Ann N Y Acad Sci 966:1–12

75. Mastorakos G, Chrousos GP, Weber J (1993) Recombinant interleukin-6 activates the hypothalamic-pituitary-adrenal axis in humans. J Clin Endocrinol Metab 77:1690–1694

76. Mountjoy KG, Robbins LS, Mortrud MT, et al (1992) The cloning of a family of genes that encode the melanocortin receptors. Science 257:1248–1251

77. Munck A, Guyre PM, Holbrook NJ (1984) Physiological functions of glucocorticoids in stress and their relation to pharmacological actions. Endocr Rev 5:25–44

78. Naitoh Y, Fukata J, Tominaga T, et al (1988) Interleukin-6 stimulates the secretion of adrenocorticotropin hormone in conscious freely moving rats. Biochem Biophys Res Commun 155:1459–1463

79. Oki S, Nakao K, Tanaka I, et al (1981) Concomitant secretion of adrenocorticotropin, β-endorphin and γ-melanotropin from perfused pituitary tumor cells of Cushing's disease. J Clin Endocrinol Metab 52:42–49

80. Orth DN (1992) Corticotropin-releasing hormone in humans. Endocr Rev 13:164–191

81. Pasquali R, Cantobelli S, Casimirri F, et al (1993) The hypothalamic-pituitary-adrenal axis in obese women with different patterns of body fat distribution. J Clin Endocrinol Metab 77:341–346

82. Plotsky PM (1986) Opioid inhibition of immunoreactive corticotropin-releasing factor secretion into the hypophysial-portal circulation of rats. Regul Pept 30:235–242

83. Potter E, Behan DP, Fischer WH, et al (1991) Cloning and characterization of the cDNAs for human and rat corticotropin-releasing factor-binding proteins. Nature 349:423–426

84. Potter E, Behan DP, Linton EA, et al (1992) The central distribution of a corticotrophin releasing factor (CRF)-binding protein predicts multiple sites and modes of interaction with CRF. Proc Natl Acad Sci USA 89:4192–4196

85. Pratt WB (1990) Glucocorticoid receptor structure and the initial events in signal transduction. Prog Clin Biol Res 322:119–320

86. Rabin D, Gold PW, Margioris A, et al (1988) Stress and reproduction: Interactions between the stress and reproductive axis. In: Chrousos GP, Loriaux DL, Gold PW (eds) Mechanisms of physical and emotional stress. Plenum Press, New York, pp 377–390

87. Rabin D, Schmidt P, Gold PW, et al (1990) Hypothalamic-pituitary-adrenal function in patients with the premenstrual syndrome. J Clin Endocrinol Metab 71:1158–1162

88. Reichlin S (1993) Neuroendocrine-immune interactions. N Engl J Med 329:1246–1253

89. Richard D, Lin Q, Timofeeva E (2002) The corticotropin-releasing factor family of peptides and CRF receptors: Their roles in the regulation of energy balance. Eur J Pharmacol 12:189–197

90. Risher-Flowers D, Adinoff B, Ravitz B, et al (1988) Circadian rhythms of cortisol during alcohol withdrawal. Adv Alcohol Subst Abuse 7:37–41

91. Rittmaster RS, Cutler GB Jr, Brandon D, et al (1987) The relationship of saline-induced changes in vasopressin secretion to basal and corticotropin-releasing hormone-stimulated adrenocorticotropin and cortisol secretion in man. J Clin Endocrinol Metab 64:371–376

92. Rivier C, Plotsky PM (1986) Mediation by corticotropin-releasing factor (CRF) of adenohypophysial hormone secretion. Ann Rev Physiol 48:475–494

93. Rivier C, Rivest S (1991) Effect of stress on the activity of the hypothalamic-pituitary-gonadal axis: Peripheral and central mechanisms. Biol Reprod 45:523–532

94. Rivier C, Rivier J, Mormede P, et al (1984) Studies on the nature of the interaction between vasopressin and corticotropin-releasing factor on adrenocorticotropin release in the rat. Endocrinology 115:882–886

95. Rivier C, Rivier J, Vale W (1986) Stress-induced inhibition of reproductive function: Role of endogenous corticotropin releasing factor. Science 231:607–609

96. Rivier C, Vale W (1985) Involvement of corticotropin-releasing factor and somatostatin in stress induced inhibition of growth hormone secretion in the rat. Endocrinology 117:2478–2482

97. Roth KA, Weber E, Barchas JD, et al (1983) Immunoreactive dynorphin-(1–8) and CRH in subpopulation of hypothalamic neurons. Science 219:189–191

98. Saffran M, Schally AV (1955) The release of corticotropin by anterior pituitary tissue in vitro. Can J Biochem Physiol 33:408–415

99. Salas MA, Evans SW, Levell MJ, et al (1990) Interleukin-6 and ACTH act synergistically to stimulate the release of corticosterone from adrenal gland cells. Clin Exp Immunol 79:470–473

100. Sanchez ER, Faber LE, Henzel WJ, et al (1990) The 56–59-kilodalton protein identified in untransformed steroid receptor complexes is a unique protein that exists in cytosol in a complex with both the 70 and 90 kilodalton heat shock proteins. Biochemistry 29:5145–5152

101. Saper CB, Loewy AD, Swanson LW, et al (1979) Direct hypothalamoautonomic connections. Brain Res 117:305–312

102. Sapolsky R, Rivier C, Yamamoto G, et al (1987) Interleukin-1 stimulates the secretion of hypothalamic corticotropin releasing factor. Science 238:522–524

103. Sasaki A, Shinkawa O, Margioris AN, et al (1987) Immunoreactive corticotropin releasing hormone in human plasma during pregnancy, labor and delivery. J Clin Endocrinol Metab 64:224–229

104. Selye H (1950) Stress. Acta Medical, Montreal, Quebec

105. Sirinathsinghji DJ, Rees LH, Rivier J, et al (1983) Corticotropin-releasing factor is a potent inhibitor of sexual receptivity in the female rat. Nature 305:232–235

106. Smith AI, Funder JW (1988) Proopiomelanocortin processing in the pituitary, central nervous system, and peripheral tissues. Endocr Rev 9:159–179

107. Smith DF, Toft DO (1993) Steroid receptors and their associated proteins. Mol Endocrinol 7:4–11

108. Smith GW, Aubry JM, Dellu F, et al (1998) Corticotropin releasing factor receptor 1-deficient mice display decreased anxiety, impaired stress response, and aberrant neuroendocrine development. Neuron 20:1093–1102

109. Sternberg EM, Chrousos GP, Wilder RL, et al (1992) The stress response and the regulation of inflammatory disease. Ann Intern Med 117:854–866

110. Sutton RE, Koob GF, Le Moal M, et al (1982) Corticotropin-releasing factor produces behavioral activation in the rat. Nature 297:331–333

111. Tait SAS, Schulster D, Okamoto M, et al (1970) Production of steroids by in vitro superfusion of endocrine tissue: II. Steroid output from whole, capsular and decapsulated adrenals of normal intact, hypophysectomized and hypophysectomized-nephrectomized rats as a function of time of perfusion. Endocrinology 86:360–382

112. Torpy DJ, Tsigos C, Lotsikas AJ, Defensor R, Chrousos GP, Papanicolaou DA (1998) Acute and delayed effects of a single-dose injection of interleukin-6 on thyroid function in healthy humans. Metabolism 47:1289–1293

113. Tsigos C, Arai K, Hung W, et al (1993) Hereditary isolated glucocorticoid deficiency is associated with abnormalities of the adrenocorticotropin receptor gene. J Clin Invest 92:2485–2561

114. Tsigos C, Chrousos GP (1994) Physiology of the hypothalamic-pituitary-adrenal axis in health and dysregulation in psychiatric and autoimmune disorders. Endocrinol Metab Clin North Am 23:451–466

115. Tsigos C, Crosby SR, Gibson S, et al (1993) Proopiomelanocortin is the predominant ACTH related peptide in human cerebrospinal fluid. J Clin Endocrinol Metab 76:620–624

116. Tsigos C, Kyrou I, Chala E, Tsapogas P, Stavridis JC, Raptis SA, Katsilambros N (1999) Circulating tumor necrosis factor alpha concentrations are higher in abdominal versus peripheral obesity. Metabolism 48:1332–1335

117. Tsigos C, Papanicolaou DA, Defensor R, Mitsiadis CS, Kyrou I, Chrousos GP (1997) Dose-dependent effects of recombinant human interleukin-6 on anterior pituitary hormone secretion and thermogenesis. Neuroendocrinology 66:54–62

118. Tsigos C, Papanicolaou DA, Kyrou I, Defensor R, Mitsiadis CS, Chrousos GP (1997) Dose-dependent effects of recombinant human interleukin-6 on glucose regulation. J Clin Endocrinol Metab 82:4167–4170

119. Tsigos C, Papanicolaou DA, Kyrou I, Raptis SA, Chrousos GP (1999) Dose-dependent effects of recombinant human interleukin-6 on the pituitary-testicular axis. J Interferon Cytokine Res 19:1271–1276

120. Tsigos C, Young RJ, White A (1993) Diabetic neuropathy is associated with increased activity of the hypothalamic-pituitary-adrenal axis. J Clin Endocr Metab 76:554–558

121. Turnbull AV, Rivier C (1997) Corticotropin-releasing factor (CRF) and endocrine responses to stress: CRF receptors, binding protein, and related peptides. Proc Soc Exp Biol Med 215:1–10

122. Unterman TG, Phillips LS (1985) Glucocorticoid effects on somatomedins and somatomedin inhibitors. J Clin Endocrinol Metab 61:618–626

123. Vale W, Spiess J, Rivier C, et al (1981) Characterization of a 41-residue ovine hypothalamic peptide that stimulates secretion of corticotropin and beta-endorphin. Science 213:1394–1397

124. Vale W, Vaughan J, Smith M, et al (1983) Effects of synthetic ovine corticotropin-releasing factor, glucocorticoid, catecholamines, neuro-hypophyseal peptides, and other substances on cultured corticotropic cells. Endocrinology 113:1121–1131

125. Valentino RJ, Foote SL, Aston-Jones G (1983) Corticotropin-releasing hormone activates noradrenergic neurons of the locus ceruleus. Brain Res 270:363–367

126. Vamvakopoulos NC, Chrousos GP (1993) Evidence of direct estrogen regulation of human corticotropin releasing hormone gene expression: Potential implications for the sexual dimorphism of the stress response and immune/inflammatory reaction. J Clin Invest 92:1896–1902

127. Vanderpool J, Rosenthal N, Chrousos GP, et al (1991) Abnormal pituitary-adrenal responses to corticotropin-releasing hormone in patients with seasonal affective disorder: Clinical and pathophysiological implications. J Clin Endocrinol Metab 72:1382–1387

128. Veldhuis JD, Iranmanesh A, Johnson ML, et al (1990) Amplitude, but not frequency, modulation of adrenocorticotropin secretory bursts gives rise to the nyctohemeral rhythm of corticotropic axis in man. J Clin Endocrinol Metab 71:452–463

129. Wand GS, Dobs AS (1991) Alterations in the hypothalamic-pituitary-adrenal axis in actively drinking alcoholics. J Clin Endocrinol Metab 72:1290–1295

130. Weitzman ED, Fukushima D, Nogeire C, et al (1971) Twenty-four hour pattern of the episodic secretion of cortisol in normal subjects. J Clin Endocrinol Metab 33:14–22

131. Winter JS, Cow KW, Perry YS, et al (1990) A stimulatory effect of interleukin-1 on adrenocortical cortisol secretion mediated by prostaglandins. Endocrinology 127:1904–1909

132. Wong ML, Licinio J, Pasternak KI, Gold PW (1994) Localization of corticotrophin releasing hormone (CRH) receptor mRNA in adult rat brain by in situ hybridization histochemistry. Endocrinology 135:2275–2278

133. Yang-Yen HF, Chambard JC, Sun YL, et al (1990) Transcriptional interference between c-jun and the glucocorticoid receptor: Mutual inhibition of DNA binding due to direct protein-protein interaction. Cell 62:1205–1215

4 The Sympathoadrenal System

Integrative Regulation of the Cortical and the Medullary Adrenal Functions

A. Souvatzoglou

CONTENTS

In this chapter an attempt is made to show that the neuroectodermally derived adrenal medulla and the mesodermally derived adrenal cortex are organized into a single gland despite their different embryonic origin, and have achieved a phylogenetically unified function. In concert with the sympathetic nervous system they operate functionally as a coherent whole to maintain homeostasis in the resting state and to activate appropriate cellular mechanisms in response to different stresses.

4.1 The Anatomical Basis of the Interplay Between the Adrenal Cortex, the Adrenal Medulla and the Sympathetic Nervous System

4.1.1 Circulatory and Structural Relationships Between the Adrenal Cortex and Medulla

The adrenal glands, each weighing approximately 4 g in the unstressed adult, are highly vascular, having one of the highest blood flows of any tissue in the body. They receive, usually, arterial supply directly from the inferior phrenic arteries, the aorta, the renal arteries and frequently other small arteries. This may be looked upon as a protection of adrenal blood supply, as the failure of any single artery has little effect upon the total blood supply reaching the gland. Multiple small arterial branches pierce the capsule of the cortex and divide repeatedly into smaller vessels forming an extensive network in the capsule, the capsular arterial plexus, or enter the cortex to form an extensive subcapsular arterial plexus. From the capsular-subcapsular plexus the arteries which supply the entire cortex arise. The cortical arterioles feed into a complex reticular capillary network in the glomerulosa and reticularis but with straighter centripetal components in the fasciculata with more numerous cross-connecting channels in the deeper regions. All of these vessels then converge towards the smallest of the collecting veins in the medulla that empty into the central adrenal vein. Thus, the central vein collects blood from both the cortex and the medulla (Fig. 1). From the capsular-subcapsular plexus the medullary arteries arise which penetrate the cortex without branching to pass into the medulla. There they divide into arterioles and capillaries. The capillary network in the medulla feeds into smaller branches of the medullary veins or into the capillaries of the reticularis. Thus, the medulla receives two types of blood. A small fraction of its blood is supplied directly by the capsular-subcapsular plexus, via the arteriae medullae, but most, at least under conditions of stimulation, must come from the cortex [34]. Blood flow within the adrenal gland is distinctly heterogeneous. In conscious, not unduly stressed dogs [18], blood flow to the adrenal medulla is approximately fivefold greater (per unit mass) than blood flow to the adrenal cortex. But, since the medulla comprises a small portion (about 10%) of the total gland, total adrenal blood flow is only slightly greater than cortical blood flow.

At the corticomedullary border cortical and medullary tissues are closely interwoven. Chromaffin

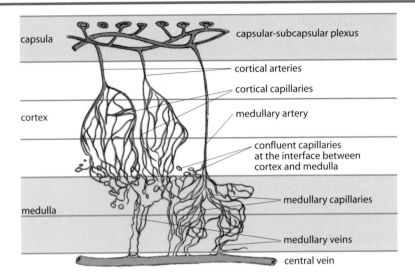

Fig. 1. Schematic drawing of the adrenal circulation. The medulla receives blood both via the cortex and from its direct supply through the medullary arteries

cell formations intruding into the cortex are observed in different mammalian species, including humans [7]. Cordlike structures in continuity with the medullary tissue, medullary rays, extend through the entire cortex up to the capsular zone. Ultrastructural studies show that there is no difference in the characteristic features of the medullary ray cells and those of the medulla [20]. Moreover, larger and smaller islets of chromaffin cells are located within all the three cortical zones and cortical tissue invades the medulla. Cytoplasmic extensions and direct contact can be seen between adjacent medullary and cortical cells, indicating a close functional relationship between the two cellular types [6, 7, 20]. In addition, the sinuses of the cortex and medulla are continuous and structurally indistinguishable; there is a continuity between vessels at the interface between cortex and medulla [34]. In this region confluent cortical and medullary capillaries feeding into collecting veins form a portal-like net (Fig. 1). This distinctive vascular connection between cortical and medullary tissue may signify a route along which medullary products could reach cortical cells.

The structure of the adrenal capillaries throughout the whole gland is sinusoidal; the capillary wall is very frail, consisting of only the endothelium and basal lamina. The extreme delicacy of the structure of the endothelium of the sinusoids throughout the gland strongly suggests that the system normally operates under low-pressure conditions, and internally the tissue is exposed to significantly lower pressures than the arterial pressure. This in turn suggests that a pressure barrier may be encountered before the internal vessels are reached. Such a barrier may be provided by the vessels of the capsural-subcapsular plexus. These vessels are the only adrenal vessels which show a suitable wall structure for adjusting blood flow over a very wide range of flow rates [34].

As will be discussed below, changes in blood flow rate are an important component of the secretory response of the whole adrenal gland. The common blood supply of the mesodermally derived cortex and the neuroectodermally derived medulla, intimately associated in one organ, as well as the ultrastructural features of neighboring cortical and medullary cells, imply functional interrelations. This may explain how the functions of these two distinct organs of diverse embryogenetic origin are interconnected.

4.1.2 Central and Peripheral Neural Pathways Involved in the Regulation of the Adrenal Cortex and Medulla

The spinal cord is the most distal site of the central nervous system generating patterns of sympathetic activity. The preganglionic cell bodies of the nerve fibers innervating both the adrenal cortex and the adrenal medulla are mainly located in the intermediolateral column of the thoracic part of the spinal cord [10]. Preganglionic cholinergic axons exiting the spinal cord pass through the lower thoracic, upper lumbar and collateral ganglia (celiac, superior mesenteric) to

reach the adrenal medulla directly via multiple pre-
vertebral plexuses, or synapses in these ganglia. Postganglionic noradrenergic fibers arising from the trunk
and the collateral ganglia form the different preverte-
bral plexuses providing the splanchnic neural innervation of the adrenal cortex (Fig. 2). As in most sym-
pathetically innervated organs, all visible small nerve
fibers toward the adrenal glands run parallel and adjacent to small arteries supplying the glands. The postganglionic catecholaminergic fibers enter the adrenal
capsule and disperse predominantly into the zona
glomerulosa along blood vessels innervating parenchymal cells and vessels [26]. Branches from the capsular-
glomerulosa catecholaminergic nerve fibers surround
the fasciculata cells or transverse the inner cortical
zones sporadically (Fig. 2). Catecholaminergic vari-
cosities are present in the zona fasciculata and reticularis [35]. Accordingly, the medulla seems to be predominantly innervated by preganglionic fibers and the
cortex essentially by postganglionic fibers mainly
associated with cortical blood vessels. However, experimental results in the rat imply a direct innervation
of the adrenal cortex by neurons present in the intermediolateral column of the spinal cord [10] and indicate that apart from the preganglionic, a postganglionic sympathetic, innervation of the medulla is
present as well [25].

It is generally acknowledged that the chromaffin
cells of the adrenal medulla are modified postganglionic sympathetic neurons. However, besides the two
types of chromaffin cells in the adrenal medulla, noradrenaline and adrenaline cells, ganglion neurons can
also be found (Fig. 2). These medullary neurons have
been thought to represent postganglionic neurons
innervating the chromaffin cells; they may also project
their axons to the cortex and retrogradely into the
splanchnic nerve (Fig. 2), thus possibly representing
a feedback system [13]. The intramedullary ganglion
neurons providing an intrinsic innervation of the
medulla and the cortex as well are of two types: type I
cells are noradrenergic and neuropeptide Y (NPY)-pos-
itive, whereas type II cells are positive for vasoactive intestinal polypeptide (VIP) and may be cholinergic [13].

The outflow of impulses from preganglionic sympathetic neurons in the intermediolateral column of
the spinal cord innervating the adrenals is regulated by
a complex system of hierarchical circuits located in
cortical and subcortical centers. There is anatomic and
functional evidence for a polysynaptic connection
between cortical and hypothalamic centers and the
adrenal glands that involves the autonomic division of
the paraventricular nucleus of the hypothalamus and

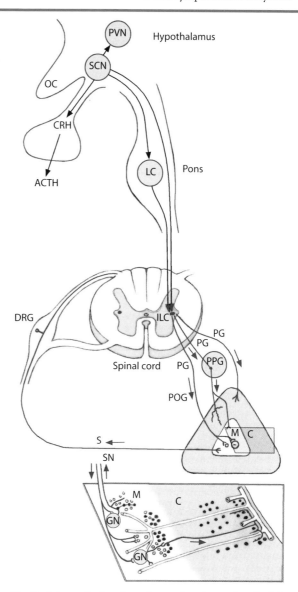

Fig. 2. Schematic drawing of neural pathways involved in
the regulative mechanisms of the sympathoadrenal system
(*C*, adrenal cortex; *DRG*, dorsal root ganglia; *GN*, ganglion
neurons; *ILC*, intermediolateral column; *LC*, locus ceruleus;
M, adrenal medulla; *OC*, optic chiasm; *PG* preganglionic
fibers; *POG*, postganglionic fibers; *PPG*, pre-, paravertebral
ganglia; *PVN*, paraventricular nucleus; *S*, sensory fibers;
SCN, suprachiasmatic nucleus; *SN*, splanchnic nerve)

the interomediolateral column of the spinal cord as
relay structures. Neurons from the medial part of the
nucleus suprachiasmaticus (Fig. 2) but also from other
hypothalamic and subcortical regions (medial pre-
optic area, arcuate nucleus, bed nucleus of the stria
terminalis, anterior hypothalamic and retrochiasmatic
area, dorsomedial and ventromedial hypothalamus,

magnocellular reticular nucleus and central amygdala) project to regions of the brainstem (rostroventrolateral medulla, locus coeruleus) and the hypothalamic paraventricular nucleus [10]. From these centers, especially from the autonomic parts of the nucleus paraventricularis, neurons project directly to the preganglionic cell bodies in the intermediolateral column of the thoracic part of the spinal cord, which, as described before, innervate the adrenal glands (Fig. 2). Similarly from the autonomic parts of the nucleus paraventricularis corticotrophin-releasing hormone (CRH) neurons project to the median eminence of the hypothalamus [10], releasing CRH (corticotrophin-releasing hormone) into the hypothalamic-hypophyseal portal system to stimulate the secretion of ACTH (adrenocorticotropic hormone) (Fig. 2).

As already mentioned, the most prominent catecholaminergic innervation is present in the capsular-zona glomerulosa area. In the inner cortical zones catecholaminergic nerve fibers are sparse. Axon terminals are primarily seen in close proximity to blood vessels but also to the glomerulosa cells without making synaptic contacts [26, 35]. The appearance of sympathetic nerves in the adrenal cortex is reminiscent of classical descriptions of autonomic innervation whereby a small number of nerves can have a widespread influence. Both sympathetic control of blood flow entering the adrenal cortex and paracrine signal are potential mechanisms by which a relatively sparse local innervation could affect the function of many cells. Many adrenal cortical cells contact their neighboring cells with distinctive cytoplasmatic formations [19]. Thus, adrenocortical cells affected by neurotransmitters released from adjacent nerve terminals may affect, in a paracrine manner, many other cortical cells that they contact. Immunocytochemical evidence [35] indicates that all catecholaminergic nerve profiles in the adrenal cortex are noradrenergic. In addition, in the cortical cells of the three zones receptors specific for β-adrenergic agonists have been demonstrated [31]. Thus, it has been suggested that the catecholaminergic innervation of the adrenal cortex may influence adrenocortical steroidogenesis.

The adrenal cortex and the adrenal medulla receive not only a spinal sympathetic motor (efferent) innervation (Fig. 2), but also a spinal sympathetic sensory (afferent) innervation. Experimental evidence is present to show that the adrenal gland of the guinea pig and the rat receives a relatively rich afferent sympathetic innervation from neurons located in the dorsal root ganglia at segments T3–L2 [29]. Furthermore, in the same animals a sensory parasympathetic, vagal, innervation of the adrenal gland has been demonstrated. Additionally, in the guinea pig, efferent motor neurons from the dorsal motor nucleus of the vagus project to the adrenal gland [11]. The sensory nerve endings are found predominantly in the adrenal medulla and ultrastructurally resemble the baroreceptors found in the carotid sinus [29]. They may serve to monitor capsular or vascular distension caused by raised arterial pressure or increased blood flow (baroreceptor function) and to monitor intramedullary concentrations of catecholamines and different vasoactive peptides (chemoreceptor function).

4.2 Functional Integration of Neural and Humoral Activity: The Sympathoadrenal System

4.2.1 Main Integrative Mechanisms

The functional integrity of the sympathoadrenal system involves hormonal messages, neural signals and cellular mechanisms acting in concordance. The primary regulatory mechanisms of this system are production and secretion of corticosteroids by the adrenal cortex, regulated by ACTH released from the pituitary and biosynthesis and release of catecholamines by the medullary chromaffin cells controlled by sympathetic nerve activity. However, for the biosynthesis of catecholamines both sympathetic nerve input and glucocorticoid secretion are concomitantly necessary. In essence, the activity of tyrosine hydroxylase, a rate limiting enzyme in the biosynthesis of catecholamines converting tyrosine to dopa, is mainly neurally controlled whereas the activity of dopamine β-hydroxylase, the enzyme converting dopamine to noradrenaline, is affected by both nerve activity and glucocorticoids. The activity of phenylethanolamine N-methyltransferase, the rate limiting enzyme converting noradrenaline to adrenaline, is controlled mainly by glucocorticoids. In acute stress the activity of tyrosine hydroxylase is rapidly elevated in the adrenal medulla but remains low if the sympathetic impulse transmission is disrupted [4]. In addition, experiments in rats [36] showed that after removal of the pituitary, adrenal weight, as well as adrenaline content and phenylethanolamine N-methyltransferase activity of the adrenals, dropped dramatically in a few days. A gradual reduction of tyrosine hydroxylase and dopamine β-hydroxylase activity in the adrenal medulla has also been observed. Thus, the chromaffin cells of the adrenal medulla constitute a target organ for the glucocorticoids elaborated by the adrenal cortex under ACTH stimulation. For the normal response of the adrenal medulla both the integrity of the hypophysial-adrenal cortex axis and the unimpaired sympathetic nerve function are essential. It seems that there are two components to the reflex response of the adrenal medulla. The rapid component requires an intact nerve supply to the adrenal gland, but is independent of adrenocortical response. The delayed component, on the other hand, requires an intact pituitary-adrenocortical axis, but is independent of the motor nerves to the adrenal gland [12].

In addition to sympathetic nerve signaling and sufficient intramedullary glucocorticoid concentration, the response of the adrenal medulla requires a minimum "permissive" concentration of circulating angiotensin II [27]. Specific angiotensin II receptors of the subtype AT1 are found predominantly in the zona glomerulosa and in moderate densities in the adrenal medulla. In the zona fasciculate and reticularis AT1 receptors occur in minimal concentrations [38]. It seems that at least in the dog a part of the stimulatory effect of angiotensin II on the adrenal medulla is indirect, through its steroid-secretagogue action on the adrenal cortex. The reflex release of catecholamines is not mediated by the activation of the renin-angiotensin system [27].

The stimulatory action of sympathetic nerves on steroidogenesis has been shown in experiments with pigs [6, 16], dogs [17, 37], and calves [15] using the isolated in-situ-perfused adrenal system. Infusion of catecholamines or sympathetic nerve activation provoked a significantly increased release of corticosteroids (cortisol, corticosterone, aldosterone, androstendione, 11-deoxycortisol) without, it should be noted, exerting any detectable effect on cortisol output in the absence of ACTH [15]. A direct selective stimulation of 11-β-hydroxylase activity by sympathetic neural impulse enhancing cortisol production has been postulated [17]. Catecholamines also influence steroidogenesis on a molecular level. Incubation of bovine adrenocortical cells with catecholamines resulted in an increase in mRNA encoding the P450 enzymes of adrenal steroidogenesis [22]. Furthermore, it has been suggested that increases in adrenal catecholamine secretion due to sympathetic neural input activation most likely results in the exposure of adrenocortical cells to increased circulating concentration of catecholamines. Catecholamines would act on the adrenal cortex to elicit a steroidogenic response. Based on experimental findings, a modulating effect on steroidogenesis by noradrenaline and dopamine

released from noradrenergic non-synaptic varicose axon terminals adjacent to steroid secreting cells has been discussed [35]. The noradrenergic varicose nerve terminals in the adrenal cortex may be able to take up, and accumulate, noradrenaline and dopamine originating from the circulation. They release noradrenaline and dopamine in the space between them and adjacent cortical cells during axonal firing stimulating β-adrenergic [31] and dopaminergic receptors of the cortical cells [35]. In addition, catecholamines released from noradrenergic nerve terminals may have local modulatory effects on the steroid producing cortical cells.

Frequency and amplitude of the normally occurring episodic bursts in the secretion of steroids by the adrenal cortex is mainly regulated by the secretory activity of the CRH-ACTH axis. The suprachiasmatic nucleus through neuronal connections with the hypothalamic CRH releasing neurons (Fig. 2) includes a circadian variation in this signal resulting in the episodic secretion of cortisol. However, the ACTH secretion patterns correspond only partly to those of cortisol. Numerous experimental observations implicate extra-pituitary mechanisms influencing the sensitivity of the adrenal cortex to ACTH. In rats, splanchnic neural activity may exert an inhibitory effect on pulse frequency of corticosterone secretion by decreasing the adrenocortical responsiveness to ACTH [23, 24]. Pituitary-adrenal cortex secretory rhythms may be affected by a suprachiasmatic nucleus-adrenal cortex pathway (Fig. 2) via preganglionic neurons in the thoracic spinal cord reaching the adrenal cortex directly [10]. This pathway may provide an explanation for the observations that depressed patients often do not show any correlation between plasma ACTH and corresponding cortisol values.

Compensatory growth of the remaining gland following unilateral adrenalectomy is mediated by a neural loop including afferent and efferent limbs between the adrenal glands and the ventromedial hypothalamus [14]. Activation of neuronal efferents from the ventromedial hypothalamus may upregulate a serine protease in the remaining adrenal after unilateral adrenalectomy. This specific protease is capable of cleaving the N-terminal fragment of pro-opiomelanocortin after its secretion from the pituitary into a potent mitogenic fragment [5]. Thus, neural impulses and hormonal secretion seem to be necessary for adrenocortical growth, illustrating a further aspect of the functional interrelation between neural and hormonal activity in the regulation of the adrenocortical function.

4.2.2 Intra-adrenal Regulatory Mechanisms

Humoral and neural regulatory mechanisms originating in the adrenal medulla significantly modulate both the adrenocortical and the medullary hormonal production and secretion. Experimental evidence indicates that the adrenal medulla may exert a paracrine control on the secretory activity of the adrenal cortex by releasing catecholamines and several other regulatory peptides that may act either directly on adrenocortical cells or on the gland vasculature. The morphological background of this paracrine mechanism may be the close proximity of medullary to the cortical cells and, in addition, the presence of abundant cytoplasmic extensions of cortical cells forming wide gap connections with sympathetic nerve terminals. Adrenergic and peptidergic nerve fibers of medullary origin traverse the cortex up to the capsule. A variety of regulatory neuropeptides have been identified in nerve endings within the adrenal cortex and the medulla and in medullary chromaffin cells as well. The medullary chromaffin cells originating from neural crest cells obviously retain a cellular machinery which is able to synthesize and release different neuro-endocrine active substances. Met-, leu-enkephalin and their precursors, neuropeptide Y [33], vasoactive interstinal peptide, oxytocin and vasopressin [3], and pro-opiomelanocortin derived peptides including ACTH, CRH and its receptor [9], have been found in medullary chromaffin cells, nerve fibers and nerve terminals in medulla and cortex. Pituitary adenylate-cyclase activating peptide [30], adrenomedullin [2], and cerebellin [1, 28] are also found in medullary cells. It seems that these peptides exert a stimulatory effect on noradrenaline and adrenaline release, which in turn may stimulate aldosterone secretion probably in a paracrine manner.

4.2.3 Blood Flow

The vascular response to stimulation is an important component of the whole secretory response of the adrenal gland. Increased blood flow influences both the rate of delivery of stimulant to the adrenal cells and the release of secretory products into the bloodstream. It has been shown that cortisol secretion rate is better correlated with the ACTH presentation rate than with the ACTH concentration in the circulation [32]. Also, flow itself can greatly influence hormonal secretion rate even when the stimulant concentration in the circulation is held constant.

ACTH has clear stimulatory effects on blood flow rates through the adrenal gland [21]. At the same time as the rate of corticosteroid production is stimulated by ACTH, blood flow through the whole gland and blood content of the gland are greatly increased. In contrast electrical splanchnic nerve stimulation and reflex stimuli selectively increased blood flow to the adrenal medulla while the blood flow to the adrenal cortex remained unchanged [8, 18]. Neural mechanisms, which influence catecholamine output, may also play an important role in regulation of blood flow to the adrenal medulla without affecting blood flow to the adrenal cortex. Large increases in secretion of catecholamines are associated with increases in blood flow to the adrenal medulla.

References

1. Albertin G, Malendowicz LK, Macchi C, Markowska A, Nussdorfer GG (2000) Cerebellin stimulates the secretory activity of the rat adrenal gland: in vitro and in vivo studies. Neuropeptides 34:7–11
2. Andreis PG, Neri G, Prayer-Galetti T, Rossi GP, Gottardo G, Malendowicz LK, Nussdorfer GG (1997) Effects of adreno-medullin on human adrenal glands: An in vitro study. J Clin Endocrinol Metab 82:1167–1170
3. Ang VTY, Jenkins JS (1984) Neurohypophyseal hormones in the adrenal medulla. J Clin Endocrinol Metab 58:688–691
4. Axelrod J, Reisine TD (1984) Stress hormones: their interaction and regulation. Science 224:452–459
5. Bicknell AB, Lomthaisong K, Woods RJ, Hutchinson EG, Bennett HP, Gladwell RT, Lowry PJ (2001) Characterization of a serine protease that cleaves pro-γ-melanotropin at the adrenal to stimulate growth. Cell 105:903–912
6. Bornstein SR, Ehrhart-Bornstein M, Sherbaum WA, Pfeiffer EF, Holst JJ (1990) Effects of splanchnic nerve stimulation on the adrenal cortex may be mediated by chromaffin cells in a paracrine manner. Endocrinology 127:900–906
7. Bornstein SR, Gonzalez-Hernandez JA, Ehrhart-Bornstein M, Adler G, Sherbaum WA (1994) Intimate contact of chromaffin and cortical cells within the human adrenal gland forms the cellular basis for important intraadrenal interactions. J Clin Endocrinol Metab 78:225–232
8. Breslow MJ, Jordan DA, Thellman ST, Traystman RJ (1987) Neural control of adrenal medullary and cortical blood flow during hemorrhage. Am J Physiol 252:H521–H528
9. Bruhn TO, Engeland WC, Antony ELP, Gann DS, Jackson IMD (1987) Corticotropin-releasing factor in the dog adrenal medulla is secreted in response to hemorrhage. J Clin Endocrinol Metab 120:25–33
10. Buijs RM, Wortel J, van Heerikhuize JJ, Fenstra MGP, Ter Horst GJ, Romijn HJ, Kalsbeek A (1999) Anatomical and functional demonstration of a multisynaptic suprachiasmatic nucleus adrenal (cortex) pathway. Eur J Neurosci 11:1535–1544

11. Coupland RE, Parker TL, Kesse WK, Mohamed AA (1989) The innervation of the adrenal gland. III. Vagal innervation. J Anat 163:173–181

12. Critchley JAJH, Ellis P, Henderson CG, Ungar A (1982) The role of the pituitary-adrenocortical axis in reflex responses of the adrenal medulla of the dog. J Physiol 323:533–541

13. Dagerlind A, Pelto-Huikko M, Diez M, Hokfelt T (1995) Adrenal medullary ganglion neurons project into the splanchnic nerve. Neuroscience 69:1019–1023

14. Dallman MF (1984) Control of adrenocortical growth in vivo. Endocr Res 10:213–242

15. Edwards AV, Jones CT (1987) The effect of splanchnic nerve stimulation on adrenocortical activity in conscious calves. J Physiol 382:385–396

16. Ehrhart-Bornstein M, Bornstein SR, Gonzalez-Hernandez J, Holst J, Waterman MR, Scherbaum WA (1995) Sympathoadrenal regulation of adrenocortical steroidogenesis. Endocr Res 21:13–24

17. Engeland WC, Gann DS (1989) Splanchnic nerve stimulation modulates steroid secretion in hypophysectomized dogs. Neuroendocrinology 50:124–131

18. Faraci FM, Chilian WM, Koudy Williams J, Heistad DD (1989) Effects of reflex stimuli on blood flow to the adrenal medulla. Am J Physiol 257:Ç590–Ç596

19. Friend DS, Gilula NB (1972) A distinctive cell contact in the rat adrenal cortex. J Cell Biol 53:148–163

20. Gallo-Payet N, Pothier P, Isler H (1987) On the presence of chromaffin cells in the adrenal cortex: their possible role in adrenocortical function. Biochem Cell Biol 65:588–592

21. Grant JK, Forrest APM, Symington T (1957) The secretion of cortisol and corticosterone by the human adrenal cortex. Acta Endocrinol (Copenh) 26:195–203

22. Guse-Behling H, Ehrhart-Bornstein M, Bornstein SR, Waterman MR, Scherbaum WA, Adler G (1992) Regulation of adrenal steroidogenesis by adrenaline: Expression of cytochrome P450 genes. J Endocrinol 135:229–237

23. Jasper MS, Engeland WC (1994) Splanchnic neural activity modulates ultradian and circadian rhythms in adrenocortical secretion in awake rats. Neuroendocrinology 59:97–109

24. Jasper MS, Engeland WC (1997) Splanchnicotomy increases adrenal sensitivity to ACTH in nonstressed rats. Am J Physiol 273:E363–E368

25. Kesse WK, Parker TL, Coupland RE (1988) The innervation of the adrenal gland I. The source of pre- and postganglionic nerve fibres to the rat adrenal gland. J Anat 157:33–41

26. Kleitman N, Holzwarth MA (1985) Catecholaminergic innervation of the rat adrenal cortex. Cell Tissue Res 241:139–147

27. MacLean MR, Ungar A (1986) Effects of the renin-angiotensin system on the reflex response of the adrenal medulla to hypotension in the dog. J Physiol 373:343–352

28. Mazzocchi G, Andreis PG, De Caro R, Aragona F, Gottardo L, Nussdorfer GG (1999) Cerebellin enhances in vitro secretory activity of human adrenal gland. J Clin Endocrinol Metal 84:632–635

29. Mohamed AA, Parker TL, Coupland RE (1988) The innervation of the adrenal gland. II. The source of spinal afferent nerve fibres to the guinea-pig adrenal gland. J Anat 160:51–58

30. Neri G, Andreis PG, Prayer-Galetti T, Rossi GP, Malendowicz LK, Nussdorfer GG (1996) Pituitary adenylate-cyclase activating peptide enhances aldosterone secretion of human adrenal gland: Evidence for an indirect mechanism, probably involving the local release of catecholamines. J Clin Endocrinol Metab 81:169–173

31. Shima S, Komoriyama K, Hirai M, Kouyama H (1984) Studies on cyclic nucleotides in the adrenal gland. XI. Adrenergic regulation of adenylate cyclase activity in the adrenal cortex. Endocrinology 114:325–329

32. Urquhart J (1965) Adrenal blood flow and the adrenocortical response to corticotropin. Am J Physiol 209:1162–1168

33. Varndell IM, Polak JM, Allen JM, Terenghi G, Bloom SR (1984) Neuropeptide tyrosine (NPY) immunoreactivity in norepinephrine-containing cells and nerves of the mammalian adrenal gland. Endocrinology 114:1460–1462

34. Vinson GP, Pudney JA, Whitehouse BJ (1985) The mammalian adrenal circulation and the relationship between adrenal blood flow and steroidogenesis. J Endocr 105:285–294

35. Vizi ES, Orso E, Vinson GP, Szalay KS (1996) Local fine tuning by noradrenaline and dopamine of steroid release from glomerulosa boosted by ACTH. In: Vinson GP, Anderson DC (eds) Adrenal glands, vascular system and hypertension. J Endocrinol Ltd, Bristol, pp 293–302

36. Wurtman RJ, Axelrod J (1966) Control of enzymatic synthesis of adrenaline in the adrenal medulla by adrenal cortical steroids. J Biol Chem 241:2301–2305

37. Yamaguchi N, Lamarche L, Briand R (1991) Simultaneous evaluation of medullary secretory functions of normal and acutely denervated adrenals. Am J Physiol 260:R306–R313

38. Zhuo J, MacGregor DP, Mendelsohn FAO (1996) Comparative distribution of angiotensin II receptor subtypes in mammalian adrenal glands. In: Vinson GP, Anderson DC (eds) Adrenal glands, vascular system and hypertension. J Endocrinol Ltd, Bristol, pp 53–68

5   The Value of Adrenal Imaging in Adrenal Surgery

Bruno Niederle, Gertraud Heinz-Peer, Klaus Kaczirek, Amir Kurtaran

CONTENTS

5.1   Introduction

Clinically inapparent adrenal masses (incidentaloma, adrenaloma) are discovered inadvertently during abdominal imaging for several clinical conditions not related to adrenal disease. By definition, the term incidentaloma excludes patients undergoing localization for suspected hormonal excess or those undergoing a staging work-up for previously diagnosed cancer [26].

When detected, these adrenal tumors raise challenging questions for physicians and patients. Not all incidentalomas are of clinical importance and therefore candidates for treatment. After a careful clinical, biochemical and radiological evaluation patients need to be selected for surgery. The indication for surgical treatment and the type of surgical approach depend on hormonal activity, tumor size, localization and suspected malignancy.

Independent of their size, functioning or subclinically autonomous adrenal tumors are candidates for surgery, while non-functioning tumors are not (Fig. 1). According to the literature the indication for the surgical treatment of non-functioning adrenal lesions depends on their size and indirect signs of malignancy. *Non-functioning tumors smaller than 30 mm* are usually followed up. In instances of radiologically documented growth they become candidates for operation. *Non-functioning tumors between 30 and 50 mm* present a relative indication for surgery, since malignancy rarely occurs. The patient's age, co-morbidities and the patient's concern influence therapy. *Non-functioning tumors larger than 50 mm* need a total histological work-up since malignancy increases dramatically with size.

5.2   Fine-Needle Aspiration

The poor prognosis of adrenocortical carcinoma (ACC) makes early diagnosis very important. A reliable histopathological diagnosis from adrenal biopsy, by *fine-needle aspiration (FNA)* or *adrenal core biopsy,* would be desirable but is controversial because of its questionable accuracy and its risks. Whereas sensitivity is high with adrenal metastases (particularly lung, breast and kidney), its accuracy is questionable in the context of primary adrenal tumors (adenomas versus ACC). An overall sensitivity for malignancy of 94.6% and specificity of 95.3% was documented in a recently published ex vivo adrenal core biopsy study [67], when sufficient biopsy specimens were obtained. Comparing the sensitivity and specificity in detection of malignancy of ^{75}Se-selenonocholesterol scintigraphy (^{75}Se-NCS; for further details see below), computed tomography (CT), magnetic resonance im-

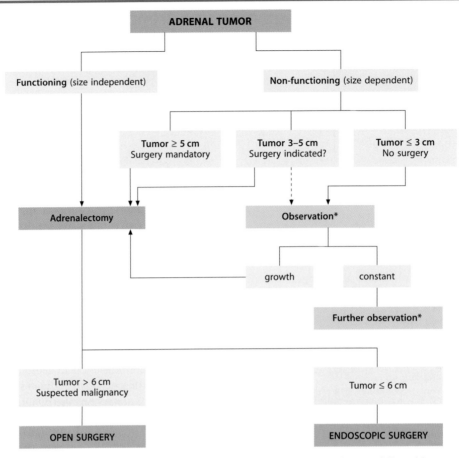

Fig. 1. Treatment algorithm of adrenal tumors depending on hormone function and size (*followed by CT or MRI every 6 months for 2 years)

aging (MRI) and FNA, ^{75}Se-NCS and FNA were more sensitive than CT and MRI [13, 46]. However, in clinical practice it remains to be shown whether the benefits of FNA outweigh the risks of the procedure. Pheochromocytoma must always be excluded before FNA of any adrenal mass is attempted in order to avoid the risk of a life-threatening hypertensive crisis. A benign FNA cytological diagnosis does not exclude malignancy because of the high rate of false-

negative rates. FNA has well-documented side effects such as hemorrhage, pneumothorax or needle track seeding.

The development of semiquantitative adrenal imaging techniques (CT, MRI) has reduced the necessity for cytological differentiation of adrenal lesions [9]. They may help to differentiate between benign and malignant adrenal lesions. Therefore their results strongly influence further treatment (observation or

Table 1. Endoscopic adrenalectomy: indications and contraindications

Indication Functioning/ non-functioning tumors	Relative indication Functioning/ non-functioning tumors	Contraindication Adrenocortical cancer
≤6 cm	≥6 cm Metastasis Very obese patients Major upper abdominal surgery in history	Suspected malignancy

extirpation) and the surgical strategy (open or endoscopic) in patients selected for surgery.

Endoscopic adrenalectomy represents the "New Golden Standard" in the surgical treatment of benign adrenal lesions up to 60 mm [51, 62]. Open adrenalectomy is recommended for patients with suspected malignant disease and for tumors larger than 60 mm (Fig. 1, Table 1). Whether endoscopic adrenalectomy should be proposed for larger (>60 mm) or potentially malignant tumors remains controversial [12, 15, 29].

5.3 Angiography

Angiography has lost its former importance [16] in classifying adrenal tumors and assessing their relationship to adjacent tissue. Angiography of an unknown pheochromocytoma can cause life-threatening hypertensive crisis [16]. Several morphological (ultrasonography, computed tomography, magnetic resonance imaging) and functional imaging studies (selective hormonal venous sampling, scintigraphic techniques) may be applied. In specific clinical situations a combination of morphological and functional adrenal imaging studies is mandatory to answer the following important questions which influence the therapeutic strategy.

5.4 Questions Regarding Adrenal Imaging

1. What is the size of the tumor?
2. Is the lesion solitary or multiple in the affected adrenal gland?
3. Is the contralateral adrenal gland normal or affected?
4. Are there indirect signs of malignancy (prediction of the status by taking into account the appearance of the lesion (homogeneous? inhomogeneous? necrotic areas? fat content? enhancement of the contrast medium?)?
5. Are there direct signs of malignancy (rapid growth in follow-up examinations? infiltration of adjacent organs/structures? tumor-thrombus in the inferior vena cava or the renal vein?)?

5.5 Tumor Size and Malignancy

The size of the adrenal mass, best documented by CT or MRI, is a good but not the best indicator for the prediction of the histological status of an adrenal lesion. The prevalence of ACC is clearly related to the size of the tumor: ACC are usually large (>50 mm in diameter) and adrenal adenomas are usually small (≤50 mm); nevertheless relatively small adrenal cancers and large benign tumors occur with measurable frequency [2]. ACC accounts for 2% of tumors ≤40 mm, 6% of tumors from 41 to 60 mm, and 25% of lesions greater than 60 mm [26]. As shown recently, according to their biochemical profile, 144 (91%) of 158 adrenal lesions were classified as benign and 14 (9%) malignant [62]; 124 (78%) lesions were smaller than 60 mm, 34 (22%) larger than 60 mm, respectively; 25 (17%) of 144 benign lesions were larger than 60 mm; 5 (36%) of 14 malignant tumors were less than 60 mm (i.e. 4% of all lesions smaller than 60 mm); 9 (64%) of 14 malignant lesions were larger than 60 mm and 9 (26%) of 34 tumors larger than 60 mm were classified as malignant. On histopathological examination 74% of all tumors larger than 60 mm were classified as benign. Therefore, the initial size of a lesion *alone* cannot predict the biological behavior of an adrenal lesion and cannot influence the selection of the surgical strategy. Endocrine surgeons and endocrinologists must also take into account that CT and MRI at times underestimate the true size of adrenal tumors [37, 38, 41, 42]; thus the size has to be interpreted with caution [38].

Considering size alone when choosing the surgical access would lead to an endoscopic removal of up to 36% of adrenal malignant tumors [2, 10, 62], which might lead to a high recurrence rate. Therefore additional imaging criteria are mandatory [2].

5.6 Radiological Imaging

5.6.1 Ultrasonography

Ultrasonography (US) is inexpensive, detects adrenal lesions and discriminates cystic from solid lesions. However, ultrasound has a low sensitivity for detection of small masses compared to other modalities (see below). US poorly characterizes solid adrenal masses and poorly detects extension into adjacent structures or is, in the majority of situations, unable to exclude distant metastases. Therefore US seems of no value in answering the questions raised above, for follow-up, for selection of patients who need further treatment, or for planning any surgical procedure.

5.6.2 Computed Tomography

Computed tomography (CT) is generally the preferred primary modality for evaluation of the adrenal glands. CT is fast, readily available, and offers the highest spatial resolution. Helical scanning, using 3–5 mm thick slices to reduce volume averaging, improves the accuracy of density measurement of small adrenal lesions. The latest generation of CT machines (multidetector CT) allows rapid acquisition of very thin slices with excellent spatial resolution. An isotropic data set provides the basis for performance of multiplanar reconstructions and thereby viewing adrenal masses in multiple planes. In addition, anatomic details and relation of adrenal lesions to adjacent structures can be better evaluated. This proves to be extremely helpful in the current era of laparoscopic adrenalectomy.

Contrast CT and delayed images help to characterize enhancement of vessels in the region of the adrenal. Unenhanced CT, however, is often the key series in the evaluation of "incidentalomas" or potential adenomas (Figs. 2, 3). Diagnosis of adenoma when the density is <10 Hounsfield Units (HU) has a sensitivity of 74% and a specificity of 96% [35]. Since many adrenal lesions are incidentally detected on contrasted CT, enhancement patterns of adrenal lesions have been studied to help obviate the need for a separate non-contrast CT, which would require imaging at a separate visit. Immediate post-contrast density is variable and non-discriminatory. Several authors have reported high sensitivity and specificity for density readings on delayed post-contrast CT, but varying cut-off values (25–37 HU) and delay times have been used (15–60 min). In one study of 78 lesions, all adenomas had CT <37 HU and all non-adenomas had a density >41 HU with a 30 min delay after contrast [75]. This yielded both a specificity and sensitivity for adenoma of 100%, respectively. Another recent study showed that no malignant lesions had densities of less than 25 HU at a 15 min delay [43]. This allows 100% specificity with only minimal interruption of the patient flow in CT. The same study showed 96% sensitivity and 100% specificity for adenoma using a 40% washout after a 15 min delay compared to immediate post-contrast images [36].

5.6.3 Magnetic Resonance Imaging

With the advent of dynamic gadolinium enhanced and chemical shift (CSI) techniques, magnetic resonance imaging (MRI) has become a well-accepted diagnos-

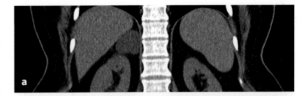

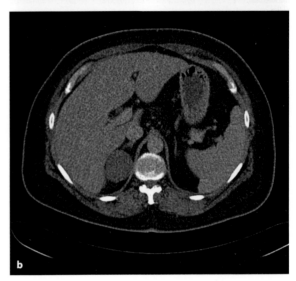

Fig. 2a, b. Benign adrenal adenoma in CT. Twenty-seven-year-old asymptomatic female patient: incidentally detected 40 mm non-functioning adrenal mass in the right adrenal gland. Density of the lesion was 4 HU on unenhanced coronal reconstructed CT scan (**a**) and 39 HU on delayed enhanced CT scan (**b**) with a percentage wash-out of >50% – typical characteristics of a benign adenoma

tic method for the characterization of adrenal masses. Many studies have shown sensitivities and specificities for differentiation of adenomas from non-adenomas ranging between 81–100%, respectively [27, 34, 39, 40, 52, 69].

Korobkin et al. [35] and Outwater et al. [58] showed that the presence of lipid in many of the examined adenomas accounted for the low attenuation on unenhanced CT, causing a loss in signal intensity on chemical shift MR imaging.

In addition, MRI has the best contrast resolution for adrenal evaluation. The spatial resolution is adequate for detection of lesions as small as 0.5–1.0 cm. MRI adrenal studies should include T1-weighted axial images for anatomic detail and T2-weighted axial images [57]. Fat suppression is used so that heavily T2-weighted images are not degraded by chemical shift artifact from the fat which surrounds the adrenals. Contrast helps to characterize enhancement patterns, and on delayed post-contrast MRI series washout

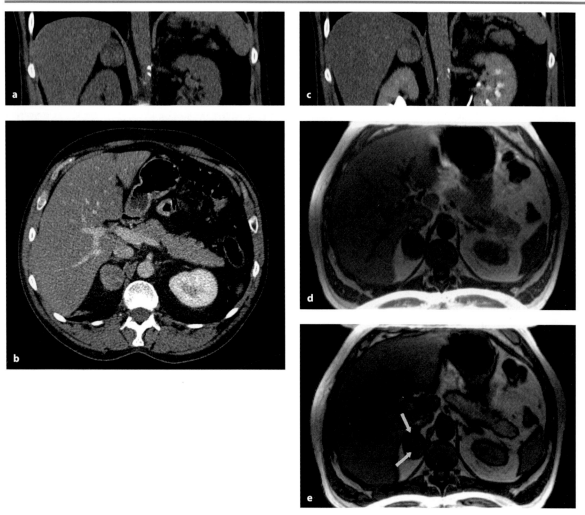

Fig. 3a–e. Benign adrenal adenoma in CT and MRI. Fifty-six-year-old male patient with lung cancer: staging examinations documented a non-functioning, 45 mm mass in the right adrenal gland. Density of the lesion was 6 HU on unenhanced coronal reconstructed CT scan (**a**). On contrast-enhanced scans (**b**) the lesion showed minor enhancement (55–88 HU) and rapid wash-out on delayed scans (**c**), indicating a benign lesion. On MRI (**d, e**) some spotty areas (*arrows*) of significantly decreased SI were demonstrated on opposed-phase images (**e**) again indicative of a benign lesion

curves similar to that on delayed post-contrast CT can be achieved.

By definition [52], an adrenocortical adenoma appears hypo- or isointense relative to the liver on T1-weighted images and hyper- or isointense to the liver on T2-weighted images, and has lost signal intensity on opposed-phase images compared with in-phase images (Fig. 3). In addition, a quick washout on gadolinium-enhanced studies is considered more typical of benign than of malignant lesions [39].

Lesions with marked enhancement on delayed gadolinium series are considered more likely to be malignant (Fig. 4). The diagnosis of carcinomas and metastases (Fig. 5) is based on findings from chemical shift and gadolinium enhanced studies rather than on the signal intensities of conventional techniques [52].

High signal intensity of homogeneous adrenal masses on T2-weighted images and no signal loss on opposed-phase images compared with in-phase images is considered to indicate a pheochromocytoma (Fig. 6) [27, 30]. In addition, an atypical pheochromocytoma may be of medium signal intensity on T2-weighted images or may appear inhomogeneous, especially when they are cystic pheochromocytomas [30].

Lesions appearing heterogeneous on T1 and heterogeneous on T2 and showing a peripheral nodular enhancement and central hypoperfusion on contrasted MRI were characterized as adrenal carcinoma. The

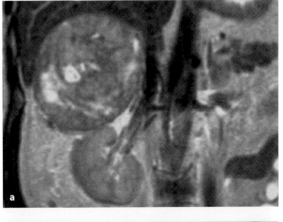

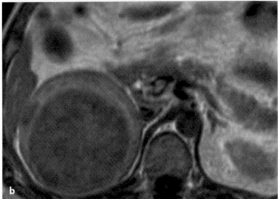

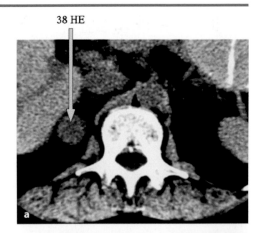

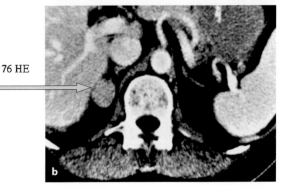

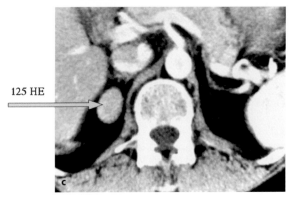

Fig. 4a, b. Adrenocortical cancer in MRI. Sixty-one-year-old male patient with an incidentally 8 cm mass in the right adrenal gland. T2-weighted images showed a sharply demarcated inhomogeneous mass (**a**). There was no evidence of a fat containing lesion and on contrast-enhanced images the mass showed a predominantly peripheral enhancement with central necrosis (**b**)

invasion of adjacent organs or the inferior vena cava was also considered typical of adrenal carcinoma [30].

The presence of fat-containing areas that showed signal intensity equal to those of subcutaneous and retroperitoneal fat at all pulse sequences was the criterion for myelolipoma. The suppression of fat-containing areas on fat-saturation MRI was also considered typical of myelolipoma. [30]. The signal intensity of cysts may depend on their content [30]; however, round adrenal masses with sharp margins in which there was no gadolinium enhancement were diagnosed as adrenal cysts.

In recently published series including a total of 229 adrenal masses in 204 patients, the sensitivity of MRI for the differentiation of benign and malignant adrenal masses was 89%, the specificity 99%, and the accuracy 93.9%. This resulted in a positive predictive value

Fig. 5a–c. Adrenal metastasis. Sixty-five-year-old female patient with breast cancer: abdominal CT scan revealed a 20 mm mass in the right adrenal gland with a density of 38 HU on unenhanced scans (**a**), an increasing enhancement on the arterial phase (**b**) and the 3 min delayed series (**c**), indicating a malignant lesion (metastasis)

(PPV) of 90.9% and in a negative predictive value (NPV) of 94.2% [27, 30].

To transfer this experience into daily surgical practice a prospective protocol was conducted to prove the suitability of gadolinium-enhanced MRI with chemical shift studies (CSI) for predicting the status of adre-

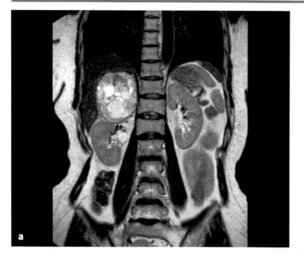

Fig. 6a–d. Benign pheochromocytoma in MRI. Forty-two-year-old female patient with severe hypertension MRI showed a 9 cm predominantly solid mass in the right adrenal gland with some cystic areas on T2-weighted sequence (**a**) and with a hypertense structure on T1-weighted sequence, indicating a hematoma (**b**). After i.v. Gd-DTPA, the mass shows only a mild inhomogeneous enhancement (**c**) and rapid wash-out (**d**)

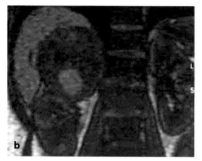 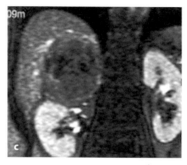 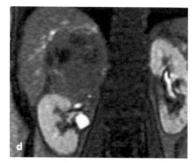

nal tumors irrespective of the tumor size [61] and for planning the surgical procedure [62].

As summarized in Table 2, gadolinium enhanced MRI with CSI diagnosed 120 of 137 tumors (88%) as benign, and 5 (3%) and 12 (9%) of 137 tumors as borderline (epithelial tumors with high malignant potential) and malignant, respectively. During staging examinations no distant metastases, or invasion into adjacent organs or vessels were diagnosed. Histopathological examinations classified 120 (88%) of 137 adrenal tumors as benign, 3 (2%) as borderline and 14 (10%) as malignant. MRI correctly predicted the dignity (benign, borderline and malignant) in 130 of 137 adrenal lesions (sensitivity: 95%). By MRI two

Table 2. Results of MRI ["gadolinium enhanced" MRI with "chemical shift imaging (CSI)"] and histopathology in a prospective study

Predicted status by MRI	n (%)	Histopathology of the adrenal tumor (size)
Benign	120 (87.6)	117 benign [98%] 2 ACC (25 mm; 50 mm) 1 malignant pheochromocytoma (90 mm)
Borderline	5 (3.6)	3 benign 2 borderline classification unclear
Malignant	12 (8.8)	1 borderline 7 ACC 3 metastasis 1 malignant pheochromocytoma
Total	137 (100)	120 benign [88%] 3 borderline [2%] 14 malignant [10%]

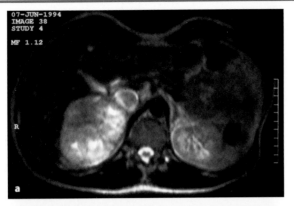

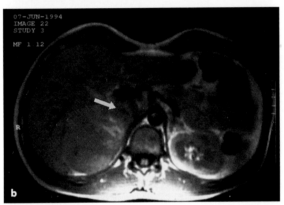

Fig. 7a, b. Malignant pheochromocytoma with tumor thrombus. Fifty-year-old male patient with right flank pain. MRI revealed a 9 cm mass in the right adrenal gland appearing very inhomogeneous on T2-weighted images (**a**) and showing an infiltration of the VCI after Gd–DTPA administration (**b**), indicating a malignant tumor

and histopathological examination proved benign disease in all patients [61].

In addition multiplanar imaging helps to detect extension of the adrenal tumor into adjacent organs and vessels (Fig. 7). These findings are very important because they definitively document malignancy. If surgery is indicated, an open approach has to be performed. MRI proves to be an adequate alternative for imaging of adrenals without radiation exposure. MRI is the first choice in patients with an allergy to iodine contrast media and in patients with renal insufficiency.

5.6.4   The Value of a Combined Use of CT and MRI in Characterizing an Adrenal Mass

To differentiate a benign adenoma from ACC or from a metastasis non-enhanced CT should be performed after appropriate biochemical testing and the attenuation of the mass should be quantified (Fig. 8). If the attenuation of the adrenal mass is 10 HU or less, the mass is an adenoma and the work-up can be stopped. If the attenuation is over 10 HU, contrast-enhanced CT should be performed and washout calculated. A washout of over 50% on a 10-min delayed CT implies an adenoma. If the mass remains indeterminate, MRI should be performed. The characteristics of benign and malignant adrenal lesions in dynamic gadolinium enhanced MRI with CSI are summarized in Table 3. Adrenal lesions suspected to be malignant have to be operated on. Adrenal biopsy could be helpful in the oncologic patient to document metastatic disease, indicating an advanced disease that is sometimes not amenable to surgical resection and potential cure.

cortisol producing ACC (25 mm; 50 mm) and one malignant pheochromocytoma (90 mm) were misdiagnosed as benign tumors. Both patients with the ACC underwent an uneventful transperitoneal laparoscopic adrenalectomy. The patient with the malignant pheochromocytoma was operated on using an open approach. All three patients are free of disease at 12, 38 and 48 months, respectively. One further tumor (80 mm) diagnosed as benign on MRI had a borderline tumor on histopathological examination and was removed by open adrenalectomy. Three tumors (55 mm; 65 mm; 90 mm) were diagnosed as borderline on MRI. Histopathology revealed adenomas with degeneration. With improving endoscopic experience nine patients with adrenal masses (five pheochromocytomas, three non-functioning adenomas, one schwannoma) larger than 6 cm and benign characteristics on MRI were operated on laparoscopically. All of these patients had an uneventful postoperative course

5.6.5   Adrenal Venous Sampling

In 15–25% of patients hypercortisolism is ACTH independent (Cushing's syndrome). In the majority the cause is a primary adrenal neoplasm, usually a benign adenoma rarely a carcinoma, greater than 20 mm in diameter. In a small group of patients bilateral micro- or macronodular hyperplasia is present.

Once the diagnosis of primary aldosteronism (Conn's syndrome) is confirmed the different therapeutic strategies make it important to separate patients with unilateral adrenal tumors (60–80%) from those with unilateral and bilateral adrenal hyperplasia (idiopathic aldosteronism). Primary aldo-

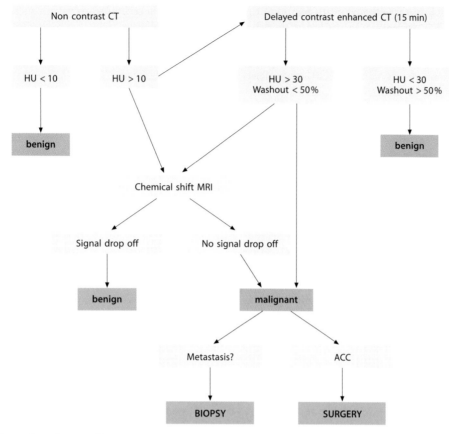

Fig. 8. Work-up algorithm to differentiate benign and malignant adrenal tumors (*HU*, Hounsfield units; *CT*, computed tomography; *MRI*, magnetic resonance imaging)

Table 3. Characteristics of benign and malignant adrenal lesions in dynamic gadolinium enhanced MRI with CSI (*SI*, signal intensity)

	Malignant lesion	Benign lesion
Enhancement of gadolinium	Strong	Moderate
Wash-out phenomenon	Moderate	Quick
CSI: decrease of SI on opposed phase images	Weak	Strong

steronism has uncommonly been associated with ACC [44].

Appropriate treatment depends on a correct morphological diagnosis. Therefore it is necessary to employ radiological and/or scintigraphic localization techniques. The final diagnosis of bilateral hyperplasia in Cushing's syndrome and in Conn's syndrome depends on the determination of cortisol or aldosterone in adrenal venous sampling [11]. In Conn's syndrome this is not only the oldest but also the most precise localization technique available [47, 82], because the solitary lesions causing aldosteronism are smaller than 10 mm in the majority of patients. Magilli [47] and Rossi [66] demonstrated that neither adrenal CT nor MRI is a reliable method to differentiate primary aldosteronism from other adrenal tumors. Adrenal vein sampling seems essential to establish the correct diagnosis of primary aldosteronism [78].

5.7 Nuclear Medicine Imaging

Radiological imaging modalities such as CT and MRI give excellent anatomic details due to their high image resolution, which is very important in planning the operation [5] but provides no information on the function of an adrenal mass.

Both adrenomedullary and adrenocortical scintigraphy of adrenal glands using specific radiopharmaceuticals have the advantage of providing functional metabolic information for lesion characterization [24, 50].

Scintigraphic imaging may help to discriminate between benign and malignant lesions [1]. In patients with bilateral adrenal masses scintigraphy is able to differentiate between unilateral cortical/medullary tumors and bilateral hyperplasia [24, 25]. Finally, when a malignancy is present, scintigraphic techniques have the advantage of providing unique information concerning the entire body with only one administration of tracer without an additional radiation dose to the patient [59].

Based on their different natures, radiological as well as scintigraphic techniques should be considered complementary and both are necessary in the investigation of the patients [24, 59].

5.7.1 Adrenocortical Scintigraphy with ^{131}I-6β-iodomethyl-norcholesterol (NP-59), ^{131}I-19-iodocholesterol or ^{75}Se-selenocholesterol

Adrenocortical scintigraphy with NP-59 provides functional characterization of the adrenal glands due to the uptake of the radiotracer by functioning adrenal cortical tissue (Fig. 9). After intravenous injection this tracer is bound to low-density lipoproteins, which are transported by the circulation to specific low-den-

sity lipoprotein receptors on tissues such as liver and adrenocortical cells. Following the receptor mediated uptake by adrenocortical cells, NP-59 is etherified and stored in the intracellular lipid droplets but is not further metabolized [1, 22, 23]. NP-59 is well recognized to evaluate both hypersecreting and non-hypersecreting adrenal abnormalities. The main clinical questions for NP-59 scintigraphy in patients with hypercortisolism, hyperaldosteronism and hyperandrogenism are whether the disease is due to adenoma, or to bilateral hyperplasia or whether there is evidence of malignancy [7, 18, 19, 21, 64].

The imaging pattern of NP-59 scintigraphy can be compared with that of a thyroid scan, i.e. hormonally hypersecretory and non-hypersecretory adrenocortical adenomas demonstrate NP-59 accumulation and thus scintigraphic visualization on the side of the radiologically known adrenal mass. This is based on the fact that an adrenal adenoma is thought to represent non-malignant proliferation of adrenocortical cells able to accumulate greater amounts of NP-59. Nonfunctioning malignancies (primary or secondary) as well as other expansive lesions of the adrenal glands demonstrate decreased or an absent uptake by the affected gland [1, 7, 24, 56]. Bilaterally symmetrical NP-59 uptake is considered normal [14], while bilaterally increased uptake is consistent with bilateral hyperactive disease [22, 25, 53]. A number of studies have indicated that the degree of adrenocortical NP-59 uptake correlates with the level of hormonal hypersecretion [22, 24].

In patients with primary aldosteronism the overall sensitivity of combined NP-59 scan and CT was 100% [46]. Thus norcholesterol scintigraphy and CT seem necessary to confirm exclusive unilateral adrenal hyperfunction and, subsequently, establish the appropriate treatment [46].

Apart from NP-59, several other adrenocortical radiopharmaceuticals such as ^{131}I-19-iodocholesterol and ^{75}Se-selenomethyl-norcholesterol which have a similar uptake mechanism are used for adrenocortical imaging [25]. As shown recently [45], ^{75}Se-selenomethyl-norcholesterol represents the most sensitive and specific method of adrenal imaging study in patients with Cushing's syndrome compared to CT and MRI.

5.7.1.1 Patient Premedication

Thyroid Blockade ▶ Uptake of free ^{131}I derived from in vivo deiodination should be inhibited by oral adminis-

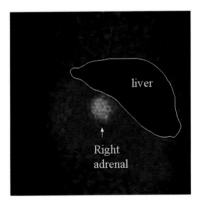

Fig.9. ^{131}I-NP59 (norcholesterol) scintigraphy in a patient with primary aldosteronism demonstrating a focally increased tracer accumulation in right adrenal gland (dorsal view)

tration of saturated potassium iodide (100–200 mg/day, orally) starting 24 h prior to and throughout the imaging sequences and should be continued for about 1 week. Inadequate thyroid blockade leads to scintigraphic visualization of the thyroid gland and a substantial radiation exposure [7, 20, 24].

Laxatives ► To reduce potentially non-specific colonic radioactivity, 2 days before the 1st day of planned imaging, a mild laxative (10 mg bisacodyl) can be given [7, 22, 24, 70].

5.7.1.2 Interfering Drugs

Administration of drugs that might interfere with scintigraphic studies have to be interrupted before and during scintigraphy to avoid misinterpretation of the scintigraphic findings. This includes glucocorticoids, diuretics, spironolactone, beta- and calcium channel blockers, alpha-blockers and agents which interfere with the hypothalamic-pituitary adrenal axis and the renin-angiotensin–aldactone-system [7, 20, 22, 24, 53, 71].

In the case of aldosteronism, dexamethasone suppression is necessary to optimize the sensitivity of NP-59 scintigraphy. Dexamethasone suppresses the normal ACTH sensitive adrenal cortical function of corticoid production and has two important advantages: firstly, and most importantly, is the distinction between hyperplasia and adenoma, and, secondly, the reduction of radiation exposure to the normal adrenal gland. Dexamethasone is given at a dose of 0.5–1 mg 4 times a day starting 7 days prior to the tracer dose until the last day of the scintigraphy [7, 33, 64].

5.7.1.3 Scintigraphy

The usual dose of NP-59 is 1 mCi (37 MBq) administered by slow intravenous injection. Scintigraphic evaluation is possible 3–7 days after NP-59 application depending on the clinical situation. Planar images of a posterior view with a 256×256 matrix (high-energy collimator, 50,000–100,000 cts per image) are obtained on day 3 or 4 in patients with hyperaldosteronism and on day 5 after NP-59 administration in other clinical scenarios. If needed, additional images can be obtained on day 6 and 7 post NP-59 injection to give additional anatomical information. In some patients, additional acquisitions in a lateral projection may be required to assist in adrenocortical localization. Like-

wise, ^{99m}Tc-DTPA or ^{99m}Tc-DMSA scintigraphy of the kidneys may be necessary for a better anatomic identification of the tumor location, which can be done on the 5th or 7th day of the study. If ectopic adrenocortical tumor or tissue remnants are suspected, whole-body imaging has to be performed [7, 33, 64].

Although adrenocortical scintigraphy is able to provide an important contribution to identifying functional behavior of adrenal lesions, adrenocortical scanning is a laborious, time-consuming investigation and its results are dependent on the tumor size [81]. This method has a high overall sensitivity and specificity, although it is not able to give 100% true positive results [22, 33, 68, 83].

5.7.2 Adrenomedullary Imaging with ^{131}I- or ^{123}I-labeled Metaiodobenzylguandine

Chromaffin tumors can affect one or both adrenals (pheochromocytoma) or are localized outside the adrenal gland (paragangliomas). Paragangliomas can be found from the base of the skull to the pelvic diaphragm [59, 77]. They can appear as sporadic lesions or hereditary as part of the multiple endocrine neoplasia syndromes type 2A and 2B, Recklinghausen's neurofibromatosis, von-Hippel-Lindau disease or with the Sturge-Weber syndrome [59, 64, 76].

Most sporadic adrenomedullary tumors are benign, and are mostly localized in one adrenal [59]. Hereditary tumors are very often found in both adrenal glands.

Since appropriate therapy is highly dependent upon reliable exclusion of multifocality or metastatic disease, preoperative localization by scintigraphy is mandatory. For this reason and because of the introduction of minimal invasive surgery in recent years, accurate clinical staging of the disease is now of utmost importance. Of these nuclear medicine modalities, ^{123}I- or ^{131}I-labeled metaiodobenzylguanidine (MIBG) is a well-established radiopharmaceutical sensitive and specific for localization of phechromocytoma and paraganglioma since its initial clinical introduction in 1981 [5, 72].

MIBG is a functional and structural analog of the neurotransmitter norepinephrine that exploits the amine precursor uptake mechanism and is incorporated into vesicles or neurosecretory granules in the cytoplasm [31, 72, 74, 79, 80]. MIBG intensity in MIBG-avid tissue is a balance between uptake, storage capacity as well as tracer turnover. These properties of MIBG have led to the use of labeled MIBG to visualize chromaffin tumors (Fig. 10). This technique permits non-invasive and safe localization of pheochromocy-

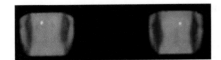

Fig. 10. ^{123}I-MIBG scintigraphy in a patient with a pheochromocytoma in the left adrenal gland. *Left* dorsal view, *right* ventral view

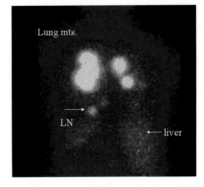

Fig. 11. ^{123}I-MIBG scintigraphy in a 77-year-old female patient with a malignant pheochromocytoma 17 years after primary surgery. Note the multiple MIBG-avid lesions in the thorax and abdomen (LNN metastases). Patient selected for ^{131}I-MIBG therapy

toma and paraganglioma with several advantages over anatomical radiological images. One significant advantage of MIBG scintigraphy over radiological imaging techniques is the possibility of whole body evaluation with a single administration of the radiotracer. Other advantages of MIBG scintigraphy are the low rate of false-positive, and when labeled with ^{123}I, the low rate of false-negative, results, and its high sensitivity and specificity in postoperative patients with distorted anatomy [59]. After intravenous injection, MIBG is distributed throughout the body. The normal MIBG biodistribution includes depiction of salivary glands, lacrimal glands, heart and spleen based on the extensive sympathetic innervation of these tissues. The distribution of radiolabeled MIBG within the limbs shows modest diffuse activity within the muscles and none within the long bones. Excretory organs such as the kidneys, urinary bladder, liver and intestine are also visualized. Of the radiolabeled MIBG, 55–60% is excreted through the kidneys in the first 24 h. The normal adrenal medulla may be seen with ^{123}I-labeled MIBG; it is, however, only rarely visualized with ^{131}I-labeled MIBG [54, 55, 72]. Any focal MIBG accumulation at sites not described above is strongly suspicious for MIBG-avid abnormal tissue.

The main clinical questions for MIBG scintigraphy in patients with adrenomedullary hypersecretion are whether the secreting tumor is localized in or outside the adrenal gland, whether the tumor site is uni- or bilateral or whether there is evidence of malignancy (Fig. 11).

5.7.2.1 Patient Premedication

Thyroid Blockade ▸ To avoid uptake of free iodine in the thyroid, there is a need for thyroid blockade because of the iodine content of the radiolabeled MIBG. Starting 2 days before administration of ^{131}I-MIBG, 100–200 mg saturated potassium iodine/day should be administered for 1 week. If ^{123}I-MIBG is administered for adrenomedullar scintigraphy, a thyroid blockade for only 2 days starting the day before MIBG injection

can also be done with saturated potassium iodine (100–200 mg/orally, daily).

Laxatives ▸ For better evaluation of the abdomen, the intake of laxatives (e.g. bisacodyl 10 mg) 1 or better still 2 days before scintigraphy is recommended.

5.7.2.2 Interfering Drugs

It is known that MIBG uptake is hampered by a large number of drugs. Thus drugs known to interfere with MIBG uptake have to be interrupted to prevent drug interference. These drugs include tricyclic antidepressants (amitriptyline, imipramine), sympathomimetics (phenylephrine, phenylpropanolamine, pseudoephrine, ephedrine and cocaine), and antihypertensive/cardiovascular drugs (labetolol, reserpine and calcium channel blockers). Another group of drugs which in principle may also interfere with MIBG has not yet been confirmed clinically or experimentally [7, 32, 33, 72, 74].

5.7.2.3 ^{123}I-MIBG Scintigraphy

^{123}I has better physical characteristics and higher photon efficiency with consequently better image quality than ^{131}I-MIBG and thus is the radiopharmaceutical of choice. Due to the shorter physical half-life and lower number of particulate emissions, ^{123}I-MIBG has a more favorable radiation dosimetry, and approximately 20 times higher diagnostic doses can be administered when compared with ^{131}I-MIBG [7]. ^{123}I-MIBG permits better localization and clearer delineation of small lesions and also allows SPECT (single photon emission computer tomography) imaging. ^{123}I-MIBG scintigraphy is performed 24 h after administration of 185–370 MBq ^{123}I-MIBG, which should be administered as a slow intravenous injection to avoid potential side effects such as hypertensive crises or tachycardia. If non-specific tracer accumulation is suspected in the kidneys and/or in the intestine, a delayed image may be necessary up to 72 hours postinjection. Although ^{123}I-MIBG is the radiopharmaceutical of choice, its use is limited because of the higher costs and due to the fact that ^{123}I-MIBG is not commercially available in all countries [7, 33, 64, 72]. ^{131}I-MIBG which is commercially available also gives very good results despite its suboptimal physical properties.

For better orientation whole-body acquisition (10 cm/min) in anterior and posterior views with a low-energy collimator is helpful. Thoracic and abdominal planar projections (anterior and posterior, matrix 256x256) are obligatory. For each acquisition 300–800 Kcts are needed. The additional SPECT technique of the abdomen and/or other suspected regions is important for recognition of small lesions and for better correlation with radiological techniques.

5.7.2.4 ^{131}I-MIBG

Clinical imaging is performed 1, 2, and 3 days after ^{131}I-MIBG administration of 17–37 MBq by intravenous injection. Gamma camera procedures have to be performed with planar views of the pelvis, abdomen, thorax and skull in anterior and posterior projections (matrix 265×265) with a high energy collimator. A quantity of 50–100 Kcts is needed for each planar acquisition. In some cases, lateral views of a region are important to define overlapping of organs. If the anatomical localization of the lesions depicted is not possible with ^{131}I-MIBG alone, simultaneous scintigraphies such as those of bone scan; renogram; or cardiac or liver scans may be helpful. Due to the long half-life of ^{131}I, scintigraphic evaluation is possible up to 5–7 days after injection of ^{131}I-MIBG, and this is occasionally useful [72].

5.7.3 Positron Emission Tomography

[18]F-Fluorodeoxyglucose (FDG) positron emission tomography (PET) has been proposed in nuclear oncology to evaluate tumor metabolism, especially providing functional information to characterize adrenal masses [65]. However, limited dates are available regarding the role of FDG and ^{11}C-metomidate PET in patients with adrenal masses [6, 49]. Further studies must be performed to define the role of PET in the diagnostic algorithm of adrenal lesions.

5.8 The Value of Imaging Studies for the Surgeon

The radiological work-up of diseases affecting the adrenal gland should start with appropriate biochemical screening tests followed by thin-collimation CT. If the results of CT are not diagnostic, MRI and in selected cases nuclear medicine imaging examinations should be performed.

The probability of an adrenal mass being malignant has been shown to increase significantly with its size (greatest diameter). But not all growing lesions are malignant [3, 4, 8, 48, 73]. A malignant-to-benign ratio of 8:1 has been reported in masses greater than 4 cm in diameter, thus prompting the recommendation for the systematic removal of a mass above that size and for enlarging lesions on follow-up examinations. Management strategies based on adrenal tumor size alone are neither sensitive nor specific, and tend to miss smaller and perhaps more surgically amenable lesions. Recommendations have been made that all lesions greater than 4 cm should be removed [45]. This approach would have the consequence that many more benign than malignant masses would be subjected to surgery, with attendant cost and risks. Many studies show that (multidetector) CT and dynamic gadolinium enhanced MRI with CSS are useful single investigations to predict the status of adrenal tumors in up to 95%. At least one of these investigations should be applied prior to planning the surgical strategy (minimally invasive adrenal versus open adrenal surgery) independent of the tumor size and function for planning surgery. Unforeseen conversion to open surgery and intraoperative complications (laceration of tumor capsule) can be reduced or prevented [28]. Tumor size alone is not suitable to predict the status of adrenal lesions. Taking into account tumor size and the results of preoperative imaging (CT or MRI), up to 70% of patients selected for surgery are suitable for endoscopic adrenalectomy [62]. Even tumors larger than 6 cm, classified as benign by CT or MRI, may be removed laparoscopically by endocrine surgeons experienced in endoscopic adrenalectomy [15, 29, 60].

In selected cases adrenocortical or adrenomedullary scintigraphic imaging of the adrenal glands is mandatory to localize the tumor within the gland, to exclude extra adrenal disease, multifocality or distant spread in a single procedure [17, 59, 63].

References

1. Arnaldi G, Masini AM, Giacchetti G, Taccaliti A, Faloia E, Mantero F (2000) Adrenal incidentaloma. Braz J Med Biol Res 33:1177–1189

2. Barnett CC Jr, Varma DG, El-Naggar AK, Dackiw AP, Porter GA, Pearson AS, Kudelka AP, Gagel RF, Evans DB, Lee JE (2000) Limitations of size as a criterion in the evaluation of adrenal tumors. Surgery 128:973–982; discussion 982–983

3. Barry MK, van Heerden JA, Farley DR, Grant CS, Thompson GB, Ilstrup DM (1998) Can adrenal incidentalomas be safely observed? World J Surg 22:599–603; discussion 603–604

4. Barzon L, Scaroni C, Sonino N, Fallo F, Paoletta A, Boscaro M (1999) Risk factors and long-term follow-up of adrenal incidentalomas. J Clin Endocrinol Metab 84:520–526

5. Berglund S, Hulthen UL, Manhem P (2001) Metaiodobenzylguanidine (MIBG) scintigraphy and computed tomography (CT) in clinical practice. J Intern Med 249:247–251

6. Bergstrom M, Juhlin C, Bonasera TA, Sundin A, Rastad J, Akerstrom G, Langstrom B (2000) PET imaging of adrenal cortical tumors with the 11beta-hydroxylase tracer 11C-metomidate. J Nucl Med 41:275–282

7. Biersack HJ, Grunwald F (1995) Endocrinological applications in nuclear medicine. Semin Nucl Med 25:92–110

8. Brunt LM, Moley JF (2001) Adrenal incidentaloma. World J Surg 25:905–913

9. Choyke PL (1998) From needles to numbers: can noninvasive imaging distinguish benign and malignant adrenal lesions? World J Urol 16:29–34

10. Dackiw AP, Lee JE, Gagel RF, Evans DB (2001) Adrenal cortical carcinoma. World J Surg 25:914–926

11. Doppman JL (1996) Hyperaldosteronism: Sampling the adrenal veins. Radiology 198:309–312

12. Duh QY (2002) Adrenal incidentalomas. Br J Surg 89:1347–1349

13. Favia G, Lumachi F, Basso S, D'Amico DF (2000) Management of incidentally discovered adrenal masses and risk of malignancy. Surgery 128:918–924

14. Freitas JE, Thrall JH, Swanson DP, Rifai A, Beierwaltes WH (1975) Normal adrenal asymmetry: explanation and interpretation. J Nucl Med 19:149–154

15. Gagner M, Pomp A, Heniford BT, Pharand D, Lacroix A (1997) Laparoscopic adrenalectomy: lessons learned from 100 consecutive procedures. Ann Surg 226:238–246; discussion 246–247

16. Geelhoed GW, Druy EM (1983) Adrenal radiography: problems and pitfalls in adrenal localization. World J Surg 7:209–222

17. Glazer GM (1988) MR imaging of the liver, kidneys, and adrenal glands. Radiology 166:303–312

18. Gross MD, Freitas JE, Swanson DP, Brady T, Beierwaltes WH (1979) The normal dexamethasone-suppression adrenal scintiscan. J Nucl Med 20:1131–1135

19. Gross MD, Thrall JH, Beierwaltes WH (1980) The adrenal scan: a current status report on radiotracers, dosimetry and clinical utility. Nucl Med Annual, Raven Press, New York, pp 27–175

20. Gross MD, Valk TW, Swanson DP, Thrall JH, Grekin RJ, Beirewaltes WH (1981) The role of pharmacologic manipulation in adrenal cortical scintigraphy. Semin Nucl Med 11:128–148

21. Gross MD, Shapiro B, Grekin RJ, Freitas JE, Glazer G, Beierwaltes WH, Thompson NW (1984) Scintigraphic localization of adrenal lesions in primary aldosteronism. Am J Med 77:839–844

22. Gross MD, Shapiro B, Bouffard JA, Glazer GM, Francis IR, Wilton GP, Khafagi F, Sonda LP (1988) Distinguishing benign from malignant euadrenal masses. Ann Intern Med 109:613–618

23. Gross MD, Shapiro B (1989) Scintigraphic studies in adrenal hypertension. Semin Nucl Med 19:122–143

24. Gross MD, Shapiro B, Francis IR, Glazer GM, Bree RL, Arcomano MA, Schteingart DE, McLeod MK, Sanfield JA, Thompson NW (1994) Scintigraphic evaluation of clinically silent adrenal masses. J Nucl Med 35:1145–1152

25. Gross MD, Shapiro B, Francis IR, Bree RL, Korobkin M, McLeod MK, Thompson NW, Sanfield JA (1995) Scintigraphy of incidentally discovered bilateral adrenal masses. Eur J Nucl Med 22:315–321

26. Grumbach MM, Biller BM, Braunstein GD, Campbell KK, Carney JA, Godley PA, Harris EL, Lee JK, Oertel YC, Posner MC, Schlechte JA, Wieand HS (2003) Management of the clinically inapparent adrenal mass ("incidentaloma"). Ann Intern Med 138:424–429

27. Heinz-Peer G, Honigschnabl S, Schneider B, Niederle B, Kaserer K, Lechner G (1999) Characterization of adrenal masses using MR imaging with histopathologic correlation. AJR Am J Roentgenol 173:15–22

28. Henry JF, Defechereux T, Gramatica L, Raffaelli M (1999) Should laparoscopic approach be proposed for large and/or potentially malignant adrenal tumors? Langenbecks Arch Surg 384:366–369

29. Henry JF, Sebag F, Iacobone M, Mirallie E (2002) Results of laparoscopic adrenalectomy for large and potentially malignant tumors. World J Surg 26:1043–1047

30. Hönigschnabl S (2002) How accurate is MR imaging in characterisation of adrenal masses: update of a long-term study. Eur J Radiol 41:113–122

31. Kaltsas G, Korbonits M, Heintz E, Mukherjee JJ, Jenkins PJ, Chew SL, Reznek R, Monson JP, Besser GM, Foley R, Britton KE, Grossman AB (2001) Comparison of somatostatin analog and meta-iodobenzylguanidine radionuclides in the diagnosis and localization of advanced neuroendocrine tumors. J Clin Endocrinol Metab 86:895–902

32. Khafagi FA, Shapiro B, Fig LM, Mallette S, Sisson JC (1989) Labetalol reduces iodine-131 MIBG uptake by pheochromocytoma and normal tissues. J Nucl Med 30:481–489

33. Kloos RT, Gross MD, Francis IR, Korobkin M, Shapiro B (1995) Incidentally discovered adrenal masses. Endocr Rev 16:460–484

34. Korobkin M, Lombardi TJ, Aisen AM, Francis IR, Quint LE, Dunnick NR, Londy F, Shapiro B, Gross MD, Thompson NW (1995) Characterization of adrenal masses with chemical shift and gadolinium-enhanced MR imaging. Radiology 197:411–418

35. Korobkin M, Giordano TJ, Brodeur FJ, Francis IR, Siegelman ES, Quint LE, Dunnick NR, Heiken JP, Wang HH (1996) Adrenal adenomas: relationship between histologic lipid and CT and MR findings. Radiology 200:743–747

36. Korobkin M, Brodeur FJ, Francis IR, Quint LE, Dunnick NR, Londy F (1998) CT time-attenuation washout curves of adrenal adenomas and nonadenomas. AJR Am J Roentgenol 170:747–752

37. Kouriefs C (1999) Surgical implications of underestimation of adrenal tumour size by computed tomography. Br J Surg 86:385–387

38. Kouriefs C, Mokbel K, Choy C (2001) Is MRI more accurate than CT in estimating the real size of adrenal tumours? Eur J Surg Oncol 27:487–490

39. Krestin GP, Steinbrich W, Friedmann G (1989) Adrenal masses: evaluation with fast gradient-echo MR imaging and Gd-DTPA-enhanced dynamic studies. Radiology 171:675–680

40. Krestin GP, Freidmann G, Fishbach R, Neufang KF, Allolio B (1991) Evaluation of adrenal masses in oncologic patients: dynamic contrast-enhanced MR vs CT. J Comput Assist Tomogr 15:104–110

41. Lau H, Lo CY, Lam KY (1999) Surgical implications of underestimation of adrenal tumour size by computed tomography. Br J Surg 86:385–387

42. Linos DA, Stylopoulos N (1997) How accurate is computed tomography in predicting the real size of adrenal tumors? A retrospective study. Arch Surg 132:740–743

43. Lockhart ME, Smith JK, Kenney PJ (2002) Imaging of adrenal masses. Eur J Radiol 41:95–112

44. Ludvik B, Niederle B, Roka R, Längle F, Neuhold N, Templ M, G. S (1993) Isolated primary aldosteronism in adrenocortical carcinoma: a case report and review of the literature. Acta Chir Austriaca 25:212–216

45. Lumachi F, Zucchetta P, Marzola MC, Bui F, Casarrubea G, Angelini F, Favia G (2002) Usefulness of CT scan, MRI and radiocholesterol scintigraphy for adrenal imaging in Cushing's syndrome. Nucl Med Commun 23:469–473

46. Lumachi F, Borsato S, Tregnaghi A, Basso SM, Marchesi P, Ciarleglio F, Fassina A, Favia G (2003) CT-scan, MRI and image-guided FNA cytology of incidental adrenal masses. Eur J Surg Oncol 29:689–692

47. Magill SB, Raff H, Shaker JL, Brickner RC, Knechtges TE, Kehoe ME, Findling JW (2001) Comparison of adrenal vein sampling and computed tomography in the differentiation of primary aldosteronism. J Clin Endocrinol Metab 86:1066–1071

48. Mantero F, Terzolo M, Arnaldi G, Osella G, Masini AM, Ali A, Giovagnetti M, Opocher G, Angeli A (2000) A survey on adrenal incidentaloma in Italy. Study Group on Adrenal Tumors of the Italian Society of Endocrinology. J Clin Endocrinol Metab 85:637–644

49. Maurea S, Mainolfi C, Bazzicalupo L, Panico MR, Imparato C, Alfano B, Ziviello M, Salvatore M (1999) Imaging of adrenal tumors using FDG PET: comparison of benign and malignant lesions. AJR Am J Roentgenol 173:25–29

50. Maurea S, Klain M, Mainolfi C, Ziviello M, Salvatore M (2001) The diagnostic role of radionuclide imaging in evaluation of patients with nonhypersecreting adrenal masses. J Nucl Med 42:884–892

51. Miccoli P, Raffaelli M, Berti P, Materazzi G, Massi M, Bernini G (2002) Adrenal surgery before and after the introduction of laparoscopic adrenalectomy. Br J Surg 89:779–782

52. Mitchell DG, Crovello M, Matteucci T, Petersen RO, Miettinen MM (1992) Benign adrenocortical masses: diagnosis with chemical shift MR imaging. Radiology 185:345–351

53. Nacaudie-Calzade M, Huglo D, Lambert M (1999) Efficacy of iodine-131–6β-methyl-iodo-19-norcholesterol scintigraphy and computed tomography in patients with primary aldosteronismus. Eur J Nucl Med 26:1326–1332

54. Nakajo M, Shapiro B, Copp J, Kalff V, Gross MD, Sisson JC, Beierwaltes WH (1983) The normal and abnormal distribution of the adrenomedullary imaging agent m-[I-131]iodobenzylguanidine (I-131 MIBG) in man: evaluation by scintigraphy. J Nucl Med 24:672–682

55. Nakajo M, Shapiro B, Glowniak J, Sisson JC, Beierwaltes WH (1983) Inverse relationship between cardiac accumulation of meta-[131I]iodobenzylguanidine (I-131 MIBG) and circulating catecholamines in suspected pheochromocytoma. J Nucl Med 24:1127–1134

56. Niederle B, Winkelbauer FW, Frilling A (1995) Inzedentaloma der Nebenniere – eine Übersicht. Chir Gastroenterol 11:34–41

57. Outwater EK, Siegelman ES, Radecki PD, Piccoli CW, Mitchell DG (1995) Distinction between benign and malignant adrenal masses: value of T1-weighted chemical-shift MR imaging. AJR Am J Roentgenol 165:579–583

58. Outwater EK, Siegelman ES, Huang AB, Birnbaum BA (1996) Adrenal masses: correlation between CT attenuation value and chemical shift ratio at MR imaging with in-phase and opposed-phase sequences. Radiology 200:749–752

59. Pattou FN, Combemale FP, Poirette JF, Carnaille B, Wemeau JL, Huglo D, Ernst O, Proye CA (1996) Questionability of the benefits of routine laparotomy as the surgical approach for pheochromocytomas and abdominal paragangliomas. Surgery 120:1006–1011; discussion 1012

60. Prager G, Heinz-Peer G, Passler C, Kaczirek K, Schindl M, Scheuba C, Niederle B (2002) Surgical strategy in adrenal masses. Eur J Radiol 41:70–77

61. Prager G, Heinz-Peer G, Passler C, Kaczirek K, Schindl M, Scheuba C, Vierhapper H, Niederle B (2002) Can dynamic gadolinium-enhanced magnetic resonance imaging with chemical shift studies predict the status of adrenal masses? World J Surg 26:958–964

62. Prager G, Heinz-Peer G, Passler C, Kaczirek K, Scheuba C, Niederle B (2004) Applicability of laparoscopic adrenalectomy in 150 consecutive patients – a prospective study. Arch Surg 139:46–49

63. Quint LE, Glazer GM, Francis IR, Shapiro B, Chenevert TL (1987) Pheochromocytoma and paraganglioma: comparison of MR imaging with CT and I-131 MIBG scintigraphy. Radiology 165:89–93

64. Reiners C (1994) Nebennierenrinde. In: Büll U, Schicha H, Biersack HJ, Knapp WH, Reiners C, Schober O (eds) Nuklearmedizin. Thieme, Stuttgart

65. Rigo P, Paulus P, Kaschten BJ, Hustinx R, Bury T, Jerusalem G, Benoit T, Foidart-Willems J (1996) Oncological applications of positron emission tomography with fluorine-18 fluorodeoxyglucose. Eur J Nucl Med 23:1641–1674

66. Rossi GP, Sacchetto A, Chiesura-Corona M, De Toni R, Gallina M, Feltrin GP, Pessina AC (2001) Identification of the etiology of primary aldosteronism with adrenal vein sampling in patients with equivocal computed tomography and magnetic resonance findings: results in 104 consecutive cases. J Clin Endocrinol Metab 86:1083–1090

67. Saeger W, Fassnacht M, Chita R, Prager G, Nies C, Lorenz K, Barlehner E, Simon D, Niederle B, Beuschlein F, Allolio B, Reincke M (2003) High diagnostic accuracy of adrenal core biopsy: results of the German and Austrian adrenal network multicenter trial in 220 consecutive patients. Hum Pathol 34:180–186

68. Salam Z, Lubbos H, Martinez C, Mozley PD, Miller JL, Rose LI (1996) Case report: failure of adrenal scintigraphy to exhibit 131I cholesterol uptake in a CT-demonstrated, surgically proven aldosteronoma. Am J Med Sci 312:130–132

69. Semelka RC, Shoenut JP, Lawrence PH, Greenberg HM, Maycher B, Madden TP, Kroeker MA (1993) Evaluation of adrenal masses with gadolinium enhancement and fat-suppressed MR imaging. J Magn Reson Imaging 3:337–343

70. Shapiro B, Nakajo M, Gross MD, Freitas J, Copp J, Beierwaltes WH (1983) Value of bowel preparation in adrenocortical scintigraphy with NP-59. J Nucl Med 24:732–734

71. Shapiro B, Grekin RJ, Gross MD, Freitas JE (1994) Interference of spironolactone on adrenocortical scintigraphy and other pitfalls in the location of adrenal abnormalities in primary aldosteronismus. Clin Nucl Med 19:441–445

72. Shapiro B, Fig LM, Gross MD, Shulkin BL, Sisson JC (1998) Neuroendocrine tumors. In: Aktolun C, Tauxe WN (eds) Nuclear oncology. Springer, Tokyo, pp 3–31

73. Siren J, Tervahartiala P, Sivula A, Haapiainen R (2000) Natural course of adrenal incidentalomas: seven-year follow-up study. World J Surg 24:579–582

74. Solanki KK, Bomanji J, Moyes J, Mather SJ, Trainer PJ, Britton KE (1992) A pharmacological guide to medicines which interfere with the biodistribution of radiolabelled meta-iodobenzylguanidine (MIBG). Nucl Med Commun 13:513–521

75. Szolar DH, Kammerhuber F (1997) Quantitative CT evaluation of adrenal gland masses: a step forward in the differentiation between adenomas and nonadenomas? Radiology 202:517–521

76. Van der Harst E, De Herder WW, Bruining HA (2001) Metaiodobenzylguanidine and In-111-Octreotide uptake in benign and malignant pheochromocytomas. J Clin Endocrinol Metab 86:685–693

77. Whalen RK, Althausen AF, Daniels GH (1992) Extra-adrenal pheochromocytoma. J Urol 147:1–10

78. Wheeler MH, Harris DA (2003) Diagnosis and management of primary aldosteronism. World J Surg 27:627–631

79. Wieland DM, Wu J, Brown LE, Mangner TJ, Swanson DP, Beierwaltes WH (1980) Radiolabeled adrenergic neuron-blocking agents: adrenomedullary imaging with [131I]iodobenzylguanidine. J Nucl Med 21:349–353

80. Wieland DM, Brown LE, Tobes MC, Rogers WL, Marsh DD, Mangner TJ, Swanson DP, Beierwaltes WH (1981) Imaging the primate adrenal medulla with [123I] and [131I] meta-iodobenzylguanidine: concise communication. J Nucl Med 22:358–364

81. Young WF Jr, Hogan MJ, Klee GG, Grant CS, van Heerden JA (1990) Primary aldosteronism: diagnosis and treatment. Mayo Clin Proc 65:96–110

82. Young WF Jr, Stanson AW, Grant CS, Thompson GB, van Heerden JA (1996) Primary aldosteronism: adrenal venous sampling. Surgery 120:913–919; discussion 919–920

83. Yu KC, Alexander HR, Ziessman HA, Norton JA, Doppman JL, Buell JF, Nieman LK, Cutler GB Jr, Chrousos GP, Fraker DL (1995) Role of preoperative iodocholesterol scintiscanning in patients undergoing adrenalectomy for Cushing's syndrome. Surgery 118:981–986; discussion 986–987

6 Cushing's Syndrome

Alejandro Ayala, George Chrousos

6.1 Introduction

Originally described by Harvey Cushing early in the last century, Cushing's syndrome is a multisystem disorder that results from sustained exposure to glucocorticoids, that when untreated results in a fivefold elevation in the relative cardiovascular mortality risk [12, 22]. The clinical spectrum of Cushing's syndrome is broad and although certain signs and symptoms suggest its presence, most clinical manifestations are nonspecific and are seldom pathognomonic. Furthermore, conditions of high prevalence such as hypertension, osteoporosis, depression and obesity may present with laboratory abnormalities of the hypothalamic-pituitary-adrenal axis (i.e., increased cortisol urinary excretion rates and abnormal responses to dexamethasone suppression) that do not reflect sustained pathologic hypercortisolemia ("pseudo-Cushing's states").

6.2 Etiology and Pathophysiology

Cortisol secretion is the result of an integrated response involving suprahypothalamic centers, the hypothalamus, the anterior pituitary and adrenal glands. CRH released into hypophysial portal blood in the median eminence is carried to the anterior pituitary gland, where it stimulates the synthesis and pulsatile release of ACTH. Cortisol, in turn, is secreted from the zonae fasciculata and reticularis of both adrenal glands under ACTH stimulation. ACTH and cortisol secretion are highest in the early morning hours and reach a nadir at midnight. Patients with Cushing's syndrome have elevated nocturnal cortisol levels. A characteristic loss of the circadian hormonal rhythm is the pathophysiologic hallmark of Cushing's syndrome and results in chronic sustained exposure to excessive circulating cortisol levels [23].

Cushing's syndrome can be caused by *exogenous* administration of glucocorticoids or by excessive *endogenous* production of cortisol. In exogenous Cushing's syndrome, ACTH secretion is suppressed *(ACTH-independent)* while in cases of endogenous Cushing's syndrome excess cortisol secretion may be *ACTH-dependent* or *-independent* (Table 1).

Exogenous administration of glucocorticoids, mostly iatrogenic, accounts for the majority of cases of ACTH-independent Cushing's syndrome. Prolonged oral and injected administration of glucocorticoids often causes Cushing's syndrome while topical and inhaled glucocorticoids rarely do so. Surreptitious or factitious (self-induced) intake of a glucocorticoid can occur and should be considered in the early stages of the diagnostic process. The detection of synthetic glucocorticoids in the plasma or urine by high-pres-

Table 1. Classification of Cushing's syndrome

Exogenous
  ACTH-independent
    Iatrogenic
    Factitious
Endogenous
  ACTH-dependent (85%)
    Pituitary adenoma (80%)
    Ectopic ACTH (20%)
    Ectopic CRH (very rare)
  ACTH-independent (15%)
    Adrenal adenoma
    Adrenal carcinoma
    Micronodular adrenal disease (rare)
    Massive macronodular adrenal disease (rare)
    Ectopic adrenal adenoma (very rare)
    Cortisol hypersensitivity (very rare)

sure liquid chromatography is helpful in the diagnosis of this disorder.

Once the diagnosis of endogenous Cushing's syndrome is made, a determination of whether the patient has primary adrenal disease or an ACTH-secreting tumor (ACTH-dependent vs. ACTH-independent)

should be made (Table 1). ACTH-dependent Cushing's syndrome accounts for about 85% of endogenous cases. Approximately 80% of the cases of ACTH-dependent Cushing's syndrome are caused by autonomous pituitary ACTH secretion (referred to as *Cushing's disease*). In the remaining 20% the source of ACTH (or rarely CRH) secretion is ectopic [28]. The molecular pathophysiology of ACTH-secreting tumors remains elusive. Unlike the case of growth hormone secreting adenomas, abnormalities of the G-proteins are not frequent in corticotropinomas. Nonetheless, approximately 50% of these tumors overexpress the cytoplasmic form of the p53 tumor suppressor gene.

ACTH-independent Cushing's syndrome accounts for approximately 15% of endogenous cases and is more often caused by benign cortisol-secreting adrenal adenomas, adrenocortical carcinomas and, rarely, ectopic (extra-adrenal) adrenocortical tumors [16]. Cortisol-secreting adrenal tumors are monoclonal in origin but their pathogenesis remains largely unknown [10]. Abnormalities of the p53 tumor suppressor gene or of the inhibitory subunit of G-proteins and overexpression of insulin-like growth factor II were

Table 2. Adrenal tumors and genetic syndromes

	Clinical presentation	Inheritance	Genetic defect
Multiple endocrine neoplasia (Type 1)[a]	Hyperparathyroidism Pituitary tumors Enteropancreatic tumors Adrenal tumors (rare)	Dominant	Mutations of the menin gene
Carney's syndrome[a]	Mucocutaneous lentigines Multiple endocrine tumors Adrenal hyperplasia (common) Myxomas	Dominant	Mutations of PRKAR1A
Li Fraumeni syndrome	Soft tissue sarcomas Osteosarcomas Leukemias Brain tumors Adrenal tumor Breast cancer	Dominant	Mutations *TP53* gene and the *CHK2* gene
Beckwith-Wiedemann syndrome	Exomphalos Macroglossia Gigantism in the neonate Hemihypertrophy	Variable	Microduplication of chromosome 11p15
McCune-Albright syndrome[a]	Fibrous dysplasia Café au lait spots Sexual precocity	Sporadic	An activating somatic Arg201Cys or Arg201His mutation of the alpha-subunit of Gs

[a] Can cause Cushing's syndrome.

identified in a subset of these neoplasms and might be implicated in their pathogenesis. Several genetic syndromes have been associated with adrenocortical tumors, including *Carney's complex*, the *multiple endocrine neoplasia type 1* syndrome, the *Li-Fraumeni syndrome, Beckwith's syndrome* and the *McCune-Albright syndrome* (Table 2).

6.3   Clinical Features

The typical clinical presentation of Cushing's syndrome results primarily from excess glucocorticoids (hypercortisolism) and to a lesser extent from excess mineralocorticoids (hypermineralo-corticoidism) and adrenal androgens (hyperandrogenism). The nature and severity of symptoms depends on the degree and duration of hypercortisolism and the underlying cause of excess cortisol secretion.

The characteristic somatic changes include weight gain and accumulation of visceral fat which results from excess cortisol and insulin secretion and is associated with the full expression of metabolic syndrome X (hyperlipidemia, hypertension, insulin resistance) and its long-term sequelae. Therefore, even when subtle, excesses of cortisol may have significant effects on glycemic control and blood pressure, and may therefore be an important cause of cardiovascular morbidity. Malignant adrenal and ectopic ACTH-secreting tumors can cause symptoms such as weight loss instead of weight gain. Other signs and symptoms include facial plethora, menstrual irregularities, hirsutism, hypertension, ecchymoses, depression, mucosal hyperpigmentation, muscle weakness and osteoporosis [25]. Hyperpigmentation is caused by increased secretion of ACTH, and androgen excess occurs only in women with adrenal tumors because hypercortisolism per se does not cause hirsutism or acne. Thromboembolic phenomena, including deep venous thrombosis and pulmonary embolism, may occur and can be part of the initial presentation of Cushing's syndrome.

Establishing the differential diagnosis of Cushing's syndrome merely on clinical grounds can be challenging. Hypertension and obesity are commonly found in the general population. Patients with HIV-related lipodystrophy have physical and laboratory findings that can easily be indistinguishable from Cushing's syndrome but do not have hypercortisolemia. Moreover, depressed patients can present with weight gain and osteopenia.

6.4   Laboratory Diagnosis

6.4.1   Screening: Establishing the Diagnosis of Cushing's Syndrome

Because signs and symptoms of Cushing's are not specific, appropriate documentation and verification of sustained endogenous hypercortisolemia is the cornerstone for the detection and diagnosis of Cushing's syndrome. The 1 mg overnight dexamethasone suppression test (DST), the 24-h urinary free cortisol excretion rate, and the measurement of a late evening serum cortisol are all reliable screening tests when appropriately performed [17].

The 1 mg overnight dexamethasone suppression test (DST) is a simple screening tool for Cushing's syndrome, with a reported sensitivity of 95–98% and specificity of 87% [8]. During this procedure, a 0900 hours plasma cortisol following a single dose of 1 mg dexamethasone taken at midnight is obtained. An alternative screening method involves the determination of single plasma or serum cortisol level following 48 h of dexamethasone 0.5 mg 6 hourly. Overall, the 2-day test and the overnight 1 mg DST can be done in outpatients and appear to have comparable sensitivities. False-positive results can occur following weight loss and after sleep deprivation, in patients with obsessive-compulsive disorder, Alzheimer's dementia, or during acute alcohol withdrawal. Moreover, false negatives occur in those treated with medications that enhance the hepatic metabolism of dexamethasone such as phenytoin, barbiturates, rifampicin and carbamazepine.

A *24-hour UFC collection* produces an integrated measure of serum cortisol and has a 95–100% sensitivity and 94–98% specificity for the diagnosis of Cushing's syndrome. This test has superseded the measurement of urinary cortisol metabolites (17-hydroxycorticosteroids or 17-oxogenic steroids [24]). To confirm abnormal results, two or three 24-h urine samples should be obtained. Values consistently in excess of 300 µg/day are highly suggestive of Cushing's syndrome. Appropriate urine collection and determination of the creatinine excretion rate are essential for the interpretation of this test. However, if a correction for size needs to be made, one should correct for body surface area. Additionally, UFC may be higher than the normal limits in up to 40% of patients with depression, anxiety disorder, obsessive-compulsive disorder, sleep apnea, morbid obesity, polycystic ovary syndrome, poorly controlled diabetes mellitus, familial resistance to glucocorticoids, hyperthyroidism and alcoholism.

Urinary cortisol excretion may also be falsely elevated in those patients treated with cortisone or hydrocortisone.

A measurement of *late evening serum cortisol* (plasma cortisol between 11:00 P.M. and 12:00 P.M.) documents the loss of the normal circadian rhythm of cortisol secretion in patients with Cushing's syndrome. The sensitivity and specificity of this test in distinguishing subjects with pseudo-Cushing's states from patients with Cushing's syndrome varies from 95%, to 89% and 97–100% respectively [20, 21]. Normal subjects who have irregular sleeping patterns or who have recently crossed many time zones may have abnormal results (false positives). An alternative to the serum midnight cortisol test is the bedtime salivary cortisol (which measures the free hormone fraction) which a sensitivity of ~93% and specificity of ~100% and the advantage of being an outpatient procedure.

As previously stated, the diagnosis of Cushing's syndrome may be difficult given that hypercortisolism can occur in several disorders other than Cushing's syndrome (Table 3). *The dexamethasone-CRH stimulation test* distinguishes patients with pseudo-Cushing's syndrome from those with Cushing's syndrome. Thus, most patients with Cushing's syndrome (80–90%) show inadequate suppression to low-dose (0.5 mg every 6 h for 2 days) dexamethasone, in contrast to the normal responses of pseudo-Cushing's patients. In addition, patients with Cushing's disease (85%) have a "normal" or exaggerated ACTH response to CRH. When these tests are considered individually their diagnostic accuracy in the differential diagnosis of mild hypercortisolism does not exceed 80%. However, when utilized sequentially, dexamethasone suppression (0.5 mg every 6 h for 2 days) and the ovine CRH (Dex-CRH) stimulation test can distinguish Cushing's disease from pseudo-Cushing's state. The criterion used for the diagnosis of Cushing's disease is a 15-min cortisol level of greater than 38 nmol per liter after the CRH injection. In a limited number of patients with Cushing's syndrome sensitivity and specificity for the dexamethasone-CRH test were found to be 100%. However, the sensitivity was lower (90%) when comparing normals to patients with Cushing's syndrome. Moreover, the accuracy of the dexamethasone-CRH test in patients with episodic hormonogenesis has not been tested. Therefore, this test should be reserved for those patients with mild hypercortisolemia who fail to suppress to 1 mg of overnight dexamethasone. Finally, glucocorticoid resistance is a rare familial or sporadic

Table 3. Differential diagnosis of Cushing's syndrome

Physiologic (adaptive) states
  Stress
  Pregnancy
  Chronic strenuous exercise
  Malnutrition
Pathophysiologic states
  Psychiatric disorders
    Melancholic depression
    Obsessive-compulsive disorder
    Chronic active alcoholism
    Panic disorder
    Anorexia nervosa
    Narcotic withdrawal
  Complicated diabetes mellitus
  Glucocorticoid resistance
  Obesity

condition caused by mutations of the glucocorticoid receptor that results in generalized or partial end-organ insensitivity to physiologic glucocorticoid concentrations. The diagnosis should be considered in patients with elevated urine and plasma cortisol and ACTH levels that are not suppressed by dexamethasone. Plasma cortisol has a circadian rhythm similar to that of normal subjects, albeit at elevated concentrations, and responds normally to stress tests such as insulin-induced hypoglycemia. In addition these patients frequently have elevated plasma and urinary adrenal androgens and mineralocorticoids resulting in hyperandrogenism and hypertension.

In summary, Cushing's syndrome is generally excluded if the response to the single-dose dexamethasone suppression test and appropriately collected 24-h urinary free cortisol measurements is normal. One should bear in mind, however, that cortisol hypersecretion may be intermittent and periodic in 5–10% of patients with Cushing's syndrome of any etiology. Documenting the loss of diurnal variation of plasma cortisol would support the diagnosis of Cushing's syndrome and vice versa. Obtaining more than a single morning and evening blood sample increases the diagnostic value of the test, since a significant variability of cortisol levels may be present. Another strategy involves close monitoring of the patient over the course of a few months. While true hypercortisolism will persist and possibly produce further symptomatology, the hypercortisolism of pseudo-Cushing's states will be corrected spontaneously or with anti-depressant therapy (Fig. 1) [2].

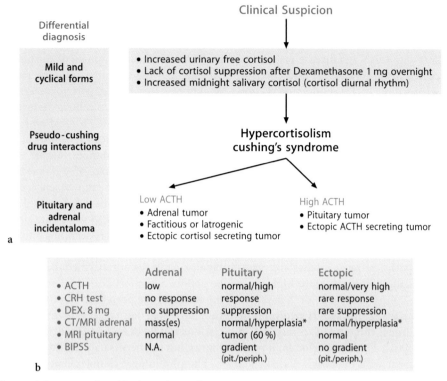

Fig. 1. **a** Differential diagnosis of Cushing's syndrome. **b** Diagnostic tests in Cushing's syndrome

6.4.2 Establishing the Cause: Differential Diagnosis of Cushing's Syndrome: ACTH-Dependent vs. ACTH-Independent

Once the diagnosis of endogenous Cushing's syndrome has been made, the source of excess cortisol should be found. The *plasma ACTH level* distinguishes ACTH-dependent from ACTH-independent Cushing's syndrome [9]. Because they may compromise the diagnostic accuracy of the tests, all adrenal-blocking agents should be discontinued for at least 6 weeks prior to testing. Circulating ACTH is typically suppressed in adrenal cortisol-secreting tumors, micronodular adrenal disease and autonomously functioning macronodular adrenals. In contrast, plasma ACTH concentrations are normal or elevated in Cushing's disease and in those patients with ectopic ACTH and CRH secretion. Serum CRH levels should be measured if ectopic CRH secretion is suspected. Although the determination of plasma ACTH level is often helpful, normal ACTH levels can be found in a subset of patients with Cushing's disease, ectopic ACTH secretion, and in those with adrenal tumors. Similar overlap of baseline ACTH levels may also be seen in children and adolescents with Cushing's syndrome.

The discrepancies in the diagnostic value of plasma ACTH in the differential diagnosis of Cushing's syndrome are probably a reflection of different assay techniques.

6.4.3 Differential Diagnosis of ACTH-Dependent Cushing's Syndrome: Pituitary vs. Ectopic

The vast majority of ACTH-dependent Cushing's syndrome is caused by ACTH-secreting pituitary neoplasms and less often by an ectopic neuroendocrine (thoracic or intra-abdominal) tumor. The strategies used to differentiate the subtypes of ACTH-dependent Cushing's syndrome include biochemical tests, imaging tests (MRI, CT, radionuclide scans) and venous angiography with sampling of the inferior petrosal sinuses for ACTH before and after CRH administration. Because of its low prevalence, the pre-test probability of ectopic ACTH secretion is low. Therefore, one must consider confirming the diagnosis with at least two biochemical tests prior to proceeding with imaging studies intended to localize the tumor. The CRH stimulation test, the high dose dexamethasone suppression test (Liddle's test), and the overnight 8-mg dexamethasone suppression test (see below) are used for this purpose.

The CRH stimulation test is based on the finding that most patients with Cushing's disease respond to CRH with increases in plasma ACTH and cortisol, while patients with ectopic ACTH production do not. A mean cortisol increase at 30 and 45 min of greater than 20% following a bolus infusion of ovine CRH (1 µg/kg i.v.) has a sensitivity of 91% sensitivity and 88% specificity. Similarly, an increase of mean ACTH concentrations at 15 and 30 min after CRH by at least 35% above the mean basal values achieves a sensitivity of 91% and a specificity of nearly 100 [5].

The "standard" *high dose dexamethasone suppression* test (Liddle's test) has been used extensively in the differential diagnosis of ACTH-dependent Cushing's syndrome. Patients with Cushing's disease are sensitive to glucocorticoid inhibition only at the high doses of dexamethasone (2.0 mg every 6 h for 2 days). In contrast, patients with the ectopic ACTH syndrome or cortisol-secreting adrenal tumors fail to respond to the same dose. The classic Liddle criterion for a positive response consistent with Cushing's disease is a greater than 50% fall in 17-hydroxysteroid excretion on day 2 of high-dose dexamethasone (80% diagnostic accuracy). The diagnostic accuracy of the test, however, increases to 86% by measuring both urine free cortisol and 17-hydroxysteroid excretion and by requiring greater suppression of both steroids (greater than 64% and 90%, respectively, for 100% specificity).

A simple, reliable, and inexpensive alternative to the Liddle's dexamethasone suppression test is the *overnight 8-mg dexamethasone suppression test*. The advantages are its outpatient administration and the avoidance of errors due to incomplete urine collections. The diagnostic accuracy of this overnight test may be similar to that of the standard Liddle dexamethasone suppression test.

6.4.4 Unusual Presentations of Cushing's Syndrome

Occasionally, cortisol production in Cushing's syndrome may not be constantly increased but may fluctuate in a "periodic" infradian pattern, ranging in length from days to months. This relatively rare phenomenon of periodic, cyclic, or *episodic hormonogenesis* (periodic Cushing's syndrome) has been described in patients with Cushing's disease, ectopic ACTH-secreting tumors, cortisol-secreting adrenal tumors and micronodular adrenal disease.

Patients with periodic hormonogenesis may have consistently normal 24-h urine free cortisol and paradoxically "normal" responses to dexamethasone in the presence of clinical stigmata of Cushing's syndrome. To establish the diagnosis in such patients, several weekly 24-h urinary free cortisol determinations for a period of 3–6 months may be necessary.

The *occult ectopic ACTH syndrome* can mimic the clinical and biochemical behavior of Cushing's disease. In some circumstances, despite extensive localization studies, the source of ACTH secretion remains elusive. In such cases, the absence of a central to peripheral ACTH gradient before and after administration of oCRH in BIPSS rules out Cushing's disease. After excluding an ACTH-secreting pituitary adenoma, imaging studies with special emphasis on the lungs, thymus, pancreas, adrenal medulla, and thyroid should be obtained, as most described ectopic ACTH-secreting tumors have been found in these organs. Thymic vein sampling for measurement of ACTH concentrations can be of help in localizing the tumor to the thorax, but not necessarily the thymus.

The physiologic changes that occur during *pregnancy* may make the diagnosis of Cushing's syndrome more complicated. In normal pregnancy human placental CRH mRNA transcription and CRH plasma levels increase significantly during the third trimester of pregnancy. A small progressive rise in plasma ACTH and a two- to threefold increase in plasma total and free cortisol also occur. Urinary free cortisol is also elevated during pregnancy, especially between the 34th and 40th weeks of gestation and the suppression of cortisol by dexamethasone may be blunted. Nonetheless, the diurnal rhythm in serum cortisol is maintained.

The *glucocorticoid hypersensitivity syndrome (non-hypercortisolemic endogenous Cushing's syndrome)* characterized by increased tissue sensitivity to cortisol has been reported in two patients harboring the phenotype of Cushing's syndrome but with normal or low cortisol secretion in whom iatrogenic corticosteroid administration was excluded. However, the molecular mechanisms underlying this entity remain elusive since mutational analysis of the glucocorticoid receptor did not reveal any abnormalities.

6.5 Imaging Evaluation

Imaging techniques can help clarify the etiology of hypercortisolism. These include usually MRI of the pituitary and CT scanning of the adrenal glands. CT and MRI scans of the chest and abdomen and isotope scans are also employed when tumors secreting ectopic ACTH are sought.

Computed tomography is the preferred diagnostic method in the detection of adrenal tumors. Most adrenal adenomas causing hypercortisolism are larger than 2 cm in diameter. An attenuation value of more than 10 Hounsfield units (HU) in non-enhanced CT is helpful in differentiating adrenal adenomas from non-adenomas ("incidentalomas") [18]. Tumors with diameters greater than 6 cm, those containing areas of necrosis and those with local spread should raise the suspicion of malignancy.

MRI is as sensitive as CT for the visualization of both normal and enlarged adrenal glands. T2-weighted magnetic resonance images may prove helpful in differentiating between malignant and benign adrenocortical neoplasms. Bilateral enlargement of the adrenal gland with preservation of a relatively normal overall glandular configuration is observed in both Cushing's disease and ectopic ACTH production. Approximately 10–15% of patients with ACTH-dependent Cushing's syndrome demonstrate bilateral nodules (macronodular hyperplasia).

Although the diagnostic accuracy of *radionuclide scanning with iodocholesterol* is questionable, it can occasionally be useful in localizing ectopic adrenal tissue (adrenal rest) or an adrenal remnant causing recurrent hypercortisolism after bilateral adrenalectomy.

MRI scanning is the imaging procedure of choice to visualize pituitary adenomas. The large majority of pituitary ACTH-secreting tumors are microadenomas with a diameter less than 10 mm. The ACTH-secreting adenomata are best demonstrated on coronal T1-weighted images as foci of reduced signal intensity within the pituitary gland. On unenhanced scans, however, ACTH-producing adenomas are detected in only 40% of patients with Cushing's disease. An additional 15–20% of microadenomas are visualized with injection of contrast material (gadolinium-DTPA) and repeat T1-weighted coronal scan immediately after the injection (combined MRI sensitivity 55–60%). Although still experimental, spoiled gradient recalled acquisition MRI might be superior to conventional postcontrast spin echo MRI for detection of adrenocorticotropin-secreting pituitary tumors. CT scanning with infusion of contrast demonstrates pituitary microadenomas in less than 20% of patients with bona fide lesions on subsequent surgery. Thus, pituitary CT should be performed if necessary only to demonstrate bony anatomy prior to transsphenoidal surgery.

If suppression and/or stimulation tests are suggestive of ectopic ACTH production, radiologic imaging of the chest and abdomen should be undertaken. ACTH-producing thymic carcinoids and pheochromocytomas are generally found by CT at the initial presentation of the patient. Patients with a negative CT should undergo MRI of the chest and abdomen using T2-weighted images. A body scan following the injection of the radiolabeled somatostatin analogue octreotide might disclose the tumor site, which can be re-examined by CT or MRI. However, a significant number of small ectopic tumors may remain elusive. In these cases, 3 to 6 monthly reassessments with MRI of the chest are indicated.

Distinguishing Cushing's disease from the ectopic ACTH syndrome frequently presents a major diagnostic challenge. Both pituitary microadenomas and ectopic ACTH-secreting tumors may be radiologically occult and may have similar clinical and laboratory features. *Bilateral inferior petrosal venous sinus* and peripheral vein catheterization with simultaneous collection of samples for measurement of ACTH before and after CRH administration is one of the most specific tests available to localize the source of ACTH production.

Venous blood from the anterior pituitary drains into the cavernous sinus and subsequently into the superior and inferior petrosal sinuses. Catheters are led into each inferior petrosal sinus via the ipsilateral femoral vein. Samples for measurement of plasma ACTH are collected from each inferior petrosal sinus and a peripheral vein both before and after injection of 1 µg/kg body weight of ovine or human CRH. Patients with ectopic ACTH syndrome have no ACTH concentration gradient between either of the inferior petrosal sinuses and the peripheral sample. A ratio greater than or equal to 2.0 in basal ACTH samples between either or both of the inferior petrosal sinuses and a peripheral vein is highly suggestive of Cushing's disease (95% sensitivity, 100% specificity). Stimulation with CRH during the procedure with the resulting outpouring of ACTH increases the sensitivity of BIPSS for detecting corticotroph adenomas to 100% when peak ACTH central to peripheral ratio is greater than or equal to 3.0. Petrosal sinus sampling must be performed bilaterally and simultaneously, because the sensitivity of the test falls to less than 70% with unilateral catheterization [26].

BIPSS is technically difficult and, like all invasive procedures, can never be risk-free even in the most experienced hands. It should be reserved only for patients with a clear diagnosis of hypercortisolism and a negative or equivocal MRI of the pituitary or for those with positive pituitary MRI but equivocal dynamic endocrine testing.

6.6   Medical Treatment

6.6.1   Chemical Adrenolysis

Ketoconazole blocks adrenal steroidogenesis at several levels by inhibiting C17–20 lyase, 11β-hydroxylase, 17-hydroxylase and 18-hydroxylase. Reversible side effects, including elevations of hepatic transaminases and gastrointestinal irritation, may occur and may be dose-limiting. In this case, metyrapone can be added to achieve normocortisolemia. Hypercortisolism is usually easily controlled within a few days with 200–400 mg ketoconazole per day and/or 250–750 mg of metyrapone three times a day. Other blocking agents that may be used alone or in combination with ketoconazole and/or metyrapone include aminoglutethamide and mitotane. Etomidate, a hypnotic imidazole derivative, may also be used safely as a parenteral agent [1, 15].

6.6.2   Radiotherapy

For patients who are not cured by transsphenoidal resection or in those in whom a tumor is not found, *pituitary irradiation* is the next treatment option [4]. Although data on long-term follow-up is still scant, stereotactic radiotherapy provides less irradiation to neuronal tissues, and may offer similar or superior results when compared to conventional radiotherapy. A conventional linear accelerator with 4,500–5,000 rad delivered over a period of 6 weeks will correct the hypercortisolism in approximately 45% of adults and 85% of children, usually within 3–12 months of administration. Addition of the adrenolytic agent mitotane improves the correction of hypercortisolism produced by pituitary radiotherapy. Pituitary irradiation also decreases the occurrence of Nelson's syndrome in patients not cured by irradiation that require bilateral adrenalectomy. If irradiation fails to normalize cortisol secretion, adrenal enzyme inhibitors (medical adrenalectomy) can be used to ameliorate the hypercortisolism. Surgical bilateral total adrenalectomy with lifelong daily glucocorticoid and mineralocorticoid replacement therapy is the final definitive cure.

6.7   Surgery

The treatment of choice for Cushing's disease is selective *transsphenoidal microadenomectomy,* a procedure with a remission rate approaching 95% at major specialized centers on the first exploration by expert pituitary neurosurgeons [14, 19]. Failure of surgery at the first exploration may be followed by a repeat procedure with a 50% chance of cure [11]. Success is defined as a drop of serum cortisol and urinary free cortisol to an undetectable level in the immediate postoperative period. A successful outcome can also be predicted by lack of cortisol response to oCRH, when the test is performed 7–10 days after surgery.

Unilateral or bilateral benign tumors of the adrenals should be surgically resected. Laparoscopic adrenalectomy is the procedure of choice. Aggressive and repetitive open surgery provides the only chance for cure or prolonged survival in adrenal carcinomas [13]. An anterior transabdominal approach with careful examination of the liver and the pararenal structures should be performed [6]. Mitotane may be added to maximally tolerated levels or toxicity when complete resection of the tumor is unsuccessful [27].

In cases of ectopic ACTH-secreting tumors, surgery is warranted except in cases of widely metastatic malignant tumors. If surgery is contraindicated, medical therapy with adrenal enzyme inhibitor is the treatment of choice. If the source of ACTH secretion is not localized, repeat searches for the tumor should be undertaken every 6–12 months. If by 2 years the tumor has escaped detection, bilateral adrenalectomy could be considered [7]. This may have to be done earlier in developing children in whom ketoconazole and the other medications may interfere with growth and pubertal progression.

Glucocorticoid replacement should be started after a successful pituitary adenomectomy or a complete resection of an ACTH-secreting ectopic or a unilateral cortisol-producing adrenal tumor. Hydrocortisone should be replaced at a rate of 10–12 mg/m^2/day by mouth with appropriate increases in minor stress (twofold) and major stress (tenfold) for appropriate lengths of time. The recovery of the suppressed HPA axis can be monitored with a short ACTH test every 3 months. When the 30 min plasma cortisol exceeds 18 μg/dl, hydrocortisone can be discontinued. After a bilateral adrenalectomy, corticosteroid replacement will be necessary for life and includes both glucocorticoids and mineralocorticoids.

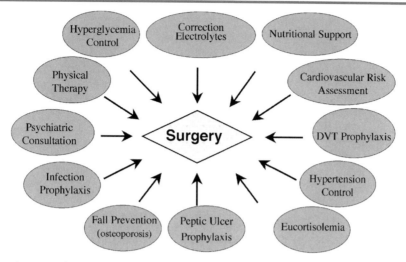

Fig. 2. Cushing's syndrome: perioperative considerations

6.8   Perioperative Considerations (Fig. 2)

Early recognition and treatment of the metabolic, immune, musculoskeletal, psychiatric and cardiovascular complications of Cushing's syndrome are essential to minimize surgical complications (Fig. 1). Uncontrolled hypercortisolemia, electrolyte abnormalities (i.e., hypokalemia), poorly controlled diabetes mellitus and hypertension can increase surgical morbidity and prolong recovery and should be corrected prior to surgery. Adrenal insufficiency often results as a consequence of a successful surgical intervention. In such cases, close monitoring of serum cortisol levels and appropriate glucocorticoid replacement in the early postoperative period is warranted. The patient with Cushing's syndrome should be treated as an immunocompromised host and receive appropriate antimicrobial prophylaxis. Deep venous thrombosis prophylaxis should be considered given that thromboembolic phenomena occur more frequently in patients with Cushing's syndrome than in the general population [3]. Appropriate assessment of cardiovascular risks should be undertaken in light of the fact that Cushing's syndrome is associated with the full expression of metabolic syndrome X (hyperlipidemia, hypertension, insulin resistance) and its long-term sequelae, including coronary artery disease. The high prevalence of mood and cognition disorders in patients with Cushing's syndrome warrants psychiatric consultation. Finally, given early in patients with significant muscle wasting and gait abnormalities, physical therapy may accelerate recovery.

6.9   Conclusions

Cushing's syndrome is suspected on a clinical basis and confirmed with laboratory tests. In mild cases, distinction from the hypercortisolism of pseudo-Cushing states may prove difficult. Surgery is the treatment of choice for all types of Cushing's syndrome. Early recognition and treatment of the metabolic, immune and cardiovascular complications of Cushing's syndrome are essential to minimize surgical complications. Serum cortisol levels and electrolyte abnormalities should be normalized prior to surgery. Appropriate antibiotic prophylaxis and deep venous thrombosis prevention should be instituted. Radiation therapy, radiosurgery and medical adrenalectomy with adrenolytics and adrenal enzyme inhibitors are effective adjuvant treatments. Bilateral adrenalectomy is reserved for those patients who have failed all other forms of treatment.

References

1. Allolio B, Schulte HM, et al. (1988) Nonhypnotic low-dose etomidate for rapid correction of hypercortisolaemia in Cushing's syndrome. Klin Wochenschr 66:361–364
2. Bornstein SR, Stratakis CA, et al. (1999) Adrenocortical tumors: recent advances in basic concepts and clinical management. Ann Intern Med 130:759–71
3. Boscaro M, Sonino N, et al. (2002) Anticoagulant prophylaxis markedly reduces thromboembolic complications in Cushing's syndrome. J Clin Endocrinol Metab 87: 3662–6
4. Estrada J, Boronat M, et al. (1997) The long-term outcome of pituitary irradiation after unsuccessful transsphenoidal surgery in Cushing's disease. N Engl J Med 336: 172–177

5. Findling JW, Raff H (2001) Diagnosis and differential diagnosis of Cushing's syndrome. Endocrinol Metab Clin North Am 30:729–747

6. Godellas CV, Prinz RA (1998) Surgical approach to adrenal neoplasms: laparoscopic versus open adrenalectomy. Surg Oncol Clin N Am 7:807–17

7. Ilias I, Nieman LK (2002) Cushing syndrome due to ectopic ACTH secretion: two decades' experience at a single center. The Endocrine Society 84th Annual Meeting, San Francisco, California

8. Invitti C, Giraldi FP, et al. (1999) Diagnosis and management of Cushing's syndrome: results of an Italian multicentre study. Study Group of the Italian Society of Endocrinology on the Pathophysiology of the Hypothalamic-Pituitary-Adrenal Axis. J Clin Endocrinol Metab 84:440–448

9. Klose M, Kofoed-Enevoldsen A, et al. (2002) Single determination of plasma ACTH using an immunoradiometric assay with high detectability differentiates between ACTH-dependent and -independent Cushing's syndrome. Scand J Clin Lab Invest 62:33–7

10. Lacroix A, N'Diaye N, et al. (2000) The diversity of abnormal hormone receptors in adrenal Cushing's syndrome allows novel pharmacological therapies. Braz J Med Biol Res 33:1201–1209

11. Laws ER, Reitmeyer M, et al. (2002) Cushing's disease resulting from pituitary corticotrophic microadenoma. Treatment results from transsphenoidal microsurgery and gamma knife radiosurgery. Neurochirurgie 48:294–9

12. Lindholm J, Juul S, et al. (2001) Incidence and late prognosis of Cushing's syndrome: a population-based study. J Clin Endocrinol Metab 86:117–23

13. Linos DA, Stylopoulos N, et al. (1997) Anterior, posterior, or laparoscopic approach for the management of adrenal diseases? Am J Surg 173:120–125

14. Ludecke DK, Flitsch J, et al. (2001) Cushing's disease: a surgical view. J Neurooncol 54:151–66

15. Morris D, Grossman A (2002) The medical management of Cushing's syndrome. Ann N Y Acad Sci 970:119–33

16. Newell-Price J, Grossman AB (2001) The differential diagnosis of Cushing's syndrome. Ann Endocrinol (Paris) 62:173–9

17. Nieman LK (2002) Diagnostic tests for Cushing's syndrome. Ann N Y Acad Sci 970:112–8

18. Nwariaku FE, Champine J, et al. (2001) Radiologic characterization of adrenal masses: the role of computed tomography-derived attenuation values. Surgery 130:1068–71

19. Oldfeld EH (2003) Cushing disease. J Neurosurg 98: 948–51; discussion 951

20. Papanicolaou DA, Mullen N, et al. (2002) Nighttime salivary cortisol: a useful test for the diagnosis of Cushing's syndrome. J Clin Endocrinol Metab 87:4515–4521

21. Papanicolaou DA, Yanovski JA, et al. (1998) A single midnight serum cortisol measurement distinguishes Cushing's syndrome from pseudo-Cushing states. J Clin Endocrinol Metab 83:1163–1167

22. Pikkarainen L, Sane T, et al. (1999) The survival and wellbeing of patients treated for Cushing's syndrome. J Intern Med 245:463–8

23. Raff H, Findling JW (2003) A physiologic approach to diagnosis of Cushing syndrome. Ann Int Med 138:980–991

24. Taylor RL, Grebe SK, et al. (2003) Diagnosis of Cushing's syndrome with a sensitive and specific LC-MS/MS method for late night salivary cortisol. ENDO 2003: 85th Annual Meeting of the American Endocrine Society, June 19–22, Philadelphia, PA

25. Torpy DJ, Mullen N, et al. (2002) Association of hypertension and hypokalemia with Cushing's syndrome caused by ectopic ACTH secretion: a series of 58 cases. Ann N Y Acad Sci 970:134–44

26. Tsigos C, Papanicolaou DA, et al. (1995) Advances in the diagnosis and treatment of Cushing's syndrome. Baillieres Clin Endocrinol Metab 9:315–36

27. van Heerden JA, Young WFJ, et al. (1995) Adrenal surgery for hypercortisolism-surgical aspects. Surgery 117:466–472

28. Wajchenberg BL, Mendonca B, et al. (1995) Ectopic ACTH syndrome. J Steroid Biochem Mol Biol 53:139–51

7 Subclinical Cushing's Syndrome

Felix Beuschlein, Martin Reincke

CONTENTS

7.1 Introduction

Clinically inapparent adrenal masses are discovered incidentally in the course of diagnostic testing for other conditions and, thus, are commonly termed incidentalomas. By definition, clinical signs or symptoms of such an adrenal tumor have to be absent. However, a substantial percentage of these incidentally detected adrenal tumors are hormonally active, with up to 20% of the tumors producing glucocorticoids (Fig. 1).

Autonomous glucocorticoid production lacking specific signs and symptoms of Cushing's syndrome is termed subclinical or preclinical Cushing's syndrome (SCCS). Glucocorticoid production in these patients is low resulting in no or only mild symptoms which may not be clinically recognized as Cushing's syndrome (Fig. 2a).

On the contrary, overt Cushing's syndrome, the consequence of longstanding excess of circulating glucocorticoids, is characterized by typical signs and symptoms of hypercortisolism like plethora, moon face, buffalo hump, central obesity, easy bruising, deep-purple striae, proximal muscle weakness, menstrual irregularities, acne, hirsutism, osteoporosis, and glucose intolerance (Fig. 2b). Classical Cushing's syndrome is a rare disease with an estimated incidence of 1:500,000 [34].

Pre- or subclinical Cushing's syndrome has become more recently the focus of a steadily increasing number of original reports and reviews [32]. Preclinical and subclinical Cushing's syndrome have often been used interchangeably in the literature. However, whereas subclinical Cushing's syndrome relates to a biochemical abnormality which most likely will not become clinically manifest, pre-clinical Cushing's syndrome implicates progression to overt Cushing's syndrome. Since progression to overt Cushing's syndrome occurs in a minority of patients, subclinical Cushing's syndrome better describes the metabolic consequences of this condition and will be used throughout this article.

7.2 Epidemiology

The prevalence of classical, overt Cushing's syndrome in the general population is not known with certainty [34]. Approximately 85% of cases are ACTH dependent, mainly due to pituitary dependent Cushing's syndrome (Cushing's disease). ACTH independent, adrenal Cushing's syndrome accounts for 15% of all cases of Cushing's syndrome. Assuming a mean period of 5 years before diagnosis, the prevalence of overt

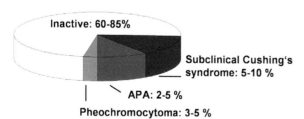

Fig. 1. Prevalence of subclinical endocrine activity in patients with adrenal incidentalomas

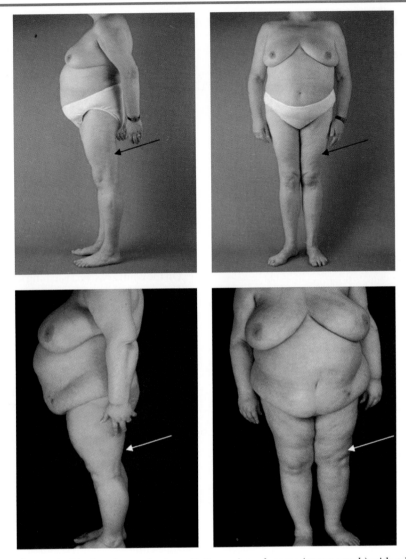

Fig. 2. Comparison of overt Cushing' syndrome due to a pituitary microadenoma (*upper panels*) with subclinical Cushing's syndrome (*lower panels*) in a 45-year-old female with an incidentally detected right adrenal mass measuring 3 cm. In contrast to the more diffuse type of obesity in this patient, the patient with overt Cushing's syndrome has central obesity with thin legs and arms (*arrows*) and more pronounced rubeosis (especially of the breasts)

adrenal Cushing's syndrome has been estimated to be 0.7 per 100,000 in Japan [33], and that of pituitary dependent Cushing's syndrome to be 3.9 per 100,000 in Spain [14].

The prevalence of subclinical Cushing's syndrome is much higher than that of overt Cushing's syndrome. Subclinical Cushing's syndrome is found in 5–20% of patients with incidentally detected adrenal masses, accounting for a mean of 7.8% (Table 1). Depending on the imaging modality used and the age of the subjects the prevalence of incidentally detected adrenal masses ranges from 0.6% to 7% [33, 21, 18]. Assuming a pop-

ulation prevalence of 1% and a prevalence of subclinical Cushing's syndrome of 7.8% in incidentaloma patients, the population prevalence would be 78 per 100,000. A relatively high prevalence of subclinical Cushing's syndrome is also supported by studies in diabetic and obese subjects (Table 2).

7.3   Clinical Presentation

By definition, no clinical signs or symptoms of Cushing's syndrome should be present in patients

Table 1. Prevalence of subclinical Cushing's syndrome in patients with adrenal incidentalomas. Subclinical Cushing's syndrome was diagnosed by variable biochemical means. (Adapted from [32])

Author	Patients with incidentally detected adrenal mass (n)	Patients with subclinical Cushing's syndrome (n, %)
Hensen 1990 [19]	50	4 (8%)
McLeod 1990 [25]	122	6 (5%)
Reincke 1992 [30]	67	8 (12%)
Siren 1993 [35]	36	2 (6%)
Corsello 1993 [13]	17	3 (18%)
Caplan 1994 [10]	26	3 (12%)
Orsella 1994 [27]	45	7 (16%)
Fernandez-Real 1994 [16]	21	3 (14%)
Ambrosi 1995 [1]	29	4 (14%)
Seppel 1996 [34]	85	5 (6%)
Terzolo 1996 [37]	20	4 (20%)
Mantero 1997 [24]	786	49 (6%)
Bondanelli 1997 [8]	38	4 (11%)
Terzolo 1998 [38]	53	8 (15%)
Barzon 1999 [4]	75	5 (7%)
Total	1,475	115 (8%)

Table 2. Subclinical Cushing's syndrome in patients with diabetes and obesity

	Leibowitz et al. 1996 [22]	Contreras et al. 2000 [10]	Ness-Abramof et al. [26] 2002
Patient cohort	Patients with NIDDM and poor metabolic control	Overweight patients with NIDDM	Overweight patients with simple obesity, diabetes, hypertension, PCOS
Patients with SCCS	3/90 (3.3%)	1/48 (2.1%)	5/86 (5.8%)
Origin of SCCS	Pituitary CS: $n=2$ Adrenal CS: $n=1$	Pituitary CS: $n=1$	Pituitary CS: $n=4$ Unclear: $n=1$

with incidentally detected adrenal tumors. However, more detailed questioning and careful second physical examination may reveal subtle evidence for hormone excess (such as recent weight gain, skin atrophy, increased facial fullness).

7.4 Subclinical Cushing's Syndrome: Cause or Manifestation of the Metabolic Syndrome?

Arterial hypertension and obesity are significantly more prevalent in patients with incidentally detected adrenal masses than in the general population. In 1997 Angeli et al. reported for the Adrenal Incidentaloma National Italian Study Group, that of 887 patients 42% were hypertensive, 28% obese and 10% diabetics. In a more recent study [35] 50 consecutive patients with incidentally detected adrenal adenomas were prospectively evaluated. In comparison to patients with non-functional adrenal incidentalomas patients with subclinical Cushing's syndrome were more often affected with hypertension (92% vs 48%), type-2 diabetes (42% vs 24%), hyperlipidemia (50% vs 28%) and obesity (50% vs 36%). In another cross-sectional study (Tauchmanova et al. 2002) the cardiovascular risk profile was assessed in 28 consecutive patients with subclinical Cushing's syndrome. All cardiovascular risk factors were more prevalent in patients than in controls with 86% patients having multiple risk factors. Mean carotid artery intima-media thickness was increased, and atherosclerotic plaques were more frequent (39%). These data suggest that chronic mild endogenous cortisol excess is paralleled by a cardiovascular risk profile similar to that described in overt Cushing's syndrome. Whether these findings have

Table 3. The spectrum of biochemical findings in subclinical Cushing's syndrome. (Adapted from Reincke 2000 [32])

Blunted diurnal variation of cortisol secretion

Low 8 A.M. to 12 P.M. cortisol ratio

Elevated midnight salivary cortisol

Low DHEA-S concentrations

Low or suppressed plasma ACTH

Blunted response of ACTH to stimulation with CRH

Missing cortisol suppression after 1 mg overnight dexamethasone suppression test

Missing cortisol suppression after standard low dose dexamethasone suppression

Missing cortisol suppression after high dose dexamethasone suppression

Elevated UFC

impact on long-term cardiovascular morbidity of patients with subclinical Cushing's syndrome has not been determined.

Incidentaloma patients with subclinical Cushing's syndrome also have higher markers of bone turnover [1, 28] and lower bone mass [40], which may be the result of subtle hypercortisolism. However, whether there is a major bone loss remains controversial [29, 35].

7.5   Biochemical Evaluation (Table 3)

The rationale for screening patients with adrenal incidentalomas for the presence of subclinical Cushing's syndrome is twofold: detection of subclinical (or even mildly symptomatic) Cushing's syndrome for early detection and prevention of disease and exclusion of subclinical Cushing's syndrome in patients with adrenal incidentaloma scheduled for unilateral adrenalectomy. In the latter, postoperative adrenal crisis (in some cases with fatal outcome [20, 25]) has been reported in patients with unrecognized subclinical Cushing's syndrome. In these patients, ACTH suppression via the negative glucocorticoid feedback resulted in atrophy of the contralateral adrenal with consecutive hypocortisolism after surgery. A diagnostic evaluation for hypercortisolism should be part of the routine work-up of patients with incidentally detected adrenal lesions as recently emphasized by the recent NIH consensus statement [18] (Figs. 3, 4).

Depending on the amount of glucocorticoids secreted by the tumor the biochemical significance of subclinical Cushing's syndrome ranges from slightly attenuated diurnal cortisol rhythm to complete atrophy of the contralateral adrenal with lasting adrenal insufficiency after unilateral adrenalectomy (Fig. 3). The diagnostic criteria and biochemical features of subclinical Cushing's syndrome used in the literature vary accordingly. As expected, higher cortisol concentrations after dexamethasone are correlated with lower plasma ACTH concentrations, lower DHEA-S levels and higher midnight cortisol concentrations in patients with adrenal incidentalomas [42], reflecting the continuous spectrum of subclinical hypercortisolism. The best means to uncover autonomous cortisol secretion is the short (overnight) dexamethasone suppression test, which rarely fails to detect subclinical Cushing's syndrome [42]. A suppressed serum cortisol (<5 μg/dl or 180 nmol/l) excludes significant cor-

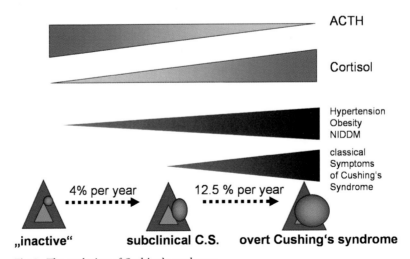

Fig. 3. The evolution of Cushing's syndrome

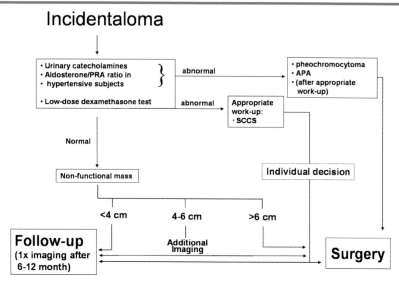

Fig. 4. Diagnostic and therapeutic considerations for the treatment of patients with adrenal incidentalomas following the recommendations of the National Institutes of Health State-of-the-Science Statement of 4–6 February 2002 [18]

tisol secretion although lower cut-off levels of cortisol (<3 μg/dl) have been emphasized by some investigators. Serum cortisol >5 μg/dl requires further investigation (Table 4) including a confirmatory high-dose dexamethasone suppression test (8 mg), a corticotropin releasing hormone (CRH) test and analysis of the diurnal cortisol rhythm. If serum cortisol concentrations are not suppressible by high-dose dexamethasone, the diagnosis of subclinical Cushing's syndrome is established. Subtle changes in glucocorticoid secretion like abnormalities in the diurnal rhythm or a blunted ACTH response to CRH in the presence of normal suppressibility by dexamethasone preclude the diagnosis of subclinical Cushing's syndrome since these changes may be non-specific. Determination of urinary free cortisol as a screening test for subclinical Cushing's syndrome is less useful, as increased values

Table 4. Stepwise endocrinological investigation of subclinical Cushing's syndrome in patients with adrenal incidentalomas

Step I: Screening test
  Serum cortisol after dexamethasone suppression
  (3 mg dexamethasone at 2300 hours orally)

Step II: confirmatory test
  Confirmation by high dose (8 mg) dexamethasone
  suppression

Step III: evaluation of the degree of hypercortisolism
  Plasma ACTH during CRH testing, UFC,
  diurnal rhythm of cortisol secretion

are a late finding usually associated with emerging clinical signs of Cushing's syndrome [29]. Patients with low plasma ACTH concentrations not responding to CRH are likely candidates for adrenal insufficiency after surgery and require adequate substitution therapy [31].

7.6   Adrenal Scintigraphy

Visualization of the adrenal mass by means of ^{131}J-norcholesterol scintigraphy has been advocated by several groups to screen for subclinical Cushing's syndrome [21]. The rationale of this approach is based on the observation that significant glucocorticoid production by the tumor will lead to unilateral tracer uptake whereas the contralateral adrenal will be scintigraphically silent due to atrophy. Moreover, adrenal scintigraphy seems to allow differentiation between benign and malignant lesion to some degree [21]. Two recent studies evaluated the use of adrenal scintigraphy in the evaluation of patients with incidentally detected adrenal masses. In the first prospective study by Bardet et al. 1996 [3], the prevalence of unilateral ^{131}I-methylnorcholesterol uptake (tumor uptake with no visualization of the contralateral adrenal gland) and bilateral uptake (uptake in both the tumoral and the contralateral adrenal glands) was investigated in patients with unilateral incidentaloma. The scan showed unilateral uptake in 46% patients (group A) and bilateral uptake in 54% (group B). Patients in group A exhibited lower

ACTH values at 0800 hours and higher cortisol values after an overnight dexamethasone suppression test, than did patients in group B. In addition, three patients in group A failed the overnight and the low-dose dexamethasone suppression tests. These data provide evidence that unilateral uptake is related to functioning adenomas with various degrees of autonomy and suggest that the ^{131}I-methylnorcholesterol scan could be a valuable tool for screening of subclinical Cushing's syndrome. In the study by Barzon et al. [4], hormonal and morphological data were investigated in 202 consecutive patients with adrenal incidentaloma in an attempt to assess subclinical hyperfunction or malignancy. In addition to the classical hormonal evaluation, adrenal scintigraphy with ^{75}Se-methylnorcholesterol was carried out. ^{75}Se-Methylnorcholesterol scintigraphy depicted malignant, space-occupying lesions as decreased or absent radiotracer uptake by the mass, and cortical adenomas as increased or normal uptake. In cortical adenomas, again a good relationship between radiocholesterol uptake and degree of functional autonomy was demonstrated. The authors concluded that, although hormonal assessment is mandatory to clarify the functional activity of adrenal incidentalomas, morphofunctional examination by ^{75}Se-methylnorcholesterol scanning seems to provide more data about the likelihood of malignancy.

7.7 Progression to Overt Cushing's Syndrome

The natural course of subclinical autonomous glucocorticoid production and the risk that such conditions will evolve towards overt Cushing's syndrome are still largely unknown (Fig. 3). Barzon and colleagues reported on the long-term outcome of 75 patients with incidentally detected adrenal masses which were initially hormonally inactive [5]: 5 patients developed subclinical Cushing's syndrome which progressed to overt Cushing's syndrome in two patients after 8 and 9 years of follow-up. In a more extended series of the same group [6], 130 consecutive patients with adrenal incidentaloma with a follow-up of at least 1 year were studied. Eight had subclinical hypercortisolism at diagnosis. Four patients developed overt Cushing's syndrome after 1–3 years of follow-up. Only one of these patients had subclinical hypercortisolism at first diagnosis. The estimated cumulative risk of a nonsecreting adrenal incidentaloma developing subclinical hyperfunction was 3.8% after 1 year and 6.6% after 5 years. For patients with masses with subclinical

autonomous glucocorticoid overproduction the estimated cumulative risk of developing overt Cushing's syndrome was 12.5% after 1 year. These data demonstrate that patients with incidentalomas are at risk of progression towards overt Cushing's syndrome. A careful biochemical and hormonal follow-up is advisable in all patients who do not need surgery at first presentation.

7.8 Surgery in Patients with SCCS

As a general rule hormonally active incidentally detected adrenal masses are surgically removed to prevent serious morbidity [11, 18, 21, 30]. This strategy is undisputed for aldosterone-producing adrenal tumors and pheochromocytoma [33]. As autonomous cortisol secretion by the tumor may range from a small percentage of the daily requirements to frank cortisol hypersecretion with suppression of the contralateral adrenal, it is evident that the metabolic benefits of surgery will vary accordingly. Adrenal surgery has a significant morbidity and mortality which has to be taken into account if surgery is considered [23]. The newly developed endoscopic adrenalectomy with its lower morbidity may justify earlier intervention [13, 16, 17].

The NIH consensus conference on the management of the clinically inapparent adrenal mass concluded that both adrenalectomy and careful observation can be suggested as treatment options, but that the long-term outcome and quality of life after surgery are unknown [18]. In our opinion, surgery should be considered in patients with subclinical Cushing's syndrome who have suppressed plasma ACTH and elevated UFC because progression to overt Cushing's syndrome is imminent. Patients with normal plasma ACTH and UFC should undergo adrenalectomy if they are young (age <50) or have metabolic disease of recent onset possibly related to Cushing's syndrome (hypertension, obesity, diabetes). In our own series of eight patients with subclinical Cushing's syndrome, surgery resulted in permanent weight loss >5 kg in all four obese patients [31]. Three of six hypertensive patients were able to reduce the antihypertensive medication, and one patient had normal blood pressure after adrenalectomy. Both patients with diabetes mellitus had improvement of glycemic control and could be switched to dietary treatment. A recent report highlights the difficulties in assessing the benefits of surgery in patients with SCCS. Six patients with SCCS and nine with nonfunctioning adenomas were followed for 12 months after adrenalectomy [7]. A high frequency of overweight/obesity (67%), hypertension (67%) and impaired glucose profile (27%) was present before surgery, with a greater prevalence of these cardiovascular risk factors in the subclinical Cushing's syndrome group. After surgery, values normalized or improved in eight out of ten hypertensive patients and in three out of four patients with impaired glucose profile. In the whole group, a marginal decrease in body weight (0.9 kg), in blood pressure (mean 135/84 mmHg vs 146/91 mmHg preoperatively) and in glucose levels in response to OGTT (mean 106 mg/dl vs 128 mg/dl) was observed. The effects were not more pronounced in patients with subclinical Cushing's syndrome. The study was lacking a non-surgical control group.

7.9   Peri- and Postoperative Management

Peri- and postoperatively, glucocorticoid replacement therapy is required in patients with subclinical Cushing's syndrome, until adrenocortical function is reassessed and rules out adrenocortical insufficiency. Especially patients with suppressed plasma ACTH levels are likely candidates for postoperative adrenal insufficiency and should be monitored closely. The best test in the postoperative period is the standard ACTH stimulation test. In our experience, glucocorticoid therapy cannot be withdrawn earlier in patients with subclinical Cushing's syndrome than in patients with overt adrenal Cushing's syndrome [31]. Mean duration of adrenocortical insufficiency in our series was 17 ± 15 months vs. 19 ± 8 months in overt Cushing's syndrome.

References

1. Ambrosi B, Peverelli S, Passini E, Ferrario R, Colombo P, Sartorio A, Faglia G (1995) Abnormalities of endocrine function in patients with clinically silent adrenals masses. Eur J Endocrinol 132:419–21
2. Angeli A, Osella G, Ali A, Terzolo M (1997) Adrenal incidentaloma: An overview of clinical and epidemiological data from the National Italian Study Group. Horm Res 47:279–283
3. Bardet S, Rohmer V, Murat A, et al. (1996) 131J-6 beta-iodomethylnorcholesterol scintigraphy: an assessment of its role in the investigation of adrenocortical incidentalomas. Clin Endocrinol 44:587–96
4. Barzon L, Scaroni C, Sonino N, et al. (1998) Incidentally discovered adrenal tumors: endocrine and scintigraphic correlates. J Clin Endocrinol Metab 83:55–62
5. Barzon L, Scaroni C, Sonino N, et al. (1999) Risk factors and long term follow up of adrenal incidentalomas. J Clin Endocrinol Metab 84:520–526
6. Barzon L, Fallo F, Sonino N, Boscaro M (2002) Development of overt Cushing's syndrome in patients with adrenal incidentaloma. Eur J Endocrinol 146:61–6
7. Bernini G, Moretti A, Iacconi P, Miccoli P, Nami R, Lucani B, Salvetti A (2003) Anthropometric, haemodynamic, humoral and hormonal evaluation in patients with incidental adrenocortical adenomas before and after surgery. Eur J Endocrinol 148:213–9
8. Bondanelli M, Campo M, Transforini G, Ambrosio MR, Zatelli MC, Franceschetti P, Valentini A, Pansini R, degli Uberti EC (1997) Evaluation of hormonal function in a series of incidentally discovered adrenal masses. Metabolism 46:1078–113
9. Caplan RH, Strutt PJ, Wickus GG (1994) Subclinical hormone secretion by incidentally discovered adrenal masses. Arch Surg 129:291–96
10. Contreras LN, Cardoso E, Lozano MP, Pozzo J, Pagano P, Claus-Hermbeg H (2000) [Detection of preclinical Cushing's syndrome in overweight type 2 diabetic patients] Medicina (B Aires) 60:326–30
11. Copeland PM (1983) The incidentally discovered adrenal mass. Ann Intern Med 98:940–945
12. Corsello SM, Della-Casa S, Bollanti L, Rufini V, Rota CA, Danza F, Colasanti S, Vellante C, Troncone L, Barbarino A (1993) Incidentally discovered adrenal masses: A functional and morphological study. Exp Clin Endocrinol 101:131–137
13. Dralle H, Scheumann GFW, Nashan B, Brabant G (1994) Review: recent developments in adrenal surgery. Acta Chir Belg 94:137–140
14. Extabe J, Vazques JA (1994) Morbidity and mortality in Cushing's syndrome: An epidemiologic approach. Clin Endocrinol 40:479–484
15. Fernandez-Real J-M, Ricart-Engel W, Simo R (1994) Preclinical Cushing's syndrome: Report of three cases and literature review. Horm Res 41:230–235
16. Fletcher DR, Beiles CB, Hardy KY (1994) Laparoscopic adrenalectomy. Aust N Z Surg 64:427–430
17. Gnazzoni G, Montorsi F, Bergamaschi F, Rigatti P, Cornaggia G, Lanzi R, Pontiroli AE (1994) Effectiveness and safety of laparoscopic adrenalectomy. J Urol 152:1375–1378
18. Grumbach MM, Biller BM, Braunstein GD, Campbell KK, Carney JA, Godley PA, Harris EL, Lee JK, Oertel YC, Posner MC, Schlechte JA, Wieand HS (2003) Management of the clinically inapparent adrenal mass ("incidentaloma"). Ann Intern Med. 138:424–9
19. Hensen J, Buhl M, Oelkers W (1990) Diagnostisches und therapeutisches Vorgehen bei Patienten mit hufällig entdeckten Nebennierentumoren. In: Allolio B, Schulte HM (eds) Moderne Diagnostik und therapeutische Strategien bei Nebennierenerkrankungen. Schattauer, Stuttgart, pp 210–215
20. Huiras CM, Pehling GB, Caplan RH (1989) Adrenal insufficiency after operative removal of apparently nonfunctioning adrenal adenomas. JAMA 261:894–898

21. Kloos RT, Gross MD, Francis IR, Korobkin M, Shapiro B (1995) Incidentally discovered adrenal masses. Endocr Rev 16:460–484

22. Leibowitz G, Tsu A, Chayen SD, Saloameh M, Raz I, Cerase E, Gross DJ (1996) Pre-clinical Cushing's syndrome: an unexpected frequent cause of poor glycaemic control in obese diabetic patients. Clin Endocrinol 44:717–22

23. Mancini F, Mutter D, Peix JL, Chapuis Y, Henry JF, Proye C, Cougard P, Marescaux J (1999) [Experiences with adrenalectomy in 1997. Apropos of 247 cases. A multicenter prospective study of the French-speaking Association of Endocrine Surgery]. Chirurgie 124:368–74

24. Mantero F, Masini AM, Opocher G, Giovagnetti M, Arnaldi G (1997) Adrenal incidentaloma: An overview of hormonal date from the National Italian Study Group. Horm Res 47:284–289

25. McLeod MK, Thompson NW, Gross MD, Bondeson L (1990) Sub-clinical Cushing's syndrome in patients with adrenal incidentalomas. Pitfalls in diagnosis and management. Ann Surg 56:398–403

26. Ness-Abramof R, Nabriski D, Apovian CM, Niven M, Weiss E, Shapiro MS, Shenkman L (2002) Overnight dexamethasone suppression test: a reliable screen for Cushing's syndrome in the obese. Obes Res 10:1217–21

27. Osella G, Terzolo M. Boretta G, Magro G, Ali A, Piovesan A, Pacotti P, Angeli A (1994) Endocrine evaluation of incidentally discovered adrenal masses (incidentalomas). J Clin Endocrinol Metab 79:1532–1539

28. Osella G, Terzolo M, Reimondo G, et al. (1997) Serum markers of bone and collagen turnover in patients with Cushing's syndrome and in subjects with adrenal incidentalomas. J Clin Endocrinol Metab 82:3303–7

29. Osella G, Reimondo G, Peretti P, Ali A, Paccotti P, Angeli A, Terzolo M (2001) The patients with incidentally discovered adrenal adenoma (incidentaloma) are not at increased risk of osteoporosis. J Clin Endocrinol Metab 86:604–7

30. Reincke M, Allolio B (1995) Das Nebennereninzidentalom: Die Kunst der Beschränkung in Diagnostik und Therapie. Dtsch Ärzteblatt 92:764–770

31. Reincke M, Nieke J, Krestin GP, Saeger W, Allolio B, Winkelmann W (1992) Preclinical Cushing's syndrome in adrenal "incidentalomas": comparison with adrenal Cushing's syndrome. J Clin Endocrinol Metab 75:826–832

32. Reincke M (2000) Subclinical Cushing's syndrome. Endocrinol Metab Clin North Am 29:43–56

33. Ross NS, Aron DC (1990) Hormonal evaluation of the patient with an incidentally discovered adrenal mass. N Engl J Med 323:1401–1405

34. Ross NS (1994) Epidemiology of Cushing's syndrome and subclinical disease. Endocrinol Metab Clin North Am 23:539–46

35. Rossi R, Tauchmanova L, Luciano A, Di Martino M, Battista C, Del Viscovo L, Nuzzo V, Lombardi GJ (2000) Subclinical Cushing's syndrome in patients with adrenalincidentaloma: clinical and biochemical features. J Clin Endocrinol Metab 85:1440–8

36. Seppel T, Schlaghecke R (1996) Subklinischer Hypercortisolismus bei zufällig entdeckten Nebennierentumoren. Dtsch Med Wochenschr 121:503–508

37. Siren JE, Haapiainen RK, Huikuri KT, Sivula AH (1993) Incidentalomas of the adrenal gland: 36 operated patients and review of literature. World J Surgery 17:634–639

38. Terzolo M, Osella G, Ali A, et al (1998) Subclinical Cushing's syndrome in adrenal incidentalomas. Clin Endocrinol 48:89–97

39. Torlonto M, Zingrillo M, D'Aloiso L, et al. (1997) Pre-Cushing's syndrome not recognized by conventional dexamethasone suppression test in an adrenal incidentaloma patient. J Endocrinol Invest 20:501–04

40. Tauchmanova L, Rossi R, Nuzzo V, del Puente A, Esposito-del Puente A, Pizzi C, Fonderico F, Lupoli G, Lombardi G (2001) Bone loss determined by quantitative ultrasonometry correlates inversely with disease activity in patients with endogenous glucocorticoid excess due to adrenal mass. Eur J Endocrinol 145:241–7

41. Tauchmanova L, Rossi R, Biondi B, Pulcrano M, Nuzzo V, Palmieri EA, Fazio S, Lombardi G (2002) Patients with subclinical Cushing's syndrome due to adrenal adenoma have increased cardiovascular risk. J Clin Endocrinol Metab 87:4872–8

42. Tsagarakis S, Roboti C, Kokkoris P, et al. (1998) Elevated post-dexamethasone suppression cortisol concentrations correlate with hormonal alterations of the hypothalamic-pituitary axis in patients with adrenal incidentalomas. Clin Endocrinol 49:165–71

8 Ectopic Cushing's Syndrome

D. Vassiliadi, S. Tsagarakis, N. Thalassinos

CONTENTS

Ectopic Cushing's syndrome refers to endogenous hypercortisolism originating from adrenal stimulation by ACTH produced inappropriately by a variety of extrapituitary tumors. On very rare occasions ectopic Cushing's syndrome is due to pituitary ACTH secretion driven by ectopic CRH secretion. Although the first extrapituitary tumor associated with hypercortisolism was reported as early as in 1928, it was in 1962 when ectopic Cushing's syndrome was characterized as a disorder of ACTH production by neoplastic cells [44]. In the following years it became evident that there are two types of ectopic ACTH syndrome (EAS). One is associated with overt malignancies, the prototype being small-cell lung cancer (SCLC) and the other with more indolent neoplasms, represented mainly by bronchial and other carcinoid tumors. Although EAS is rare, it is the underlying cause in a substantial proportion (10–20%) of patients presenting with ACTH-dependent Cushing's syndrome [57, 86]. Differentiation of ectopic ACTH secretion from "eutopic" overproduction by pituitary corticotroph adenomas is of paramount importance and represents, on many occasions, one of the most challenging problems in clinical endocrinology. In recent years efforts have been directed to understanding the pathophysiology of EAS and developing effective diagnostic tests to differentiate between EAS and Cushing's disease. Our current knowledge related to these issues is summarized in this chapter.

8.1   Pathophysiology

Elucidation of the mechanisms involved in the transcription and processing of the POMC gene and its products provided the background for a better understanding of the various disturbances observed in ectopic ACTH secretion [61]. The POMC gene is located in the short arm of chromosome 2p23 and consists of three exons and two introns [68].

It is unusual in that it contains at least three distinct promoters giving rise to three different length mRNA transcripts. In corticotroph cells, a mature POMC mRNA of 1,072 nucleotides (nt) is generated [14], which is translated into a pre-POMC molecule starting with a 26 amino acid signal peptide. The signal peptide is rapidly cleaved leaving the 241 amino acid POMC molecule that is then engaged in the secretory pathway. Apart from the pituitary, POMC mRNA is also expressed in many other normal tissues [18]. In most of these tissues, POMC gene expression is quantitatively and qualitatively different from that in the pituitary; the tissue concentration of POMC mRNA is extremely low, and the generated mRNAs are short, truncated, transcripts of 800 nt. These transcripts are non-functional and cannot be efficiently translated into POMC [36]. In the vast majority of pituitary corticotroph adenomas leading to Cushing's disease (CD), gene transcription shows no gross abnormality and the POMC transcripts in pituitary tumors are similar to those in the normal pituitary [7]. In non-pituitary tumors, altered POMC gene expression is frequent. Most ACTH-secreting tumors contain various types of messengers: a large mRNA transcript of about 1,450 nt, the normal-sized (pituitary-like) 1,072 nt POMC mRNA, and a small 800 nt mRNA transcript [15]. The absolute amount and molecular forms of POMC mRNA differ among the various tumors. In bronchial carcinoids associated with the ectopic ACTH syndrome, the pituitary messenger is highly predominant and present in high amounts. In endocrine tumors not associated with the ectopic ACTH syndrome, the short 800 nt mRNA is predominant and the total amount of POMC mRNA is low. In general the ectopic ACTH syndrome occurs with tumors capable of generating high amounts of the pituitary-like message [71].

In a given tissue the nature of the POMC end products depends on the differential expression of enzymes, known as prohormone convertases (PCs), which are involved in its proteolysis [63, 66]. When only PC1 is present, as in normal and most neoplastic pituitary corticotrophs, proteolytic action is limited and ACTH is the major end product [29]. When both PC1 and PC2 are present their coordinate or synergistic actions lead to a more extensive proteolysis generating smaller hormonal fragments [92]. An abnormal maturation pattern of POMC is a classic feature of the ectopic ACTH syndrome [7, 89]. In many cases intact POMC is predominantly secreted; in other cases, abnormal fragments such as CLIP and human βMSH

may be generated [83]. Recent studies [60] demonstrated that aggressive, poorly differentiated tumors (e.g. SCLCs) preferentially release intact POMC most likely because of a general defect in both PC1 and PC2. It should be noted, however, that this form of abnormal processing of POMC is not specific to non-pituitary tumors since it is also occasionally present in rare pituitary macroadenomas and in some exceptional pituitary cancers [61]. Thus defective POMC processing actually indicates an impaired state of neuroendocrine differentiation in aggressive tumors, independently of their pituitary or non-pituitary origin. In contrast, carcinoid tumors usually overprocess the precursor, releasing ACTH and smaller peptides like CLIP most likely because they are heavily loaded with PC2.

The above findings led several investigations to suggest that ectopic ACTH syndrome is made up of two distinct entities including (a) neoplasms, like carcinoid tumors, that achieve a process of corticotroph differentiation being able to express and process the POMC gene correctly to release large amounts of intact ACTH, and (b) rapidly progressive malignancies, like SCLCs, that process POMC in an aberrant way releasing high concentrations of ACTH precursors and less intact ACTH in the circulation. In fact the term

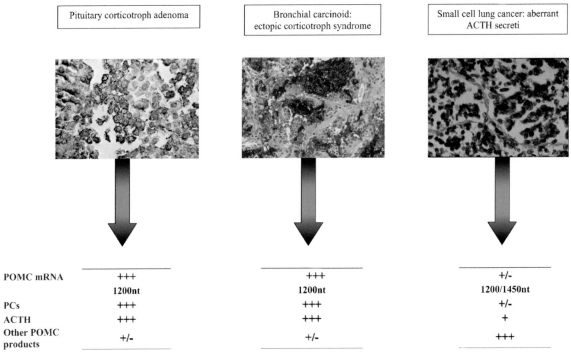

	Pituitary corticotroph adenoma	Bronchial carcinoid: ectopic corticotroph syndrome	Small cell lung cancer: aberrant ACTH secreti
POMC mRNA	+++ 1200nt	+++ 1200nt	+/- 1200/1450nt
PCs	+++	+++	+/-
ACTH	+++	+++	+
Other POMC products	+/-	+/-	+++

Fig. 1. Different POMC (proopiomelanocortin) processing in Cushing's disease, "ectopic corticotroph syndrome" and "aberrant ACTH secretion syndrome". (Modified from [17])

"ectopic corticotroph syndrome" has been introduced to better delineate the former and "aberrant ACTH secretion syndrome" the latter category of these tumors [17] (Fig. 1).

However, despite the progress made in understanding the molecular changes in tumors associated with EAS the intimate mechanisms that trigger POMC gene transcription are not well understood [88]. Recently, based on data derived from experiments with SCLC cell lines, a possible mechanism for the upregulation of POMC gene transcription has emerged. This relies on the enhanced activation of the binding site for the E2F transcription factors [59]. This promoter site is situated upstream from the pituitary promoter and its activity is inhibited by the retinoblastoma protein (RB) [42]. Because inactivation of RB occurs frequently in SCLCs it has been speculated that the loss of RB repression of E2F transcriptional activation might contribute to the aberrant POMC gene expression in these tumors [31]. On the other hand, bronchial carcinoids adopt a corticotroph phenotype. The best marker of such a phenotype seems to be the expression of the pituitary type vasopressin (V3) receptors [16].

8.2   Tumor Types Associated with EAS

The widespread expression of POMC derived peptides in tissues such as lung, adrenal glands, testis, spleen, ovary, thyroid, liver, thymus, placenta, skin, mononuclear leukocytes and colon explains the growing list of tumors that can be the cause of ectopic ACTH syndrome [55]. The relative frequencies of the various tumor types associated with EAS are listed in Table 1 [8]. Lung tumors (SCLCs and bronchial carcinoids) constitute the vast majority (48–66%) of all cases. In earlier series small cell lung carcinomas represented the largest proportion of cases, whereas in more recent series bronchial carcinoids seem to predominate (36–46%) in part because of the increased detection of

small bronchial carcinoids and the decreased reporting of Cushing's syndrome due to oat cell carcinomas [3, 41].

Amongst patients with SCLCs only a small proportion have been reported to be associated with hypercortisolism [38,64]. In one large series of 840 patients with SCLC only 14 (1.6%) had ectopic corticotropin production [19]. However, it should be mentioned that in very aggressive tumors with vigorous symptoms due to the primary disease, or in cases with only subtle abnormalities of cortisol production, the syndrome is often underdiagnosed. Bronchial carcinoids arise from the Kulchitsky cells of the lung. In the majority they are perihilar, but they can also be found in the periphery. Although they are considered to have a low potential of malignancy, metastases, usually in mediastinal lymph nodes, and less frequently in liver, bone, or skin, have been reported in a small proportion (less than 15% of patients) [41]. Bronchial carcinoids associated with clinically overt hypercortisolemia seem to be more aggressive than those with no hormone overproduction [65]. Frequently their detection can be very difficult. Because of their small size they do not cause local symptoms and are often hard to detect with imaging studies. This is particularly true in those rare cases when ectopic ACTH production is due to carcinoid tumorlets. Tumorlets are multiple microscopic nests of neuroendocrine cells in the lungs; they are either isolated or surround a bronchial carcinoid tumor. In some cases [4] they were identified many years after the initial presentation of Cushing's syndrome.

The thymus is another organ associated with tumors leading to ectopic ACTH production [62]. Most cases involve thymic carcinoids that despite their term are in fact malignant neuroendocrine neoplasms. In addition small cell neuroendocrine carcinoma of the thymus and benign thymic hyperplasia have been reported as the source of ACTH-dependent hypercortisolism. Carcinoid tumors of the thymus are extremely

Table 1. Tumors associated with ectopic ACTH syndrome [8]

Tumor origin	%	Tumor origin	%
Lung	48–66	Adrenal	6
Small cell carcinoma	20–27	Pheochromocytoma	5
Bronchial carcinoids	21–46	Neuroblastoma	0.8
Pancreatic islet cells	16	Ovarian uterine cervix carcinomas	2
Thymus	10	Prostate cancer	1
Medullary thyroid carcinoma	5	Other sporadic cases	7

rare in children but when present they are usually associated with Cushing's syndrome.

Ectopic adrenocorticotropic hormone-producing islet cell tumors of the pancreas are a rare cause of Cushing's syndrome with a severe and rapidly progressive clinical course [12, 22]. Pancreatic islet cell tumors are usually large and have already produced metastases to the liver by the time overt hypercortisolism is established. Multiple hormone production by the cancer cells is the cause of the common coexistence of hypercortisolism with the Zollinger-Ellison syndrome in these patients [35, 45]. Their presence is significant because it seems to aggravate the prognosis. Among 42 reported cases of pancreatic islet cell tumors and Cushing's syndrome, the 5-year survival was 16% [12].

Other reported tumors are medullary thyroid carcinomas (5%), adrenal pheochromocytomas (5%), ovarian and uterine cervix carcinomas (2%), and prostate cancers (1%) [3, 86]. Sporadic cases involve renal, breast, liver, gastrointestinal cancers, adrenal neuroblastoma, mediastinal paraganglioma, and even lymphoma and melanoma. Production of corticotrophin by inflammatory [25] leukemic cells has also been encountered in a few case reports [46]. It is of note that no tumor arising from mesoderma, i.e. sarcomas, has been reported to induce ectopic Cushing's syndrome.

So far the number of well-characterized cases of CRH secreting tumors is very small. Most involve differentiated bronchial carcinoids. In these cases ectopic secretion of CRH stimulates pituitary ACTH secretion leading to a clinical and biochemical profile indistinguishable from that observed in Cushing's disease [57].

8.3   Clinical Features

Patients of all ages have been reported with the syndrome, although it has been reported very rarely in children. Mean age at presentation is around 41 years, with patients harboring small cell lung cancer tending to be older and those with thymic carcinoids younger [8]. From the reported cases it is evident that EAS does not show the striking female predisposition of Cushing's disease; both sexes are affected almost equally (male: female ratio 1:1.2–1.4); albeit small cell lung cancer and thymic carcinoids involve men slightly more frequently [86].

Depending on the type of tumor responsible for the ectopic ACTH secretion, the development of Cushing's syndrome may precede, be apparent simultaneously or even be delayed for many years after the clinical presentation of the tumor [90, 93]. For instance, most patients with medullary carcinoids develop Cushing's syndrome late in the course of the cancer [3]. In these cases attention is required as the symptoms of hypercortisolism may be attributed to the progress of the malignancy. However, in other instances, Cushing's syndrome may precede the tumor's manifestation. On the other hand, more benign and indolent tumors with ectopic ACTH secretion may remain undetected for a long time, even longer than 10 years from the initial clinical presentation of Cushing's syndrome [79]. For these cases, with an unknown source of ACTH secretion despite an extensive diagnostic evaluation, the term "occult ectopic ACTH syndrome" has been used [32].

The clinical characteristics of patients with ectopic Cushing's syndrome differ in frequency and severity depending on the type of the tumor responsible for the ACTH overproduction [70]. Generally, patients with advanced and aggressive cancer often present with a rapid onset of usually severe symptoms including hypokalemic metabolic alkalosis and hyperpigmentation, whereas those with benign lesions, such as bronchial carcinoids, usually have a clinical picture identical to those with Cushing's disease (obesity, moon facies, hypertension, buffalo hump, purple striae, impaired glucose tolerance/diabetes, muscle atrophy, psychiatric disturbances, osteoporosis, ecchymoses, acne). It has been suggested that several clinical manifestations seem to be more common in patients with EAS than in patients with other forms of CS. Thus, almost three-quarters of the patients with EAS present with hypertension and hypokalemia [8, 32]. However, neither the presence nor the absence of the aforementioned clinical features should be considered as either suggesting or excluding the existence of EAS.

8.4   Laboratory Diagnosis

During the evaluation of a patient presenting with Cushing's syndrome it is important to establish the presence of hypercortisolism; otherwise the tests employed in the differential diagnosis may be misleading or uninterpretable. This is particularly relevant for those patients with cyclic Cushing's syndrome, characterized by intermittent periods of remission of cortisol excess during the course of the disease [80]. In our experience cyclic Cushing's syndrome is rather common in patients with EAS; in our series of seven histologically confirmed bronchial carcinoids, cyclicity was observed in over 50% of the cases. The principal biochemical indices of cortisol excess are the loss of the normal feedback of the hypothalamo-pituitary-adrenal axis (HPA) (demonstrated by the failure of suppression of cortisol levels by dexamethasone administration), the excessive endogenous integrated cortisol secretion (expressed by increased urinary free cortisol) and the disturbance of the normal diurnal variation of cortisol secretion (resulting in increased midnight cortisol levels) [52].

Once the presence of hypercortisolism has been confirmed, elevated ACTH levels exclude the adrenal origin of hypercortisolism, and further investigation for the differentiation between the pituitary (eutopic) and non-pituitary (ectopic) source of ACTH-dependent Cushing's syndrome is required. Basal cortisol and ACTH levels are usually higher than in patients with Cushing's disease (>28 μg/dl and >200 pg/ml, respectively) [32, 86]. These findings, however, are not always diagnostic since a considerable overlap between the two groups exists [40]. While the diagnosis may be straightforward in patients with highly aggressive ACTH secreting tumors, in all other cases ectopic ACTH-dependent Cushing's syndrome often mimics Cushing's disease both clinically and biochemically, owing to the high degree of neuroendocrine differentiation of these tumors and specific tests are required to elucidate the origin of ACTH.

8.4.1 High Dose Dexamethasone Suppression Test

In most patients with CD (80–90%), cortisol levels are suppressed to >50% from baseline levels whereas poorly differentiated ectopic tumors are resistant to feedback inhibition. However, a substantial proportion of benign differentiated neuroendocrine tumors (carcinoid tumors of bronchus, thymus, pancreas) can suppress their ACTH secretion similarly to CD. Several versions of high dose dexamethasone suppression, including the standard 2-day oral high dose test (2 mg every 6 h for eight doses), the 8-mg overnight oral test and intravenous tests, have been used [20]. The reported sensitivity and specificity of this test for the diagnosis of Cushing's disease versus the ectopic ACTH syndrome are 80–88% and 88–100% respectively [73]. This clearly does not allow accurate determination of the source of ACTH in all cases. A recent study analyzing the various forms of the HDDST per-formed at multiple centres revealed that overall, the test had a sensitivity of 81% and specificity of only 67% in discriminating Cushing's disease from EAS [6]. Although, on the basis of this evidence, it has been suggested that the HDDST should be abandoned, most authors tend to still use this test since when combined with the CRH test (see below) it provides the best discrimination between CD and EAS. Shifting the criteria to a greater level of cortisol suppression can only increase the specificity with a loss of sensitivity to diagnose CD [52].

8.4.2 CRH Stimulation Test

Most pituitary, but few ectopic, ACTH-secreting tumors have CRH receptors and increased plasma ACTH and cortisol levels following CRH administration. A meta-analysis suggested that an increase in cortisol of 20% or more above baseline or of ACTH 50% or more above baseline excludes EAS with high accuracy [39]. However, these criteria vary widely between centers depending on previous experience and the type of CRH used for stimulation. The majority of series report the use of ovine CRH. However, human CRH is currently more widely available worldwide [34]. Therefore, the exact criterion to use depends on the type of CRH used and at what center, and should be used with caution, as there will undoubtedly be patients with the ectopic ACTH syndrome who may respond outside the established cut-offs. Estimates on the performance of the CRH test also vary widely between centers. Overall the test has a sensitivity of 60–80% and a specificity of 90–100% in discriminating CD from EAS [30, 52]. Importantly, a lack of response in both HDDST and CRH was reported to have a sensitivity of 100% and a diagnostic specificity of 98% for ectopic Cushing's syndrome [53].

8.4.3 The Desmopressin Test

It has recently been suggested that a test based on desmopressin administration may be useful in differentiating patients with CD and EAS [47]. In fact initial studies reporting patients with CD but only few patients with EAS showed that most patients with CD responded while patients with EAS were unresponsive to desmopressin administration [77]. However, in recent studies [5, 69] it was found that this test is of no value since there was a significant overlap of responses between CD and patients with EAS due to the frequent expression of the V2 along with V3 receptors [78] in these ectopic ACTH secreting tumors. We also provided evidence that a combined test using both CRH and desmopressin, which has been shown in one study [51] to provide a far better discrimination than either test alone, is also of limited value since it failed to completely discriminate patients with CD and EAS [78].

8.4.4 Bilateral Inferior Petrosal Sinus Sampling

For patients with ACTH-dependent Cushing's syndrome whose clinical, biochemical, or radiological studies are discordant or equivocal, inferior petrosal sinus sampling for ACTH should be recommended [28]. A central (inferior petrosal) to peripheral (C/P) plasma ACTH gradient is consistent with a pituitary origin of ACTH secretion (Cushing's disease) while lack of such a gradient points to an extrapituitary and thus ectopic origin of ACTH. There is unequivocal evidence that, due to the intermittent secretion of ACTH, basal ACTH IPS/P gradients are not sensitive enough to demonstrate pituitary origin of ACTH hypersecretion [56]. Currently CRH stimulation of ACTH secretion during bilateral inferior petrosal sinus sampling (BIPSS) is used in most centers. However, although CRH stimulation grossly improves the sensitivity of the procedure, false-negative results have been increasingly recorded. Thus, with the exception of the study of Oldfield et al (1991) [56], in most other series a false-negative rate of 4–15% has been reported [33]. It has been suggested that apart from incorrect placement of catheters or the rare occurrence of a hypoplastic inferior petrosal sinus, insufficient ACTH stimulation due to CRH unresponsiveness may explain some of the false-negative cases [21]. As mentioned 10–15% of patients with Cushing's disease do not demonstrate positive ACTH and cortisol responses in peripheral blood samples during routine CRH testing. While many of these patients still demonstrate diagnostic ACTH gradients during BIPSS with CRH stimulation, others may fail to demonstrate diagnostic IPS/P ACTH gradients. In an effort to decrease the false-negative rate due to CRH unresponsiveness we have recently introduced the use of a combined stimulus with CRH plus desmopressin during BIPSS [76]. By this method we succeeded in increasing BIPSS sensitivity in our patients. A crucial issue, however, is whether such an amplified stimulation may affect the specificity of the procedure. All our six patients

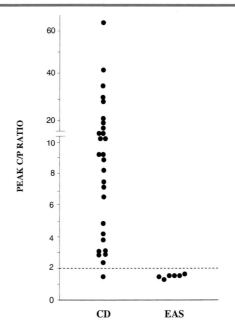

Fig. 2. Peak central to peripheral ratios during BIPSS with combined CRH/desmopressin stimulation in 6 consecutive patients with EAS and 28 patients with confirmed Cushing's disease. (S. Tsagarakis et al., unpublished observations)

with EAS undergoing stimulation with CRH plus desmopressin failed to demonstrate a C/P gradient (Fig. 2, S. Tsagarakis et al., unpublished observations). These data indicate that the combined CRH/desmopressin administration may become the preferred stimulation method during BIPSS.

8.5 Localization

An extensive radiological and hormonal work-up is necessary to detect an extrapituitary source of ACTH. Visualizing an ectopic ACTH source can be a challenge, but in general patients should begin with imaging of the chest and abdomen with CT and/or MRI, bearing in mind that these are the most likely sites of EAS secreting tumors (Table 1). Although small cell lung carcinomas and pancreatic tumors are generally easily visualized, small bronchial carcinoid tumors that can be less than 1 cm in diameter often prove more difficult [24, 85]. Fine-cut high-resolution CT scanning with both supine and prone images can help differentiate between tumors and vascular shadows. MRI can identify chest lesions that are not evident on CT scanning, and characteristically show a high signal on T2-weighted and short-inversion time inversion-recovery images [23, 50].

8.5.1 Somatostatin Receptor Scintigraphy

The majority of EAS tumors are of neuroendocrine origin and therefore may express somatostatin receptor subtypes [43]. Therefore radiolabeled somatostatin analog (^{111}In-pentetreotide) scintigraphy may be useful to show either functionality of identified tumors, or to localize radiologically unidentified tumors [58, 75, 87, 94]. The diagnostic utility of SRS, however, has been questioned by two recent studies [67, 72]. In these studies the diagnostic yield of SRS was inferior to conventional imaging and no patient with an initial negative scan became positive during follow-up. This latter finding led to the suggestion that repeated SRS is of no value when the initial scan is negative. In contrast to the above findings we recently reported data indicating that SRS is a useful method in localizing small bronchial carcinoids during the follow-up of these patients since it may become positive even years after initial presentation despite negative previous scans [74].

8.6 Therapeutic Approach

Curative resection of the tumor responsible for the ACTH production is the optimal treatment of ectopic Cushing's syndrome, a goal that cannot always be achieved because of extensive metastatic disease or the inability to locate the tumor. Patients with small cell lung cancer and Cushing's syndrome have a poorer prognosis and are more resistant to chemotherapy. Bronchial carcinoids are more indolent and slow growing and only a small number are associated with metastases usually in mediastinal lymph nodes, liver, bone, or skin. Complete resection can cure the patient. However, approximately one-third of pulmonary carcinoids have atypical histologic features and are more aggressive, with a much higher incidence of metastases and a poorer prognosis (5-year survival rate 40–60%) [41, 91]. Postoperative irradiation of the mediastinum is mandatory especially in patients with positive lymph node disease. Islet cell tumors associated with Cushing's syndrome are usually large and malignant and have usually metastasized to the liver by the time the syndrome is diagnosed [2, 22]. Hepatic metastases from carcinoids tend to grow more slowly and have a better prognosis than other adenocarcinomas. Therefore aggressive management is justified. Resection of solitary metastases or of those confined to one lobe may improve the survival period or the quality of life of the patient [86]. Hepatic arterial embolization is another adjunctive therapeutic option especially in cases where surgical treatment is not indicated or has already failed [9]. Several combination chemotherapy schemes have also been used [1, 10, 49] with moderate results and even immunotherapy with a-interferon has been proposed [26, 54]. Thymic carcinoids have also a poor prognosis and aggressive management with surgical removal followed by irradiation and chemotherapy is warranted.

When treatment directed to tumor ablation is not efficient to control hypercortisolism, additional means to diminish cortisol excess and its associated morbidity are required. Pharmacological treatment with inhibitors of adrenal steroid synthesis (ketoconazole, metyrapone, mitotane) [48], alone or in combination, provide a reasonable first line option [13, 27]. The long-acting somatostatin analog octreotide is used in the therapy of a spectrum of neuroendocrine tumors to control hypersecretion by its action on somatostatin receptors. Not surprisingly, many ectopic ACTH producing tumors of neuroendocrine origin also express somatostatin receptors, and octreotide has been shown to be effective in the hypercortisolism induced by such tumors [11, 37, 81]. Assessment with pentetreotide scintigraphy may help predict which tumors might respond to treatment [58]. Octreotide may also have a role in combination therapy, as when combined with ketoconazole it successfully normalized hypercortisolism in three of four patients with Cushing's disease or the ectopic ACTH syndrome, whereas monotherapy with either agent alone had failed [84]. Nevertheless, when with these pharmacological means, severe side effects and/or failure to completely control the cortisol excess occur, bilateral adrenalectomy is indicated. The recent introduction of laparoscopic adrenalectomy [82] has made this procedure safe and life saving for such patients.

References

1. Ajani JA, Legha SS, Karlin DA, Stratton Hill C (1983) Combination chemotherapy of metastatic carcinoid tumors with 5-FU, adriamycin, mitomycin and methyl-CCNU. Proc Am Assoc Clin Oncol 2:124 (Abstract C-486)
2. Amikura K, Alexander HR, Norton JA, Doppman JL, Jensen RT, Nieman L, Cutler G, Chrousos G, Fraker DL (1995) Role of surgery in management of adrenocorticotropic hormone-producing islet cell tumors of the pancreas. Surgery 118:1125–1130
3. Aniszewski JP, Young WF Jr, Thompson GB, Grant CS, van Heerden JA (2001) Cushing syndrome due to ectopic adrenocorticotropic hormone secretion. World J Surg 25:934–940

4. Arioglu E, Doppman J, Gomes M, Kleiner D, Mauro D, Barlow C, Papanicolaou DA (1998) Cushing's syndrome caused by corticotropin secretion by pulmonary tumorlets. N Engl J Med 24;339:883–886

5. Arnaldi G, de Keyzer Y, Gasc JM, Clauser E, Bertagna X (1998) Vasopressin receptors modulate the pharmacological phenotypes of Cushing's syndrome. Endocr Res 24: 807–816

6. Aron DC, Raff H, Findling JW (1997) Effectiveness versus efficacy: the limited value in clinical practice of high dose dexamethasone suppression testing in the differential diagnosis of adrenocorticotropin-dependent Cushing's syndrome. J Clin Endocrinol Metab 82:1780–1785

7. Bertagna X (1994) Proopiomelanocortin-derived peptides. Endocrinol Metab Clin North Am 23:467–485

8. Beuschlein F, Hammer GD (2002) Ectopic proopiomelanocortin syndrome. Endocrinol Metab Clin North Am 31:191–234

9. Blumgart LH, Allison DJ (1982) Resection and embolization in the management of secondary hepatic tumors. World J Surg 6:32–45

10. Bukowski RM, John KG, Peterson RF, Stephens RL, Rivkin SE, Neilan B, Costanzi JH (1987) A phase II trial of combination chemotherapy in patients with metastatic carcinoid tumors. A Southwest Oncology Group Study. Cancer 60:2891–2895

11. Christin-Maitre S, Chabbert-Buffet N, Mure A, Boukhris R, Bouchard P (1996) Use of somatostatin analog for localization and treatment of ACTH secreting bronchial carcinoid tumor. Chest 109:845–846

12. Clark ES, Carney JA (1984) Pancreatic islet cell tumor associated with Cushing's syndrome. Am J Surg Pathol 8:917–924

13. Comi RJ, Gorden P (1998) Long-term medical treatment of ectopic ACTH syndrome. South Med J 91:1014–1018

14. De Keyzer Y, Bertagna X, Lenne F, Girard F, Luton JP, Kahn A (1985) Altered proopiomelanocortin gene expression in adrenocorticotropin-producing nonpituitary tumors. Comparative studies with corticotropic adenomas and normal pituitaries. J Clin Invest 76:1892–1898

15. De Keyzer Y, Bertagna X, Luton JP, Kahn A (1989) Variable modes of proopiomelanocortin gene transcription in human tumors. Mol Endocrinol 3:215–223

16. De Keyzer Y, Lenne F, Auzan C, Jegou S, Rene P, Vaudry H, Kuhn JM, Luton JP, Clauser E, Bertagna X (1996) The pituitary V3 vasopressin receptor and the corticotroph phenotype in ectopic ACTH syndrome. J Clin Invest 97:1311–1318

17. De Keyzer Y, Raffin-Sanson ML, Picon A, Bertagna X (2001) Syndromes of ectopic ACTH secretion: recent pathophysiological aspects. In: Margioris AN, Chrousos GP (eds) Adrenal disorders. Humana Press, Totowa, NJ, pp 165–178

18. DeBold CR, Menefee JK, Nicholson WE, Orth DN (1988) Proopiomelanocortin gene is expressed in many normal human tissues and in tumors not associated with ectopic adrenocorticotropin syndrome. Mol Endocrinol 2:862–870

19. Delisle L, Boyer MJ, Warr D, Killinger D, Payne D, Yeoh JL, Feld R (1993) Ectopic corticotropin syndrome and small-cell carcinoma of the lung. Clinical features, outcome, and complications. Ann Intern Med 153:746–752

20. Dichek HL, Nieman LK, Oldfield EH, Pass HI, Malley JD, Cutler GB Jr (1994) A comparison of the standard high dose dexamethasone suppression test and the overnight 8-mg dexamethasone suppression test for the differential diagnosis of adrenocorticotropin-dependent Cushing's syndrome. J Clin Endocrinol Metab 78:418–422

21. Doppman JL, Chang R, Oldfield EH, Chrousos G, Stratakis CA, Nieman LK (1999) The hypoplastic inferior petrosal sinus: a potential source of false-negative results in petrosal sampling for Cushing's disease. J Clin Endocrinol Metab 84:533–540

22. Doppman JL, Nieman LK, Cutler GB Jr, Chrousos GP, Fraker DL, Norton JA, Jensen RT (1994) Adrenocorticotropic hormone-secreting islet cell tumors: are they always malignant? Radiology 190:59–64

23. Doppman JL, Pass HI, Nieman LK, Findling JW, Dwyer AJ, Feuerstein IM, Ling A, Travis WD, Cutler GB Jr, Chrousos GP, Loriaux DL (1991) Detection of ACTH-producing bronchial carcinoid tumors: MR imaging vs CT. AJR 156:39–43

24. Doppman JL (1994) Somatostatin receptor scintigraphy and the ectopic ACTH syndrome. The solution or just another test? Am J Med 96:303–304

25. Du Pont AG, Somers G, Van Steiterghem AC, Warson F, Vanhaelst L (1984) Ectopic adrenocorticotropin production: disappearance after removal of inflammatory tissue. J Clin Endocrinol Metab 58:654–658

26. Eriksson B, Oberg K, Alm G, Karlsson A, Lundqvist G, Andersson T, Wilander E, Wide L (1986) Treatment of malignant endocrine pancreatic tumors with human leucocyte interferon. Lancet 2:1307–1309

27. Farwell AP, Devlin JT, Stewart JA (1988) Total suppression of cortisol excretion by ketoconazole in the therapy of the ectopic adrenocorticotropic hormone syndrome. Am J Med 84:1063–1066

28. Findling JW, Kehoe ME, Shaker JL, Raff H (1991) Routine inferior petrosal sinus sampling in the differential diagnosis of adrenocortical (ACTH)-dependent Cushing's syndrome: early recognition of the occult ectopic ACTH syndrome. J Clin Endocrinol Metab 73:408–413

29. Friedman TC, Loh YP, Birch NP (1994) In vitro processing of proopiomelanocortin by recombinant PC1 (SPC3). Endocrinology 135:854–862

30. Grossman AB, Howlett TA, Perry L, Coy DH, Savage MO, Lavender-P, Rees LH, Besser GM (1988) CRF in the differential diagnosis of Cushing's syndrome: a comparison with the dexamethasone suppression test. Clin Endocrinol (Oxf) 29:167–178

31. Harbour JW, Lai SL, Whang-Peng J, Gazdar AF, Minna JD, Kaye FJ (1988) Abnormalities in structure and expression of the human retinoblastoma gene in SCLC. Science 241:353–357

32. Howlett TA, Drury PL, Perry L, Doniach I, Rees LH, Besser GM (1986) Diagnosis and management of ACTH-dependent Cushing's syndrome: comparison of the features in ectopic and pituitary ACTH production. Clin Endocrinol (Oxf) 24:699–713

33. Invitti C, Giraldi FP, Cavagnini F (1999) Inferior petrosal sinus sampling in patients with Cushing's syndrome and contradictory responses to dynamic testing. Clin Endocrinol (Oxf) 51:255–257

34. Invitti C, Giraldi FP, de Martin M, Cavagnini F (1999) Diagnosis and management of Cushing's syndrome: results of an Italian multicentre study. Study Group of the Italian Society of Endocrinology on the Pathophysiology of the Hypothalamic-Pituitary-Adrenal Axis. J Clin Endocrinol Metab 84:440–448

35. Ishido H, Yamashita N, Kitaoka M, Tanaka Y, Ogata E (1994) A case of ectopic ACTH syndrome associated with Zollinger-Ellison syndrome: long-term survival with chemical adrenalectomy. Endocr J 41:171–176

36. Jeannotte L, Burbach JP, Drouin J (1987) Unusual proopiomelanocortin ribonucleic acids in extrapituitary tissues: intronless transcripts in testes and log poly(A) tails in hypothalamus. Mol Endocr 1:749–757

37. Kaltsas T, Krassas GE, Pontikides N, Tsotsia E, Tsagarakis S (2003) Cyclical Cushing syndrome caused by intermittent ectopic ACTH hormonogenesis responsive to somatostatin analogues. Endocrinologist 13:7–11

38. Kato Y, Ferguson TB, Bennett DE, Burford TH (1969) Oat cell carcinoma of the lung. A review of 138 cases. Cancer 23:517–524

39. Kaye TB, Crapo L (1990) The Cushing syndrome: An update on diagnostic tests. Ann Intern Med 112:434–444

40. Kuhn JM, Proeschel MF, Seurin DJ, Bertagna XY, Luton JP, Girard FL (1989) Comparative assessment of ACTH and lipotropin plasma levels in the diagnosis and follow-up of patients with Cushing's syndrome: a study of 210 cases. Am J Med 86:678–684

41. Kulke MH, Mayer RJ (1999) Carcinoid tumors. N Engl J Med 340:858–868

42. Lam EW, La Thangue NB (1994) DP and E2F proteins: coordinating transcription with cell cycle progression. Curr Opin Cell Biol 6:859–866. Review

43. Lamberts SWS, Krenning EP, Reubi JC (1991) The role of somatostatin and its analogue in the diagnosis and treatment of tumors. Endocr Rev 12:450–482

44. Liddle GW, Island DP, Meador CK (1962) Normal and abnormal regulation of corticotropin secretion in man. Recent Prog Horm Res 18:125–166

45. Lyons DF, Eisen BR, Clark MR, Pysher TJ, Welsh JD, Kem DC (1984) Concurrent Cushing's and Zollinger-Ellison syndromes in a patient with islet cell carcinoma. Case report and review of the literature. Am J Med 76: 729–733

46. Makita M, Maeda Y, Hashimoto K, Nakase K, Takenaka K, Shinagawa K, Ishimaru F, Ikeda K, Niiya K, Ogura T, Harada M (2003) Acute lymphoblastic leukemia with large molecular ACTH production. Ann Hematol 82: 448–451

47. Malerbi DA, Mendonca BB, Liberman B, Toledo SP, Corradini MC, Cunha-Neto MB, Fragoso MC, Wajchenberg BL (1993) The desmopressin stimulation test in the differential diagnosis of Cushing's syndrome. Clin Endocrinol (Oxf) 38:463–472

48. Miller JW, Crapo L (1993) The medical treatment of Cushing's syndrome. Endocr Rev 14:443–458

49. Moertel CG, Kvols LK, O'Connell MJ, Rubin J (1991) Treatment of neuroendocrine carcinomas with combined etoposide and cisplatin: evidence of major therapeutic activity in the anaplastic variants of these neoplasms. Cancer 68:227–232

50. Naidich DP (1990) CT/MR correlation in the evaluation of tracheobronchial neoplasia. Radiol Clin North Am 28: 555–571

51. Newell-Price J, Perry L, Medbak S, Monson J, Savage M, Besser M, Grossman A (1997) A combined test using desmopressin and corticotropin-releasing hormone in the differential diagnosis of Cushing's syndrome. J Clin Endocrinol Metab 82:176–181

52. Newell-Price J, Trainer P, Besser M, Grossman A (1998) The diagnosis and differential diagnosis of Cushing's syndrome and pseudo-Cushing's states. Endocr Rev 19: 647–672

53. Nieman LK, Chrousos GP, Oldfield EH, Avgerinos PC, Cutler GB Jr, Loriaux DL (1986) The ovine corticotropin-releasing hormone stimulation test and the dexamethasone suppression test in the differential diagnosis of Cushing's syndrome. Ann Intern Med 105:862–867

54. Oberg K, Norheim I, Alm G (1989) Treatment of malignant carcinoid tumors: a randomized controlled study of streptozotocin plus 5-FU and human leucocyte interferon. Eur J Cancer Clin Oncol 25:1475–1479

55. Odell WD (1991) Ectopic ACTH secretion: a misnomer. Endocrinol Metab Clin North Am 20:371–379

56. Oldfield EH, Doppman JL, Nieman LK, Chrousos GP, Miller DL, Ktaz DA, Cutler GB Jr, Loriaux DL (1991) Petrosal sinus sampling with and without corticotropin-releasing hormone for the differential diagnosis of Cushing's syndrome. N Engl J Med 325:896–905

57. Orth DN (1995) Cushing's syndrome. N Engl J Med 332:791–803

58. Phlipponneau M, Nocaudie M, Epelbaum J, De Keyzer Y, Lalau JD, Marchandise X, Bertagna X (1994) Somatostatin analogs for the localization and preoperative treatment of an adrenocorticotropin-secreting bronchial carcinoid tumor. J Clin Endocrinol Metab 78:20–24

59. Picon A, Bertagna X, de Keyzer Y (1999) Analysis of the human proopiomelanocortin gene promoter in a small cell lung carcinoma cell line reveals an unusual role for E2F transcription factors. Oncogene 18:2627–2633

60. Raffin-Sanson ML, Massias JF, Dumont C, Raux-Demay MC, Proeschel MF, Luton JP, Bertagna X (1996) High plasma proopiomelanocortin in aggressive adrenocorticotropin-secreting tumors. J Clin Endocrinol Metab 81: 4272–4277

61. Raffin-Sanson ML, de Keyzer Y, Bertagna X (2003) Proopiomelanocortin, a polypeptide precursor with multiple functions: from physiology to pathological conditions. Eur J Endocrinol 149:79–90

62. Rena O, Filosso PL, Maggi G, Casadio C (2003) Neuroendocrine tumors (carcinoid) of the thymic gland. Ann Thorac Surg 75:633

63. Seidah NG, Marcinkiewicz M, Benjannet S, Gaspar L, Beaubien G, Mattei MG et al. (1991) Cloning and primary sequence of a mouse candidate prohormone convertase PC1 homologous to PC2, furin, and Kex2: distinct chromosomal localization and messenger RNA distribution in brain and pituitary compared to PC2. Mol Endocrinol 5:111–122

64. Shepherd FA, Laskey J, Evans WK, et al. (1992) Cushing's syndrome associated with ectopic corticotropin production and small-cell lung cancer. J Clin Oncol 10:21–27

65. Shrager JB, Wright CD, Wain JC, Torchiana DF, Grillo HC, Mathisen DJ (1997) Bronchopulmonary carcinoid tumors associated with Cushing's syndrome: a more aggressive type of typical carcinoids. J Thorac Cardiovasc Surg 114:367–375

66. Smeekens SP, Steiner DF (1990) Identification of a human insulinoma cDNA encoding a novel mammalian protein structurally related to the yeast dibasic processing protease Kex 2. J Biol Chem 265:2997–3000

67. Tabarin A, Valli N, Chanson P, Bachelot Y, Rohmer V, Bex-Bachellerie B, Catargi B, Roger P, Laurent F (1999) Usefulness of somatostatin receptor scintigraphy in patients with occult ectopic adrenocorticotropin syndrome. J Clin Endocrinol Metab 84:1193–1202

68. Takahashi H, Hakamata Y, Watanabe Y, Kikuno R, Miyata T, Numa S (1983) Complete nucleotide sequence of the human corticotropin-beta-lipotropin precursor gene. Nucleic Acids Res 11:6847–6858

69. Terzolo M, Reimondo G, Ali A, Borretta G, Cesario F, Pia A, Paccotti P, Angeli A (2001) The limited value of the desmopressin test in the diagnostic approach to Cushing's syndrome. Clin Endocrinol (Oxf) 54:609–616

70. Terzolo M, Reimondo G, Ali A, Bovio S, Daffara F, Paccotti P, Angeli A (2001) Ectopic ACTH syndrome: molecular bases and clinical heterogeneity. Ann Oncol 12 Suppl 2:S83–87

71. Texier PL, De Keyzer Y, Lacave R, Vieau D, Lenne F, Rojas-Miranda A, Verley JM, Luton JP, Kahn A, Bertagna X (1991) Proopiomelanocortin gene expression in normal and tumoral human lung. J Clin Endocrinol Metab 73:414–420

72. Torpy DJ, Chen CC, Mullen N, Doppman JL, Carrasquillo JA, Chrousos GP, Nieman LK (1999) Lack of utility of 111In-Pentetreotide scintigraphy in localizing ectopic ACTH producing tumors: follow-up of 18 patients. J Clin Endocrinol Metab 84:1186–1192

73. Trainer PJ, Grossman A (1991) The diagnosis and differential diagnosis of Cushing's syndrome. Clin Endocrinol (Oxf) 34:317–330

74. Tsagarakis S, Christoforaki M, Giannopoulou H, Rondogianni F, Housianakou I, Malagari C, Rontogianni D, Bellenis I, Thalassinos N (2003) A reappraisal of the utility of somatostatin receptor scintigraphy in patients with ectopic adrenocorticotropin Cushing's syndrome. J Clin Endocrinol Metab 88:4754–4758

75. Tsagarakis S, Giannakenas C, Vassilakos PJ, Platis O, Belenis I, Kaskarelis J, Rontoyianni D, Thalassinos N (1995) Successful localization of an occult ACTH-secreting bronchial carcinoid tumour with 111 indium-DTPA labelled octreotide. Clin Endocrinol (Oxf). 43:763–767

76. Tsagarakis S, Kaskarelis IS, Kokkoris P, Malagari C, Thalassinos N (2000) The application of combined stimulation with CRH and desmopressin during bilateral petrosal sinus sampling in patients with Cushing's syndrome. Clin Endocrinol (Oxf) 52:355–361

77. Tsagarakis S, Thalassinos N (2001) The desmopressin test: a new tool in the functional evaluation of the pituitary-adrenal axis in patients with Cushing's syndrome? In: Margioris AN, Chrousos GP (eds) Adrenal disorders. Humana Press, Totowa, NJ, pp 193–202

78. Tsagarakis S, Tsigos C, Vasiliou V, Tsiotra P, Kaskarelis J, Sotiropoulou C, Raptis SA, Thalassinos N (2002) The desmopressin and combined CRH-desmopressin tests in the differential diagnosis of ACTH-dependent Cushing's syndrome: constraints imposed by the expression of V2 vasopressin receptors in tumors with ectopic ACTH secretion. J Clin Endocrinol Metab 87:1646–1653

79. Vaidya B, Richardson D, Hilton CJ, Kendall-Taylor P (1997) Adrenocorticotropin-secreting carcinoid tumour identified and treated 12 years after presentation with Cushing's syndrome. Postgrad Med J 73:737–739

80. Van Coevorden A, Laurent E, Rickaert F, van Reeth O, Van Cauter E, Mockel J (1990) Cushing's syndrome with intermittent ectopic ACTH production. J Endocrinol Invest 13:317–326

81. Van den Bruel A, Bex M, Van Dorpe J, Heyns W, Bouillon R (1998) Occult ectopic ACTH secretion due to recurrent lung carcinoid: long-term control of hypercortisolism by continuous subcutaneous infusion of octreotide. Clin Endocrinol (Oxf) 49:541–546

82. Vella A, Thompson GB, Grant CS, van Heerden JA, Farley DR, Young WF Jr (2001) Laparoscopic adrenalectomy for adrenocorticotropin-dependent Cushing's syndrome. J Clin Endocrinol Metab 86:1596–1599

83. Vieau D, Seidah NG, Mbikay M, Chretien M, Bertagna X (1994) Expression of the prohormone convertase PC2 correlates with the presence of corticotropin-like intermediate lobe peptide in human adrenocorticotropin-secreting tumors. J Clin Endocrinol Metab 79:1503–1506

84. Vignati F, Loli P (1996) Additive effect of ketoconazole and octreotide in the treatment of severe adrenocorticotropin-dependent hypercortisolism. J Clin Endocrinol Metab 81:2885–2890

85. Vincent JM, Trainer PJ, Reznek RH, Marcus AJ, Dacie JE, Armstrong P, Besser GM (1993) The radiological investigation of occult ectopic ACTH-dependent Cushing's syndrome. Clin Radiol 48:11–17

86. Wajchenberg BL, Mendonca BB, Liberman B, Pereira MA, Carneiro PC, Wakamatsu A, Kirschner MA (1994) Ectopic adrenocorticotropic hormone syndrome. Endocr Rev 15:752–787

87. Weiss M, Yellin A, Husza'r M, Eisenstein Z, Bar-Ziv J, Krausz Y (1994) Localization of adrenocorticotropic hormone-secreting bronchial carcinoid tumor by somatostatin-receptor scintigraphy. Ann Intern Med 121:198–199

88. White A, Clark AJL (1993) The cellular and molecular basis of the ectopic ACTH syndrome. Clin Endocrinol (Oxf) 39:131–141

89. White A, Gibson S (1998) ACTH precursors: biological significance and clinical relevance. Clin Endocrinol (Oxf) 48:251–255

90. Winocour PH, Tong P, White J, Edwards A, White A, Gibson GJ, Clark F (1993) Unusual presentation and course of Cushing's syndrome due to ectopic ACTH secretion by a bronchial carcinoma. Respir Med 87:149–151

91. Zeiger MA, Pass HI, Doppman JD, Nieman LK, Chrousos GP, Cutler GB Jr, Jensen RT, Norton JA (1992) Surgical strategy in the management of non-small cell ectopic adrenocorticotropic hormone syndrome. Surgery 112: 994–1000

92. Zhou A, Bloomquist BT, Mains RE (1993) The prohormone convertases PC1 and PC2 mediate distinct endoproteolytic cleavages in a strict temporal order during proopiomelanocortin biosynthetic processing. J Biol Chem 268:1763–1769

93. Zhu L, Domenico DR, Howard JM (1996) Metastatic pancreatic neuroendocrine carcinoma causing Cushing's syndrome. ACTH secretion by metastases 3 years after resection of nonfunctioning primary cancer. Int J Pancreatol 19:205–208

9 Cushing's Syndrome in Children and Adolescents

George Mastorakos, Christina Kanaka-Gantenbein

CONTENTS

9.1 Definition and Etiology

Cushing's syndrome is a clinical syndrome caused by chronic glucocorticoid excess [3, 30, 31, 42, 44, 45]. The latter may be *exogenous,* as a result of chronic, long-standing exposure of the organism to the exogenous administration of glucocorticoids or ACTH [30, 31, 44, 45], or *endogenous,* due to the hypersecretion of cortisol, ACTH or CRH. The endogenous hypersecretion of ACTH of pituitary origin is called Cushing's disease.

The commonest cause of Cushing's syndrome in children and adolescents is by far the *exogenous administration* of glucocorticosteroids (iatrogenic Cushing's syndrome) as treatment of several chronic diseases, such as steroid-responsive, steroid-dependent nephrotic syndrome, juvenile chronic arthritis or severe asthma bronchiale [2, 31, 44]. Rarely, chronic local use of steroids in the form of inhaled steroids, dermatological creams or ointments, or even eye or nasal drops, has been reported to induce iatrogenic Cushing's syndrome [2, 10, 16, 17, 43].

Endogenous Cushing's syndrome is the result of excessive pituitary ACTH (Cushing's disease) or ectopic ACTH secretion (extremely rare in pediatric patients) [30, 31, 42, 44, 45, 48, 49]. These causes constitute *ACTH-dependent Cushing's syndrome,* accounting for about 75–85% of endogenous Cushing's syndrome cases in mostly peripubertal patients [4, 31, 48, 49]. A very small number of ACTH-dependent cases are due to ectopic CRH-secreting tumors, mainly reported in older (adult) patients. Furthermore, endogenous Cushing's syndrome can be the result of autonomous cortisol secretion by a cortisol-secreting adrenal tumor, bilateral micronodular or macronodular adrenal hyperplasia [5, 20, 30, 44, 45, 54] or other autonomous adrenal processes. These causes constitute *ACTH-independent Cushing's syndrome.* In children younger than 7 years ACTH-independent Cushing's syndrome, mainly due to adrenal carcinomas, is more frequently seen than ACTH-dependent Cushing's syndrome [20, 29, 30, 44, 45, 47] and is quite often accompanied by oversecretion of adrenal androgens. It is estimated that adrenocortical tumors account for about 70% of endogenous Cushing's syndrome in young children [20, 29, 44, 47]. Finally, rare cases of ACTH-independent Cushing's syndrome are due to activating mutations of the ACTH-receptor coupled Gs alpha subunit leading to cortisol hypersecretion in the broader spectrum of McCune-Albright syndrome [12, 23].

9.2 Incidence

Endogenous Cushing's syndrome is rare in childhood and adolescence. The incidence of endogenous Cushing's syndrome, in general, is two to five new cases per million of general population per year, with a 9:1

female to male ratio [30, 31, 42, 44]. About 10% of these new cases occur in childhood or adolescence. However, this female to male (F/M) preponderance observed in adulthood is not seen in pediatric patients [6, 31, 49]. In the long series of the National Institutes of Health (NIH) experience we found that in prepubertal children the F/M ratio was 1/5 whereas for adolescents this ratio was 3/1, indicating that there was a shift towards female preponderance after the onset of puberty and, therefore, the sexual dimorphism of the incidence of Cushing's syndrome in adulthood is clearly associated with puberty. Due to the rarity of endogenous Cushing's syndrome such young patients should optimally be managed by a multidisciplinary team consisting of a pediatric endocrinologist, an adult endocrinologist, a neuroradiologist, a neurosurgeon with special experience in transphenoidal surgery in young age as well as a specialized surgeon on adrenals and a radiotherapist [6, 26, 31, 48, 49].

9.3   Clinical Presentation

The main clinical features of pediatric patients with Cushing's syndrome differ somewhat from those observed in adult Cushing's patients (Fig. 1). The predominant features according to different series are reported in Table 1. They comprise weight gain usually with round moon facies, growth failure, fatigue, pubertal delay or arrest, hypertension, hirsutism, acne and striae [6, 26, 31, 34, 49, 50, 55]. It is noteworthy that striae are more frequent among older patients than among younger ones [55]. Further presenting symptoms are headache, emotional lability and features of pseudoprecocious puberty in young patients due to the adrenal androgen excess. Mental or behavioral problems are only rarely reported in children and adolescents with Cushing's disease, in contrast to the most frequent mental changes

or job performance deterioration observed in adult patients with Cushing's disease [30, 31, 44, 49]. However, Devoe et al. reported as many as 44% of children and adolescents with Cushing's disease presenting with compulsive behavior and overachievement at school [6]. In cases of adrenocortical carcinoma various degrees of virilization due to the adrenal androgen excess may be the prevailing clinical finding [29, 31, 44, 47].

Bone Age ▶ Bone age of Cushing's patients may be retarded due to the long-standing hypercortisolism [31, 43, 48, 49]. However, if adrenal androgen excess is present, bone age may be even advanced [31, 44, 49]. Delayed bone age was found in 13% of the patients studied by Devoe et al. [6]. In the NIH series comprising predominantly adolescents, bone age was not found to be delayed [31] (Fig. 2). The combination of the retarding effect of hypercortisolism and the accelerating effect of androgens may in some cases lead to a bone age appropriate for the chronological age of the patient [31, 44, 49].

Bone Mineral Density ▶ The long-standing hypercortisolism may also have a negative effect on the bone mineral density of these patients, who may present with osteopenia or even osteoporosis [1, 6, 27].

9.4   Diagnostic Assessment: Laboratory Investigation

9.4.1   Positive Diagnosis of Endogenous Hypercortisolism

The first step in the diagnosis of endogenous Cushing's syndrome is the biochemical confirmation of hypercortisolism. The most frequently used biochemical investigations are listed below.

Table 1. Clinical features at presentation

Clinical manifestations	Savage et al. [49]	Devoe et al. [6]	Magiakou et al. [31]	Total
Weight gain	100%	92%	90%	90–100%
Growth failure	71%	84%	83%	71–84%
Hypertension	75%	63%	47%	47–75%
Pubertal delay/arrest		60%	78%	60–78%
Hirsutism	53%	46%	78%	46–78%
Striae	53%	36%		36–53%
Acne		46%	47%	46–47%
Emotional lability		44%		44%
Fatigue		67%	44%	44–67%

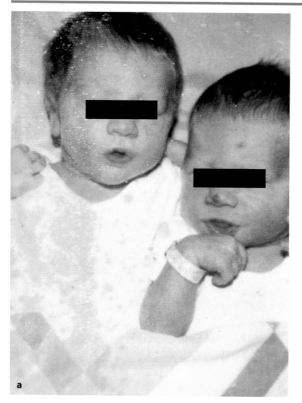
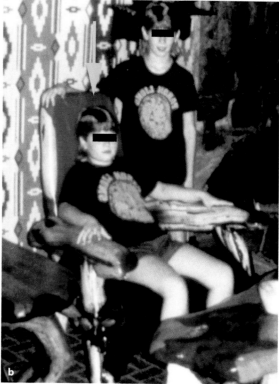
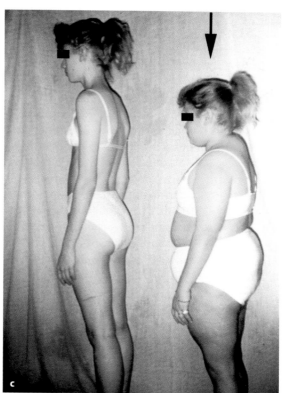

Fig. 1a–c. Chronological evolution of the clinical presentation of endogenous Cushing's syndrome in a young girl as compared to her healthy twin sister. (Courtesy of G.P. Chrousos)

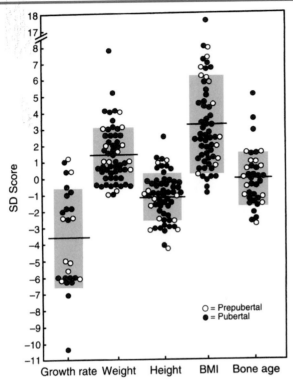

Fig. 2. Growth rate, weight, height, body mass index (*BMI*), and bone age of the NIH series as compared with expected values for age and sex [31]. The *horizontal lines* and the *shaded bars* indicate the means ± SD

9.4.1.1 Baseline Biochemical Investigations

The 24-h mean urinary free cortisol (UFC) excretion (corrected for body surface area) is an important first-line test. Values consistently in excess of 300 μg/day are virtually diagnostic for Cushing's syndrome [30]. Urinary free cortisol remains constant throughout life, when adjusted for square meter of body surface area, thus obviating establishing age-specific normal values in children or obese individuals. Normal values lie <70 μg/m²/day [30] or <80 μg/m²/day [6] according to different authors.

The 24-h Mean Urinary Excretion of 17-OH-CS (17-OH-Corticosteroids) ▶ High urinary 17-OH-CS excretion, i.e. more than 5 mg/m²/day, also suggests Cushing's disease. In the series of Devoe et al. [6], the 24-h mean urinary 17-OH-CS excretion was a more sensitive marker than UFC, since 100% of Cushing's disease patients had high urinary 17-OH-CS excretion as compared to only 86% of patients demonstrating high UFC excretion (i.e. UFC>80 μg/m²/day) [6].

Serum Cortisol and ACTH Circadian Rhythm ▶ In most cases of Cushing's disease the normal circadian rhythm of ACTH and cortisol secretion is abolished. It is therefore suggested that five consecutive morning and five consecutive evening plasma samples should be drawn for determination of diurnal variation of cortisol and ACTH secretion [30, 46, 49].

Salivary cortisol concentrations nowadays constitute an alternative to the multiple venepunctures needed for the determination of plasma cortisol variation. In a recent publication [13], measurement of salivary free cortisol by radioimmunoassay at 7.30 A.M., bedtime and midnight discriminated accurately children with Cushing's disease from healthy obese or non-obese children. Concretely, salivary cortisol was undetectable in 66% of healthy children at bedtime and in 90% of them at midnight. It has therefore been shown that, with cut-off points that excluded healthy children, a midnight salivary cortisol value of 0.27 μg/dl (7.5 nmol/l) identified 92.8% of Cushing's syndrome children, whereas a bedtime value of >1 μg/dl (≥27.6 nmol/l) detected 83.3% of Cushing's syndrome children, with the same diagnostic accuracy as the UFC per square meter body surface area [13]. Furthermore, in another study, it has been demonstrated that the combination of salivary cortisol determination at 2300 hours as well as after the dexamethasone suppression test is an easily performed and non-invasive method with high specificity and sensitivity for diagnosing Cushing's syndrome in children [35].

9.4.1.2 Dynamic Tests

Low-dose Dexamethasone Suppression Test ▶ In children 15 μg/kg body weight (maximal dose 1 mg) dexamethasone is given at midnight and blood for cortisol determination is withdrawn the next morning (8.00 A.M.). A morning plasma cortisol level of >5 mg/dl after midnight dexamethasone administration suggests hypercortisolism.

Diagnostic Value ▶ This is a screening test that is of use only when positive. The expected fall in cortisol levels may fail to occur in normal subjects because of stress, intercurrent psychiatric or other chronic or acute illnesses, states referred to as pseudocushing states [11, 30].

9.4.2 Positive Diagnosis of Endogenous Cushing's Syndrome; Diagnosis of Cushing's Disease

9.4.2.1 Dynamic Tests

Standard Low- and High-dose Dexamethasone Suppression Tests ▶ Samples of 24-h urine to determine concentrations of 17-OH-CS, free cortisol and creatinine are collected for at least 2 days before and during the entire period of dexamethasone administration, beginning at 8.00 A.M. Venous blood samples are also obtained daily at 8.00 A.M. to determine levels of cortisol. Dexamethasone is administered successively in a low dosage of 10 µg/kg body weight up to a maximum of 0.5 mg every 6 h on days 3 and 4 (standard low-dose dexamethasone suppression test), and a high dosage of 50 µg/kg body weight up to a maximum of 2 mg every 6 h on days 5 and 6 (high-dose dexamethasone suppression test). A weight-adjusted dosage of 20 µg dexamethasone/kg body weight has been recommended in pediatric patients for the standard low-dose test. Some protocols propose 3 days on low dosage and 3 days on high dosage [11, 34].

Evaluation ▶ The response to the standard low-dose dexamethasone suppression test is considered normal when serum cortisol concentrations on day 4 fall to <5 µg/dl (138 nmol/l) or to 50% of baseline levels, urinary 17-OH-CS levels decrease to <3 mg/24 h (8.3 µmol/day) or to values approaching zero and UFC levels fall to less than 50% of basal levels.

The normal response to the high-dose dexamethasone suppression test is observed when serum cortisol concentration falls to less than 1 µg/dl (27 nmol/l) and when levels of urinary 17-OH-CS or free cortisol decline to less than 90% of baseline concentration at the end of the test.

Diagnostic Value ▶ The standard low-dose test distinguishes normal subjects from patients with Cushing's syndrome in whom suppression is incomplete or never occurs. The high-dose test distinguishes patients with Cushing's disease (about 90% of these patients demonstrate suppression) from those with an adrenal adenoma, carcinoma or ectopic ACTH producing-tumors (who do not demonstrate any suppression) [11]. Suppression is incomplete in patients with adrenal incidentalomas [60].

CRH Stimulation Test ▶ During this test 1 µg CRH/kg body weight is injected i.v. Blood is withdrawn for de-termination of ACTH and cortisol 15 min before and 0, 15, 30, 60, 90, and 120 min after treatment [38, 40]. When baseline urinary steroid excretion is elevated, a CRH response is considered to be indicative of Cushing's disease if the plasma ACTH or cortisol values increase above the mean baseline value by at least 34% or 20% respectively [38, 40].

9.4.2.2 Imaging Studies

Magnetic Resonance Imaging ▶ Magnetic resonance imaging (MRI) scanning with gadolinium is the method of choice to visualize pituitary adenoma with a higher sensitivity than a computed tomography (CT) scan. However, since the majority of corticotroph micro-adenomas have a diameter of less than 5 mm, many are not visible even in the most advanced MRI scan [49].

CT Scan ▶ As already mentioned, CT scanning is not a method of choice to visualize pituitary microadenomas. In the case of ACTH-independent Cushing's syndrome, MRI or CT of the adrenals is performed to visualize the androgen secreting space-occupying lesion [29, 47].

9.4.2.3 Invasive Diagnostic Methods

Bilateral Inferior Petrosal Sinus Sampling Before and After the Administration of CRH ▶ The most direct way to demonstrate pituitary hypersecretion of ACTH is to document a central to peripheral vein ACTH gradient in blood draining the tumor [30, 41, 42, 49].

Method ▶ After a catheter is positioned in each inferior petrosal sinus, blood samples are withdrawn simultaneously from each sinus and from a peripheral vein: twice immediately before the peripheral venous injection of 1 µg of ovine CRH per kilogram of body weight and twice more, 2–3 min and 5–6 min after the injection [41]. If the sinus to peripheral vein plasma ACTH ratio for either sinus is ≥2.0 in either of the two basal sets of samples or ≥3.0 in either of the two sets of samples obtained after CRH injection, the diagnostic accuracy, sensitivity and specificity of the procedure are all 100%. The test is less reliable when the maximal ACTH concentration in the inferior petrosal sinus is less than 20 pg/ml (<4.4 pmol/l).

Diagnostic Value ▶ Central to peripheral ACTH ratios >2 indicate central ACTH secretion. The interpetrosal sinus ACTH gradient is able to indicate lateralization of

ACTH secretion that in most cases is confirmed at surgery [41, 49]. The inferior petrosal sinus sampling gives an 82% prediction of correct tumor lateralization.

9.4.2.4 Diagnostic Criteria

The diagnosis of Cushing's disease is based on several of the above-mentioned parameters. A suggested algorithm of diagnostic assessment is presented in Fig. 3. Absent diurnal cortisol rhythm was found in 100% of Cushing's patients in several studies [6, 49]. As previously mentioned, according to Devoe et al., high 24-h urinary 17-OH-CS excretion (i.e. levels >5 mg/m^2/day) was found in 100% of their Cushing's patients, while high urinary free cortisol excretion (i.e. levels >80 μg/m^2/day) was found in 86% of their Cushing's patients [6]. Failure to suppress urinary UFC under

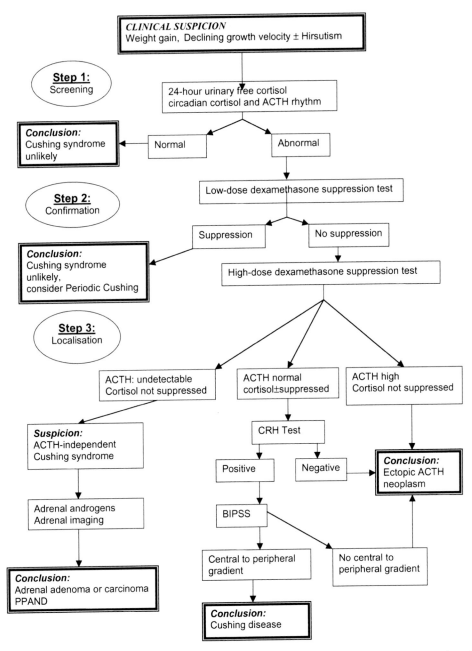

Fig. 3. Algorithm of diagnostic assessment in case of suspicion of Cushing's syndrome according to several authors [11, 34, 46]

25 µg/m^2/day or urinary 17-OH-CS under 1.5 mg/m^2/day after the standard low-dose dexamethasone suppression test was seen in 86% of their patients, while failure of suppression of UFC excretion or 17-OH-CS excretion by 50% or more was observed in 92% of their Cushing's patients [6].

Also in the study of Savage et al. [49] after the standard low-dose dexamethasone suppression test cortisol failed to suppress <50 nmol/l after 48 h in Cushing's patients. During the high-dose dexamethasone suppression test all patients with Cushing's disease showed suppression of cortisol to less than 50% of the basal pre-dexamethasone level, while no suppression was seen in one patient with an adrenal adenoma and in another with primary pigmented nodular adrenal hyperplasia (both cases of ACTH-independent Cushing's syndrome). The CRH test showed an increase of cortisol production in Cushing's disease patients, while patients with adrenal adenoma, primary pigmented nodular adrenal hyperplasia or ectopic ACTH production did not show a cortisol response to CRH [49].

9.5   Diagnosis

The diagnosis of endogenous Cushing's syndrome in children and adolescents is usually retarded. It is estimated that the elapse time between the onset of the clinical syndrome and the diagnosis is equal to or greater than 2 years [6, 26, 49], ranging from 0.5 to 10 years. A major effort must be therefore made to sensitize health care providers and specifically pediatricians to recognize Cushing's syndrome as early as possible. Thus, the deleterious and often non-reversible effects of hypercortisolism on growth and bone mineral density can be minimized, since the age of onset and duration of hypercortisolism before cure are features that contribute to the severity of growth failure and irreversible bone loss.

9.6   Treatment of Cushing's Syndrome

9.6.1 Cushing's Disease

9.6.1.1 Transphenoidal Surgery

Transphenoidal surgery with selective microadenomectomy is the worldwide accepted first-line treatment for Cushing's disease in both adults and children [6, 8, 9, 26, 31, 36, 41, 42, 49, 52]. In many centers transphe-

noidal surgery is accompanied by hemihypophysectomy [26, 31].

Preoperative Treatment ▶ In some centers [49] children and adolescents with Cushing's disease were preoperatively treated with either metyrapone or ketoconazole or a combination of both for a period of 4–8 weeks preoperatively, in order to normalize circulating cortisol levels. The dose of each drug was 0.75–2.25 g/day and 0.3–0.6 g/day for metyrapone and ketoconazole, respectively.

Complications of Transphenoidal Surgery ▶ In experienced hands, transphenoidal surgery seems to be a safe procedure with only minimal complications. About 10% of patients have postoperative complications, including cerebrospinal fluid rhinorrhea, usually transient diabetes insipidus or visual disturbances [41, 61]. In the NIH series panhypopituitarism has been reported in 19% of patients operated on [31]. Eight out of 42 operated patients (19%) presented transient diabetes insipidus that did not require medication at discharge in the series published by Devoe et al. [6], while in the series of Savage et al. [49] 1 patient out of 17 (5.9%) developed panhypopituitarism and two diabetes insipidus (11.8%). In the Mayo Clinic series, up to 6% of patients ended up with endocrine dysfunction, while 9/22 (40.9%) of patients presented transient diabetes insipidus [26].

Definition of Cure After Transphenoidal Surgery ▶ Postoperatively hydrocortisone is given for a minimum of 24 h. After transphenoidal surgery, serum cortisol levels are measured daily at 09.00 hours, at least 12 h after the last dose of hydrocortisone. Undetectable postoperative serum cortisol levels <50 nM define postoperative cure [49, 59]. However, residual pituitary function is among the criteria by which the surgical outcome is judged.

Cure and Recurrence Rates ▶ Rates of cure are reported to range from 70–95% in adult patients with Cushing's disease. In childhood cure rates are reported to reach 50–73% according to the experience of several centers [6, 8, 26, 36, 49]. It seems therefore that cure rates are much higher in adult patients when compared to childhood or adolescence Cushing's disease. This may be indicative of a more aggressive behavior of Cushing's disease at young ages or of a more conservative operative treatment at young ages [26]. However, since transphenoidal surgery, particularly in children, is a highly skilled procedure, the cure rates may also be determined by the experience and skill-fulness of the neurosurgeon [31, 41, 49]. For example, in the NIH experience cure rate after transphenoidal surgery for Cushing's disease in childhood is as high as 90% [31]. In this series 30% of the operated patients have been treated by hemihypophysectomy [26, 31]. In that cohort endocrine deficiency postoperatively was found in 19% of cases [31]. On the other hand, in the Mayo Clinic experience [26], cure rate after first transphenoidal surgery was lower, but also the per-centage of endocrine deficiency was lower, namely only 6%. Thus, more aggressive surgery improves the efficacy of treatment but increases the incidence of postoperative hypopituitarism [26, 31, 33]. Further-more, a significant number of the NIH patients have already been operated on in another center before being admitted to NIH. However, it should be empha-sized that the duration of the long-term follow-up in the reported series can significantly influence the re-currence rates [6, 26, 31, 49] since many recurrences occur only about 4 years postoperatively [26]. Follow-up of patients in the NIH series extended up to 5 years with a mean of 22 months. Thus, the low recurrence rate in that cohort may be explained by the short follow-up period in that series [31]. In accordance with that, in the Mayo Clinic series, cure rate after long-term follow-up was only 50%, since after 5 years of follow-up 21% of patients presented with recurrence, and when follow-up was extended to 10 years, recur-rence rate increased to 42.2% [26]. In the series of the University of San Francisco, follow-up was extend-ed up to 13 years [6] and the overall remission rate after transphenoidal surgery was 73%, while the mean time to recurrence was 4.2 years (ranging from 0.75–6.2 years) [6]. Finally, in the London experience the median period of follow-up was 8 years (ranging from 0.5–24 years) and cure rate after transphenoidal surgery alone was 56%. Patients with persisting hyper-cortisolemia underwent pituitary irradiation. When both therapeutic strategies were considered together (transphenoidal surgery alone or surgery followed by pituitary irradiation) the overall cure rate for the median of 8 years of follow-up was 82% [49].

9.6.1.2 Second-Line Treatment

There is no clear agreement on the optimal therapy after unsuccessful transphenoidal surgery. The options are: repeat transphenoidal surgery, pituitary radiotherapy, adrenalectomy or drug therapy such as ketoconazole [42, 49, 52, 61]. The decision is primarily taken after consideration of the experience of the neu-rosurgeon, the general surgeon, the radiotherapist and of course in consideration of possible side-effects and residual sequelae of each therapeutic modality.

Pituitary Radiotherapy ► Pituitary radiotherapy is used in specialized centers with good experience of the treatment of pediatric Cushing's disease. There is evidence that Cushing's disease in children responds to pituitary radiation treatment more readily than does Cushing's disease in adults [9, 14, 26, 49, 51]. In cases where transphenoidal surgery fails to cure the patient, pituitary irradiation may lead to complete cure. The addition of pituitary radiotherapy as second-line treatment has brought the cure rate to over 80% in centers where transphenoidal surgery resulted in 50% cure rate [49, 52]. The dose currently used is 4,500–5,000 cGy [26, 49, 52] in 25 fractions over 35 days using a 6 MV linear accelerator. Until radio-therapy becomes effective, hypercortisolemia is con-trolled with ketoconazole at a dose of 200–600 mg/day and metyrapone at a dose of 750 mg^{-3} g/day with or without aminoglutethimide (1 g/day) or o'p'DDD (3 mg/day) [49].

Definition of Cure After Pituitary Radiotherapy ► Cure of Cushing's disease after radiotherapy [52] is defined as mean serum cortisol on a 5-point day curve of less than 150 nM (5.4 µg/dl) after discontinuation of medical treatment in addition to midnight serum cortisol of less than 50 nM (1.8 µg/dl) and suppression of serum cortisol to less than 50 nM on the standard low-dose dexamethasone suppression test [52]. Ac-cording to the London experience, based on young patients who underwent radiotherapy shortly after transphenoidal surgery because of persisting postop-erative hypercortisolemia, indicating lack of cure, the mean interval from radiotherapy to cure (defined as mean serum cortisol on a 5-point day curve <150 nM) was 0.94 years, ranging from 0.25–2.86 years, while recovery of pituitary-adrenal function (defined as mean cortisol 150–300 nM) occurred at 1.16 years, ranging from 0.4–2.86 years postradiotherapy. Patients were followed up for a mean of 6.9 years (ranging from 1.4–12 years) [49, 52].

Side Effects of Radiotherapy ► After pituitary radio-therapy, *GH deficiency* occurred in 86% of patients. However, long-term follow-up to 9.5 years postradio-therapy indicated some recovery of GH secretion and preservation of other anterior pituitary function [49, 52]. The risk of precocious puberty after cranial irradiation is a well-known phenomenon and should also be taken into consideration in the decision of radiotherapeutic intervention, since the combination of GH deficiency with precocious puberty can significantly compromise final height [25, 39, 49, 52].

9.6.1.3 Third-Line Treatment

Bilateral Adrenalectomy ▶ This option has been most usually considered in older studies [18, 22, 37, 58]. However, the higher incidence of Nelson's syndrome after adrenalectomy in childhood renders this treatment modality not a preferred one [18, 26, 37, 58].

9.6.1.4 Fourth-Line Treatment

Drug Therapy: Metyrapone or o,p DDD ▶ These treatment modalities are rarely considered for Cushing's disease but may be helpful in cases of adrenocortical carcinoma [47].

9.6.2 Adrenocortical Adenoma or Carcinoma

The treatment of choice for an adrenocortical adenoma or carcinoma is the surgical resection of the adrenals by an experienced surgeon [29, 47]. In cases of adrenocortical carcinoma, surgical resection may be followed by chemotherapy such as mitotane treatment. Rarely, adrenocortical carcinoma may rupture and constitute a cause of pediatric acute abdomen [28]. The long-term prognosis of adrenocortical carcinoma is poor, when metastases are already present at diagnosis and when complete resection of the tumor is impossible. On the other hand, patients with completely resected tumor of small size or adrenocortical adenoma histology have a very good prognosis. In any case, however, precise and careful preoperative planning with special attention to electrolyte balance, hypertension and steroid replacement therapy because of suppression of the contralateral adrenal are required [29, 47].

9.7 Long-Term Consequences

9.7.1 Long-Term Consequences on Growth

9.7.1.1 Growth During Cushing's Syndrome

Growth retardation to complete growth arrest is one of the main clinical characteristics of children and adolescents with Cushing's syndrome [50] (Figs. 1, 2). Glucocorticoid excess is well known to induce growth impairment, exerting various effects at various levels of the GH-IGF-1-target organ axis [15]. First of all, at the level of arcuate nucleus glucocorticoid excess downregulates the Ghrelin receptors, while, at the hypothalamic level, it enhances somatostatin release. Patients with Cushing's disease have been shown to have both decreased spontaneous mean plasma 24-h GH concentration and subnormal GH levels after various provocative tests [15, 32]. Another possible mechanism of growth arrest in cases of glucocorticoid excess has been suggested to be mediated by a glucocorticoid-induced target tissue resistance to IGF-1 and other growth factors [15]. Finally, there is a lot of evidence that glucocorticoid excess has a direct deleterious effect on the growth plate cartilage and bone by downregulating GH receptor expression, by suppressing local IGF-1 generation, by accelerating hypertrophic cell apoptosis and inhibiting vascular invasion [15].

9.7.1.2 Growth After Cure of Cushing's Disease

Earlier studies on the natural course of the final height of such patients have reported a compromised final height of successfully treated young patients compared to their midparental or target height [33]. Growth velocity after cure of Cushing's disease has been reported to be abnormally low or to range from 1.8–7.6 cm/year [25, 32, 33, 49]. The abnormally low post-cure growth velocity with lack of catch-up growth has been considered to be responsible for the compromised final height. It has been shown that spontaneous as well as L-arginine or L-dopa stimulated growth hormone secretion is suppressed in Cushing's disease patients until 12 months after surgical treatment even in cases where a better post-cure growth rate has been documented and despite a normalization of body mass index after their surgical treatment [32]. It has specifically been suggested that early onset of Cushing's syndrome might be more critical for growth and that deficits occurring at that critical time might not be self-corrected by an adequate post-cure catch-up growth [33]. However, earlier studies on stimulation of GH secretion by insulin-induced hypoglycemia 3–6 and 6–12 months after transphenoidal surgery in Cushing's patients have demonstrated normalization of GH secretory capacity [24, 56]. Of course, insulin-induced hyperglycemia is a stronger stimulus for GH secretion than L-arginine or L-dopa. Whether this fact could explain the different results in those studies remains just a plausible explanation. Moreover, recent studies from the London group have demonstrated that GH secretion after cure of Cushing's disease may be either deficient, or subnormal or even normal in several cases [25, 49]. As far as bone age is concerned, it is noteworthy that many children and adolescents with Cushing's disease have no bone age retardation as should have been expected from the glucocorticoid excess, but bone age appropriate for chronological age or even advanced, mainly due to the concurrent adrenal androgen excess. The lack of retarded bone age in such patients constitutes a further negative prognostic factor for their final height [33, 49]. A recent analysis of the GH status following treatment of Cushing's disease either by transphenoidal surgery alone or in combination with pituitary radiotherapy [19, 51], demonstrated that as many as 59% of surgically treated patients assessed within 2 years following remission had severe GH deficiency while this percentage dropped to 22% when assessed beyond 2 years following remission, suggesting that some patients demonstrated recovery of GH secretory status. Among the radiotherapy-treated patients 36% showed severe GH deficiency at a mean time of 99 months following remission. In conclusion, some surgically treated patients with Cushing's disease may have a recovery of their GH secretory capacity at a mean time of 19 months postoperatively and they may therefore be reassessed 2 years after surgery, while, on the contrary, radiotherapy treated patients may not demonstrate severe GH deficiency until many years (up to 8 years after radiotherapy) and should therefore be closely monitored for a long period of time [9, 19, 25].

9.7.1.3 GH Treatment in Cushing's Disease

Recent data on young patients with Cushing's syndrome, who have been successfully treated for their main disease and have been subsequently substituted with recombinant GH, with or without GnRH analogue to delay puberty, reported normal adult height of these patients, providing reassuring results [25, 49].

9.7.2 Impact on Other Hormonal Axes

9.7.2.1 Thyroid Function

It has been shown that endogenous or exogenous hypercortisolism can affect the hypothalamic-pituitary-thyroid axis at various levels [53]. Notably, TSH pulsatility and the nocturnal TSH surge are suppressed during Cushing's disease or after exogenous dexamethasone administration. Furthermore, glucocorticoids inhibit thyroid hormone 5'-deiodinase, resulting in decreased serum triiodothyronine (T_3) and increased serum reverse T_3. Furthermore, transphenoidal surgery can per se lead to disruption of the hypothalamic-pituitary function and can lead to transient or permanent complete or partial hypopituitarism. TSH deficiency after transphenoidal surgery is reported to range between 16% and 40% of cases [53]. Furthermore, resolution of hypercortisolism after treatment for adrenocortical adenoma has been reported to induce an exacerbation of autoimmune thyroid disease [57].

9.7.2.2 Puberty

Puberty is usually retarded or arrested during Cushing's syndrome and progresses normally after treatment of the underlying disease [27]. On the other hand, puberty may even be precocious after pituitary irradiation for Cushing's disease [9, 39, 49, 52].

9.7.2.3 Diabetes Insipidus

Diabetes insipidus is a possible, most usually transient, postoperative complication of transphenoidal surgery for Cushing's disease [6, 26, 49, 61].

9.7.3 Bone Mineral Density: Effect of Glucocorticoids on Bone

It is known that excess hypercortisolism negatively affects bone density, leading to osteopenia or even osteoporosis, depending on the duration of hypercortisolism until final cure. In the series of Devoe et al., there was a dramatic improvement in bone mineral density in the years following cure of hypercortisolism [6], while reports from the NIH experience pointed to a long-lasting deficit of bone mineral density despite cure of Cushing's disease [1, 27]. The underlying mechanisms leading to bone loss are complex: Glucocorticoid excess hinders osteoblast function, decreasing bone formation, while the number of osteoclasts increases. It seems that the loss of bone mineral density is primarily the result of glucocorticoid suppression of osteoblast function [27]. Glucocorticoid excess further diminishes matrix collagen mineralization. Therefore, glucocorticoid excess leads to a relatively smaller trabecular bone volume and to a smaller bone mineral content. At the level of calcium metabolism, glucocorticoids diminish intestinal calcium absorption and reduced renal calcium reabsorption, leading to secondary hyperparathyroidism. Supplementation of vitamin D improves the intestinal calcium absorption [7, 15]. It is noteworthy that even after successful treatment of Cushing's disease patients may never recover normal bone density, since glucocorticoid excess during adolescence may induce a long-standing persistent deficit in bone mass [1, 7].

9.8   Conclusions

In conclusion, childhood obesity of recent origin or change in facial characteristics in comparison to older photos, especially when accompanied by growth deceleration, warrant special attention because of the possibility of Cushing's syndrome. When such a possibility is evoked it should be always ruled out. Screening tests should be initially performed, and, when suspicion becomes a real possibility, more laborious investigations should be promptly undertaken in order to make the diagnosis early enough to prevent the long-lasting deleterious effects of hypercortisolemia.

The overall diagnostic and therapeutic modalities, as well as the long-term follow-up of such patients, should be guided by a multidisciplinary experienced team in order to provide the best possible outcome devoid of further morbidity.

References

1. Abad V, Chrousos GP, Reynolds JC, Nieman LK, Hill SC, Weinstein RS, Leong GM (2001) Glucocorticoid excess during adolescence leads to a major persistent deficit in bone mass and an increase in central body fat. J Bone Miner Res 16:1879–1885
2. Covar RA, Leung DYM, McCormick D, Steelman J, Zeitler P, Spahn JD (2000) Risk factors associated with glucocorticoid-induced adverse effects in children with severe asthma. J Allergy Clin Immunol 106:651–659
3. Cushing H (1912) The pituitary body and its disorders. Lippincott, Philadelphia, pp 219
4. Damiani D, Aguiar CH, Crivellaro CE, Galvao JA, Dichtchekenian V, Setian N (1998) Pituitary macroadenoma and Cushing's disease in pediatric patients: patient report and review of the literature. J Pediatr Endocrinol Metab 11:665–669
5. De Leon DD, Lange BJ, Walterhouse D, Moshang T (2002) Long-term (15 years) outcome in an infant with metastatic adrenocortical carcinoma. J Clin Endocrinol Metab 87:4452–4456
6. Devoe DJ, Miller WL, Conte FA, Kaplan SL, Grumbach MM, Rosenthal SM, Wilson CB, Gitelman SE (1997) Long-term outcome in children and adolescents after transphenoidal surgery in Cushing's disease. J Clin Endocrinol Metab 82:3196–3202
7. Di Somma C, Pivonello R, Loche S, Faggiano A, Klain M, Salvatore M, Lombardi G, Colao A (2003) Effect of 2 years of cortisol normalization on the impaired bone mass and turnover in adolescent and adult patients with Cushing's disease: a prospective study. Clin Endocrinol 58:302–308
8. Dyer EH, Civit T, Visot A, Delande O, Derome P (1994) Transphenoidal surgery for pituitary adenomas in children. Neurosurgery 34:207–212
9. Estrada J, Boronat M, Mielgo M, Magallon R, Millan I, Diez S, Lucas T, Barcelo B (1997) The long-term outcome of pituitary irradiation after unsuccessful transphenoidal surgery in Cushing's disease. N Engl J Med 336:172–177
10. Findlay CA, Macdonald JF, Wallace AM, Geddes N, Donaldson MDC (1998) Childhood Cushing's syndrome induced by betamethasone nose drops and repeat prescriptions. BMJ 317:739–740
11. Forest MG (2003) Adrenal function tests. In: Ranke MB (ed) Diagnostics of endocrine function in children and adolescents. Karger Verlag, Basel, pp 372–427
12. Fragoso MCBV, Domenice S, Latronico AC, Martin RM, Pereira MAA, Zerbini MCN, Lucon AM, Mendonca BB (2003) Cushing's syndrome secondary to adrenocorticotropin-independent macronodular adrenocortical hyperplasia due to activating mutations of GNAS1 gene. J Clin Endocrinol Metab 88:2147–2151
13. Gafni RI, Papanicolaou DA, Nieman LK (2000) Nighttime salivary cortisol measurement as a simple, noninvasive outpatient screening test for Cushing's syndrome in children and adolescents. J Pediatr 137:30–35
14. Grigsby PW, Thomas PR, Simpson JR, Fineberg BB (1988) Long-term results of radiotherapy in the treatment of pituitary adenomas in children and adolescents. Am J Clin Oncol 11:607–611
15. Hochberg Z (2002) Mechanisms of steroid impairment of growth. Horm Res 58(Suppl 1):33–38
16. Hollman GA, Allen DB (1988) Overt glucocorticoid excess due to inhaled corticosteroid therapy. Pediatrics 81:452–5
17. Homer JJ, Gazis TG (1999) Cushing's syndrome induced by betamethasone nose drops. BMJ 318:1355
18. Hopwood NJ, Kenny FM (1977) Incidence of Nelson's syndrome after adrenalectomy for Cushing's disease in children. Am J Dis Child 131:1351–1356

19. Hughes NR, Lissett CA, Shalet SM (1999) Growth hormone status following treatment for Cushing's syndrome. Clin Endocrinol (Oxf) 51:61–66

20. Icard P, Goudet P, Charpenay C, Andreassian B, Carnaille B, Chapuis Y, Cougard P, Henry JF, Proye C (2001) Adrenocortical carcinomas: surgical trends and results of a 253-patient series from the French Association of Endocrine Surgeons study group. World J Surg 25:891–897

21. Johnston LB, Grossmann AB, Plowman PN, Besser GM, Savage MO (1998) Normal final height and apparent cure after pituitary irradiation for Cushing's disease in childhood: long-term follow-up of anterior pituitary function. Clin Endocrinol 48:663–667

22. Kernick L, Pieters G, Hermus A, Smals A, Kloppenborg P (1994) Patient's age is a simple predictive factor for the development of Nelson's syndrome after total adrenalectomy for Cushing's disease. J Clin Endocrinol Metab 79:887–889

23. Kirk JM, Brain CE, Carson DJ, Hyde JC, Grant DB (1999) Cushing's syndrome caused by nodular adrenal hyperplasia in children with McCune-Albright syndrome. J Pediatr 134:789–792

24. Kuwayama A, Kageyama N, Nakane T, Watanabe M, Kanie N (1981) Anterior pituitary function after transphenoidal selective adenomectomy in patients with Cushing's disease. J Clin Endocrinol Metab 53:165–173

25. Lebrethon MC, Grossman AB, Afshar F, Plowman PN, Besser GM, Savage MO (2000) Linear growth and final height after treatment for Cushing's disease in childhood. J Clin Endocrinol Metab 85:3262–3265

26. Leinung MC, Kane LA, Scheithauer BW, Carpenter PC, Laws ER, Zimmerman D (1995) Long-term follow-up of transphenoidal surgery for the treatment of Cushing's disease in childhood. J Clin Endocrinol Metab 80: 2475–2479

27. Leong GM, Marcado-Asis LB, Reynolds JC, Hill SC, Oldfield EH, Chrousos GP (1996) The effect of Cushing's disease on bone mineral density, body composition, growth and puberty: a report of an identical twin pair. J Clin Endocrinol Metab 81:1905–1911

28. Leung LY, Leung WY, Chan KF, Fan TW, Chung KW, Chan CH (2002) Ruptured adrenocortical carcinoma as a rare cause of paediatric acute abdomen. Pediatr Surg Int 18:730–732

29. Liou LS, Kay R (2000) Adrenocortical carcinoma in children: review and recent innovations. Urol Clin North Am 27:403–421

30. Magiakou MA, Mastorakos G, Chrousos GP (1997) Cushing syndrome. Differential diagnosis and treatment. In: Wierman ME (ed) Contemporary endocrinology, vol 3: diseases of the pituitary: diagnosis and treatment. Humana Press, Totowa, NJ, pp 179–202

31. Magiakou MA, Mastorakos G, Oldfield EH, Gomez MT, Doppman JL, Cutler GB, Nieman LK, Chrousos GP (1994) Cushing's syndrome in children and adolescents – presentation, diagnosis and therapy. N Engl J Med 331: 629–636

32. Magiakou MA, Mastorakos G, Gomez MT, Rose SR, Chrousos GP (1994) Suppressed spontaneous and stimulated growth hormone secretion in patients with Cushing's disease before and after surgical cure. J Clin Endocrinol Metab 78:131–137

33. Magiakou MA, Mastorakos G, Chrousos GP (1994) Final stature in patients with endogenous Cushing's syndrome. J Clin Endocrinol Metab 79:1082–1085

34. Magiakou MA, Chrousos GP (2002) Cushing's syndrome in children and adolescents: current diagnostic and therapeutic strategies. J Endocr Invest 25:181–194

35. Martinelli CE Jr, Sader SL, Oliveira EB, Daneluzzi JC, Moreira AC (1999) Salivary cortisol for screening of Cushing's syndrome in children. Clin Endocrinol (Oxf) 51:67–71

36. Mathivon L, Carel JC, Coutant R, Derome P, Adamsbaum C, Bougneres P, Chaussain JL (1997) Cushing disease in children and in adolescents. Therapeutic results. Arch Pediatr 4:521–528

37. McArthur R, Hayles A, Salassa R (1979) Childhood Cushing disease: results of bilateral adrenalectomy. J Pediatr 95:214–219

38. Newell-Price J, Morris D, Drake W, Korbonits M, Monson JP, Besser GM, Grossman AB (2002) Optimal response criteria for the human corticotrophin-releasing hormone test in the differential diagnosis of ACTH-dependent Cushing's syndrome. J Clin Endocrinol Metab 87:1640–1645

39. Nicholl RM, Kirk JMW, Grossman AB, Plowman PN, Besser GM, Savage MO (1993) Acceleration of pubertal development following pituitary radiotherapy for Cushing's disease. Clin Oncol 5:393–394

40. Nieman LK, Oldfield EH, Wesley R, Chrousos GP, Loriaux DL, Cutler GB (1993) A simplified morning ovine corticotropin-releasing hormone stimulation test for the differential diagnosis of adrenocorticotropin-dependent Cushing's syndrome. J Clin Endocrinol Metab 77:1308–1312

41. Oldfield EH, Doppman JL, Nieman LK, Chrousos GP, Miller DL, Katz DA, Cutler GB Jr, Loriaux DL (1991) Petrosal sinus sampling with and without corticotropin-releasing hormone for the differential diagnosis of Cushing's syndrome. N Engl J Med 325:897–905

42. Orth DN (1995) Cushing's syndrome. N Engl J Med 332:791–803

43. Ozerdem U, Levi L, Cheng L, Song M-K, Scher C, Freeman WR (2000) Systemic toxicity of topical and periocular corticosteroid therapy in an 11-year old male with posterior uveitis. Am J Ophthalmol 130:240–241

44. Raux-Demay MC, Girard F (1993) Adrenal hyperfunction. In: Bertrand J, Rappaport R, Sizonenko PC (eds) Pediatric endocrinology, 2nd edn. Williams and Wilkins, Baltimore, pp 342–350

45. Raux-Demay MC, Girard F (1993) Cushing syndrome in children. Ann Pediatr (Paris) 40:453–462

46. Rogol AD, Hochberg Z (1999) Cushing syndrome. In: Hochberg Z (ed) Practical algorithms in pediatric endocrinology. Karger Verlag, Basel, pp 46–47

47. Sandrini R, Ribeiro RC, De Lacerda L (1997) Childhood adrenocortical tumors. J Clin Endocrinol Metab 82: 2027–2031

48. Savage MO, Besser GM (1996) Cushing's disease in childhood. Trends Endocrinol Metab 7:213–216
49. Savage MO, Lienhardt A, Lebrethon M-C, Johnston LB, Huebner A, Grossman AB, Afshar F, Plowman PN, Besser GM (2001) Cushing's disease in childhood: presentation, investigation, treatment and long-term outcome. Horm Res 55(Suppl 1):24–30
50. Savage MO, Scommegna S, Carroll PV, Ho JTF, Monson JP, Besser GM, Grossman AB (2002) Growth in disorders of adrenal hyperfunction. Horm Res 58(Suppl 1):39–43
51. Shalet SM (1986) Pituitary adenomas in childhood. Acta Endocrinol 279(Suppl):434–439
52. Storr HL, Nicholas Plowman P, Carroll PV, Francois I, Krassas GE, Afshar F, Besser GM, Grossman AB, Savage MO (2003) Clinical and endocrine responses to pituitary radiotherapy in pediatric Cushing's disease: an effective second line treatment. J Clin Endocrinol Metab 88:34–37
53. Stratakis Ca, Mastorakos G, Magiakou MA, Papavasiliou E, Oldfield EH, Chrousos GP (1997) Thyroid function in children with Cushing's disease before and after transphenoidal surgery. J Pediatr 131:905–909
54. Stratakis Ca, Kirschner LS (1998) Clinical and genetic analysis of primary bilateral adrenal diseases (micro- and macronodular disease) leading to Cushing syndrome. Horm Metab Res 456–463
55. Stratakis Ca, Mastorakos G, Mitsiades NS, Mitsiades CS, Chrousos GP (1998) Skin manifestations of Cushing disease in children and adolescents before and after the resolution of hypercortisolemia. Pediatr Dermatol 15:253–258
56. Suda T, Demura H, Demura R, Jibiki K, Tozawa F, Shizume K (1980) Anterior pituitary hormones in plasma and pituitaries from patients with Cushing's disease. J Clin Endocrinol Metab 51:1048–1053
57. Takasu N, Komiya I, Nagasawa Y, Asawa T, Yamada T (1990) Exacerbation of autoimmune thyroid dysfunction after unilateral adrenalectomy in patients with Cushing's syndrome due to an adrenocortical adenoma. N Engl J Med 322:1708–1712
58. Thomas CG, Smith AT, Benson M et al. (1984) Nelson's syndrome after Cushing's disease in childhood: a continuing problem. Surgery 96:1066–1067
59. Trainer PJ, Lawrie HS, Verhelst J, Howlett TA, Lowe DG, Grossman AB, Savage MO, Afshar F, Besser GM (1993) Transphenoidal resection in Cushing's disease: undetectable serum cortisol as the definition of successful treatment. Clin Endocrinol (Oxf) 38:73–78
60. Tsagarakis S, Kokoris P, Roboti C, Malagari C, Kaskarelis J, Vlassopoulou A, Alevizaki C, Thalassinis N (1998) The low-dose dexamethasone suppression test in patients with adrenal incidentalomas: Comparisons with clinically euadrenal subjects and patients with Cushing's syndrome. Clin Endocrinol (Oxf) 48:627–633
61. Utiger R (1997) Treatment and retreatment of Cushing's disease. N Engl J Med 336:215–217

10 Classic Congenital Adrenal Hyperplasia

Evangelia Charmandari, George Chrousos, Deborah P. Merke

CONTENTS

10.1 Introduction

Congenital adrenal hyperplasia (CAH) is a group of autosomal recessive disorders resulting from deficiency of one of the five enzymes required for synthesis of cortisol in the adrenal cortex. The most frequent form of the disease is steroid 21-hydroxylase deficiency, which accounts for 90–95% of all cases of CAH [1–4]. Deletions or mutations of the cytochrome P450 21-hydroxylase gene result in decreased synthesis of glucocorticoids and often mineralocorticoids. This leads to increased secretion of corticotropin releasing hormone (CRH) and adrenocorticotropin hormone (ACTH) from the hypothalamus and anterior pituitary, respectively, adrenal hyperplasia, and excessive production of adrenal androgens and steroid precursors prior to the enzymatic defect [1–5] (Fig. 1). The present review will focus on the most common form of CAH, 21-hydroxylase deficiency.

10.2 Clinical Manifestations

The clinical spectrum of 21-hydroxylase deficiency is quite broad, ranging from most severe to mild forms, depending on the degree of 21-hydroxylase activity. Accordingly, three main clinical phenotypes have been described: (1) *classic salt-wasting,* which accounts for 75% of all cases of classic CAH and represents the most severe form characterized by both cortisol and aldosterone deficiency, excess adrenal androgen production early in fetal life, and virilization of the external genitalia in affected females. The aldosterone deficiency results in renal salt-wasting, hyponatremia, hyperkalemia, high plasma renin activity and intravascular volume depletion, a constellation that may result in life-threatening hypovolemic shock. (2) *Classic simple virilizing,* which is characterized by progressive virilization, accelerated growth velocity and advanced bone age but no or mild evidence of mineralocorticoid deficiency; and (3) *nonclassic,* a mild form that may be asymptomatic or associated with signs of postnatal androgen excess only [1, 3–5]. The prevalence of classic 21-hydroxylase deficiency is approximately 1 in 16,000 births in most populations [6], while that of nonclassic is 0.2% in the general white population but higher (1–2%) in certain populations, such as Ashkenazi Jews [7].

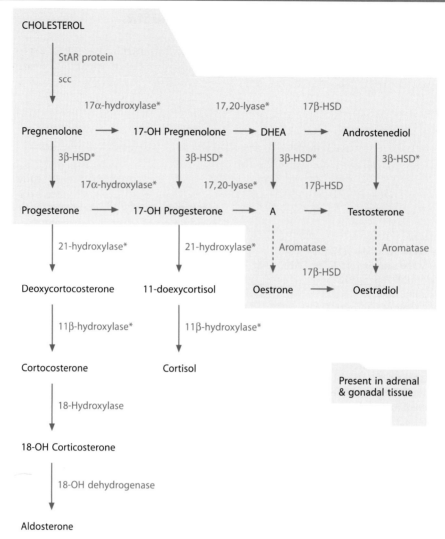

Fig. 1. Schematic representation of adrenal steroidogenesis (*solid line*, major pathway; *dotted line*, major pathway in ovaries and minor in adrenals; * deficient enzymatic activity results in CAH; *A*, androstenedione; *DHEA*, dehydroepiandrosterone; *3β-HSD*, 3β-hydroxysteroid dehydrogenase; *17β-HSD*, 17β-hydroxysteroid dehydrogenase; *SCC*, cholesterol side-chain cleavage enzyme; *StAR*, steroidogenic regulatory protein)

10.3   Clinical Manifestations of Classic CAH

10.3.1   Prenatal Virilization

Patients with classic 21-hydroxylase deficiency are exposed to elevated serum androgen concentrations from the first trimester of pregnancy. As a result, affected females present at birth with ambiguous genitalia, including enlarged clitoris, rugated and partially fused labia majora, and a common urogenital sinus, while the most severely affected patients may present with male-appearing external genitalia with perineal hypospadias, chordee and undescended testes, and

may rarely be erroneously assigned a male gender. The severity of virilization is often quantitated using a five-point scale developed by Prader [8]. The uterus, fallopian tubes, and ovaries develop normally. Affected males are normal appearing at birth, but may have variable degrees of hyperpigmentation and penile enlargement.

10.3.2   Salt-Wasting

Patients with salt-wasting CAH have severe 21-hydroxylase deficiency leading to decreased synthesis of aldosterone, while the elevated concentrations of progesterone and 17-hydroxyprogesterone (17-OHP) may antagonize the mineralocorticoid receptor directly, further exacerbating mineralocorticoid deficiency [9]. The combined glucocorticoid and mineralocorticoid deficiency in untreated or inadequately treated patients may cause hyponatremic dehydration and shock. The latter may be further exacerbated by the concurrent catecholamine deficiency [10].

Salt-wasting may manifest with non-specific symptoms, such as poor appetite, vomiting, lethargy and failure to thrive. Severely affected individuals usually present during the first 2–3 weeks of life with adrenal crises (hyponatremia, hyperkalemia, metabolic acidosis, hyperreninemia, hypovolemic shock) that are potentially fatal. This problem is particularly critical in male infants who have no genital ambiguity to alert physicians to the possibility of CAH.

Patients with simple virilizing 21-hydroxylase deficiency usually preserve adequate mineralocorticoid secretion. Although affected females are often diagnosed shortly after birth due to genital ambiguity, affected males may go undetected for several years, until symptoms and signs of androgen excess develop. Delayed diagnosis is associated with greater difficulty in achieving hormonal control and a more compromised adult height compared to that attained in patients with the salt-wasting form of the disease.

10.3.3   Postnatal Signs of Androgen Excess

Symptoms and signs of postnatal virilization may vary considerably depending on the degree of enzymatic deficiency, compliance with medical therapy, and inter-patient variation in the conversion of steroid precursors to more potent androgens or in androgen receptor expression. Ongoing increased adrenal androgen secretion results in accelerated linear growth, advanced skeletal maturation, premature fusion of the epiphyses and compromised final height compared to the target height [11, 12]. Even with close therapeutic monitoring, the adult height of patients with classic CAH lies approximately 1.4 SD (10 cm) below the population mean [13]. Undertreatment and overtreatment further increase the risk for compromised final height, because of premature epiphyseal closure and glucocorticoid-induced inhibition of growth, respectively [11, 14].

Other signs of increased adrenal androgen production include premature pubic and axillary hair, increased penile size without testicular enlargement in males, and progressive clitoral enlargement in females.

Inadequately controlled adolescent females may present with acne, hirsutism, menstrual irregularities and ovarian dysfunction. Long-term exposure to elevated androgen concentrations may activate the hypothalamic-pituitary-gonadal axis and lead to central precocious puberty in both sexes [1, 4].

10.3.4   Reproductive Function

In females with classic CAH, reproductive problems usually develop in adolescence and include oligo-amenorrhea, oligoanovulation, menstrual irregularities and polycystic appearance of the ovaries on ultrasound scanning [15]. In inadequately treated females, menarche occurs later than in their healthy counterparts [16, 17]. Fertility rates are also lower in females with CAH compared to the general population owing to oligoamenorrhea/oligoanovulation and heterosexual inactivity. The latter is due to an inadequate introitus [18] and the psychosexual effects of prenatal and postnatal virilization, which may prevent patients from establishing heterosexual relationships [19, 20]. Recent advances in surgical, medical, and psychological management have enabled more women with 21-hydroxylase deficiency to complete pregnancies successfully and give birth, typically by cesarean section. Approximately 60% of females with salt-wasting CAH and 80% of those with the simple virilizing form of the disease are fertile [21, 22].

Males with CAH have impaired gonadal function less frequently than affected females. Most have normal sperm counts and are fertile. Inadequate steroid replacement and high corticotropin levels have been associated with activation and growth of ectopic adrenal rest tissue, most commonly found in the testes. The clinical significance of testicular adrenal rest tissue is unknown, but its presence may lead to infertility. Adult males with classic CAH should be counseled that compliance with steroid replacement is important to enhance normal fertility and reduce the risk of a palpable testicular mass [23, 24].

10.3.5   Neuropsychology

Psychosexual identification has been a major area studied in female subjects with CAH. Psychosexual identification is evaluated by studying *gender identity, gender role, sexual orientation* and *parenting.*

Gender identity, the awareness of oneself as male, female or ambiguous, has been uniformly reported to be female in early-treated girls with CAH. *Gender role,* however, which refers to gender-stereotyped behaviors, has been found by most investigators to be more masculine, as suggested by an increased tomboyish behavior and more outdoor activities in girls or a more career-oriented outlook in young women [25, 26]. Parenting rehearsal, such as doll play and baby care, is also decreased [27]. The majority of women with CAH are heterosexual, although homosexual fantasy appears to be increased [28–30]. Females with CAH differ from their healthy counterparts in several aspects of psychosexual identification: many have a disturbed image of their body, feel less feminine or attractive, are unable to establish a partnership or marry, and have significantly fewer children [19, 20].

Interestingly, however, the overall *quality of life in CAH* is not reduced compared to control population. Patients develop coping strategies and cognitive appraisals that enable them to accept their life and view it as very satisfactory. These forms of compensatory efforts are well-documented in psychological research studies of adaptation [20].

10.3.6 Tumors

10.3.6.1 Adrenal

Patients with CAH and carriers of 21-hydroxylase deficiency have higher incidence of adrenal tumors, including adenoma, myelolipoma and hemangioma, than healthy subjects [31]. Steroid-responsive hyperplastic adrenal nodules may present in previously undiagnosed patients late in life and can be mistakenly diagnosed as virilizing adrenal adenomas. Given that these tumors often regress with glucocorticoid therapy, it may not be necessary to resect them provided careful follow-up is in place. Most adrenal masses in children with CAH are benign [32].

10.3.6.2 Testicular

Affected males often develop testicular adrenal rests, which are detected ultrasonographically before they become palpable [23, 33]. Approximately 30% of males with classic CAH have ultrasonic evidence of testicular adrenal rest tissue [34], and testicular masses have been detected in boys with CAH as early as age 3 years [35]. Characteristic radiologic features have been described [34, 36]. The majority of masses surround the mediastinum testes, are bilateral, intratesticular and hypoe-

choic [2, 34, 36]. The preferred mode of therapy is adequate hypothalamic-pituitary-adrenal (HPA) axis suppression with higher dose glucocorticoid therapy, since most of these tumors are responsive to corticotropin. However, the clinical significance of small (<5 mm) testicular adrenal rest tissue, which is detected only by screening ultrasonography, is unknown [2]. The clinician should balance the need for shrinkage of testicular adrenal rest tissue with the iatrogenic side effects of increased glucocorticoid therapy. These tumors, although almost invariably benign, have prompted biopsies and even partial orchiectomy [37]. When they are large and the patient is symptomatic or infertile, and the response to medical therapy is inadequate, testis-sparing surgery may be performed [37].

10.3.6.3 Pituitary

Despite the supraphysiologic cortisol concentrations attained following standard glucocorticoid replacement therapy in patients with CAH, elevated CRH and ACTH concentrations may persist and result in the development of pituitary tumors. Although symptomatic pituitary tumors have not been reported in this population, in one study, four out of seven patients with CAH undergoing brain MRI scanning were found to have pituitary abnormalities (microadenomas: 3, empty sella: 1) [38].

10.3.7 Clinical Manifestations of Nonclassic CAH

Patients with the nonclassic form of the disease are able to synthesize cortisol and aldosterone normally, however, at the expense of mild-to-moderate overproduction of adrenal androgens and steroid precursors. Patients may be asymptomatic or present with premature pubic and axillary hair, advanced skeletal age, hirsutism, acne and/or oligomenorrhea [39]. Decreased fertility is an indication for glucocorticoid treatment in both males and females with the condition [23, 24].

10.4 Diagnosis of 21-Hydroxylase Deficiency

10.4.1 Evaluation of Ambiguous Genitalia

Classic 21-hydroxylase deficiency is the most common cause of ambiguous genitalia in an XX infant. Girls with classic CAH are exposed to high levels of androgens in utero starting at approximately the 7th week gestation. The high level of adrenal androgens affects the formation of the external genitalia, while the internal female reproductive organs are normally formed. The effects may include: clitoral enlargement, rugated and partially fused labia majora, and the fusion of the urethra and vagina into one opening, a urogenital sinus.

In the evaluation of ambiguous genitalia, physical examination should identify the urethral meatus and include careful palpation for gonads in the inguinal canals and labia or scrotum. Standard diagnostic tests include basal serum 17-OHP concentrations, karyotype and pelvic/abdominal ultrasound scan. Plasma renin activity (PRA) and aldosterone are elevated in many normal infants and do not usually add much useful information during the first days of life [40]. Internal genitalia are normal and ovaries are in the normal pelvic location. Therefore, palpable gonads suggest an undervirilized XY infant or other less common causes of ambiguous genitalia.

10.4.2   Newborn Screening

CAH is a condition suitable for newborn screening because it is a potentially fatal childhood disease, it is diagnosed easily by a simple hormonal measurement in blood and its early recognition and treatment can prevent serious morbidity and mortality. The diagnosis is suspected if there is a marked elevation of filter paper blood 17-OHP concentration [4]. Normative values for filter paper assays vary in different laboratories. These assays use the same 'Guthrie' cards that are used for screening of phenylketonuria and hypothyroidism. Subsequent measurement of serum 17-OHP is performed to confirm the diagnosis. Ill or stressed newborns tend to have higher concentrations of 17-OHP and may generate many false positive results unless higher normal cut-off values are used. Similar problems with interpretation arise as a result of screening of preterm neonates, who also have elevated 17-OHP concentrations compared to term infants, particularly around the 29th week of gestation, when the function of several adrenal steroidogenic enzymes reaches its nadir [41].

Neonatal screening not only reduces the time to diagnosis [4, 6, 42], but also decreases morbidity and mortality, given that infants with the salt-wasting form of the disease are diagnosed more promptly. Since undiagnosed infants who die suddenly may not be ascertained, it is difficult to demonstrate a benefit of screen-

ing by direct comparison of death rates from CAH in non-screened and screened populations. Males with salt-wasting CAH are more likely than females to suffer from delayed or incorrect diagnosis because there is no genital ambiguity. Thus, a relative paucity of salt-wasting males in a patient population may indicate unreported deaths from salt-wasting crises. Indeed, females outnumbered males in some [43] but not all [44] retrospective studies, in which CAH was diagnosed clinically. By contrast, cases with salt-wasting CAH ascertained through screening programs are equally or more likely to be males rather than females [41, 45]. In addition, infants ascertained through screening have less severe hyponatremia and tend to be hospitalized for shorter periods of time [41]. Furthermore, males with simple virilizing CAH may otherwise not be diagnosed until rapid growth and accelerated skeletal maturation are detected later in childhood, at which time final height may already be adversely affected.

10.4.3   Biochemical Evaluation

Classic 21-hydroxylase deficiency is characterized by markedly elevated serum levels of 17-OHP. Basal 17-OHP values usually exceed 10,000 ng/dl (300 nmol/l) in affected infants (normal values <100 ng/dl or 3 nmol/l) [1, 4]. In cases where neonatal screening is not available and 21-hydroxylase deficiency is suspected on clinical grounds, an ACTH stimulation test with measurements of cortisol, 17-OHP and androgens before and 1 h after exogenous administration of ACTH (0.25-mg intravenous bolus of cosyntropin) should be performed after the first 24–48 h of life. Patients with the salt-wasting form of the disease have the highest stimulated 17-OHP concentrations [up to 100,000 ng/dl (3,000 nmol/l)]. Patients with simple virilizing CAH usually have lower stimulated concentrations [10,000–30,000 ng/dl (300–1,000 nmol/l)], while patients with nonclassic disease have smaller elevations [1,500–10,000 ng/dl (50–300 nmol/l)] [1, 4, 46]. Measurements of basal serum 17-OHP concentrations are often normal in patients with nonclassic disease unless samples are obtained early in the morning.

Progesterone, androstenedione, and, to a lesser extent, testosterone may also be elevated in patients with 21-hydroxylase deficiency [47]. Several other diagnostic biochemical assays have been proposed but few are widely available. The main urinary metabolite of 17-OHP, pregnanetriol, can be also used to diagnose

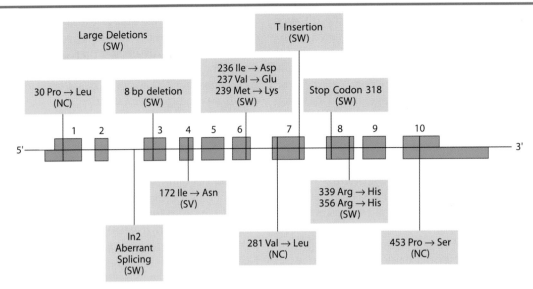

Fig. 2. Schematic representation of the 21-hydroxylase gene structure, the most common reported mutations, and their expected phenotype (*SW*, salt-wasting; *SV*, simple virilizing; *NC*, nonclassic). *Numbers in the mutant allele boxes* indicate codon numbers; *numbers above the shaded boxes* indicate exon numbers. (Adapted from [2])

21-hydroxylase deficiency. Urinary steroid metabolites can be analyzed by urine gas chromatography/mass spectrometry and several relevant markers for CAH and other disorders of steroid metabolism can be assayed simultaneously [48, 49].

10.4.4   Molecular Genetic Analysis

10.4.4.1   Mutations

The 21-hydroxylase gene (*CYP21*) is located in the human leukocyte antigen gene cluster region on the short arm of chromosome 6 [50]. The functional gene (*CYP21*) and its homologue, the non-functional pseudogene (*CYP21P*), consist of ten exons each, and share 98% sequence homology in exons and approximately 96% sequence homology in introns [51, 52]. In most cases, the mutations responsible for 21-hydroxylase deficiency are the result of unequal crossing over or gene conversion events between *CYP21* and *CYP21P* [4, 53–55], whereas novel mutations or unique point mutations not present in the pseudogene have been identified in few cases only [4]. The most frequently reported mutations include gene deletions, large gene conversions involving the promoter region, P30L in exon 1, an intron 2 splice site mutation (In2), an 8-bp deletion in exon 3 (8-bp del), I172 N in exon 4, a cluster of mutations (I236 N, V237E, M239 K) in exon 6 (E6 cluster), V281L and 1762T insertion in exon 7, and

Q318X and R356 W in exon 8 (Fig. 2). Since 1–2% of affected alleles represent spontaneous mutations not carried by either parent, it is particularly important to ascertain parental genotypes for prenatal counseling [56].

10.4.4.2   Genotype-Phenotype Correlation

Correlations between the *CYP21* genotype and phenotype have been studied in various ethnic and racial groups. *CYP21* mutations can be grouped into three categories according to the level of enzymatic activity predicted from in vitro studies [57, 58]. The first group consists of mutations that confer no 21-hydroxylase activity (gene deletions, large gene conversions, 8 bp del, E6 cluster, Q318X, R356W). These are most often associated with salt-wasting disease. The second group consists mainly of the missense mutation I172N, which results in approximately 2% of residual enzymatic activity in vitro. These mutations permit adequate aldosterone synthesis and are usually associated with the simple virilizing form of the disease. The third group includes mutations such as V281L and P30L that confer 20–60% of normal enzymatic activity and are associated with nonclassic CAH [1, 4, 58, 59].

The clinical expression of CAH is reported to correlate with the less severely mutated allele and, consequently, with the residual activity of 21-hydroxylase.

A number of studies suggest high concordance rates between genotype and phenotype in patients with the most severe and mildest forms of the disease, but considerably less genotype-phenotype correlation in moderately affected patients [56, 60–64]. This genotype-phenotype discordance has been attributed to the variable 21-hydroxylase activity conferred by the In2 and I172N mutations as well as the variety of mutations often observed in patients who are compound heterozygotes, the possibility of additional not yet identified mutations, and genetic variations in extra-adrenal 21-hydroxylase activity or sensitivity to glucocorticoids [4, 65–67].

We have recently investigated the association between adrenomedullary function, disease severity and genotype in children with classic CAH and showed that both measurement of plasma free metanephrine (a metabolite of epinephrine) concentrations and determination of molecular genotype were well correlated with the clinical severity of the disease and were similarly accurate in predicting clinical phenotype [68].

10.5 Treatment

Current treatment of classic CAH aims to provide adequate glucocorticoid and, when necessary, mineralocorticoid substitution to prevent adrenal crises and to suppress the abnormal secretion of androgens and steroid precursors from the adrenal cortex.

10.5.1 Glucocorticoid Replacement

Patients with classic 21-hydroxylase deficiency and symptomatic patients with non-classic disease are treated with glucocorticoids in an attempt to suppress the excessive secretion of CRH and ACTH and to reduce the circulating concentrations of adrenal androgens. In children and adolescents, the preferred glucocorticoid option is hydrocortisone, because its short half-life minimizes growth suppression and other adverse side effects of more potent, longer acting glucocorticoids [69, 70].

Most children have satisfactory control of androgen with doses of hydrocortisone of 10–18 mg/m^2/day in three divided doses. Higher doses of approximately 20 mg/m^2/day may be required in the neonatal period. These doses exceed physiologic cortisol secretion (6–7 mg/m^2/day in children and adolescents) [71]. Older adolescents and adults may be treated with modest doses of prednisone or dexamethasone that do not exceed the equivalent of 20 mg/m^2 of hydrocortisone daily, but should be monitored carefully for signs of iatrogenic Cushing's syndrome. Males with testicular adrenal rests may require higher doses of dexamethasone to suppress ACTH. Treatment efficacy is assessed by monitoring growth velocity, rate of skeletal maturation (bone age) and weight gain, as well as by determining the 0800 h concentrations of 17-OHP and androstenedione [72]. Testosterone may also be useful in females and prepubertal males.

Since patients with classic CAH are not able to mount a normal cortisol response to stress, pharmacologic doses of hydrocortisone are required during febrile illnesses and minor or major surgery under general anesthesia. Treatment doses should approximate typical endogenous adrenal secretion in critically ill and perioperative patients [73, 74]. For febrile illnesses, patients are advised to triple the normal maintenance dose of oral hydrocortisone. For major surgery, intravenous hydrocortisone up to 100 mg/m^2/day in four divided doses is recommended for at least 24–48 h perioperatively before tapering to the maintenance dose. Intravenous hydrocortisone is preferred over methylprednisolone or dexamethasone because its mineralocorticoid activity is able to substitute for oral fludrocortisone.

10.5.2 Mineralocorticoid Replacement

Patients with salt-wasting CAH require mineralocorticoid (9α-fludrocortisone, 0.1–0.3 mg/day) in addition to glucocorticoid replacement. During infancy sodium chloride supplements are also added (1–2 g sodium chloride) because the sodium content of breast milk as well as most infant formulae (~8 mEq/l) is only sufficient for maintenance sodium requirements in healthy infants [1, 4]. Although patients with simple virilizing CAH do not manifest mineralocorticoid deficiency, they are nevertheless often treated with fludrocortisone, which can aid in adrenocortical suppression, thus reducing the maintenance dose of glucocorticoid. The adequacy of mineralococorticoid substitution therapy is monitored by measuring PRA levels.

10.5.3 Other Therapeutic Approaches

10.5.3.1 Pharmacological

Limitations of standard medical therapy with glucocorticoid and/or mineralocorticoid substitution in classic CAH include: (a) inability to replicate physiologic cortisol production with exogenous administration of glucocorticoid; (b) hyperresponsiveness of the adrenal glands to ACTH; and (c) difficulty in suppressing ACTH secretion from the anterior pituitary [75]. The latter is due to the decreased sensitivity of glucocorticoid feedback inhibition possibly secondary to the hyperactive HPA axis, as well as the fact that glucocorticoid feedback is only one of the mechanisms governing ACTH secretion [76]. Therefore, achieving and maintaining adrenal androgen suppression is far more challenging than preventing adrenal crises, and often necessitates supraphysiologic doses of glucocorticoid. Iatrogenic Cushing's syndrome and hyperandrogenism may develop in tandem and represent the main problems encountered in the clinical management of classic CAH [1–5]. Patients with absent or minimal 21-hydroxylase activity are particularly vulnerable to these difficult management issues.

Alternative approaches to standard medical therapy include: (a) a four-drug treatment regimen of flutamide (an androgen-receptor blocking drug), testolactone (an aromatase inhibitor), reduced hydrocortisone dose, and 9α-fludrocortisone, which has been shown to achieve normal growth and development after 2 years of therapy; however, longer follow-up data are required before safe recommendations for such therapy are made [77]; (b) intra-adrenal blockade of adrenal androgen production with a steroidogenesis inhibitor, such as ketoconazole; (c) administration of a corticotropin-releasing hormone antagonist [78]; and (d) gene therapy. The last three therapeutic options have yet to be tried in patients with the classic form of the disease [1–4, 24, 75].

10.5.3.2 Adrenalectomy

Bilateral adrenalectomy has been suggested as an alternative to medical therapy in patients with severe salt-wasting disease who had ongoing virilization despite adequate doses of standard replacement regimens and/or patients with mutations predicting absent or minimal 21-hydroxylase activity [75, 79]. Bilateral surgical adrenalectomy provides an efficient elimination of excess adrenal androgens and steroid precursors, and should be considered in patients with severe CAH, in whom conventional therapy has failed. This invasive treatment has become more accessible because of the introduction of laparoscopic adrenalectomy, a safe and well-tolerated approach. Laparoscopic adrenalectomy may not reduce the operative time, but significantly reduces bleeding, postoperative hospitalization time, and postoperative pain [80–83]. The majority of patients with CAH who undergo bilateral adrenalectomy report an improved quality of life following surgery [79].

Potential advantages of adrenalectomy include: (a) control of hyperandrogenism and progressive virilization, which may prevent premature epiphyseal closure, sexual precocity, acne, hirsutism, and fertility problems; (b) protection of the patient from the undesirable effects of iatrogenic hypercortisolism (granted that physiologic doses of glucocorticoid are given postoperatively), including obesity, insulin resistance and compromised final height; and (c) prevention of salt-losing crises, because the adrenal androgens and steroid precursors are removed. These intermediate steroids interact with the glucocorticoid and mineralocorticoid receptors, thereby acting as potent inhibitors and inducing resistance to both systemic effects of glucocorticoids and the salt-retaining effects of aldosterone [84]. During illness or other stressful occurrences, patients with classic CAH are more prone to rapid salt loss and collapse compared to healthy subjects [84, 85].

Concerns surrounding bilateral adrenalectomy include:

1. *Risk of surgery and anesthesia:* Provided that the appropriate stress doses of steroid are administered perioperatively, the surgical risk associated with adrenalectomy should be negligible and similar to that of anesthesia. A laparoscopic procedure will further reduce postoperative bleeding, hospitalization time and postoperative pain.

2. *Theoretic loss of protective adrenomedullary function:* This protective function may already be absent in the most severe cases, given that patients with classic 21-hydroxylase deficiency also have compromised adrenomedullary function [10]. This is due to developmental defects in the formation of the adrenal medulla, which result in depletion of epinephrine stores and decreased production of metanephrine, the O-methylated metabolite of epinephrine. The significant positive correlation between plasma free metanephrine concentrations and the expected 21-hydroxylase activity based on

genotype further suggests that patients with absent or minimal 21-hydroxylase activity would also demonstrate minimal adrenomedullary function [68].

3. *Risk of Nelson's syndrome:* Following bilateral adrenalectomy, patients may develop hyperpigmentation because of the lower doses of glucocorticoid substitution. Although Nelson's syndrome has not been described in adrenalectomized patients with classic CAH, the longstanding CRH, arginine vasopressin and/or other ACTH secretagogue hypersecretion may lead to the development of ACTH-secreting tumors similar to those described in Addison's disease [86–88], glucocorticoid resistance [89] or untreated/undertreated CAH [90].

4. *Activation of adrenal rests or ectopic adrenal tissue:* Recurrent virilization due to activation of ovarian or testicular adrenal rests may be observed secondary to the increased ACTH secretion and can be managed with increased doses of glucocorticoid treatment. Periodic monitoring with ovarian/-testicular ultrasound scans may be helpful in identifying the problem and assessing response to treatment. While ablation of ectopic adrenal rests could possibly be performed laparoscopically if required, ectopic ovarian adrenal rests may be difficult to remove completely without risking damage to the remaining ovary. The propensity for developing hyperpigmentation is also likely to be greater after bilateral adrenalectomy because of the expected decrease in the glucocorticoid dose.

5. *Complete dependency on substitution therapy:* The complete dependency of patients on exogenous administration of glucocorticoid requires life-long adherence to medical therapy. Therefore, bilateral adrenalectomy should not be performed in patients with erratic compliance to treatment.

6. *Limitations of adrenalectomy:* Bilateral adrenalectomy will have no effect on prenatal and prior to the procedure virilization. Female patients will still require feminizing genitoplasty during the first 6 months of life and possibly further vaginal reconstruction later in life. Furthermore, adrenalectomy may bear very little if any effect on the psychosexual differentiation of affected females because of the prior exposure of the brain to androgens. Finally, the irreversibility of the procedure will eliminate the option of new therapeutic approaches.

10.5.4 Management of Ambiguous Genitalia

In CAH, the typical gender assignment and rearing is that of the genetic/gonadal sex. XX patients with virilized external genitalia due to 21-hydroxylase deficiency have normal internal genital structures and the potential for childbearing. Moreover, CAH females with severe virilization and/or behavioral masculinization are typically well adjusted. There is insufficient evidence to support rearing a 46XX infant at Prader stage 5 as a male.

Surgical correction of the external genitalia mainly involves feminizing genitoplasty, which should be performed in infancy [91], while vaginal reconstruction is usually postponed until late adolescence and before the age of expected sexual activity [92,93]. Single-stage corrective surgery at the age of 2–6 months, when the tissues are most pliable and psychological trauma to the patient minimal, has been performed in a few cases [94], but long-term outcome is awaiting evaluation. Surgery between the age of 12 months and adolescence is not recommended [24].

10.5.5 Psychological Counseling

Parents of patients with CAH should be offered psychological counseling as soon as the diagnosis is confirmed particularly if the patient involved is a female requiring genital reconstruction. Intermittent assessment of family functioning is suggested to assess the family dynamics and predict future problems. Children should be informed about their condition by their parents and physicians in a sensitive and age-appropriate manner. Parents of female patients with classic CAH may be prepared that their affected daughters will be more likely to exhibit tomboyish behavior, masculine play preferences and a preference for a career over domestic activities [26]. The effectiveness of the genital repair in adolescent and adult women needs to be assessed and counseling regarding sexual matters is indicated.

10.5.6 Prenatal Diagnosis and Treatment

Prenatal genetic counseling should be offered to all affected families. Administration of dexamethasone to the mother during pregnancy has been advocated for fetuses at risk for classic CAH and ameliorates genital ambiguity in affected female fetuses [95]. It is not appropriate for female fetuses at risk for nonclassic

CAH. When both parents are known carriers of CAH and treatment is desired, the recommended dose is 20 µg/kg of body weight per day given in three divided doses starting as soon as pregnancy is confirmed and no later than 9 weeks after the last menstrual period.

Given the autosomal recessive mode of inheritance of the disease, it is important to note that only one of eight fetuses will be an affected female when both parents are known carriers, and seven out of eight pregnancies will be treated unnecessarily, albeit for a short period of time. Therefore, prompt and accurate genetic diagnosis is mandatory in all cases.

The long-term safety of prenatal treatment remains uncertain. No congenital malformations or fetal deaths have been associated with the treatment [96, 97]. Maternal complications, on the other hand, may vary. Overt Cushing's syndrome, excessive weight gain, and hypertension have been reported in approximately 1% of all women with treated pregnancies, usually those who were treated throughout pregnancy [98]. Thus, women must be fully informed of the potential risks to themselves and their fetus and the possible lack of benefit to an affected female. Treatment should be carried out in specialized centers with the use of approved protocols [24].

References

1. Speiser PW, White PC (2003) Congenital adrenal hyperplasia. N Engl J Med 349:776–88
2. Merke DP, Bornstein SR, Avila NA, Chrousos GP (2002) NIH conference. Future directions in the study and management of congenital adrenal hyperplasia due to 21-hydroxylase deficiency. Ann Intern Med 136:320–34
3. Merke DP, Cutler GB Jr (2001) New ideas for medical treatment of congenital adrenal hyperplasia. Endocrinol Metab Clin North Am 30:121–35
4. White PC, Speiser PW (2000) Congenital adrenal hyperplasia due to 21-hydroxylase deficiency. Endocr Rev 21:245–91
5. Newfield RS, New MI (1997) 21-Hydroxylase deficiency. Ann N Y Acad Sci 816:219–29
6. Therrell BL (2001) Newborn screening for congenital adrenal hyperplasia. Endocrinol Metab Clin North Am 30:15–30
7. Speiser PW, Dupont B, Rubinstein P, Piazza A, Kastelan A, New MI (1985) High frequency of nonclassical steroid 21-hydroxylase deficiency. Am J Hum Genet 37:650–667
8. Prader A (1954) Der Genitalbefund beim Pseudohermaphroditismus Femininus der kengenitalen andrenogenitalen Syndroms. Helv Paediatr Acta 9:231–248
9. Oelkers WK (1996) Effects of estrogens and progestogens on the renin-aldosterone system and blood pressure. Steroids 61:166–171
10. Merke DP, Chrousos GP, Eisenhofer G, Weise M, Keil MF, Rogol AD, Van Wyk JJ, Bornstein SR (2000) Adrenomedullary dysplasia and hypofunction in patients with classic 21-hydroxylase deficiency. N Engl J Med 343:1362–1368
11. Jaaskelainen J, Voutilainen R (1997) Growth of patients with 21-hydroxylase deficiency: an analysis of the factors influencing adult height. Pediatr Res 41:30–33
12. New MI, Gertner GM, Speiser PW, del Balzo P (1988) Growth and final height in classical and nonclassical 21-hydroxylase deficiency. Acta Paediatr Jpn 30 [Suppl]:79–88
13. Eugster EA, Dimeglio LA, Wright JC, Freidenberg GR, Seshadri R, Pescovitz OH (2001) Height outcome in congenital adrenal hyperplasia caused by 21-hydroxylase deficiency: a meta-analysis. J Pediatr 138:26–32
14. Yu AC, Grant DB (1995) Adult height in women with early-treated congenital adrenal hyperplasia (21-hydroxylase type): relation to body mass index in earlier childhood. Acta Paediatr 84:899–903
15. Barnes RB, Rosenfield RL, Ehrmann DA, Cara JF, Cuttler L, Levitsky LL, Rosenthal IM (1994) Ovarian hyperandrogynism as a result of congenital adrenal virilizing disorders: evidence for perinatal masculinization of neuroendocrine function in women. J Clin Endocrinol Metab 79:1328–33
16. Helleday J, Siwers B, Ritzen EM, Carlstrom K (1993) Subnormal androgen and elevated progesterone levels in women treated for congenital virilizing 21-hydroxylase deficiency. J Clin Endocrinol Metab 76:933–936
17. London DR (1987) The consequences of hyperandrogenism in young women. J R Soc Med 80:741–745
18. Azziz R, Mulaikal RM, Migeon CJ, Jones HW, Rock JA (1986) Congenital adrenal hyperplasia: long term results following vaginal reconstruction. Fertil Steril 46:1011–1014
19. Kuhnle U, Bullinger M, Schwarz HP, Knorr D (1993) Partnership and sexuality in adult female patients with congenital adrenal hyperplasia. First results of a cross-sectional quality – of – life evaluation. J Steroid Biochem 45:123–126
20. Kuhnle U, Bullinger M, Schwarz HP (1995) The quality of life in adult female patients with congenital adrenal hyperplasia: a comprehensive study of the impact of genital malformations and chronic disease on female patients' life. Eur J Pediatr 154:708–716
21. Lo JC, Grumbach MM (2001) Pregnancy outcomes in women with congenital virilizing adrenal hyperplasia. Endocrinol Metab Clin North Am 30:207–229
22. Premawardhana LD, Hughes IA, Read GF, Scanlon MF (1997) Longer term outcome in females with congenital adrenal hyperplasia (CAH): the Cardiff experience. Clin Endocrinol (Oxf) 46:327–332
23. Stikkelbroeck NM, Otten BJ, Pasic A, Jager GJ, Sweep CG, Noordam K, Hermus AR (2001) High prevalence of testicular adrenal rest tumors, impaired spermatogenesis, and Leydig cell failure in adolescent and adult males with congenital adrenal hyperplasia. J Clin Endocrinol Metab 86:5721–8

24. Clayton PE, Miller WL, Oberfield SE, Ritzen EM, Sippell WG, Speiser PW (2002) Consensus Statement on 21-Hydroxylase Deficiency from The Lawson Wilkins Pediatric Endocrine Society and The European Society for Paediatric Endocrinology. J Clin Endocrinol Metab 87:4048–4053

25. Fedderman DD (1987) Psychosexual adjustment in congenital adrenal hyperplasia. N Engl J Med 316:209–211

26. Dittmann RW, Kappes M, Kappes ME, Berger D, Stegner H, Willig Rh, Wallis H (1990) Congenital adrenal hyperplasia I: gender-related behavior and attitudes in female patients and sisters. Psychoendocrinology 15:401–420; 421–434

27. Berenbaum SA, Duck SC, Bryk K (2000) Behavioral effects of prenatal versus postnatal androgen excess in children with 21-hydroxylase-deficient congenital adrenal hyperplasia. J Clin Endocrinol Metab 85:727–33

28. Dittmann RW, Kappes ME, Kappes MH (1992) Sexual behavior in adolescent and adult females with congenital adrenal hyperplasia. Psychoneuroendocrinology 17:153–70

29. Zucker KJ, Bradley SJ, Oliver G, Blake J, Fleming S, Hood J (1996) Psychosexual development of women with congenital adrenal hyperplasia. Horm Behav 30:300–18

30. Meyer-Bahlburg HF (2001) Gender and sexuality in classic congenital adrenal hyperplasia. Endocrinol Metab Clin North Am 30:155–71

31. Jaresch S, Kornely E, Kley HK, Schlaghecke R (1992) Adrenal incidentaloma and patients with homozygous and heterozygous congenital adrenal hyperplasia. J Clin Endocrinol Metab 74:685–689

32. Lightner ES, Levine LS (1993) The adrenal incidentaloma. A pediatric perspective. Am J Dis Child 147:1274–1276

33. Cabrera MS, Vogiatzi MG, New MI (2001) Long term outcome in adult males with classic congenital adrenal hyperplasia. J Clin Endocrinol Metab 86:3070–3078

34. Avila NA, Premkumar A, Merke DP (1999) Testicular adrenal rest tissue in congenital adrenal hyperplasia: comparison of MR imaging and sonographic findings. AJR Am J Roentgenol 172:1003–6

35. Srikanth MS, West BR, Ishitani M, Isaacs H Jr, Applebaum H, Costin G (1992) Benign testicular tumors in children with congenital adrenal hyperplasia. J Pediatr Surg 27:639–641

36. Avila NA, Premkumar A, Shawker TH, Jones JV, Laue L, Cutler GB Jr (1996) Testicular adrenal rest tissue in congenital adrenal hyperplasia: findings at Gray-scale and color Doppler US. Radiology 198:99–104

37. Walker BR, Skoog SJ, Winslow BH, Canning DA, Tank ES (1997) Testis sparing surgery for steroid unresponsive testicular tumors of the adrenogenital syndrome. J Urol 157:1460–1463

38. Speiser PW, Heier L, Serrat J, New MI, Nass R (1995) Failure of steroid replacement to consistently normalize pituitary function in congenital adrenal hyperplasia: hormonal and MRI data. Horm Res 44:241–246

39. Moran C, Azziz R, Carmina E, Dewailly D, Fruzzetti F, Ibanez L, Knochenhauer ES, Marcondes JA, Mendonca BB, Pignatelli D, Pugeat M, Rohmer V, Speiser PW, Witchel SF (2000) 21-Hydroxylase-deficient nonclassical adrenal hyperplasia is a progressive disorder: a multicenter study. Am J Obstet Gynecol 183:1468–1474

40. Grumbach MM, Conte FA (1998) Disorders of sex differentiation. In: Wilson JD, Foster DW, Kronenberg HM, Larsen PR (eds) Williams textbook of endocrinology. WB Saunders, Philadelphia, pp 1303–1426

41. Nomura S (1997) Immature adrenal steroidogenesis in preterm infants. Early Hum Dev 49:225–233

42. Brosnan PG, Brosnan CA, Kemp SF, Domek DB, Jelley DH, Blackett PR, Riley WJ (1999) Effect of newborn screening for congenital adrenal hyperplasia. Acta Pediatr Adolesc Med 153:1272–1278

43. Thompson R, Seargeant L, Winter JS (1989) Screening for congenital adrenal hyperplasia: distribution of 17α-hydroxyprogesterone concentrations in neonatal blood spot specimens. J Pediatr 114:400–404

44. Thilen A, Larsson A (1990) Congenital adrenal hyperplasia in Sweden 1969–1986. Prevalence, symptoms and age at diagnosis. Acta Pediatr Scand 79:168–175

45. Balsamo A, Cacciari E, Piazzi S, Cassio A, Bozza A, Pirazzoli P, Zappula F (1996) Congenital adrenal hyperplasia: neonatal mass screening with clinical diagnosis only in the Emilia-Romagna region of Italy, 1980–1995. Pediatrics 98:362–367

46. New MI, Lorenzen F, Lerner AJ, Kohn B, Oberfield SE, Pollack MS, Dupont B, Stoner E, Levy DJ, Pang S, Levine LS (1983) Genotyping steroid 21-hydroxylase deficiency: hormonal reference data. J Clin Endocrinol Metab 57:320–326

47. Fiet J, Gueux B, Gourmelen M, Kuttenn F, Vexiau P, Couillin P, Pham-Huu-Trung MT, Villette JM, Raux-Demay MC, Galons H, et al. (1988) Comparison of basal and adrenocorticotropin-stimulated plasma 21-deoxycortisol and 17-hydroxyprogesterone values as biological markers of late-onset adrenal hyperplasia. J Clin Endocrinol Metab 66:659–667

48. Honour JW (1997) Steroid profiling. Ann Clin Biochem 34:32–44

49. Honour JW, Brook CGD (1997) Clinical indications for the use of urinary steroid profiles in neonates and children. Ann Clin Biochem 34:45–54

50. Carroll MC, Campbell RD, Porter RR (1985) Mapping of steroid 21-hydroxylase genes adjacent to complement component C4 genes in HLA, the major histocompatibility complex in man. Proc Natl Acad Sci USA 82:521–5

51. Higashi Y, Yoshioka H, Yamane M, Gotoh O, Fujii-Kuriyama Y (1986) Complete nucleotide sequence of two steroid 21-hydroxylase genes tandemly arranged in human chromosome: a pseudogene and a genuine gene. Proc Natl Acad Sci USA 83:2841–5

52. White PC, New MI, Dupont B (1986) Structure of human steroid 21-hydroxylase genes. Proc Natl Acad Sci USA 83:5111–5

53. White PC, Tusie-Luna MT, New MI, Speiser PW (1994) Mutations in steroid 21-hydroxylase (CYP21). Hum Mutat 3:373–8

54. White PC, Vitek A, Dupont B, New MI (1988) Characterization of frequent deletions causing steroid 21-hydroxylase deficiency. Proc Natl Acad Sci USA 85:4436–40

55. Higashi Y, Tanae A, Inoue H, Fujii-Kuriyama Y (1988) Evidence for frequent gene conversion in the steroid 21-hydroxylase P-450(C21) gene: implications for steroid 21-hydroxylase deficiency. Am J Hum Genet 42:17–25

56. Speiser PW, Dupont J, Zhu D, Serrat J, Buegeleisen M, Tusie-Luna MT, Lesser M, New MI, White PC (1992) Disease expression and molecular genotype in congenital adrenal hyperplasia due to 21-hydroxylase deficiency. J Clin Invest 90:584–595

57. Higashi Y, Hiromasa T, Tanae A, Miki T, Nakura J, Kondo T, Ohura T, Ogawa E, Nakayama K, Fujii-Kuriyama Y (1991) Effects of individual mutations in the P-450(C21) pseudogene on the P-450(C21) activity and their distribution in the patient genomes of congenital steroid 21-hydroxylase deficiency. J Biochem (Tokyo) 109:638–44

58. Tusie-Luna MT, Speiser PW, Dumic M, New MI, White PC (1991) A mutation (Pro-30 to Leu) in CYP21 represents a potential nonclassic steroid 21-hydroxylase deficiency allele. Mol Endocrinol 5:685–692

59. Speiser PW, New MI (1987) Genotype and hormonal phenotype in nonclassical 21-hydroxylase deficiency. J Clin Endocrinol Metab 64:86–91

60. Wedell A, Thilen A, Ritzen EM, Stengler B, Luthman H (1994) Mutational spectrum of the steroid 21-hydroxylase gene in Sweden: implications for genetic diagnosis and association with disease manifestation. J Clin Endocrinol Metab 78:1145–52

61. Wilson RC, Mercado AB, Cheng KC, New MI (1995) Steroid 21-hydroxylase deficiency: genotype may not predict phenotype. J Clin Endocrinol Metab 80:2322–9

62. Jaaskelainen J, Levo A, Voutilainen R, Partanen J (1997) Population-wide evaluation of disease manifestation in relation to molecular genotype in steroid 21-hydroxylase (CYP21) deficiency: good correlation in a well defined population. J Clin Endocrinol Metab 82:3293–7

63. Krone N, Braun A, Roscher AA, Knorr D, Schwarz HP (2000) Predicting phenotype in steroid 21-hydroxylase deficiency? Comprehensive genotyping in 155 unrelated, well defined patients from southern Germany. J Clin Endocrinol Metab 85:1059–65

64. Deneux C, Tardy V, Dib A, Mornet E, Billaud L, Charron D, Morel Y, Kuttenn F (2001) Phenotype-genotype correlation in 56 women with nonclassical congenital adrenal hyperplasia due to 21-hydroxylase deficiency. J Clin Endocrinol Metab 86:207–13

65. Winkel CA, Casey ML, Worley RJ, Madden JD, MacDonald PC (1983) Extraadrenal steroid 21-hydroxylase activity in a woman with congenital adrenal hyperplasia due to steroid 21-hydroxylase deficiency. J Clin Endocrinol Metab 56:104–7

66. Mellon SH, Miller WL (1989) Extraadrenal steroid 21-hydroxylation is not mediated by P450c21. J Clin Invest 84:1497–502

67. Zhou Z, Agarwal VR, Dixit N, White P, Speiser PW (1997) Steroid 21-hydroxylase expression and activity in human lymphocytes. Mol Cell Endocrinol 127:11–18

68. Charmandari E, Eisenhofer G, Mehlinger SL, Carlson A, Wesley R, Keil MF, Chrousos GP, New MI, Merke DP (2002) Adrenomedullary function may predict phenotype and genotype in classic 21-hydroxylase deficiency. J Clin Endocrinol Metab 87:3031–7

69. Charmandari E, Hindmarsh PC, Johnston A, Brook CG (2001) Congenital adrenal hyperplasia due to 21-hydroxylase deficiency: alterations in cortisol pharmacokinetics at puberty. J Clin Endocrinol Metab 86:2701–8

70. Charmandari E, Johnston A, Brook CG, Hindmarsh PC (2001) Bioavailability of oral hydrocortisone in patients with congenital adrenal hyperplasia due to 21-hydroxylase deficiency. J Endocrinol 169:65–70

71. Kerrigan JR, Veldhuis JD, Leyo SA, Iranmanesh A, Rogol AD (1993) Estimation of daily cortisol production and clearance rates in normal pubertal males by deconvolution analysis. J Clin Endocrinol Metab 76:1505–1510

72. Charmandari E, Matthews DR, Johnston A, Brook CG, Hindmarsh PC (2001) Serum cortisol and 17-hydroxyprogesterone interrelation in classic 21-hydroxylase deficiency: is current replacement therapy satisfactory? J Clin Endocrinol Metab 86:4679–85

73. Lamberts SW, Bruining HA, De Jong FH (1997) Corticosteroid therapy in severe illness. N Engl J Med 337:1285–1292

74. Charmandari E, Lichtarowicz-Krynska EJ, Hindmarsh PC, Johnston A, Aynsley-Green A, Brook CG (2001) Congenital adrenal hyperplasia: management during critical illness. Arch Dis Child 85:26–8

75. Van Wyk JJ, Gunther DF, Ritzen EM, Wedell A, Cutler GB Jr, Migeon CJ, New MI (1996) The use of adrenalectomy as a treatment for congenital adrenal hyperplasia. J Clin Endocrinol Metab 81:3180–3190

76. Tajima T, Ma XM, Bornstein SR, Aguilera G (1999) Prenatal dexamethasone treatment does not prevent alterations of the hypothalamic pituitary adrenal axis in steroid 21-hydroxylase deficient mice. Endocrinology 140:3354–62

77. Merke DP, Keil MF, Jones JV, Fields J, Hill S, Cutler GB Jr (2000) Flutamide, testolactone, and reduced hydrocortisone dose maintain normal growth velocity and bone maturation despite elevated androgen levels in children with congenital adrenal hyperplasia. J Clin Endocrinol Metab 85:1114–20

78. Grammatopoulos DK, Chrousos GP (2002) Functional characteristics of CRH receptors and potential clinical applications of CRH-receptor antagonists. Trends Endocrinol Metab 13:436–44

79. Van Wyk JJ, Ritzen EM (2003) The role of bilateral adrenalectomy in the treatment of congenital adrenal hyperplasia. J Clin Endocrinol Metab 88:2993–8

80. Miccoli P, Iacconi P, Conte M, Goletti O, Buccianti P (1995) Laparoscopic adrenalectomy. J Laparoendosc Surg 5:221–6

81. Prinz RA (1995) A comparison of laparoscopic and open adrenalectomies. Arch Surg 130:489–92

82. Godellas CV, Prinz RA (1998) Surgical approach to adrenal neoplasms: laparoscopic versus open adrenalectomy. Surg Oncol Clin N Am 7:807–17

83. Wells SA, Merke DP, Cutler GB Jr, Norton JA, Lacroix A (1998) Therapeutic controversy: The role of laparoscopic surgery in adrenal disease. J Clin Endocrinol Metab 83:3041–9

84. Janowski A (1977) Naturally occurring adrenal steroids with salt losing properties; relationship to congenital adrenal hyperplasia. In: Lee P, Plotnick L, Kowarski AA, Migeon C (eds) Congenital adrenal hyperplasia. University Park Press, Baltimore, pp 99–112

85. Gunther DF, Bukowski TP, Ritzen EM, Wedell A, Van Wyk JJ (1997) Prophylactic adrenalectomy of a three-year-old girl with congenital adrenal hyperplasia: pre- and postoperative studies. J Clin Endocrinol Metab 82: 3324–7

86. Jara-Albarran A, Bayort J, Caballero A, Portillo J, Laborda L, Sampedro M, Cure C, Mateos JM (1979) Probable pituitary adenoma with adrenocorticotropin hypersecretion (corticotropinoma) secondary to Addison's disease. J Clin Endocrinol Metab 49:236–41

87. Yanase T, Sekiya K, Ando M, Nawata H, Kato K, Ibayashi H (1985) Probable ACTH-secreting pituitary tumour in association with Addison's disease. Acta Endocrinol (Copenh) 110:36–41

88. Carr DB, Fisher JE, Rosenblatt M (1986) Response to low-dose pulsatile cortisol in Addison's disease with suspected corticotropinoma. Horm Metab Res 18:569–73

89. Karl M, Lamberts SW, Koper JW, Katz DA, Huizenga NE, Kino T, Haddad BR, Hughes MR, Chrousos GP (1996) Cushing's disease preceded by generalized glucocorticoid resistance: clinical consequences of a novel, dominant-negative glucocorticoid receptor mutation. Proc Assoc Am Physicians 108:296–307

90. Horrocks PM, Franks S, Hockley AD, Rolfe EB, Van Noorden S, London DR (1982) An ACTH-secreting pituitary tumour arising in a patient with congenital adrenal hyperplasia. Clin Endocrinol (Oxf) 17:457–68

91. Newman K, Randolph J, Parson S (1992) Functional results in young women having clitoral reconstruction as infants. J Pediatr Surg 27:180–183; discussion 183–184

92. Powell DM, Newman KD, Randolph J (1995) A proposed classification of vaginal anomalies and their surgical correction. J Pediatr Surg 30:271–275; discussion 275–276

93. Alizai NK, Thomas DF, Lilford RJ, Batchelor AG, Johnson N (1999) Feminizing genitoplasty for congenital adrenal hyperplasia: what happens at puberty? J Urol 161:1588–1591

94. Schnitzer JJ, Donahoe PK (2001) Surgical treatment of congenital adrenal hyperplasia. Endocrinol Metab Clin North Am 30:137–154

95. New MI, Carlson A, Obeid J, Marshall I, Cabrera MS, Goseco A, Lin-Su K, Putnam AS, Wei JQ, Wilson RC (2001) Prenatal diagnosis for congenital adrenal hyperplasia in 532 pregnancies. J Clin Endocrinol Metab 86:5651–5657

96. Seckl JR, Miller WL (1997) How safe is long-term prenatal glucocorticoid treatment? JAMA 277:1077–1079

97. Newnham JP (2001) Is prenatal glucocorticoid administration another origin of adult disease? Clin Exp Pharmacol Physiol 28:957–961

98. Pang S, Clark AT, Freeman LC, Dolan LM, Immken L, Mueller OT, Stiff D, Shulman DI (1992) Maternal side effects of prenatal dexamethasone therapy for fetal congenital adrenal hyperplasia. J Clin Endocrinol Metab 75:249–253

11 Overview of Mineralocorticoid Excess Syndromes

Richard D. Gordon, Michael Stowasser

CONTENTS

11.1 Introduction

11.1.1 Mineralocorticoid Excess Causes Hypertension

Hypertension affects 20–30% of all adults over the age of 50 years in Western societies, with its treatment, morbidity and mortality consuming a very significant part of precious health budgets. The surgical relevance of the "Mineralocorticoid Excess Syndromes" is that ideal treatment (possible in some of them) is surgical excision of the source of mineralocorticoid excess. The most important example of this is a benign aldosterone-producing adenoma (APA) confined to one adrenal gland, where the possibility of permanent cure of the syndrome exists.

11.1.2 Surgically Curable Primary Aldosteronism Affects Possibly 3% of Hypertensive Patients

The entity of primary aldosteronism (PAL) was shown 10 years ago to be 10 times more common than previously thought [8–12], and to affect as many as 10% of the hypertensive population, up to one-third due to unilateral disease. The possibility of cure in approximately 50% achieved by unilateral adrenalectomy, and of better control with few drugs in the remainder, makes the diagnosis and effective surgical treatment of unilateral PAL extremely important for both the individual patient and the community. While approximately one-third of all patients with PAL have unilateral production of aldosterone, in the other two-thirds both adrenal glands are overproducing aldosterone. This large subgroup is usually treated initially with aldosterone-blocking drugs, most often with a very satisfactory response to this specific (as opposed to non-specific) antihypertensive therapy. However, in some of them the response to medical treatment is unsatisfactory, and consideration will then be given to unilateral adrenalectomy, significantly reducing the mass of tissue autonomously producing aldosterone, usually with gratifying results. The Greenslopes Hypertension Unit has been extremely fortunate to have the services of a skilled and dedicated surgeon, Dr. John C. Rutherford, who pioneered laparoscopic adrenal surgery in Australia, and in August 2003 completed his 300th laparoscopic adrenalectomy. Over 200 of them have been for unilateral overproduction of aldosterone [23–25]. In this chapter the steps required for the diagnosis of this surgically treatable condition will be described in detail, because attention to detail is essential for best outcomes.

11.1.3   Other Causes of Mineralocorticoid Excess May Be Surgically Treatable

Other surgically treatable causes of mineralocorticoid excess appear to be much less common, and certainly are rarely recognized. However, they are just as important for the individual patient. In essence, if the source of mineralocorticoid excess can be localized, and removed without significant perioperative risk to the patient, and its removal does not lead to reduced quality of life, this represents an ideal application for surgery. As in all other clinical situations, each patient must be treated as a unique individual, with a unique set of factors making surgery more or less attractive, including general medical condition, efficacy and side-effects of current antihypertensive therapy and psychological and philosophical attitude to surgery. Detailed explanation at each step of the diagnostic and treatment pathway

is essential for an informed, compliant patient who will be satisfied with the outcome.

11.2   Causes and Consequences of Mineralocorticoid Excess

When the mineralocorticoid receptor (MR) is activated, the epithelial sodium channel is stimulated to greater activity, and potassium is excreted into the urine. Thus mineralocorticoid excess syndromes are usually associated with the eventual development of hypokalemia. Whereas volume expansion can trigger release of atrial natriuretic peptide, and by this and other mechanisms reduce proximal sodium reabsorption, "swamping" the downstream MR-regulated sodium reabsorption with its limited capacity, the excretion of potassium which occurs at that site is relentlessly increased, leading to total body potassium depletion first affecting the cells with their normal high concentrations of potassium, and eventually the extracellular fluids including blood. Thus hypokalemia eventually develops and is a late sign of severe

Table 1. Mineralocorticoid excess syndromes

1   Aldosterone excess secondary to excessive production of renin – secondary aldosteronism
1.1   Renal artery stenosis
1.2   Renin-secreting tumor of juxtaglomerular cells (reninoma)
1.3   Renal tumors which secrete renin such as Wilm's tumor
2   DOC (11-desoxycorticosterone) excess secondary to excessive production of ACTH
2.1   Congenital adrenal hyperplasia due to 11β-hydroxylase deficiency
2.2   Congenital adrenal hyperplasia due to 17α-hydroxylase deficiency
2.3   Ectopic ACTH production by tumors. These may be benign (for example, bronchial carcinoid) or malignant (for example, small cell cancer of the lung)
2.4   Cushing's syndrome due to pituitary microadenoma or hyperplasia producing excessive ACTH
3   Aldosterone excess secondary to normal production of ACTH
3.1   Presence of an abnormal gene for steroid biosynthesis, a "hybrid" of the regulatory portion of the 11β-hydroxylase gene (CYP11B1) and the coding portion of the aldosterone synthase gene (CYP11B2), resulting in ACTH-regulated aldosterone production (familial hyperaldosteronism type I)
4   Aldosterone excess secondary to responsiveness of the mineralocorticoid receptor to cortisol
4.1   Deficiency of the enzyme 11β-hydroxysteroid dehydrogenase (11βHSD-2) which converts cortisol to cortisone (poor affinity for the mineralocorticoid receptor) in the kidney
4.2   Ingestion of licorice or carbenoxolone in sufficient quantity to inhibit 11βHSD-2
5   Primary aldosterone overproduction (primary hyperaldosteronism)
5.1   Solitary, benign adrenocortical aldosterone-producing adenoma (Conn's syndrome)
5.2   Bilateral adrenal hyperplasia, diffuse or nodular
5.3   Unilateral adrenal hyperplasia, diffuse or nodular
5.4   Adrenocortical carcinoma producing aldosterone, possibly with other steroids
6   Primary DOC overproduction
6.1   Solitary, benign DOC secreting tumor
6.2   Adrenocortical carcinoma producing DOC, possibly with other steroids
7   Ingestion of steroids with mineralocorticoid activity such as 9α-fluoro-hydrocortisone or hydrocortisone itself in high dosage

total body potassium depletion and the possibility of mineralocorticoid excess.

A list of causes of mineralocorticoid excess syndromes is shown in Table 1. Mineralocorticoid excess leads to excessive renal reabsorption of sodium leading, via secondary reabsorption of water in order to keep sodium concentration normal, to volume expansion and hypertension. While most of the filtered sodium is reabsorbed in the proximal renal tubule and loop of Henle, the fine-tuning of sodium balance occurs in the distal tubule and collecting duct under the influence of aldosterone via the MR. Cortisol, present in almost 1,000 times the concentration of aldosterone in blood, also has high affinity for the MR, but an enzyme (11β-hydroxysteroid dehydrogenase type 2, 11βHSD-2) is normally present in the renal tubular cells and converts cortisol to cortisone, which has poor affinity for the MR. Congenital absence of this enzyme, or ingestion of substances such as licorice or carbenoxolone which inhibit it, can lead to a "syndrome of apparent mineralocorticoid excess" [2]. Aldosterone is the physiological ligand for the MR and its production is regulated mainly by angiotensin II, resulting from the action of renin secreted by the juxtaglomerular apparatus in the kidney on its substrate (angiotensinogen) made by the liver. Other adrenal steroids, particularly 11 desoxycorticosterone (DOC), also can activate the MR. For example, in congenital adrenal hyperplasia due either to 11β-hydroxylase deficiency or 17α-hydroxylase deficiency, excessive DOC secretion occurs as a result of stimulation of the adrenal cortex by high circulating ACTH levels [1, 33]. Adrenal cortical adenomas or carcinomas secreting DOC are rare, but their removal will cure the mineralocorticoid excess which they caused [17]. If cortisol is present in sufficient excess to overwhelm the 11βHSD-2 enzyme, then the MR is stimulated and a form of mineralocorticoid excess develops which is indistinguishable from PAL except that aldosterone is suppressed. In "ectopic ACTH" syndromes, the MR is stimulated by both DOC and cortisol. Thus, when ACTH is secreted in excess, as in "ectopic ACTH syndromes" due, for example, to production of ACTH by bronchial carcinoid tumors or small cell cancers of the lung, excessive sodium reabsorption and volume expansion (due to very high levels of cortisol and DOC acting on the MR) leads to hypokalemia and suppression of renin (and, as a consequence, of aldosterone), and hypertension develops if the patient lives long enough and is not too ill from the effects of the neoplasm.

In a rare familial disorder, Liddle's syndrome (pseudohyperaldosteronism), the epithelial sodium channel

Table 2. Primary aldosteronism

1 Unilateral
   1.1 Aldosterone-producing adenoma (APA)
   1.2 Aldosterone-producing carcinoma
   1.3 Unilateral hyperplasia, nodular or diffuse
2 Bilateral
   2.1 Bilateral adrenal hyperplasia (BAH), nodular or diffuse

is constitutively "switched on" due to a genetic mutation, and the result is clinically indistinguishable from aldosterone excess in terms of hypertension, hypokalemia and suppressed renin [31]. However, levels of aldosterone are suppressed secondary to suppression of renin.

The surgically correctable mineralocorticoid excess syndromes include those associated with tumors of the adrenal (adenoma or carcinoma) or kidney (reninoma or renal carcinoma) or those producing ectopic ACTH hypersecretion (most commonly lung tumors). In the case of ectopic ACTH syndromes, relief from hypertension and hypokalemia is occasionally achieved by bilateral adrenalectomy, but only in situations where the source of ectopic ACTH is not suitable for resection or unresponsive to chemotherapy and other effects of the tumor apart from hypertension and hypokalemia are not overriding considerations. Mineralocorticoid excess due to renin hypersecretion in renal artery stenosis due to atheroma or fibromuscular dysplasia is treated by percutaneous transluminal renal angioplasty and stenting or by surgery in carefully selected patients, but will not be further discussed here.

The primary focus of this chapter will be on those mineralocorticoid excess syndromes which are treatable by adrenal surgery. By far the commonest of them is PAL (Table 2).

11.3 Primary Aldosteronism and Surgery of the Adrenal Gland

11.3.1 Familial Forms

There are so far two recognized familial forms of PAL. The first is a glucocorticoid-suppressible form (familial hyperaldosteronism type I – FH-I) first described clinically in 1966 [30] and genetically in 1992 [19], which can be identified by a test performed using peripheral blood DNA [16] (even at birth) and responding to low doses of dexamethasone orally which will not cause side-effects [26]. This form would not be expected to respond, except perhaps briefly, to unilateral adrenalectomy. Adrenal venous sampling, which should always be performed before adrenal surgery is contemplated, would show bilateral production of aldosterone. Adrenal adenomas have been reported at least twice in this condition [22, 27]. Hence, computerized tomographic (CT) scanning without adrenal venous sampling might have led to unhelpful unilateral adrenalectomy. Although we have studied a Queensland-based family with FH-I which has 21 affected members, over 500 living members and almost 200 tested by examination of peripheral blood DNA, this familial form of PAL is rare. We have encountered only four new patients (and subsequently families) with FH-I among more than 790 new patients with PAL diagnosed by the Brisbane Hypertension Units since 1992. During the same period we have identified 28 families with more than one member affected by PAL which is not glucocorticoid suppressible. This variety (familial hyperaldosteronism type II–FH-II) is in our experience therefore at least 5 times more common than FH-I. We are currently seeking the genetic basis of FH-II and in collaboration with Constantine Stratakis and coworkers from NIH [18] and Maria New and coworkers from New York Presbyterian Hospital [28] we have established linkage to a region on chromosome 7p22 in large families from Brisbane and Equador/Dominican Republic respectively. Using clinical and biochemical criteria, patients with FH-II are indistinguishable from patients with apparently non-familial PAL, and it is likely that FH-II will be found to be common among patients with PAL if a genetic test involving a peripheral blood sample can be established [6, 29]. Importantly from the surgical viewpoint, patients with FH-II frequently suffer from the unilateral tumorous variety of PAL [6, 29], where treatment options include unilateral adrenalectomy.

11.3.2   When to Look for Primary Aldosteronism

Since less than 50% of the more than 250 patients diagnosed with PAL who have lateralized on adrenal venous sampling and gone on to unilateral adrenalectomy in our units have been hypokalemic, many patients with potentially curable PAL will be denied the opportunity for cure if only hypokalemic hypertensives are screened for PAL (Fig. 1). The Greenslopes Hospital Unit adopted the policy in 1991 to screen all new hypertensive patients for PAL using the aldosterone to renin ratio (ARR), shown by Hiramatsu et al.

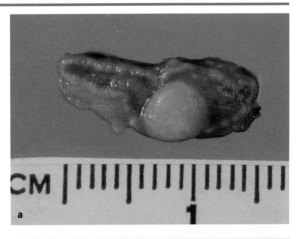

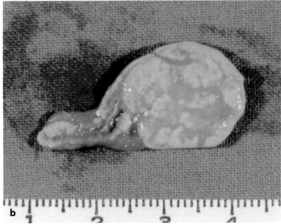

Fig. 1a, b. Examples of aldosterone-producing adenomas (APAs) removed from hypertensive patients who were found to have elevated aldosterone/renin ratios on screening, primary aldosteronism confirmed by fludrocortisone suppression testing, and lateralization of aldosterone production to the corresponding adrenal on adrenal venous sampling. In each case, unilateral laparoscopic adrenalectomy led to cure of hypertension. **a** Left adrenal 0.5 cm APA removed from a 40-year-old hypertensive, normokalemic male. This tumor was not visible on adrenal computed tomography (CT) scanning. **b** Left adrenal 1.9 cm APA, visible on CT scanning, removed from a 42-year-old hypertensive, hypokalemic female

[14] in 1981 to be capable of identifying (with only the assistance of organ imaging) nine patients with aldosterone-producing adenomas among 348 hypertensives, six of whom were normokalemic. The effects of medication on the ARR must be taken into account, and it should be repeated at least once (Table 3). Accepting a diagnosis of PAL only after failure of aldosterone to suppress with oral salt loading and fludrocortisone (despite concurrent suppression of renin), the Greenslopes Unit has been diagnosing 50–100 patients per year with PAL since 1992. The total

Table 3. Factors and conditions capable of affecting the aldosterone-renin ratio and causing loss of specificity and sensitivity due to false positives and false negatives

Factor or condition	False positive	False negative
Total body (serum) potassium	High K$^+$ – aldo $\uparrow$	Low K$^+$ – aldo $\downarrow$
Antihypertensive medications	Beta-blockers – renin $\downarrow$	Diuretics – low K$^+$, aldo $\downarrow$ renin $\uparrow$
	Alpha-methyldopa – renin $\downarrow$	ACE inhibitors – renin $\uparrow$ aldo $\downarrow$
	Clonidine – renin $\downarrow$	AII-blockers – renin $\uparrow$ aldo $\downarrow$
		Calcium blockers – renin $\uparrow$ aldo $\downarrow$
Other medications	NSAIDS – renin $\downarrow\downarrow$ aldo $\downarrow$	
Diabetic renal disease	Renin $\downarrow\downarrow$ aldo $\downarrow$	
Renal failure	Renin $\downarrow\downarrow$ aldo $\uparrow$ (high K$^+$)	
Dietary salt loading	Renin $\downarrow\downarrow$ aldo $\downarrow$	
Dietary salt restriction		Renin $\uparrow\uparrow$ aldo $\uparrow$
Ageing (>65 years)	Renin $\downarrow\downarrow$ aldo $\downarrow$	

ACE denotes angiotensin converting enzyme; *Aldo*, aldosterone; *AII*, angiotensin II; *K$^+$*, potassium; *NSAIDS*, non-steroidal anti-inflammatory drugs.

combined experience of the two Brisbane units, following establishment of a sister unit at Princess Alexandra Hospital in 2000, is now over 1,000 patients with PAL.

It is in the best interests of all hypertensive patients to be screened for PAL. A positive family history of hypertension, rather than suggesting a diagnosis of so-called "essential hypertension", makes the diagnosis of PAL no less likely. The presence of hypokalemia unprovoked by diuretics, or of severe hypokalemia provoked by diuretics, makes PAL highly likely.

11.3.3   How to Look for Primary Aldosteronism

The simultaneous measurement of plasma aldosterone and plasma renin (or plasma renin activity) is a convenient screening test. Normally, if renin is suppressed by high salt intake or reduced renal sodium excretion, aldosterone would normally follow and the ratio of aldosterone divided by renin remains normal. On the other hand, if renin is suppressed because aldosterone secretion has become autonomous and has risen above what is required, the ratio will be increased long before aldosterone rises above the wide normal range [5]. This makes it a very sensitive test for PAL, but it suffers from lack of specificity because there are a number of situations, including drug therapy, where false positive or false negative tests are possible (Table 3). For this reason, patients screened by the Brisbane Hypertension Units using ARR have at least

two measurements, and frequently more. An exception is the hypertensive patient less than 50 years of age on no medications of any sort and with unprovoked hypokalemia who will go on to have a fludrocortisone suppression test after only one ARR. Each patient must be considered an individual, and a careful history of both prescribed and over-the-counter pharmaceutical lines as well as "alternative health remedies" must be taken if misinterpretation is to be avoided (Table 3). For example, the non-steroidal anti-inflammatory drugs taken so commonly for arthritis cause salt and water retention and also inhibit prostaglandin-mediated stimulation of renin levels. Renin often falls disproportionately to aldosterone in this setting, and false positive ratios are common.

Potassium directly stimulates aldosterone secretion, so that conditions which tend to raise or lower potassium also impact on the ARR. Because hypokalemia can lower the ratio by its effect on aldosterone, hypokalemia must always be corrected using oral supplements such as slow-release potassium chloride tablets before the ratio is measured. When checking serum or plasma potassium levels (serum levels are 0.5 mmol/l higher) request that the blood be collected "without stasis". This means that, if a tourniquet is applied to distend the veins and make venesection easier, it should be deflated for 10 s before blood is carefully collected into a syringe (not under vacuum), or for 30 s if fist clenching has been employed to distend the veins. Muscle action and venous occlusion raise potassium levels by up to 1 mmol/l (that is by 20%

or more) and even small amounts of hemolysis which are not readily detected will significantly falsely elevate potassium levels.

Of the various antihypertensive drugs, beta-blockers are the worst offenders, causing false positive ratios. If the ratio is negative despite beta-blockers, this virtually excludes PAL. Patients need to be taken off beta-blockers if the ratio is positive, but this is not easy if they have been on them long-term, and is potentially dangerous if they suffer from ischemic heart disease. The increase in heart rate following beta-blocker withdrawal can aggravate angina. If contemplated in a patient with known coronary artery disease, a cardiologist should be consulted and made aware of what is planned. We reduce beta-blockers very slowly, in stages 4 weeks apart, introducing verapamil slow release, taken in two divided doses for smooth control, because it also slows heart rate. Verapamil does not stimulate renin release as much as other calcium blockers (especially amlodipine), and so is unlikely to convert a false positive to a false negative result. Drugs such as verapamil slow-release, prazosin (in three divided doses) and hydralazine (in two or three divided doses) have been the most useful replacement drugs when we have been changing drugs in order to achieve a reliable ARR. In mildly hypertensive patients it may be possible to achieve a month off medications before the ARR is measured. If treatment needs to be started at the first visit, a ratio can usually be obtained before treatment starts. If not, in our experience commencing treatment with verapamil slow release 180 or 240 mg in two divided doses, together with hydralazine 25 mg in two divided doses (increasing after 4–7 days to 50 mg in two divided doses), has proved very useful. If a negative ratio is obtained, treatment can then be changed if necessary, for example if verapamil is causing poorly tolerated constipation. If the ratio is positive, it should usually be repeated (see above) before going on to FST.

One negative ratio does not exclude PAL, and especially in patients whose hypertension is worsening, with increasing resistance to medication, repeat testing may be indicated. PAL is a disease which usually evolves slowly, but sometimes once hypertension develops it can progress rapidly and eventually enter a resistant and even accelerating phase. If hypertension is already very severe, and especially if it has enticed a "pre-malignant" or "malignant" phase, with retinal hemorrhages, exudates and papilledema, arteriolar inflammatory changes in the kidney causing edema and ischemia can lead to significantly elevated renin levels and false negative ratios.

The ARR is a screening and not a diagnostic test. Extremely low renin levels will lead to a high ratio even if aldosterone is also reduced. This has led some workers to specify a plasma aldosterone level below which they would not consider the diagnosis of PAL [21, 32], for example, 15 ng/100 ml. We prefer to consider each patient on his or her merits, taking into account all possible factors, and repeating the ARR after modifying those which can be modified.

Both plasma renin and aldosterone are subject to a diurnal rhythm and are transiently but not instantaneously responsive to postural changes [4, 11]. Thus it is important to standardize the conditions under which renin and aldosterone are measured. Aldosterone is responsive to ACTH as well as to angiotensin II, and levels will tend to fall after 8 A.M. It is our practice to collect samples for ARR midmorning, after sitting for 5 min; that is overnight recumbency is followed by ambulation for 2–4 h. We initially arbitrarily (based on retrospective analysis of patients with proven PAL) chose a value of 25 [13] or more for a positive ARR when aldosterone is measured in ng/100 ml and PRA in ng/ml/h. We subsequently raised the bar to 30 or more in an attempt to reduce false positive tests to very few. Clearly the range 20–30 is a 'gray area" and will remain so. The conversion factor to change from renin concentration (measured in mU/l) to PRA is to divide by 8.4. The conversion factor for aldosterone from pmol/l to ng/100 ml is to divide by 27.7. The ARR is merely a guide to whether the diagnosis of PAL is likely or not likely in a hypertensive patient. It does not prove or exclude the diagnosis, and to do so requires a suppression test. But it does reduce by an order of magnitude the number of patients who require a suppression test to exclude normokalemic PAL which is potentially curable, and this is very worthwhile.

11.3.4 Suppression Tests to Establish Autonomous Production of Aldosterone

By imposing conditions under which it would be normal for both renin and aldosterone to be "shut off", suppression tests aim to uncover the situation where aldosterone production continues, despite renin, the principal normal regulator of aldosterone, being suppressed. Hence it is essential to measure renin as well as aldosterone during the test, to demonstrate that it is suppressed and not responsible for any continuing aldosterone secretion. If renin is not suppressed, the test is either negative or uninterpretable; it cannot be positive. All suppression tests consist of "salt-loading";

only the means to achieve this differs. The simplest test is to give the patient a "high salt diet" (by advice or provision) and supplemental sodium chloride either as plain salt tablets or the more palatable "slow-Na" tablets, which are sugar-coated to pass the stomach and release salt slowly from a wax honeycomb matrix, similar in formulation to "slow-K". Adequacy of the salt load is checked by measuring 24 h urine sodium (should exceed 200 mmol/day) and creatinine simultaneously with aldosterone from day 3 to 4. Criteria vary, but in general the urinary aldosterone must not suppress below 12 µg/24 h [32]. There have been a variety of suppression tests involving intravenous saline infusion reported, which introduces a new, unphysiologic component which has little relevance to the conditions under which human beings function, and which may invoke mechanisms such as acute release of atrial natriuretic peptide and neural volume-responsive mechanisms which will influence renin and aldosterone secretion. We have observed situations in which aldosterone production has been suppressed without renin suppression during saline infusion, and also suppression of plasma aldosterone to extremely low levels (together with renin suppression) in patients subsequently cured by removal of an APA and in whom fludrocortisone suppression testing was positive.

Early saline infusion tests involved infusion of 2 l of normal saline daily for 2 days, with measurement of urinary aldosterone on day 2 [3]. After it became possible to measure plasma aldosterone, the most popular saline infusion test consisted of infusing 2 l in 2–4 h in the morning with the patient continuously recumbent, usually performed as an outpatient procedure [20]. We regard this protocol as not without risk in severely hypertensive patients, particularly if elderly. One of the problems with all salt loading tests is that potassium tends to fall, but more rapidly during saline infusion with a large saline load presented to the aldosterone-sensitive distal nephron. Acute falls in plasma potassium cause acute falls in aldosterone, making a false negative test likely. In the saline infusion protocols, potassium is rarely monitored, and in any event correction of falling potassium levels by potassium infusion would be difficult and not without risk. The level below which plasma aldosterone should not suppress for a positive saline infusion test has varied between 5 and 10 ng/100 ml [15, 20]. We examined saline infusion tests in detail, comparing them with fludrocortisone suppression tests in the same patients, and abandoned saline infusion because of too many false negatives, in spite of its greater ease of delivery.

A positive saline infusion test should make primary aldosteronism highly likely, and false positives are probably rare.

11.3.5 The Fludrocortisone Suppression Test

One advantage of a fludrocortisone suppression test is that the dietary salt load is progressive to maximal effectiveness, the patient being protected from acute volume overload by "renal escape", whereby sodium and chloride are rejected in the proximal tubule and loop of Henle once volume expansion has been achieved. As with intravenous saline loading, this sodium presented to the distal nephron promotes potassium excretion. The advantage over saline infusion is that this occurs more slowly, and can be anticipated (rather than corrected) by appropriate administration of slow K. With experience with this test, it is usually possible to keep potassium levels normal throughout, and certainly to correct hypokalemia by day 4 when the aldosterone, renin, potassium and cortisol levels are examined in overnight recumbent and upright samples (Table 4). A major disadvantage of the fludrocortisone suppression test is that it is best performed in hospital, requiring five nights. This makes it an expensive test and hence only performed after several positive ARRs under appropriate conditions. Hospitalization permits 6 hourly administration of fludrocortisone and slow-K, ensuring steady levels, is associated with lower blood pressure levels than in ambulatory patients and, importantly, permits control of posture so that plasma samples can be collected at 7 A.M. after overnight recumbency from midnight, and again at 10 A.M. after 3 h standing, sitting or walking. It also makes the collection of accurate 24 h urine collections possible.

It is essential to explain the FST in detail to the patient and that the nursing staff are also familiar with the protocol. Plasma potassium levels are telephoned through to the responsible doctor within an hour of collection (without stasis) so that the dosage of slow-K can be constantly adjusted. A difficult feature of this protocol for females is the enforced recumbency between midnight and 0700 hours, necessitating use of a bedpan while lying flat if micturition is necessary despite fluid restriction after the evening meal.

The diagnostic criteria for PAL are a plasma aldosterone level at 10 A.M. upright on day 4 of ≥6 ng/100 ml, provided that (1) PRA is ≤1 ng/ml/h (renin ≤ 8.4 mU/l); (2) plasma potassium is in the normal range (3.5–5 mmol/l); (3) plasma cortisol did not rise be-

Table 4. Fludrocortisone suppression test

Day –1	Admit to hospital in evening (usually Sunday). Familiarize with protocol and ward staff: avoid fluids after evening meal. Stay in bed after midnight, rolling from side to side but not sitting up
Day 1	Blood samples collected at 0700 h while still recumbent, for measurement of renin, aldosterone, cortisol and potassium, and again at 10 A.M. Blood samples for potassium also at 3 P.M. and 7 P.M. Commence fludrocortisone 0.1 mg 6 hrly at 10 A.M. after upright blood samples (standing, sitting or walking since 0700 h sample) and slow Na (10 mmol) three tablets with each meal. Also commence slow K 6 hourly at 10 A.M. in sufficient dosage to keep plasma potassium normal. Requirements increase during the test, reaching usually 18–54 tablets of slow K daily (range 12–102)
Day 2 and 3	As for day 1, except 24 h urine collection commenced at 10 A.M., on day 3 for creatinine, sodium and aldosterone
Day 4	As for days 2 and 3 except that 24 h urine collection is completed at 10 A.M. and patient can be discharged after that

tween 0700 and 1000 hours, since if it did the ACTH rise which caused it could give a false positive FST by stimulating aldosterone; and (4) 24 h urinary sodium was ≥3 mmol/kg/day in the collection completed at 10 A.M. day 4. We are still in the process of deciding a cut-off point for urinary aldosterone in that collection. It appears that a urinary aldosterone of ≥10 µg/day is highly suggestive of PAL.

While a major disadvantage of the fludrocortisone suppression test is the cost of hospital admission, if the test were performed as an outpatient procedure the patient would still have to take time off work and it would be difficult to monitor. A major advantage is the level of control and safety, and the reliability of the test. This is important as the next step, adrenal venous sampling, is invasive.

11.3.6 The Decision that the Patient Does or Does not Have Primary Aldosteronism

Experience with patients who unequivocally had primary aldosteronism in terms of hypertension, hypokalemia, suppressed renin and unsuppressed aldosterone, plus a cure of hypertension and hypokalemia following removal of a unilateral APA, leads to consideration of arbitrary limits for aldosterone levels in blood and urine before and after salt loading in PAL. Because of the variability of levels, choice of a "limit" or cut-off point will always be arbitrary and subject to debate. Based on more than 200 unilateral adrenalectomies for lateralizing PAL, our criteria (see above and Table 4) still remain the subject of constant critical examination, and are the best that we can currently come up with with our patients' best outcomes in mind. They remain subject to revision if the evidence for change is strong enough.

At present our best outcomes appear to be based on fludrocortisone suppression testing, which, if positive, leads to us offering the patient adrenal venous sampling, an invasive procedure.

11.3.7 Adrenal Venous Sampling

Adrenal venous sampling seems to be the only sure way to identify if PAL is due to a unilateral or bilateral abnormality (Table 5). If it is truly unilateral, then the contralateral gland will have suppressed aldosterone production, with aldosterone to cortisol ratio in adrenal venous effluent being the same or lower than in peripheral blood. It can be lower, because the contralateral, normal gland will be producing little aldosterone (not zero, because ACTH and potassium can still stimulate its production) together with normal, large amounts of cortisol. The cortisol gradient between the adrenal vein and a peripheral vein will be extremely high, while that for aldosterone will be much lower. Then the aldosterone/cortisol ratio in the adrenal venous effluent can be lower than peripheral (Fig. 2). When an adrenal mass or nodule is discovered by chance during abdominal organ imaging because of, for example, abdominal pain, it is called an adrenal

Fig. 2a, b. Adrenal computed tomography (**a**) and adrenal ▶ venous sampling results (**b**) from a 54-year-old hypertensive male with primary aldosteronism. Although computed tomography showed bilateral adrenal masses [right 3.9 cm (*top image*), left 2.7 cm (*bottom image*)], adrenal venous sampling demonstrated clear lateralization of aldosterone overproduction to the right adrenal, the removal of which led to cure of his hypertension and biochemical cure of primary aldosteronism (*Aldo*, aldosterone; *cort*, cortisol; *LAV*, left adrenal vein; *RAV*, right adrenal vein)

Table 5. Adrenal venous sampling

1. Patient must have a positive FST and to have tested negative for FH-I (hybrid gene test)

2. Peripheral renin activity levels must be ≤1 ng/ml/h and have been suppressed for at least 2 months. Otherwise a suppressed contralateral, normal gland in terms of aldosterone production may have become unsuppressed and lateralization will be impossible

3. Diuretics including aldosterone blocking drugs should have been ceased and replaced with other medications at least 2 months previously

4. Treatment with angiotensin-II antagonists which powerfully inhibit the negative feedback on renin and raise renin levels should have been ceased for 2 weeks, although in theory the high renin levels would be incapable of stimulating aldosterone production by the contralateral, normal adrenal

5. A CT scan (with contrast unless an allergy exists) should be performed to show adrenal anatomy and aid in localization of adrenal veins

6. The cannulation of the adrenal veins in turn via a femoral vein should take place as soon after 8 A.M. as possible after overnight recumbency from midnight has been maintained, with the patient transported supine to the radiology department. An intravenous line pre-positioned in an anticubital vein permits simultaneous sampling, in turn, from each adrenal vein and the peripheral vein. More than one set of venous samples should be collected from each adrenal because there may be multiple veins draining each adrenal (or "streaming" may occur) so that a vein draining an area of an adrenal containing an APA may give a different result from a vein draining a different pole of the same gland

7. The patient should rest following the procedure for 2 h and then slowly mobilize

8. Blood tests for procoagulant states (such as Factor V Leiden) should precede AVS and if such a state exists, treatment with heparin should commence at the conclusion of the sampling and continue for 36 h to discourage thromboembolism due to intimal trauma while placing catheters in position

APA denotes aldosterone-producing adenoma; *AVS*, adrenal venous sampling; *CT*, computed tomography; *FH-I*, familial hyperaldosteronism type I; *FST*, fludrocortisone suppression test.

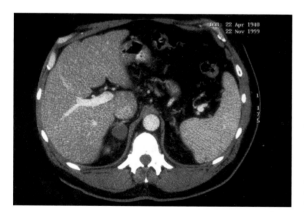

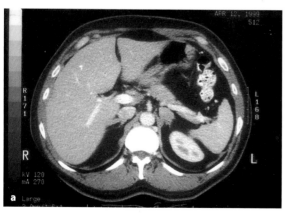

Adrenal Venous Sampling

	Aldo (ng%)	Cort (μg%)	Aldo/Cort
LAV1	147	120	1.2
Periph	71.4	12.4	5.8
LAV2	131	118	1.1
Periph	74.5	14.0	5.3
RAV1	1483	101	14.7
Periph	86.4	13.6	6.4
RAV2	3930	110	35.7
Periph	88.4	12.5	7.1

b

Adrenal Venous Sampling

	Aldo (ng%)	Cort (μg%)	Aldo/Cort
LAV	968	183	5.3
Periph	21	17	1.3
RAV	1496	1120	1.3
Periph	21	17	1.3

Fig. 3. Adrenal venous sampling results from a patient who subsequently underwent left adrenalectomy for aldosterone-producing adenoma and was cured of hypertension as a result. Although aldosterone (*Aldo*) levels were higher in the right adrenal vein (*RAV*) than in the left (*LAV*), cortisol (*Cort*) levels indicated that the LAV sample was more dilute and that Aldo production was in fact suppressed on the right side [right Aldo/Cort ratio no higher than peripheral (*Periph*)]

"incidentaloma". Such adrenal nodules are not rare. In most cases thorough investigation fails to reveal abnormal production of aldosterone, cortisol, sex steroids or catecholamines, although full suppression testing would be necessary to exclude some autonomous production. It is not unusual to encounter PAL in a patient with a nodule or mass in one adrenal who, on adrenal venous sampling, has either bilateral production of aldosterone or unilateral production by the opposite adrenal. Figure 2 represents a patient in whom CT scanning demonstrated bilateral masses, but adrenal venous sampling showed only unilateral aldosterone production. CT also lacks sensitivity, missing as many as 50% of APAs removed from patients who lateralize on adrenal venous sampling (Fig. 1) [4, 28]. These patients illustrate the importance of adrenal venous sampling. Consideration of aldosterone concentrations in the adrenal veins without correction for dilution by non-adrenal blood (by using aldosterone/cortisol ratio) can lead to false lateralization to the contralateral side (Fig. 3).

11.3.8   The Decision to Operate

Lateralization on AVS leads to consideration by the patient, after full discussion of the AVS results and the opportunities for either medical or surgical treatment, of the possibility of unilateral adrenalectomy. The type of operation will depend on the experience and preference of the surgeon. The advantages of laparoscopic adrenalectomy include speed of recovery and fewer postoperative complications [23, 24], but it is a procedure which should be performed only by a surgeon with extensive experience in laparoscopic techniques. It is preferable to remove the entire adrenal rather than to "shell out" a nodule in the hope that it might have been the sole repository of the abnormal tissue, because all the AVS tells us is which side is solely responsible, not which part of the adrenal.

11.3.9   Postoperative Care

Patients with extremely suppressed contralateral, "normal" adrenals will experience a period of hypoaldosteronism following resection of an APA with high normal or even mildly raised potassium levels despite normal serum creatinine. Depending on the duration of PAL before surgery, the suppression of renin and aldosterone can persist postoperatively for several months. Only in the presence of renal impairment is the hyperkalemia likely to be worrying, and then treatment acutely with saline infusion and chronically with 9α-fluorohydrocortisone (as in Addison's disease) should be considered, with a gradual withdrawal as recovery occurs.

We routinely perform a postoperative FST 2–6 months following surgery to assess the effects of surgery in reducing or eliminating autonomous aldosterone production [25]. We do not expect to assess the full effects of surgery on blood pressure for at least 12 months, since damage including loss of nephrons in those with long-standing hypertension will prevent achievement of normal blood pressure even when the effects of surgery on autonomous aldosterone production have been completely successful. Since many factors other than aldosterone excess collectively cause hypertension, the BP response to surgery is a poor arbiter of the appropriateness of the operation.

Patients who have had unilateral adrenalectomy for PAL do not need hormone replacement therapy and lead normal lives [7]. They should be followed long term in order to assess the need for further non-specific therapy of residual hypertension due to causes other than aldosterone excess, and to check by measurement of renin and aldosterone for persistence or recurrence of primary aldosteronism. The morphology of the remaining adrenal can be checked by periodic CT scanning.

11.4   Conclusions

The most commonly required operation for adrenal disease is unilateral adrenalectomy for aldosterone-producing adenoma. The results of this operation, these days usually performed laparoscopically, are spectacularly successful in terms of the objective, removal of the abnormal tissue, as evidenced by postoperative suppression tests. As might be predicted from other circumstances where a cause is removed but renal damage has occurred because of long-standing hypertension, the overall cure rate in terms of hypertension is approximately 50%, but approaches 80% in young females. Identification of other forms of mineralocorticoid excess due to adrenal causes is a rare event, but when present (as in DOC secreting tumors or aldosterone/DOC secreting adrenal cancers) the appropriate treatment is as for primary aldosteronism.

References

1. Biglieri EG, Herron MA, Brust N (1966) 17-Hydroxylation deficiency in man. J Clin Invest 45:1946–1954
2. Edwards CRW, Walker BR, Benediktsson R, Seckl JR (1993) Congenital and acquired syndromes of apparent mineralocorticoid excess. J Steroid Biochem Mol Biol 45:1–5
3. Espiner EA, Tucci JR, Jagger MD, et al (1967) Effect of saline infusions on aldosterone secretion and electrolyte excretion in normal subjects and patients with primary aldosteronism. N Engl J Med 277:1–7
4. Gordon RD (2001) Diagnostic investigations in primary aldosteronism. In: Zanchetti A (ed) Clinical medicine series on hypertension. McGraw-Hill International, London, pp 101–114
5. Gordon RD (2001) Mineralocorticoid excess syndromes. In: Margioris AS, Chrousos GP (eds) Contemporary endocrinology: adrenal disorders. Humana Press, Totowa NJ, pp 355–377
6. Gordon RD, Stowasser M (1998) Familial forms broaden horizons in primary aldosteronism. Trends Endocrinol Metab 9:220–227
7. Gordon RD, Hawkins PG, Hamlet SM, Tunny TJ, Klemm SA, Bachmann AW, Finn WL (1989) Reduced adrenal secretory mass after unilateral adrenalectomy for aldosterone-producing adenoma may explain unexpected incidence of hypotension. J Hypertens 7 (Suppl 6):S210– S211
8. Gordon RD, Klemm SA, Tunny TJ, Stowasser M (1992) Primary aldosteronism: hypertension with a genetic basis. Lancet 340:159–161
9. Gordon RD, Klemm SA, Stowasser M, Tunny TJ, Storie WJ, Rutherford JC (1993) How common is primary aldosteronism? Is it the most frequent cause of curable hypertension? J Hypertens 11(Suppl 5):S2–S3
10. Gordon RD, Ziesak MD, Tunny TJ, Stowasser M, Klemm SA (1993) Evidence that primary aldosteronism may not be uncommon – twelve percent incidence among antihypertensive drug trial volunteers. Clin Exp Pharmacol Physiol 20:296–298
11. Gordon RD, Stowasser M, Klemm SA, Tunny TJ (1994) Primary aldosteronism and other forms of mineralocorticoid hypertension. In: Swales JD (ed) Textbook of hypertension. Blackwell Scientific, London, pp 865–892
12. Gordon RD, Stowasser M, Tunny TJ, Klemm SA, Rutherford JC (1994) High incidence of primary aldosteronism in 199 patients referred with hypertension. Clin Exp Pharmacol Physiol 21:315–318
13. Hamlet SM, Tunny TJ, Woodland E, Gordon RD (1985) Is aldosterone/renin ratio useful to screen a hypertensive population for primary aldosteronism? Clin Exp Pharmacol Physiol 12:249–252
14. Hiramatsu K, Yamada T, Yukimura Y, Komiya I, Ichikawa K, Ishihara M, et al (1981) A screening test to identify aldosterone-producing adenoma by measuring plasma renin activity. Arch Intern Med 141:1589–1593
15. Holland OB, Brown H, Kuhnert LV, Fairchild C, Risk M, Gomez-Sanchez CE (1984) Further evaluation of saline infusion for the diagnosis of primary aldosteronism. Hypertension 6:717–723
16. Jonsson JR, Klemm SA, Tunny TJ, Stowasser M, Gordon RD (1995) A new genetic test for familial hyperaldosteronism type I aids in the detection of curable hypertension. Biochem Biophys Res Comm 207:565–571
17. Kondo K, Saruta T, Saito I, et al (1976) Benign desoxycorticosterone-producing adrenal tumor. JAMA 236:1042–1044
18. Lafferty AR, Torpy D, Stowasser M, Taymans SE, Lin JP, Huggard P, Gordon RD, Stratakis CA (2000) A novel genetic locus for low-renin hypertension: familial hyperaldosteronism type-II maps to chromosome 7 (7p22). J Med Genet 37:831–835
19. Lifton RP, Dluhy RG, Powers M, et al (1992) A chimaeric 11β-hydroxylase/aldosterone synthase gene causes glucocorticoid-remediable aldosteronism and human hypertension. Nature 355:262–265
20. Litchfield WR, Dluhy RG (1995) Primary aldosteronism. Endocrinol Metab Clin North Am 24:593–612
21. Loh K-C, Koay ES, Khaw M-C, et al (2000) Prevalence of primary aldosteronism among Asian hypertensive patients in Singapore. J Clin Endocrinol Metab 85:2854–2859
22. Pascoe L, Jeunemaitre X, Lebrethon MC, et al (1995) Glucocorticoid-suppressible hyperaldosteronism and adrenal tumors occurring in a single French pedigree. J Clin Invest 96:2236–2246

23. Rutherford JC, Gordon RD, Stowasser M, Tunny TJ, Klemm SA (1995) Laparoscopic adrenalectomy for adrenal tumours causing hypertension and for "incidentalomas" of the adrenal on CT scanning. Clin Exp Pharmacol Physiol 22:490–492

24. Rutherford JC, Stowasser M, Tunny TJ, Klemm SA, Gordon RD (1996) Laparoscopic adrenalectomy. World J Surg 20:758–760

25. Rutherford JC, Taylor WL, Stowasser M, Gordon R (1998) Success of surgery in primary aldosteronism judged by residual autonomous aldosterone production. World J Surg 22:1243–1245

26. Stowasser M, Bachmann AW, Huggard PJ, Rossetti TR, Gordon RD (2000) Treatment of familial hyperaldosteronism type I: only partial suppression of hybrid gene required to correct hypertension. J Clin Endocrinol Metab 85:3313–3318

27. Stowasser M, Gordon RD (2000) Primary aldosteronism: learning from the study of familial varieties. J Hypertens 18:1165–76

28. Stowasser M, Gordon RD (2003) Primary aldosteronism. Best Prac Res Clin Endocrinol Metab 14:310–317

29. Stowasser M, Gordon RD (in press) Primary aldosteronism: from genesis to genetics. Trends Endocrinol Metab

30. Sutherland DJA, Ruse JL, Laidlaw JC (1966) Hypertension, increased aldosterone secretion and low plasma renin activity relieved by dexamethasone. Can Med Assoc J 95:1109–1119

31. Warnock DG (1998) Liddle syndrome: an autosomal dominant form of human hypertension. Kidney Int 53:18–24

32. Young WF Jr (1997) Primary aldosteronism: update on diagnosis and treatment. Endocrinologist 7:213–221

33. Zachmann M, Tassinari D, Prade RA (1983) Clinical and biochemical variability of congenital adrenal hyperplasia due to 11β-hydroxylase deficiency. A study of 25 patients. J Clin Endocrinol Metab 56:222–229

12 Primary Aldosteronism: The Surgical Perspective

Bertil Hamberger

CONTENTS

12.1 Introduction

Primary aldosteronism was first described almost 50 years ago by Conn [2]. He predicted that aldosteronism was a common cause of hypertension. For many years internists did not consider primary aldosteronism to be common. It was thought that hypokalemia should be a prerequisite for investigating patients for primary aldosteronism. With this assumption about 0.5% of hypertensive patients had primary aldosteronism. In addition, sampling of blood with a tourniquet induces an increase in serum potassium, also contributing to the low number of patients with primary aldosteronism. However, over the last 10 years there have been an increasing number of reports from all over the world that primary aldosteronism may be much more common [4, 5, 15].

Many more patients could benefit by screening for primary aldosteronism, using the ratio plasma aldosterone/plasma renin activity or plasma renin levels. It is difficult to standardize the aldosterone/renin ratio as different laboratory methods are used and since plasma renin activity will with increasing frequency be replaced by determination of plasma renin levels. Although it may be difficult to define the exact cut-off of the aldosterone/renin ratio, it is evident that such an increased ratio once confirmed is an excellent indication for further endocrinologic workup. Several studies have shown a prevalence of primary aldosteronism of between 5% and 13% in patients with hypertension and even higher in some patients with continued high blood pressure in spite of treatment with several antihypertensive medications (see review by Young [16]). Most of these patients are not hypokalemic.

12.2 Diagnosis of Hyperaldosteronism

In a patient with hypertension, a low plasma renin value and increased plasma and urinary aldosterone remains the cornerstone in the diagnosis and evaluation. During this evaluation the patient should preferably be off all hypertensive drugs if possible. In particular spironolactone and beta blocking agents may cause diagnostic difficulties. The patient should also be normokalemic. Blood for aldosterone, renin and cortisol levels should be drawn from the patient in the morning at rest and at noon after being ambulatory. In addition, inhibitory tests by, e.g., fludrocortisol may be used to increase the accuracy of the diagnosis of primary aldosteronism [1]. The next step in the investigation, after confirmation of the diagnosis biochemically, is to obtain a high resolution computerized tomographic (CT) scan. The CT may show a unilateral enlargement, normal adrenal glands or bilateral enlargement.

12.3 Different Forms of Primary Hyperaldosteronism

- Bilateral hyperaldosteronism due to micro- or macronodular adrenocortical hyperplasia
- Aldosterone-producing adenoma
- Primary unilateral adrenal hyperplasia
- Adrenocortical carcinoma
- Familial hyperaldosteronism
  - Type I glycocorticoid remediable aldosteronism
  - Type II familial adenoma or hyperplasia

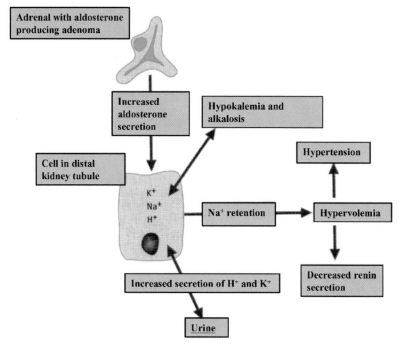

Fig. 1. Schematic drawing of the effects of an aldosterone-producing adenoma

The most common types of hyperaldosteronism are aldosterone-producing adenomas (Fig. 1) and bilateral aldosterone-producing hyperplasia. More uncommon forms are primary unilateral adrenocortical hyperplasia and the extremely rare adrenocortical carcinoma-producing aldosterone. There are two familial forms, type I, glucocorticoid remediable aldosteronism [8, 10], which is treated by oral administration of glucocorticoids, and type II, which is a recently discovered familial form with both adenoma and hyperplasia being present [7].

12.4   Differentiation Between Aldosterone-Producing Adenomas and Bilateral Hyperplasia

Patients with an aldosterone-producing adenoma should be offered surgical removal since this treatment cures the hyperaldosteronism and improves hypertension in virtually all patients [16] although about half remain hypertensive due to secondary arteriolar changes. On the other hand, patients with bilateral adrenal hyperplasia do not usually benefit from surgical removal of one adrenal unless there are large differences in aldosterone secretion between the two sides. Bilateral adrenalectomy creates more problems as a result of the need for substitution with

gluco- and mineralocorticoids and is not recommended.

As mentioned CT is the first investigation in line. A lesion of 1–2 cm in one gland and a completely normal contralateral gland may be sufficient for unilateral adrenalectomy. Magnetic resonance imaging (MRI) provides an excellent morphologic image but can also help to characterize an adrenal lesion and distinguish between a cortical and a medullary tumor [6]. However, MRI cannot give information on which steroid the cortical nodule may produce. Thus, in most cases a functional localization is required and recommended as well.

Adrenal venous sampling is the diagnostic method of choice for determining the release of aldosterone from the adrenal glands [11]. It is not an easy procedure and needs an experienced radiologist. It is essential to be able to cannulate the more difficult right adrenal vein in addition to the left adrenal vein. For experienced radiologists the success rate of this technique is greater than 90%. Samples for aldosterone and cortisol levels are taken from both adrenal veins in addition to other locations including the left renal vein, the inferior vena cava and a peripheral vein. For positive lateralization, the aldosterone/cortisol ratio must be at least four times higher from the affected gland. In addition, the cortisol level must be three times higher in both adrenal veins when compared to

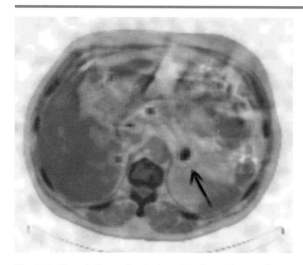

Fig. 2. Iodine cholesterol scintigraphy of a patient with primary aldosteronism showing increased activity from the left adrenal. A 1.5-cm-large tumor was also seen on computed tomography and the patient had an aldosterone-producing adenoma removed. (Courtesy of Dr. Hans Jacobsson, Dept. of Radiology, Karolinska Hospital)

peripheral blood to prove that the sample was, in fact, taken from the adrenal vein. Clear lateralization with venous sampling is an excellent indicator for adrenalectomy.

Scintigraphy after injection of iodine cholesterol may also provide an effective functional localization without invasive methods (Fig. 2 [9]). The drug is given intravenously after inhibition of adrenal cortisol secretion by dexamethasone. Clear lateralization with scintigraphy which is in accordance with the CT scan provides sufficient information for surgical intervention.

12.5   Treatment

In patients with clear lateralization by CT scanning, adrenal venous sampling or iodine cholesterol scintigraphy, there is an indication for unilateral adrenalectomy for an aldosterone-producing adenoma [13]. Usually aldosterone-producing adenomas are small (0.5–2 cm) (Fig. 3) and ideal for laparoscopic removal [11]. It is advantageous to correct hypokalemia preoperatively using spironolactone. Surgical removal of an aldosterone-producing adenoma is very cost effective especially in young patients compared to lifelong medical treatment. Cured patients should have normal serum aldosterone, renin and potassium on follow-up.

Cure of hypertension after successful removal of any aldosterone-producing adenoma ranges between 40% and 70% [14, 12] and persistent hypertension needs conventional treatment. If the patient has persisting hyperaldosteronism, it is probable that the removed nodule was not producing aldosterone and the patient may have a small adenoma in the contralateral adrenal gland or bilateral disease. Analysis of the removed tissue with in situ hybridization of steroidogenic enzymes can reveal the localization of aldosterone production [3].

Patients with bilateral hyperplasia should be treated medically. Spironolactone is the most widely used drug in combination with other hypertensive drugs. The major problem is the occurrence of side effects, particularly painful gynecomastia and impotence. A new drug, eplerenone, was introduced in 2003 to give an antimineralocorticoid effect on aldosterone receptors in the kidney [16]. This drug may be of great help in treating bilateral hyperplasia and may also prove to be useful in patients where surgical removal of an adenoma is contraindicated. In addition, primary adrenal hyperplasia and adrenal cortical carcinoma should be treated surgically. Patients with adrenocortical carcinoma and hyperaldosteronism will usually need an open adrenalectomy, as radical surgery is the only chance for permanent cure.

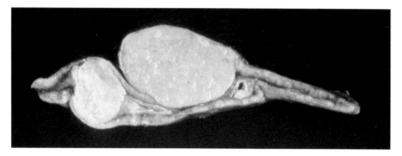

Fig. 3. A typical aldosterone-producing adenoma with a *yellow* color to the *right*. To the *left* there is a nonhyperfunctioning nodule with a pale color. The adrenal cortex has a normal appearance

References

1. Besser GM, Thorner MO (eds) (2002) Comprehensive clinical endocrinology. Mosby, St. Louis, MO
2. Conn JW (1955) Primary aldosteronism, a new clinical syndrome. J Lab Clin Med 45:3
3. Enberg U, Farnebo LO, Wedell A, Gröndal S, Höög A, Thorén M, Grimelius L, Kjellman M, Bäckdahl M, Hamberger B (2001) In vitro release of aldosterone and cortisol in human adrenal adenomas correlates to mRNA expression of steroidogenic enzymes for genes *CYP11B2* and *CYP17*. World J Surg 25:957–66
4. Gordon RD, Stowasser M, Tunny TJ, Klemm SA, Rutherford JC (1994) High incidence of primary aldosteronism in 169 patients referred with hypertension. Clin Exp Pharmacol Physiol 21:315–318
5. Gordon RD, Stowasser M, Rutherford JC (2001) Primary hyperaldosteronism: Are we diagnosing and operating too few patients? World J Surg 25:941–947
6. Hönigschnabl S, Gallo S, Niederle B, Prager G, Kaserer K, Lechner G, Heinz-Peer G (2003) How accurate is MR imaging in characterization of adrenal masses: update of a long-term study. Eur J Radiol 43:113–122
7. Lafferty AR, Torpy DJ, Stowasser M, et al. (2000) A novel genetic locus for low renin hypertension: familial hyperaldosteronism type II maps to chromosome 7 (7p22). J Med Genet 37:831–5
8. Lifton RP, Dluhy RG, Powers M, Ulick S, Lalouel JM (1992) The molecular basis of glucocorticoid-remediable aldosteronism, a Mendelian cause of human hypertension. Trans Assoc Am Physicians 105:64–71
9. Nocaudie-Calzada M, Huglo D, Lambert M, Ernst O, Proye C, Wemeau JL, Marchandise X (1999) Efficacy of iodine-131 6beta-methyl-iodo-19-norcholesterol scintigraphy and computed tomography in patients with primary aldosteronism. Eur J Nucl Med 26:1326–1332
10. Pascoe L, Curnow KM, Slutsker L, et al. (1992) Glucocorticoid-suppressible hyperaldosteronism results from hybrid genes created by unequal crossovers between *CYP11B1* and *CYP11B2*. Proc Natl Acad Sci USA 89: 8327–31
11. Rossi H, Kim A, Prinz RS (2002) Primary aldosteronism in the era of laparoscopic adrenalectomy. Am Surg 68: 253–256
12. Rutherford JC, Taylor WL, Stowasser M, Gordon RD (1998) Success of surgery for primary aldosteronism judged by residual autonomous aldosterone production. World J Surg 22:1243–5
13. Sawka AM, Young RF, Thompson GB, Grant CS, Farley DR, Leibson C, van Heerden J (2001) Primary aldosteronism: factors associated with normalization of blood pressure after surgery. Ann Intern Med 135:258–261
14. Siren J, Valimaki M, Huikuri K, Sivula A, Voutilainen P, Haapiainen R (1998) Adrenalectomy for primary aldosteronism: long-term follow-up study in 29 patients. World J Surg 22:418–21
15. Young WF (1999) Primary aldosteronism: a common and curable form of hypertension. Cardiol Rev 7:207–214
16. Young WF (2003) Primary aldosteronism – changing concepts in diagnosis and treatment. Endocrinology 144: 2208–2213

13 Primary Adrenocortical Carcinoma

Charles A.G. Proye, François N. Pattou, Jonathan Armstrong

13.1   Introduction

Primary adrenocortical carcinomas account for 0.02% of all carcinomas and rank amongst the least common malignant endocrine tumors. However, after anaplastic thyroid carcinomas they are the most malignant endocrine tumors. Twenty to 40% have metastasized at the time of presentation, and the overall 5-year survival is 19–35% [1, 2]. Early adrenalectomy is the only potential means of cure.

13.2   Incidence

Functioning adrenocortical neoplasms with clinical manifestations of hypersecretion occur in four patients per million; roughly half will be adenomas and the rest carcinomas. Adrenocortical carcinomas at autopsy account for 2.5 patients per million. Hence the suggested incidence of non-functioning adrenocortical carcinomas should be 0.6–1.7 per million of the population [3].

If these figures are matched with the prevalence of adrenal masses found incidentally (i.e. 0.6–1.3% of the ambulatory population) it is evident that, in the setting of the adrenal "incidentaloma", non-functioning adrenocortical carcinomas are an uncommon cause. Van Heerden et al. [4] reported that only 4 of 342 (1.2%) patients with incidentalomas at the Mayo Clinic had adrenocortical cancers. Our experience in Lille, France, of adrenal incidentalomas is consistent with this finding. Of 213 adrenal incidentalomas, of which 103 were operated upon, there were 5 (2%) adrenocortical carcinomas [5]. Pheochromocytomas and metastasis to the adrenal gland should really be the primary concern in this setting as they occur in 1–15% and 4–22% respectively [6].

The characteristics of our 54 adrenocortical carcinomas, among 486 patients who underwent adrenal surgery, are listed in Table 1.

Table 1. Adrenal surgery in Lille, France, during the period January 1985–December 1999

	Hyperplasia	Benign	Malignant	Total
Pheochromocytoma	–	116	35	151
Cushing	12	27	13[a]	52
Conn	5	104	–	109
Virilizing	–	6	5[a]	11
Feminizing	–	–	2[a]	2
Non-secretory	3	91	32[a]	126
Metastasis	–	–	18	18
Others	8	7	2[a]	17
Total	28	351	107	486

[a] Fifty-four malignant adrenal tumors: 46 adrenocortical carcinoma, 8 others.

13.3   Clinical Presentation

Women are affected twice as often as men. Three clinical patterns can be encountered.

13.3.1   Mass Syndrome Without Any Clinical Evidence of Hypersecretion (30%)

The patient himself notices a large, and on occasion a huge, flank tumor (Fig. 1). Alternatively, discovery is by the patient's physician when presenting with flank pain or pyrexia of unknown origin (possible tumor necrosis factor secretion), asthenia or weight loss. Subtle signs of hormonal secretion can be discovered: for instance, glycosuria or a shadow of a moustache on a woman's upper lip. Additionally there may be signs of inferior vena caval compression or obstruction (i.e. ankle edema) secondary to a neoplastic caval thrombus. Tumor rupture or hemorrhage is rarely encountered.

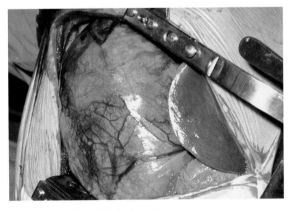

Fig. 1. Huge right-sided adrenal mass

13.3.2   Overt Clinical Syndrome of Hypersecretion (60%)

Women younger than 40 years are more often affected. In patients with malignant adrenocortical tumors, the syndrome is of almost pure hypercortisolism in 30% of patients, virilization in 22%, feminization in 10%, hyperaldosteronism in 2.5%, and mixed secretions in 35% [1, 7]. Although adrenocortical carcinomas account for 5–10% of patients with hypercortisolism, 80% of cases of hypercortisolism are in fact due to corticotropin-secreting pituitary tumors. Notably, however, 40% of patients with Cushing's syndrome and detected adrenal neoplasms do indeed have malignant tumors. Virilizing tumors are malignant in 30% of cases, feminizing tumors in male adults are virtually always malignant, and pure aldosterone-secreting tumors are malignant in less than 1% of cases [8]. Mixed hormonal secretion is highly suspicious of malignancy. Rare adrenal tumor hypersecretion syndromes that have also been noted include ectopic hyperinsulinism with hypoglycemia (Anderson's syndrome) or ectopic hyperparathyroidism with hypercalcemia. There are even case reports of these two rare hypersecretion syndromes occurring synchronously in the same patients [9].

13.3.3   Adrenal "Incidentaloma" (10%?)

The smallest reported metastasizing adrenocortical carcinoma was 3 cm in diameter and weighed 25 g [10]. Metastases occurred postoperatively. There is no evidence in the literature that solid, non-secreting adrenal incidentalomas smaller than 3 cm in diameter are malignant (i.e. metastatic at presentation). The obvious thought arises, however, that in the development of an adrenocortical carcinoma there must be a point at which mutagenesis occurs and a small island of neoplastic cells develop in a relatively normal sized adrenal gland before presumably expanding relatively rapidly in size. Must the adrenal really be more than 3 or 4 cm before malignancy can occur? The evidence, however, would tend to support this. At the same time can benign adrenocortical adenomas turn into malignant tumors with time? Current genetic and biochemical studies do not support this possibility. Most of the adrenocortical carcinomas are monoclonal, whereas the majority of adrenal adenomas are polyclonal [11]. Conversely genetic changes in the locus 11p15 are common in adrenocortical carcinomas and very rarely seen in adrenal adenomas [12]. Point mutations of ras genes are equally encountered in 12% of adrenal carcinomas and adenomas [13]. Subsequent studies may clarify whether a subset of adrenal adenomas are prone to malignant change or whether adrenocortical carcinomas begin de novo.

13.4 Determining Malignancy in an Adrenal Mass

The great challenge for the surgeon is to try preoperatively to assess the likelihood of malignancy in any referred adrenal mass.

The patient is approached in a routine fashion as for all adrenal masses. An accurate history of symptomatology is taken. An accurate family history is taken for any genetic predispositions. A full clinical examination is undertaken. Which imaging modalities have been utilized, and are they satisfactory? Is the tumor secretory or non-secretory? Have all the appropriate biochemical investigations been performed to assess adrenal hyperfunction or non-secretory status? Is there appropriate functional and morphological correlation, i.e. can a hypersecretory state be attributed to the side of the adrenal mass?

13.4.1 Clinical Factors Suggestive of Malignancy

Certain features of an adrenal mass, irrespective of size, are highly suggestive of malignancy, especially if combined. They include:
- Abrupt onset of disease
- Pyrexia
- Abdominal pain
- Abdominal mass
- Inferior vena caval compression or obstruction
- Associated breast carcinoma, osteosarcomas, or brain tumors (Li-Fraumeni syndrome)
- Mixed hormone secretion
- Mild androgenic changes (an indication of the secretion of precursors)
- Feminizing syndrome
- Ectopic secretion syndrome

13.4.2 Biochemical Factors Suggestive of Malignancy

- Urinary ketosteroid production in excess of 30–40 mg/day
- Elevated dehydroepiandrosterone (DHEA) levels (observed in 80% of patients [4])
- Inactive precursor secretion, pregnenolone and aldosterone precursors, especially 18-hydroxylated compounds [14]

13.5 Preoperative Imaging of Suspect Adrenal Lesions

In addition to distant metastases and tumor size, imaging studies can provide much information suggestive of malignancy.

Imaging findings suggestive of malignancy include the following:
- Computerized tomography (CT)
  - Stipled calcifications
  - A poorly delineated, rugged more or less square-shaped tumor, with the periodic appearance of prominent buds, very different from the round-shaped adenoma (Fig. 2)
  - Areas of necrosis (Figs. 3, 4). Benign tumors usually homogeneously enhance. Malignant tumors will inhomogeneously enhance due to areas of necrosis.
  - Aortocaval adenopathies
  - Evidence of local invasion; bearing in mind that CT is known to overestimate the extent of liver and caval invasion
- Magnetic resonance imaging (MRI)
  - Heterogeneously increased early T2-weighted signal
  - Weak and late enhancement after injection of gadolinium
  - Finding of an intravascular signal identical to the tumor signal is of paramount importance, and diagnostic of malignancy

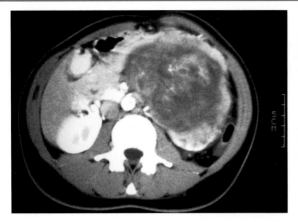

Fig. 2. CT image of left adrenocortical carcinoma showing irregular contours and central necrosis

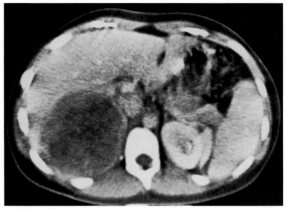

Fig. 4. CT image of right adrenocortical carcinoma illustrating heterogeneity of the cortex

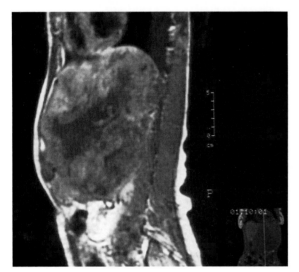

Fig. 3. Sagittal CT image of left-sided adrenocortical carcinoma

Both CT and MRI will determine if the adrenal mass is lipid-rich or lipid-poor. Lipid-rich masses have a high probability of being benign and lipid-poor adrenal masses are more likely to be malignant. There are exceptions, however, and lipid poor adrenal cortical adenomas have been described. On plain, unenhanced, CT an attenuation of <10 Hounsfield Units (HU) is likely to be benign. Lesions of >30 HU are more likely to be malignant. With contrast enhancement there are also different retention characteristics. Benign lesions exhibit >70% washout of contrast at 15 min, whereas malignant lesions wash out <20% of the contrast in a similar time. Using chemical shift MRI, lipid-rich adenomas show a decrease in relative signal intensity of 34%, whereas non-adenomas show no significant change in relative signal intensity.

The likelihood of malignancy for tumors increases with size from 1.5 to 6 cm in diameter but remains limited because only 1 in 4,000 cases (0.03%) are malignant [6]. Operating on all patients with incidentalomas would probably result in more surgical deaths than patients cured by removing small adrenocortical carcinomas. However, in young patients, lifelong observation may be unacceptable and may not be cost effective, and benign adrenocortical adenomas are less common in young patients.

For patients with adrenal tumors larger than 6 cm in diameter, adrenocortical carcinomas account for up to 15% of cases [6, 7, 15, 16]. Surgery is therefore recommended in patients with tumors of this size.

13.5.1   NP-59 Scintigraphy

Lack of, or very weak uptake in the presence of, a normal contralateral uptake [17] suggests malignancy. However, 18 instances of adrenocortical carcinomas exhibiting clear uptake of NP-59 have been described [18]. Virtually all were highly differentiated carcinomas with overt clinical hypersecretion.

13.5.2   Positron Emission Scintigraphy

A large variety of positron emitter tracers have been used for positron emission scintigraphy (PET) imaging. The most widely used tracer is 18F-fluoro-2-de-oxy-D-glucose (18F-FDG). Deoxyglucose (DG) is a glucose analog that enters the cell using specific transmembrane carrier proteins (especially GLUT-1). Once within the cytoplasm, DG is phosphorylated to FG-6-phosphate but does not appear to be further metabo-

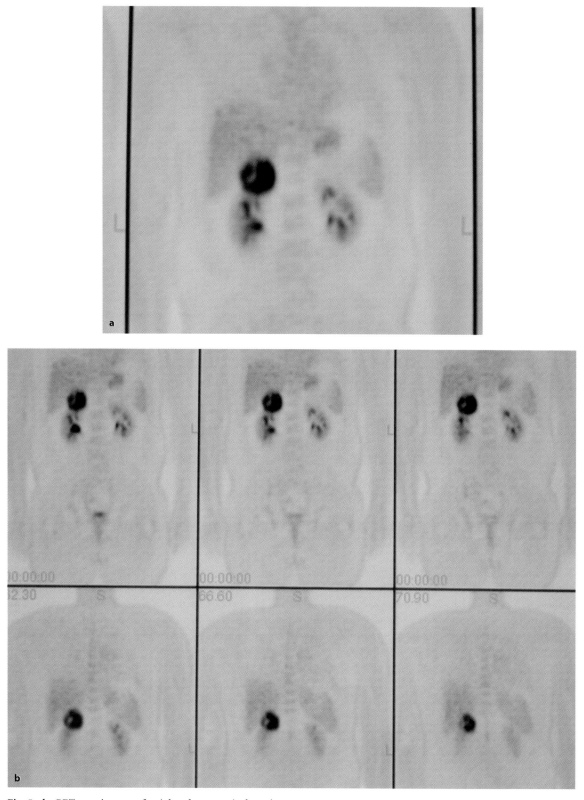

Fig. 5a, b. PET scan images of a right adrenocortical carcinoma

lized. In most malignant tumors there is an increase in the glycolytic metabolism which accounts for an increase in FDG uptake [19]. Retrospective [20] and prospective [21] studies have shown PET to be both sensitive (100%) and specific (94%) in delineating benign from malignant adrenal cortical lesions. It also has an excellent additional role in highlighting secondary metastatic adrenal disease that would have been missed on CT or MRI [21]. If available it should be included in the workup for initial staging as well as for follow-up (Fig. 5).

13.5.3   Bone Scintigraphy: Tc99

Bone scintigraphy should be performed routinely in all patients with a suspicion of adrenocortical carcinoma; it will illustrate the presence of any disseminated metastases and necessitate a palliative rather than surgical treatment.

13.5.4   The Role of Needle Biopsy for a Mass Lesion

Needle biopsy should not be routinely used because of its lack of sensitivity and the risk of a capsular tear with tumor spillage. It could, however, be utilized in some patients for diagnosis of metastatic adrenal disease from a known extra-adrenal primary.

13.6   Criteria of Malignancy of Cortical Tumors

The criteria determining whether an adrenal neoplasm is benign or malignant are not precise. Currently, the only accepted criteria are metastasis, either synchronous or metachronous, and local invasion into surrounding structures. Adrenal tumors metastasize to the lung (72%), the liver (55%), the peritoneum (33%), the bone (24%), the contralateral adrenal (15%), and the brain (10%).

Local recurrence at reoperation is not an absolute criterion of malignancy because intraoperative disruption of the capsule of a benign tumor may result in local seeding, with growth and apparent invasion.

Large adrenal neoplasms are more likely to be malignant. Critical size or weight usually ranges from 6 to 10 cm in diameter and from 40 to 100 g respectively. The size suggestive of malignant tumors may be

Table 2. Weiss criteria for malignancy (more than three features is indicative of malignancy)

High nuclear grade
Mitotic rate >5/50 high-power fields
Atypical mitoses
Eosinophilic tumor cell cytoplasm (>75% of tumor cells)
Diffuse architectural pattern (>33% of tumor) with broad fibrous and trabecular bands
Foci of confluent necrosis
Venous invasion
Sinusoidal invasion
Capsular invasion

smaller for androgen-secreting tumors than for other tumors.

A method of defining malignancy histologically has been relatively simply defined by Weiss [22]. This classification incorporates nine histological features (Table 2). The presence of three or more of these features in a specimen correlates well with a clinically malignant outcome.

The Weiss histopathological system is now the most commonly used method for assessing malignancy because of its simplicity and reliability and excellent interobserver agreement [23]. Some of the criteria are, however, less reliable than others and recently a statistically modified system of weighting has been proposed [23] (2.mitotic rate × 2.cytoplasm × abnormal mitosis × necrosis × capsular invasion) with a significant correlation with the Weiss system.

Cytological criteria are not consistent enough to predict tumor behavior: cellular atypia and abundance of mitosis are only suggestive, as is aneuploidy flow cytometry [24]. Needle biopsy is not recommended for diagnosis because it cannot differentiate between an adrenocortical adenoma and an adrenocortical carcinoma. There is also concern about rupture of the tumor capsule. A high mitotic index is perhaps more of prognostic than diagnostic significance in malignant adrenocortical cancers [25].

Major diagnostic problems arise in the evaluation of patients with tumors between 3 and 6 cm in diameter, exhibiting weak mitotic activity, with scarce areas of necrosis without obvious capsular invasion. In such cases, immunohistochemistry may prove helpful as benign tumors stain positively for vimentin (connective cell antigen) in 14% of cases versus 80–90% for malignant tumors. Synaptophysin (neuroendocrine cell antigen) is also more often expressed in malignant tumors [7]. MIB-1, another immunohistochemical marker, has also shown recent promise in delineating benign from malignant adrenal tumors [23, 26].

13.7 Staging, Surgical Indications, and Preoperative Treatment

Adrenocortical carcinomas are staged according to the stages described by MacFarlane, and modified by Sullivan (Table 3). This classification has one major drawback (i.e., malignancy in stage I is based on histological criteria only). Whether all of these tumors are malignant is unknown, so that the assumption that all are malignant may lead to an overly optimistic affirmation of the results of surgery.

All tumors at Stage I, II, III, whether diagnosed preoperatively or intraoperatively, should be resected. The need to operate on patients with Stage IV disease and distant metastases is controversial because these patients have an average postoperative survival of 3 months and a 1-year actuarial survival of 10%. Widespread metastases in elderly patients should dissuade surgical treatment. Conversely, in young patients, a solitary metastasis should not be a contraindication to surgery, and in rare cases pre- and postoperative adjunctive chemotherapy has provided long-lasting survival with complete remission.

13.8 Macroscopic Morphology, Preoperative Imaging, and Surgical Strategy

At the time of surgery, most adrenocortical carcinomas are large tumors, ranging from between 5 and 28.5 cm in diameter (average, 12.4 cm) and between 33 and 3,100 g in weight (average, 849 g) according to Javadpour [27]. In our experience the largest tumor weighed 4,600 g (see Fig. 6).

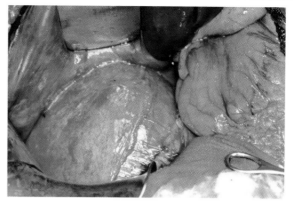

Fig. 6. A 4.6-kg right-sided adrenocortical tumor displacing the liver. Thoracoabdominal approach

The capsule of these grayish-white tumors can be thick or thin. When thin with large superficial veins, the capsule is prone to rupture and local seeding. When thick, the capsule adheres to adjacent organs, the liver or the kidney, which may be invaded. Such adhesions may lead to extensive surgery; thus it is often wiser to search for a plane of cleavage under the liver or the kidney capsule. It is necessary to bear in mind that CT scans often overestimate the local invasion.

Macroscopic venous invasion is common and more often observed on the right-hand side (20% of surgical cases), often encompassing the inferior vena cava. Surgeons should obviously be prepared for this situation. The neoplastic thrombus of an adrenocortical carcinoma invades the venous wall more frequently than a renal adenocarcinoma and can reach up to the right atrium. Assessment or exclusion of venous invasion may influence the surgical strategy and in some cases it is necessary to use cardiopulmonary bypass. Therefore, careful evaluation of the inferior vena cava, suprahepatic veins, and right atrium by MRI, Doppler flow studies, and right atrium echography is mandatory. The effectiveness of MRI has largely eliminated the need for inferior vena cava phlebography (Fig. 7).

Table 3. Staging of adrenocortical carcinomas. (Adapted from MacFarlane [43], used with permission)

Stage	Size (cm)	Weight (g)	Local extension	Lymph node extension	Distant metastasis
I	<5	and <50	None	None	None
II	>5	or >50	+None	None	None
III	–	–		or +	None
IV	–	–	+	and +	None
	or –	–	–	–	+

+, Present.

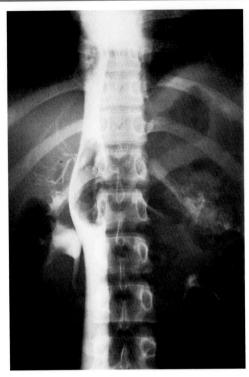

Fig. 7. Venogram illustrating a large vena caval tumor thrombus emanating from a left adrenocortical carcinoma

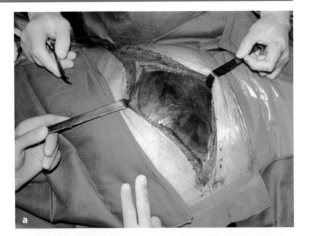

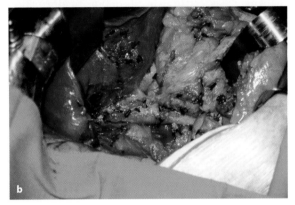

Fig. 8. a The thoracoabdominal incision for a large relatively anterior right adrenocortical carcinoma. **b** The thoracoabdominal approach provides excellent visualization of this large right adrenal mass shown here with the liver reflected superiorly. Excellent vascular access provided by the thoracoabdominal approach. Note presence of multiple resorbable clips for lymphostasis

Involved regional nodes occur in 10–45% of cases and should be resected with the tumor. They do not impede the surgical strategy [28].

13.9   Surgical Strategy and Technical Operative Risks

Wide surgical exposure is mandatory for primary vascular control, tumor removal with associated lumbar fossa clearance, and aortocaval node dissection, with a possible extension to the adjacent organs and sometimes to the inferior vena cava. Therefore, a posterior approach is not indicated in these patients with large and often invasive tumors. There currently appears to be no place for laparoscopic surgery.

In most cases, either right or left sided, an extended subcostal transverse laparotomy is the best choice, with a view to possible extension by sternotomy if extensive inferior vena cava extension is suspected or present. Access to the right adrenal vein is difficult, especially in patients with large tumors. On the left side, by contrast, it is relatively easy if Cattell's maneuver is used as a first step, combining mobilization of the right colon to the left and a Kocher's maneuver to expose the

left renal and adrenal veins at the vena cava before tumor manipulation.

Some huge right-sided tumors, creeping behind the liver, still require a thoracoabdominal approach for adequate visualization and vessel control as illustrated (Fig. 8a–c). Occasionally extremely large left sided adrenal tumors may also require a thoracoabdominal incision to allow extraction. The thoracoabdominal or thoracophrenolaparotomy incision is facilitated by the patient being placed in the lateral decubitus position with the arm supported. The incision is based on the 8th or 9th rib. Pain can be reduced by resecting the rib over which the incision is based rather than forcefully retracting the ribs and thereby causing painful fractures. The corresponding intercostal nerve is retracted and must not be entrapped at the end by the closure. Care is then taken to divide the diaphragm peripher-

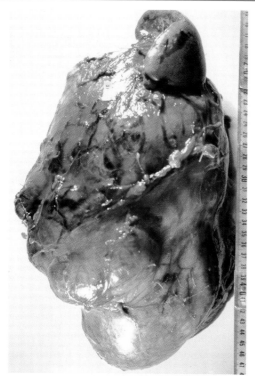

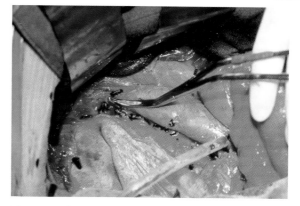

Fig. 10. Wedge resection of a small area of the wall of the vena cava after excision of a right adrenocortical carcinoma with limited caval involvement

Fig. 9. En bloc resection of left adrenocortical carcinoma with spleen and left kidney

ally 2 cm from its thoracic insertion, not radially to preserve phrenic nerve function and minimize postoperative respiratory embarrassment. The adrenal can then be approached in the routine fashion.

All adjacent invaded organs should be resected while ensuring a functioning kidney on the contralateral side. Formal liver resection is rarely needed and may require vascular exclusion of the liver. Often a cleavage plane can be found under the liver capsule. Left pancreatectomy with splenectomy is sometimes indicated on the left side for adequate resection of large invasive tumors. The adjacent kidney is rarely invaded by the tumor, but nephrectomy is often helpful, if there are dense adhesions, to obtain proper aorto-caval clearance (Fig. 9). Liberal use of resorbable clips is recommended for adequate lymphostasis and sometimes for control of the thoracic duct at its origin.

Extension to the inferior vena cava is the major surgical challenge, especially on the right side (15–20% of cases). Direct invasion, if extensive, makes resection difficult and the hope of cure unlikely. Limited invasion can be treated often by wedge resection (Fig. 10). Occasionally segmental caval resection is necessary, with or without a graft, utilizing a bypass procedure. Limited intracaval thrombus can be flushed either di-

rectly [29] or with a combination of caval clamping, vascular exclusion of the liver, and the use of a large Fogarty catheter in the atrium [30]. If the thrombus extends superiorly to the right atrium, a thoracoabdominal or combined sternotomy-laparotomy are mandatory for primary control of the inferior vena cava in the pericardium. If it invades the right atrium, cardiopulmonary bypass with cardiac arrest is required. Use of external veno-venous bypass remains controversial, but appears to be useful in selected cases [1, 31, 32]. A solitary liver metastasis should be removed when it can be done safely. Care must be taken to avoid rupturing the capsule to prevent local recurrence. We always use drains and recommend cryopreserving tumor tissue for subsequent biochemical and genetic studies.

13.10   Specific Postoperative Care

Not uncommonly, within hours after surgery, patients may exhibit hemodynamic manifestations of septic shock with negative blood cultures. This may be due to release of tumor necrosis factor (TNF) and TNF-like or other factors during tumor manipulation. Symptomatic treatment is effective. Initially stress doses and then maintenance doses of hydrocortisone are mandatory for patients with secretory tumors and for patients treated preoperatively with mitotane and ketoconazole. Drains are removed after the resumption of food intake to decrease the chances of a problematic chylous fistula.

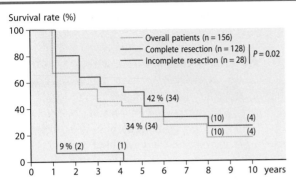

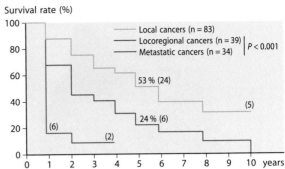

Fig. 11. Survival curves of patients overall and of patients with complete and incomplete resections. (With permission from Icard et al. [1])

Fig. 12. Survival rates in relation to extent of disease. (With permission from Icard et al. [1])

13.11   Overall Results and Prognostic Factors

Unfortunately, the intra- and postoperative mortality within 30 days of operation is about 10% [1, 4]. Most of the mortality occurs in poor-risk patients with Stage III or IV disease undergoing an extensive resection, with an occasional death from pulmonary embolism after isolated adrenalectomy.

A review of 548 patients with adrenocortical carcinomas from seven large series in the literature from 1980 to 1990 [1], of whom 290 were operated on with curative intent, revealed that:

1. Overall mean survival was 29 months, ranging from 33 to 71 months for the curative group and from 6 to 27 for the non-curative group.
2. Actuarial 5-year survival rates ranged from 16 to 34% overall and from 32 to 62% for the curative group.

The results of a French nationwide survey of 156 adrenocortical carcinoma cases during the same period (1980–1990) are illustrated (Fig. 11). The overall survival rate was 34% and for the curative group was 42%. Survival rates for patients undergoing an incomplete resection was 9% at 1 year [1].

Tumor stage was the most important factor predicting prognosis, with a 5-year actuarial survival of 53% for locally invasive carcinomas (Stage 1, 33%; and Stage II, 55%). Survival rate was 24% in patients with Stage III disease and 0% in patients with Stage IV disease (Fig. 12) [1, 4, 11].

The patients who were younger than 35 years with non-functioning tumors or with tumors that secreted androgen had a slightly better survival. Gender, tumor size, associated nehrectomy and cellular lymphadenectomy had no impact on survival [1, 7, 11].

13.12   Surgery of Metastases and Recurrences

Metachronous surgery for solitary metastases is rarely helpful, but reoperation for local recurrences is advisable when complete resection is possible. Such patients have a 5-year survival rate of 28% [1, 11, 31, 32].

13.13   Adjuvant Therapy

Mitotane, or *o,p*-DDD, is the only drug that has proven to be effective in some patients. Recommended dosages of 8–12 g/day are unfortunately associated with neurotoxicity, nausea, intractable diarrhea, and adrenal insufficiency requiring cortisol substitution. Thus, only 60–70% of patients can tolerate this therapy [33].

Preoperative treatment with mitotane (8–12 g/day) is indicated in two situations: metastatic disease and severe hypercortisolism. Mitotane successfully treats Cushing's syndrome in up to 75% of patients [34] and sometimes causes partial or dramatic shrinkage of the primary tumor and the metastases. Cortisol replacement therapy is essential as hypocortisolism results in some patients. Unfortunately, many patients cannot tolerate the nausea and other side effects of mitotane, which limits its successful application. We recommend using mitotane for 3 or 4 weeks before surgery, and patients who respond to mitotane have a more favorable prognosis.

Mitotane has a long half-life, and monitoring of serum levels can allow a lower maintenance dose for better tolerance. Alternatively, ketoconazole (400 mg/day) can be used to control the hypercortisolism.

Numerous studies have shown that mitotane fails to improve overall survival [1, 2, 4, 35–38] and that no

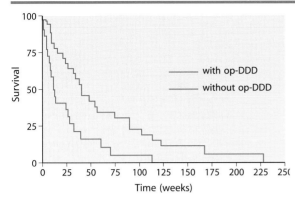

Fig. 13. Stage IV survival. Effect of mitotane (*o,p*-DDD). (With permission from Icard et al. [1])

more than 20% of patients respond in terms of tumor growth. In patients with metastases, however, mitotane can improve survival. In a French retrospective study of 253 patients with adrenocortical carcinoma, mitotane was given as an adjuvant therapy in 53.8% of the cases. The survival advantage of mitotane was only apparent in Stage IV disease (Fig. 13).

Each of the above series also includes more than a few anecdotal cases of tumor recurrences and metastases shrinking impressively for 1–2 years with survival up to 8 years and even a few cases of surgically verified disappearance of metastases in patients who received mitotane [1, 32, 35, 39]. We are also aware of unpublished data of overgrowth or reappearance of metastases when mitotane was discontinued after years of response to the drug. The only long-term survivors after surgery for metastatic adrenocortical carcinoma have received mitotane therapy. Personally, even after surgery for Stage I and II adrenocortical carcinoma, we would recommend lifelong treatment with mitotane if it is tolerated because it is the best hope for long-term survival.

Various other combination chemotherapy regimens are currently under evaluation. In one phase II trial using a combination of mitotane with infusional doxorubicin, vincristine, and etoposide in patients with metastatic adrenocortical carcinoma, responses were obtained in 22% of patients [40]. The superiority of this regime over single-agent mitotane is debatable however. More effective P-glycoprotein antagonists are needed.

Radiation therapy is usually ineffective [2, 41].

13.14 Adrenocortical Carcinoma in Childhood

Patients younger than 16 years with adrenal neoplasms are more likely to have malignant tumors than adults. A survey of the English literature between 1956 and 1986 provided 209 cases of children with adrenocortical neoplasms [42], 66% of which were malignant. Average size and weight of malignant versus benign tumors were 9 cm versus 4 cm and 466 g versus 43 g respectively. Female-male ratio was 2.2 to 1, and the mean age at presentation was 4.6 years (range 5 days–16.5 years). Hirsutism was the most common presenting symptom (51%) followed by hypercortisolism (30%) and feminization (10%): 8% of the tumors were non-functional. Of interest is the association with congenital abnormalities such as hemihypertrophy, Beckwith-Weidemann syndrome, vascular malformations, urological abnormalities, and tumors of the central nervous syndrome. Adrenal neoplasms have also been reported in patients with salt-losing congenital hyperplasia [42].

The biochemical profile in children is similar to that in adults. Surgery is the only means offering cure. The role of adjuvant therapy is unproven. Average survival is 24 months but can reach up to 8 years. It should also be kept in mind that 40% of neuroblastomas are located in the adrenals and are now commonly diagnosed by antenatal ultrasound.

13.15 Summary

Adrenocortical carcinoma is a rare tumor, and, unfortunately, patients with this neoplasm have a grim prognosis. Early detection and surgical removal offer the only chance of cure. Further studies must be done first to detect and then treat patients with small malignant tumors and to develop new forms of adjuvant therapy.

References

1. Icard P, Chapuis Y, Andreasssian B, et al. (1992) Adrenocortical carcinoma in surgically treated patients: A retrospective study on 156 cases by the French Association of Endocrine Surgery. Surgery 112:972
2. Venkatesh S, Hickey RC, Sellin RV, et al. (1989) Adrenal cortical carcinoma. Cancer 64:765
3. Copeland PM (1984) The incidentally discovered adrenal mass. Ann Surg 199:116
4. van Heerden JA, Grant CS, Weaver AL (1993) Primary carcinoma of the adrenal cortex: An institutional surgical perspective. Acta Chir Aust 25:216

5. Proye C, Jafari Manjili M, Combemale F, et al. (1998) Experience gained from operation of 103 adrenal incidentalomas. Langenbecks Arch Surg 383:330–333

6. Mcleod MK (1993) Adrenal incidentaloma. Acta Chir Aust 25:202

7. Chapuis Y, Icard P (1994) Cortico-surrénalomes malins: In: Chapuis Y, Peix JL (eds) Chirurgie des glandes surrénales. Arnette, Paris, p 61

8. Ludwig, Nierderle B, Roka R, et al. (1993) Isolieter primärer Aldosterismus bei Nebennierenkarzinom. Kasuitik und Leteraturübersicht. Acta Chir Aust 25:212

9. Proye C, Fossati P, Ben Soussan D, et al. Syndrome d'Anderson avec pseudo-hyperparathyroïdisme. Chirurgie (Paris) 111:364

10. Gicquel C, Lelond-Rrancillard M, Bertagna W, et al. (1994) Clonal analysis of human adrenocortical carcinomas and secreting adenomas. Clin Endocrinol 40:465

11. Icard P, Louvel A, Chapuis Y (1992) Survival rates and prognostic factors in adrenocortical carcinoma. World J Surg 16:453

12. Gicquel C, Bertagna X, Schneid H, et al. (1994) Rearrangements at the 11p15 locus and overexpression of insulin-like growth factor-II gene in sporadic adrenocortical tumors. J Clin Metab 78:1444

13. Yashiro T, Hara H, Fulton NC, et al. (1994) Point mutations of ras-genes in human adrenal cortical tumors: Absence in adrenocortical hyperplasia. World J Surg 18:455

14. Aupetit-Faisant B, Tabarin A, Battaglia C, et al. (1991) Incohérence de la voie des minéralocorticoïdes dans les carcinomes surrénaliens: Un signe de malignité? Ann Endocrinol (Paris) 52:149

15. Khafagi FA, Gross MD, Shapiro B, et al. (1991) Clinical significance of the large adrenal mass. Br J Surg 78:828

16. Peix JL (1994) Incidentalomes. In: Chapuis Y, Peix JL (eds) Chirurgie des glandes surrénales. Arnette, Paris, p 115

17. Gross MD, Shapiro B, Francis IR, et al. (1994) Scintigraphic evaluation of clinically silent adrenal mass. J Nucl Med 35:1145

18. Pasieka JL, McLeod MK, Thompson NW, et al. (1992) Adrenal scintigraphy of well-differentiated (functioning) adrenocortical carcinomas: Potential surgical pitfalls. Surgery 112:884

19. Rubello D, Ruffini V, Casara D, et al. (2002) Clinical role of positron emission tomography (PET) in endocrine tumors. Panminerva Med 44:185–196

20. Yun M, Kim W, Alnafisi N, et al. (2001) 18F-FDG PET in characterizing adrenal lesions detected on CT or MRI. J Nucl Med 42:1795–9

21. Becherer A, Vierhapper H, Potzi C, et al. (2001) FDP-PET in adrenocortical carcinoma. Cancer Biother Radiopharm 16:289–95

22. Weiss LM (1995) Comparative histological study of 43 metastasizing and nonmetastasizing adrenocortical tumors. Am J Surg Pathol 8:163–169

23. Aubert S, Wacrenier A, Leroy X, et al. (2002) Weiss system revisited: a clinicopathological and immunohistochemical study of 49 adrenocortical tumors. Am J Surg Pathol 26:1612–9

24. Hosaka Y, Rainwater LM, Grant CS, et al. (1987) Adrenal carcinoma: Nuclear DNA study by flow cytometry. Surgery 102:1027

25. Weiss LM, Medeiors LJ, Vickery AL (1989) Pathological features of prognostic significance in adrenocortical carcinoma. Am J Surg Pathol 13:202

26. Vargas MP, Vargas HI, Kleiner DE, et al. (1997) Adrenocortical neoplasms: role of prognostic markers MIB-1, P53, and RB. Am J Surg Pathol 21:556–562

27. Javadpour N (1987) Principles and management of adrenal cancer. Springer-Verlag, Berlin

28. Icard P, Louvel A, Chapuis Y (1990) Fréquence et valeur pronostique de l'extension ganglionnaire et rénale dans les corticosurrénalomes. Lyon Chir 86:151

29. Ritchey M, Kinard R, Novicki DE (1987) Adrenal tumors: Involvement of the inferior vena cava. J Urol 138:1134

30. Benoit G, Darteville P (1990) Ablation d'un thrombus cave retro-hépatique sans abord thoracique. Ann Urol (Paris) 24:384

31. Pommier RF, Brennan MF (1992) An eleven year experience with adrenal carcinoma. Surgery 112:963

32. Decker RA, Kuehner ME (1991) Adrenocortical carcinoma. Am Surg 57:502

33. Decker RA, Elson P, Hogan TF, et al. (1991) Eastern cooperation oncology group study 1879: Mitotan and Adriamycin in patient with advanced adrenocortical carcinoma. Surgery 111:1006

34. Lack EE, Travis WD, Oertel JE (1990) Adrenal cortical neoplasms. In: Lack EE (ed) Pathology of the adrenal glands. Churchill Livingstone, Edinburgh, p 115

35. Luton JP, Cerdas S, Billaud L, et al. (1990) Adrenocortical carcinoma: Clinical features, prognostic factors and therapeutic results in 105 patients from a single centre (1967–1987). N Eng J Med 322:1195

36. Henley DJ, van Heerden JA, Grant CS, et al. (1983) Adrenal cortical carcinoma: A continuing challenge. Surgery 94:926

37. Cohn K, Gottesman L, Brennan MF (1986) Adrenocortical carcinoma. Surgery 100:1170

38. Icard P, Goudet P, Charpenay C, et al. (2001) Adrenocortical carcinomas: surgical trends and results of a 253-patient series from the French association of endocrine surgeons study group. World J Surg 25:891–897

39. Boven E, Vermoken JB, Slotten HV, et al. (1984) Complete response of metastasized adrenal cortical carcinoma with o.p'-DDD: Case report and literature review. Cancer 53:26

40. Abraham J, Bakke S, Rutt A, et al. (2002) A phase II trial of combination chemotherapy and surgical resection for the treatment of metastatic adrenocortical carcinoma: continuous infusion of doxorubicin, vincristine, and etoposide with daily mitotane as a P-glycoprotein antagonist. Cancer 94:2333–43

41. Percarpio B, Knowlton AH (1976) Radiation therapy of adrenal cortical carcinoma. Acta Radiother 15:288

42. Scott HW Jr (1987) Experience with adrenocortical neoplasms in children. Am Surg 53:117

43. MacFarlane D (1958) Cancer of the adrenal cortex: the natural history, prognosis, and treatment in a study of 55 cases. Ann R Coll Surg Engl 23:155

14 Recurrent Adrenocortical Carcinoma

Paolo Miccoli, Pietro Iacconi

One of the reasons that make this tumor such a threatening disease (actually the second most lethal endocrine neoplasm after anaplastic thyroid carcinoma) is its proneness to both recurrences and distant metastases, very often synchronous with the recurrence itself. In spite of the most careful surgery at the time of first operation in more than 60% of the cases, adrenocortical carcinoma (ACC) recurs involving several adjacent and even distant organs. Since it is well known that medical therapy has very poor efficacy (if any) in treating these patients [14], surgery remains the only option, if not for cure, for an acceptable survival in the presence of a recurrent disease.

14.1 Epidemiology

According to the Memorial Sloan-Kettering Cancer Center experience [21], resection of a local or distant recurrence was performed in 47 of 113 patients, with almost half undergoing a third operation; one patient underwent a seventh resection! Similar experiences have been quoted by most surgeons who are familiar with this often fatal illness. The high number of repeat operations is an important point to focus on because it expresses the growth of the tumor. As in any other malignancy the possibility of recurrence is related to the stage of the disease at presentation. In fact, Sulli-

van, who introduced a Staging System which is widely used [22], reported a 5-year survival rate of 100% for Stage I disease, an 80% rate in Stage II, 20% in Stage III and 0% in Stage IV. According to others [7], even in the presence of a complete resection of the carcinoma as many as 68% of the patients will develop a local recurrence. It is easy to understand that survival is linked in most of the cases with recurrence, which is generally the crucial occurrence in the natural history of treated disease.

The relapse time between first surgery and recurrence is also an important factor because it is an expression of the aggressiveness of the disease; a very early recurrence is often related to a poor prognosis. Most authors [2, 9, 18] agree that recurrence occurs most often 1–2 years after the operation. Late recurrences have also been described from 5 to even 14 years after the first operation [13].

The organs more often involved are respectively the kidney, liver, great vessels, spleen, pancreas and stomach together with retroperitoneal fat tissue and diaphragm (Figs. 1, 2). A very common site is unfortunately the peritoneal serosa, where several nodules can be found: this constitutes a dreadful situation because it makes surgical radicality a very difficult challenge. Port site metastases are a common site as well and they will be more thoroughly discussed when discussing laparoscopic access [8].

As for distant metastases repeat resection is performed in more than 50% of the cases for lung metastases, in one-third for liver and more rarely for bones [21]. Other sites such as skin or brain are exceptional.

14.2 Clinical Features

The clinical pattern of recurrent disease differs in accordance with the functional status of the primary tumor. The onset in the case of a functioning malignancy is generally, if not always, unveiled by the presence

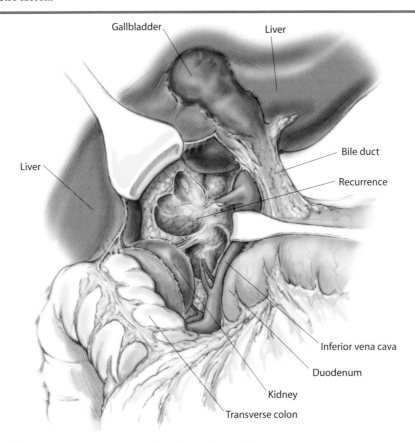

Fig. 1. Recurrent right adrenocortical carcinoma involving the liver, right kidney

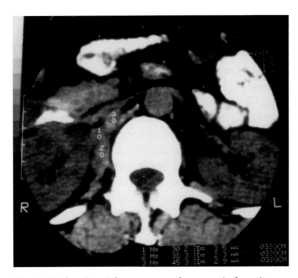

Fig. 2. CT showing right recurrent adrenocortical carcinoma infiltrating the diaphragm

of characteristic stigmata that can be divided into three types according to the type of hormone in excess: steroid, sexual and mineralocorticoid hormones. The patients usually recognize quite easily their symptoms and stigmata having experienced them before. This can be very simple in the first two instances but not in the third (mineralocorticoid) because the latter, which is exceptionally rare in malignant tumors, may cause minimal symptoms. The clinical suspicion will be confirmed by adequate hormonal serum and urinary measurements addressed by the morphologic changes which have occurred. In these patients the diagnosis is easily achieved and there is no need for measurements of hormonal markers of malignancy such as DHEA-S [17]. In contrast imaging studies should be initiated immediately to determine the exact site of the recurrence or distance metastasis. Although abdomen ultrasonography can be an excellent tool initially in particular when the liver is involved, computed tomography (CT) [12] must be considered the procedure of choice to determine the presence and the extension of a recurrence. A contrast-enhanced CT of abdomen and chest is mandatory and it will give important information about the functioning status of the contralateral kidney, since the homolateral kidney is often affected by the recurrence and thus may have to be included in the resection [21, 15].

When dealing with nonfunctioning tumors the recurrence is more often revealed by imaging studies routinely performed during follow-up because a tight surveillance by means of echography and CT is highly recommended in these patients, in particular during the first 3–5 years after primary operation. In these cases symptoms can be completely absent or nonspecific such as fever, anemia or unexplained weight loss. Pain in the flank or palpable masses are only present if the recurrent mass is very large or is invading surrounding structures and in particular nerve trunks in the retroperitoneum. In these patients the most accurate imaging workup must be accomplished before repeat surgery. Magnetic resonance imaging (MRI) might be complementary to CT when an intravascular extension of the mass is suspected: in these cases MRI is probably irreplaceable [15] and it has reduced the role for venography, which should be reserved only for patients with large masses on the right side either if some doubt about great vessels involvement still exists [19] or if a venous bypass has to be planned before operation [1]. As for fine-needle aspiration biopsy, probably everyone agrees that if it is not useful in ACC it should be excluded from the preoperative workup in these patients, having no role at all in a disease, such as recurrent ACC, where the nature of the lesion cannot be misunderstood.

14.3 Surgical Treatment

At present reoperative surgery remains the most effective, if not the only, therapeutic option for these patients. This is true for both the palliation of symptoms induced by hormonal hypersecretion in functioning tumors and to prolong the survival in all cases. In fact it is well demonstrated in all the largest series dealing with repeat surgery for ACC that surgical treatment proved to be superior in terms of life expectancy in comparison to any medical treatment [7, 18, 9, 4]. Pommier [18] demonstrated that, in his cohort of 73 cases treated in a single institution, mean survival time was 56 months for patients reoperated versus 19 months for patients who had undergone only medical therapy. Furthermore in the Cleveland Clinic's experience mitotane proved to be as efficacious as no therapy at all in treating locoregional recurrences [3].

Unfortunately, in spite of certain efficacy, repeat surgery falls short in curing these patients: Jensen et al. evaluated the NIH series of 32 cases, concluding that none of them was cured, only 20% had a 5-year survival and median survival from the time of diagnosis was less than 2 years [11]. The same authors assume that the results do not change even in the presence of the most extensive surgery. These disappointing conclusions though must not refrain surgeons from an aggressive operative attitude: there is a general agreement [21, 18, 9, 19, 4, 11] that surgery is able to improve survival dramatically and may thereby control the adverse effects of hormonal excess better than mitotane.

Thus, the decision to operate on these patients should be made in all the patients where no important medical contraindications exist: surgical contraindications consist either of extensive metastatic disease or of involvement of major arterial vessels [21]. In all other cases large debulking attempts are justified. In spite of such aggressive approaches the perioperative mortality is surprisingly low, ranging from 0% [2, 11] to 3.6% [21]. Morbidity of course cannot be negligible in such complex surgery: the complications occurring more often are bleeding and abdominal abscesses, but they are very rarely life-threatening [11].

Another characteristic indicating the difficulty of this surgery is the high rate of incomplete resections: one-third of the cases in the Memorial Sloan-Kettering Cancer Center series [21] and 36% of the patients in our institution underwent a resection that was not complete. More often the metastases' resection (69% in the same series) appeared to be radical, thus confirming the high tendency of this tumor to infiltrate locally. The natural consequences of the phenomenon are the different outcome of the patients according to the completeness of the resection: a median survival of 74 months among those undergoing a complete resection and only 16 months among those undergoing an incomplete removal of the recurrence [21].

Laparotomic access is generally the favorite access for large debulking operations, particularly on the right side, where the presence of the liver makes the thoraco-phreno-abdominal approach not particularly useful. Furthermore, it does not violate the pleural cavity and is less limiting in operating on the opposite side of the peritoneal cavity where synchronous metastases can occur (e.g. liver metastases in a recurrence on the left side). We favor bilateral subcostal incisions versus midline incisions, but sometimes the first operative incision might restrict the surgeon's choice. In our opinion it offers an optimal view of the contralateral side with the above-mentioned advantages and a better exposure of the upper abdomen, where generally the regional recurrences, more difficult to approach, are located. This is the case for infiltrations of the spleen, stomach, diaphragm, kidneys, pancreas and left colon flexure. Thoracoabdominal access remains mandatory when venous bypass is required and the superior vena cava must be approached; access to chest can also be obtained extending superiorly the abdominal incision to the sternum (sternotomy).

14.4   Medical Therapy

The very limited efficacy of medical treatment has already been stressed in this and in other specific chapters. The only drug which has been utilized widely is mitotane, but its value as adjuvant therapy in the patients operated for ACC was excluded [24] and its important side-effects were prohibitive. In recurrences where surgery cannot be accomplished though, this drug is still used. If its response could be objectively demonstrated in terms of real mass reduction (CT measurement, autopsies, etc.), its results would be even more disappointing and there is no demonstration that this supposed response correlates with prolonged survival [25]. The intended efficacy in nonoperable patients is by consequence in terms of partial control of endocrine symptoms and it must be associated with a replacement therapy with corticosteroids. It seems that in no more than one-third of these patients can medical therapy really palliate functional symptoms.

14.5   Prognosis

It has already been stated that prognosis is dismal in these patients and very prolonged survivals, if not real cures, are so exceptional as to be considered more as episodic reports rather than as a matter of discussion. In fact, long-term survivors (from 15 to even 20 years) have been described [11, 16, 20], but this is not enough to induce optimistic hopes when operating on these patients. We have already seen that a better prognosis can be expected when the operation has accomplished a complete resection. In the same way resections seem to have a better outcome in patients with a longer disease-free interval [11].

The overall median survival from the time of diagnosis is less than 2 years [11]. In a series by The Italian National Registry for Adrenal Cortical Carcinoma, 23% of the patients who underwent reoperation were alive 3 years after the recurrence diagnosis [2]. This confirms that repeat surgery should in any case be regarded as an absolute indication, being the only valid therapeutic option.

14.6   Recurrence and Laparoscopic Surgery

It should not be necessary to repeat that no role can exist for laparoscopic surgery when treating ACC, let alone when treating its recurrences. Thoracoscopy might be useful if an isolated lung metastasis has to be removed, but this represents an exceptional and episodic situation.

Vice versa this is a good opportunity to stress once again the responsibilities of laparoscopic adrenalectomies in the occurrence of peritoneal implants which must be regarded as real disasters. Although peritoneal recurrences can be present after traditional surgery, trocar port site seeding and the fair number of reports of such a situation [5, 6, 8, 10, 23] leave no doubt that this complication must be considered as a specific complication of laparoscopic removal of ACC. One of the characteristics of this kind of recurrence is their tendency to present quite early after first surgery [10]; this is a further confirmation of our concern about this dreadful occurrence. The greatest caution should be taken when deciding to operate laparoscopically on patients who present even a faint suspicion of malignancy.

14.7   Case Report

A 34-year-old female patient was admitted to our department in October 2000 with a history of recent appearance of hirsutism and a cushingoid appearance. On US, the left adrenal gland was 7×5×5 cm. CT confirmed the US report (Fig. 3). With the suspicion of adrenal carcinoma the patient underwent a traditional open approach. Histology confirmed ACC. In July 2001, for recurrent symptoms and stigmata a CT showed a locoregional recurrence involving the spleen and the left lobe of the liver (Fig. 4a, b). The mass was removed "en bloc" with apparent radicality. The following October the patient underwent an exploration with the suspicion of a uterine myomatoma (Fig. 5). The mass proved to be an ovarian metastasis. In February 2002 the third recurrence involving the left kidney and part of the left diaphragm was removed. In March 2003 the patient underwent a fifth operation

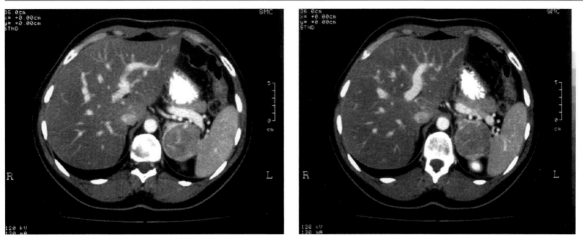

Fig. 3. CT showing a left adrenal tumor measuring up to 7 cm maximum diameter

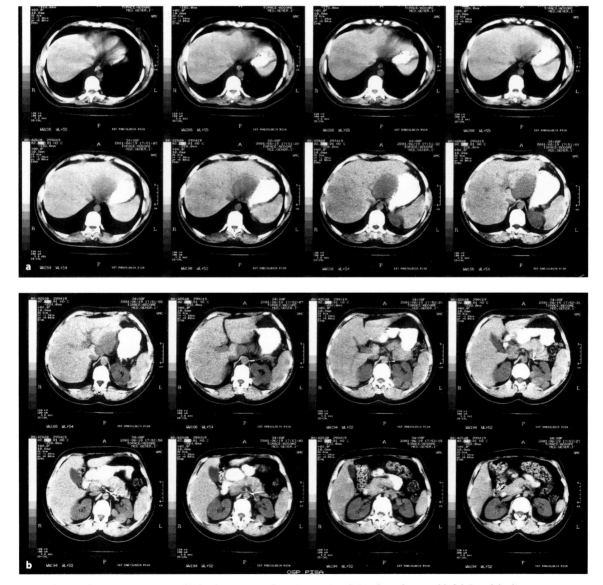

Fig. 4a, b. CT showing recurrence of left adrenocortical carcinoma involving the spleen and left lobe of the liver

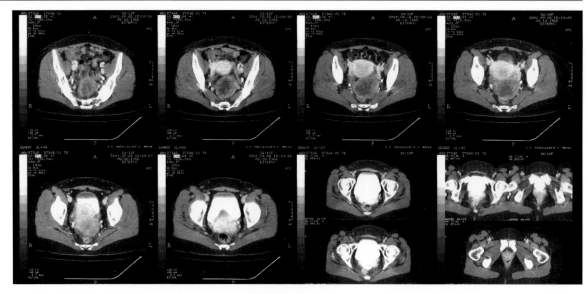

Fig. 5. CT showing an ovarian metastasis of a previously operated recurrent adrenocortical carcinoma

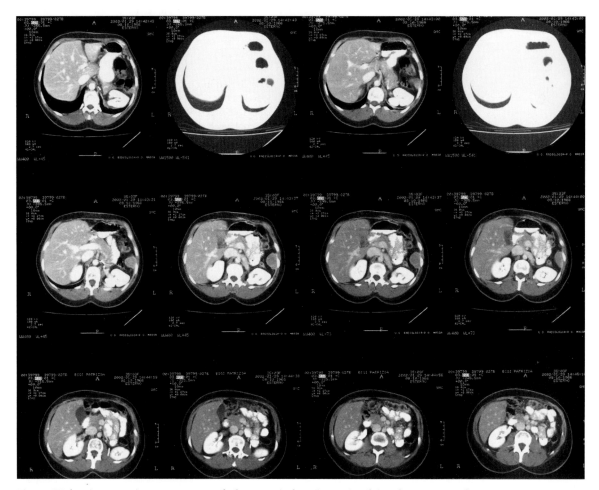

Fig. 6. CT showing extensive re-recurrence of adrenocortical carcinoma involving the psoas muscle

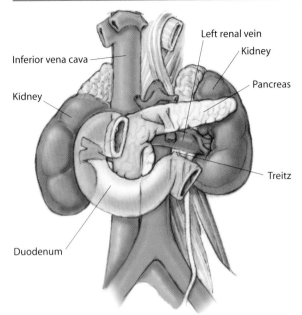

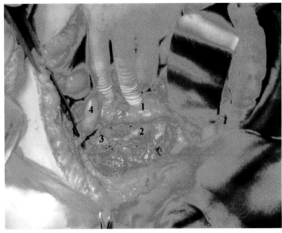

Fig. 8

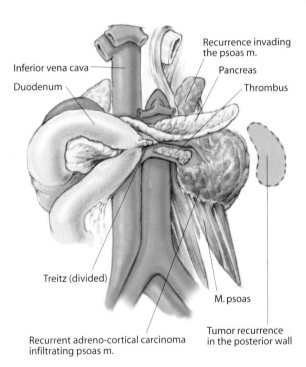

Recurrent adreno-cortical carcinoma
infiltrating psoas m.

Fig. 7

(Fig. 6) to remove a recurrence involving the psoas muscle and the stump of the renal vein (with a thrombus reaching the vena cava) (Figs. 7, 8). The patient died in July 2002, with symptoms of hypercortisolism and cerebral and pulmonary metastases. She refused any medical therapy.

References

1. Baumgartner F, et al. (1996) Modified venous bypass for resection of renal and adrenal carcinomas with involvement of the inferior vena cava. Eur J Surg 162:59–62

2. Bellantone R, et al. (1997) Role of reoperation in recurrence of adrenal cortical carcinoma: results from 189 cases collected in the National Italian Registry for Adrenal Cortical Carcinoma. Surgery 122:1212–18

3. Bodie B, et al. (1989) The Cleveland Clinic experience with adrenal cortical carcinoma. J Urol 141:257–60

4. Crucitti F, et al. (1996) The Italian Registry for Adrenal Cortical Carcinoma: analysis of a multiinstitutional series of 129 patients. Surgery 119:161–70

5. Deckers S, et al. (1999) Peritoneal carcinomatosis following laparoscopic resection of an adrenocortical tumor causing primary hyperaldosteronism. Horm Res 52: 97–100

6. Dackiw AP, et al. (2001) Adrenal cortical carcinoma. World J Surg 25:97–100

7. Didoklar MS, et al. (1981) Natural history of adrenal cortical carcinoma: a clinicopathologic study of 42 patients. Cancer 47:2153–61

8. Iacconi P, et al. (1999) Re: A case of Cushing's syndrome due to adrenocortical carcinoma with recurrence 19 months after laparoscopic adrenalectomy. J Urol 161: 1580–1

9. Icard P, et al. (1992) Adrenocortical carcinoma in surgically treated patients: a retrospective study of 156 cases by The French Association of Endocrine Surgery. Surgery 112:972–80

10. Iino K, et al. (2000) A case of adrenocortical carcinoma associated with recurrence after laparoscopic surgery. Clin Endocrinol 53:243–48

11. Jensen CJ, et al. (1991) Recurrent or metastatic disease in select patients with adenocortical carcinoma. Arch Surg 126:457

12. Korobkin M, et al. (1996) Differentiation of adrenal adenomas from nonadenomas using CT attenuation values. Am J Roentgenol 166:531–36

13. Kunieda K, et al. (2000) Recurrence of giant adrenocortical carcinoma in the contralateral adrenal gland 6 years after surgery: report of a case. Surg Today 30: 294–97

14. Luton J, et al. (1990) Clinical features of adrenocortical carcinoma, prognostic factors, and the effect of mitotane therapy. N Engl J Med 322:1195–01

15. Miccoli P, Bernini GP (2001) Adrenocortical carcinoma. In: Doherty GM, Skogseid B (eds) Surgical endocrinology. Lippincott, Williams and Wilkins, Philadelphia

16. Orlando R, et al. (2003) Adrenocortical carcinoma: a 15-year survival after complete resection and repeated resection. A retrospective study in a patient with an expected poor prognosis. Anticancer Res 23:2929–31

17. Osella G, et al. (1994) Endocrine evaluation of incidentally discovered adrenal masses (incidentalomas). J Clin Endocrinol Metab 79:1532–38

18. Pommier RF, Brennam MF (1992) An eleven-year experience with adrenocortical carcinoma. Surgery 112:963–71

19. Pommier RF, Brennan MF (19921) Management of adrenal neoplasms. Curr Probl Surg 28:677–96

20. Sakamoto K, et al. (1995) Metastatic adrenocortical carcinoma treated by repeat resection: a case report of long-term survival over 18 years. Int J Urol 2:50–2

21. Schulick RD, Brennan MF (1999) Long-term survival after complete resection and repeat resection in patients with adrenocortical carcinoma. Ann Surg Oncol 6:719–26

22. Sullivan M, et al. (1978) Adrenal cortical carcinoma. J Urol 120:660–65

23. Ushiyama T, et al. (1997) Case of Cushing's syndrome due to adrenocortical carcinoma with recurrence 19 months after laparoscopic adrenalectomy. J Urol 157:2239

24. Vassilopoulou-Sellin R, et al. (1993) Impact of adjuvant mitotane on the clinical course of patients with adrenocortical cancer. Cancer 71:3119–23

25. Wooten MD, King KD (1993) Adrenal cortical carcinoma. Cancer 72:3145–55

15 Metastatic Adrenocortical Carcinoma

D. E. Tsakayannis, Dimitrios A. Linos

15.1 Epidemiology

Metastatic tumor is the most common lesion in the adrenal gland at postmortem [1]. The common occurrence of this adrenal lesion is related to its rich sinusoidal blood supply. With continuing progress in imaging techniques, particularly computed tomography (CT), an increasing number of adrenal metastases can be detected incidentally during follow-up or at the time of presentation of extra-adrenal malignancy. The most frequent types of malignancy that manifest adrenal metastases in Western countries are primary malignancies of the lung, kidney, breast, melanoma and gastrointestinal tract [2,3]. Metastases to the adrenals have also been reported for hepatocellular carcinoma [4,5], carcinoma of the bladder [6], lymphoma [7], testicular seminoma [8], osteogenic sarcoma [9], ovarian cancer [10] and thyroid cancer [11]. About one-third of patients dying from lung cancer have adrenal metastases at autopsy [12]. Preoperative staging with a CT scan will reveal adrenal lesions in 7.5% of patients with non-small cell lung carcinoma [13]. Among patients with lung cancer, 4.1% of those who have operable disease will be found to have a coexistent unilateral adrenal lesion [14].

In a large series from Hong Kong, 464 patients with metastatic disease to the adrenal glands, over a 30-year period, were reviewed. A high prevalence of gastric, esophageal and liver/bile duct metastases was noted, which was explained by the high prevalence of these tumors in Hong Kong as compared to Western countries. Most adrenal metastases were discovered within a short period after the detection of the primary tumor (median latent period of 7 months) and less than 2% were detected more than 5 years after diagnosis of the primary tumors [15]. In the literature, late presentation of adrenal metastases, occurring after a latent period of 15 years, has been reported for renal cancer [16, 17], colorectal cancer and lymphoma [15]. Thus the presence of an adrenal mass in a patient with a history of previous malignancy should be regarded as potentially metastatic, even though the primary tumor may have been adequately treated many years previously.

15.2 Clinical Presentation

The clinical presentation of adrenal metastasis is often quite indolent. The majority of lesions are asymptomatic and are discovered on initial staging or routine follow-up. When symptomatic, pain seems to be the most common presenting symptom in up to 25% of patients and can alert the physician to investigate for possible metastatic disease [16]. Addison's disease is not a frequent clinical manifestation. Fewer than 100 cases have been reported in the literature and the prevalence of adrenal metastases in patients with Addison's disease ranges from 2% to 6% [19, 20], with the exception of one series, where it was reported to be 42% [15]. This low incidence may be attributed to the fact that more than 90% of the adrenal gland must be destroyed before there is clinical adrenal insufficiency, which usually requires bilateral adrenal involvement, by the tumor. In some cases adrenal insufficiency is caused by unilateral adrenal destruction by the cancer and concurrent pituitary metastasis [21]. Clinically significant hemorrhage secondary to metastasis is exceedingly rare and only 11 such cases have been reported; with the exception of 2 patients all had a primary lung cancer. Acute severe pain was the presenting symptom and must be recognized promptly, because decisive surgical intervention might be necessary. Many of these patients can be stabilized hemodynamically and there have been reports where there was response to radiation therapy [22, 23] following hemorrhage.

15.3   Diagnosis

The characterization of an adrenal lesion as benign or malignant (primary or metastatic) preoperatively can be very difficult. Imaging techniques and fine-needle aspiration (FNA) are the usual diagnostic tools. The size of the adrenal lesion has been used by many centers as a predictor of malignant potential and a size of greater than 5 cm correlates with a 35–98% risk of malignancy [24]. But size represents by no means definitive diagnosis. In addition, in an analysis of 76 patients with incidentalomas, Linos et al. found that CT scanning underestimated the true size of adrenal tumors by an average of 25% [25].

15.3.1   Imaging Techniques

The most widely used and accepted imaging techniques for the detection of metastatic adrenal tumors are *computed tomography (CT) and magnetic resonance imaging (MRI)*. However, they are not accurate enough to diagnose or to exclude primary or metastatic adrenal tumors preoperatively. Allard et al reviewed 91 patients with lung cancer who were examined by CT scan to assess for adrenal metastases. In all these patients at postmortem, all adrenal glands underwent histopathological examination for metastatic lesions. The calculated sensitivity and specificity of the CT scan for the detection of adrenal metastases was 41% and 99% respectively [12]. Porte et al. studied the use of combined CT scan and MRI in 443 patients with resectable non-small cell lung cancer, of whom 32 had an adrenal lesion. Sensitivity and specificity of the combination of both tests in detecting the adrenal lesions was 80% and 100% respectively. Despite the fact that adrenal metastases tended to be larger and less well defined on CT scan, their imaging characteristics were non-specific. Furthermore the authors showed that size alone was not sufficient to discriminate between metastatic adrenal lesion and non-functioning adenomas [26]. Burt et al. prospectively evaluated the accuracy of MRI in distinguishing a benign from a malignant adrenal mass in patients with otherwise operable non-small cell lung cancer. They found that MRI had a high false-positive rate of 67% and could not replace CT-guided percutaneous needle biopsy of the adrenal mass [27].

Iodocholesterol adrenal scan has been used for the detection of adrenal metastases. The reasoning is based on the fact that any metastatic tissue replacing normal adrenal tissue will not accumulate iodocholesterol, which will be shown as a lack of uptake during scanning. This technique has not been widely used, has shown some promising results, but more studies are necessary to evaluate its true sensitivity, specificity and accuracy [28].

Positron emission tomography (PET) scanning is a promising novel diagnostic modality that can be very helpful in characterizing adrenal masses. The major utility of PET in the evaluation of patients with lung cancer is staging of the entire body. PET is more accurate than the conventional imaging modalities of CT and bone scans in the detection of metastatic disease. PET is accurate in the staging of the mediastinum, adrenal glands and skeletal system [29]. In particular PET scan can either identify lesions in the adrenals that could not be detected on CT or MRI, or can help differentiate an adrenal mass as being metastatic or benign (Fig. 1). Yun et al. studied 50 adrenal lesions in patients with proven or suspected primary cancers with FDG-PET scan and found that increased FDG uptake by the adrenal gland, which signified high glucose tumor metabolism, was characteristic of adrenal metastatic involvement. FDG-PET scan showed a sensitivity of 100%, a specificity of 94% and an accuracy of 96% [30]. Therefore PET scan will soon become a very useful tool in confirming isolated metastatic disease and selecting patients for adrenalectomy. However, even though the preliminary results are promising, more studies evaluating its accuracy will be necessary [31–33]. PET scan could also be cost effective because it has the additional advantage of evaluating not only the adrenal mass, but at the same time can be used to stage the whole body by identifying extra-adrenal tumor sites in cancer patients.

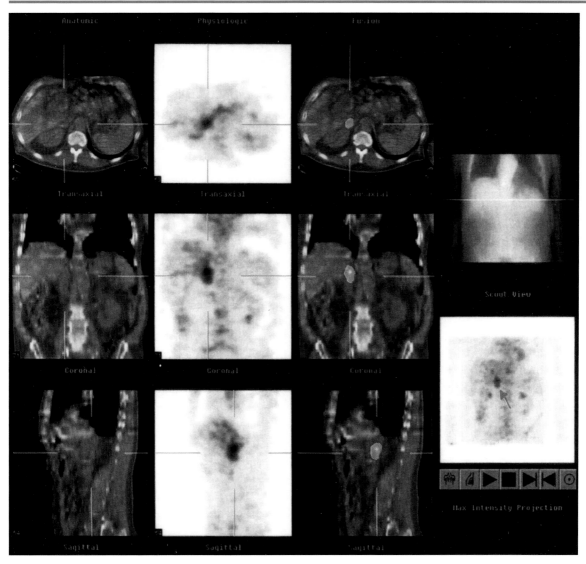

Fig. 1. A PET scan detected a small isolated adrenal metastasis (with a concurrent negative CT scan) in this 69-year-old male patient treated for mesothelioma. Laparoscopic adrenalectomy of this single metastasis was performed

15.3.2   Fine-Needle Aspiration

Fine-needle aspiration (FNA) biopsy of a non-functioning adrenal tumor is inaccurate in differentiating between a primary adrenal carcinoma and a benign lesion, has a risk of disruption of the tumor capsule and potential dissemination of cancer cells and is therefore not recommended [24]. Nevertheless it may be of great value in the diagnosis of adrenal metastases since many studies have shown that the accuracy of FNA in this situation is excellent. The combination of CT and aspiration cytology can provide a conclusive diagnosis of metastatic adrenal tumors and it seems reasonable that all patients with known malignant disease and an adrenal mass should undergo FNA cytology to determine if the lesion is a metastasis or a non-functioning adenoma [34, 35] (Fig. 2). In patients with resectable non-small cell lung cancer who present with synchronous or metachronous isolated adrenal masses, CT-guided biopsy has shown to have an up to 100% accuracy, sensitivity and specificity and is required to select patients for adrenalectomy with a potentially curative intent [14, 26, 36].

Aspiration cytology under CT or ultrasound guidance should be regarded as the procedure with the highest diagnostic yield in evaluating a possible metastasis to the adrenal gland from another primary malignancy.

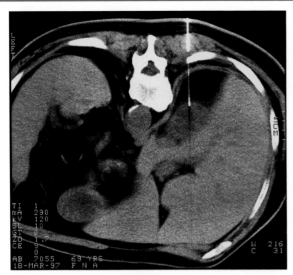

Fig. 2. CT-guided fine-needle aspiration disclosed a metastatic right adrenal carcinoma

15.4   Treatment

In most cases an adrenal metastasis occurs in the face of multiple synchronous metastases in other sites. The prognosis for these patients is dismal, with few reports of survivors past 5 years. A broad range of treatments, including chemotherapy, hormonal therapy and radiation therapy, have failed to impact significantly on their survival. A few studies using immunotherapy for melanoma and renal cell carcinoma are encouraging, but, once again, 5-year survival with metastatic disease remains an unusual event [37].

Isolated adrenal metastasis is rare and presents a therapeutic dilemma. The discovery of an isolated adrenal metastasis is considered synonymous with systemic carcinomatosis and therefore many clinicians do not consider these patients as candidates for adrenal resection [14, 38]. The stated reasons are that adrenalectomy has appreciable risks and, if the resection is bilateral, commits a patient to lifelong therapy. It remains unclear whether the survival benefits for these patients outweigh the risks of adrenalectomy.

Evidence is, however, accumulating that adrenalectomy for patients with isolated adrenal metastases may be curative [39–43]. Individual case reports and small series are available but few large series have been published [42]. Lo et al. reported the Mayo Clinic experience over a 10-year period in 52 patients undergoing adrenalectomy for metastatic disease. In this study, open surgical resection was associated with rare mortality and low morbidity rates and overall survival rates were 73% at 1 year and 40% at 2 years [39]. Kim et al. from the Memorial Sloan Kettering Cancer Center conducted a retrospective review of 37 patients who had undergone open adrenalectomy for isolated metastatic disease over a 10-year period. Five-year survival for the entire group was 24% (median, 21 months) with acceptably low mortality and morbidity. In their study, the only predictors of improved survival were complete resection and a disease free interval of greater than 6 months [41]. Given that the highest reported median overall survival in patients treated non-surgically for solitary adrenal metastasis was only 8.5 months [44] and that no long-term survivors appeared in any other series [45, 46], the authors argued that resection could alter the natural history of this disease. Long-term survival could be achieved in selected patients where complete resection was achieved and with a disease-free interval of more than 6 months. Heniford et al. reviewed 40 cases of unilateral or bilateral adrenal resections for isolated metastases from non-small cell lung carcinoma; the estimated 5-year survival for these patients was approximately 45% [37]. Porte et al. retrospectively studied 43 patients with solitary adrenal metastasis from non-small cell lung cancer treated in eight centers with curative intent. The metastases were discovered synchronously in 32 patients and metachronously in 11. Median survival was 11 months and three patients survived more than 5 years. There was no difference in survival and recurrence between the synchronous and metachronous groups [43]. Paul et al. did a meta-analysis of published series and case reports reported in the literature and identified 77 patients with isolated metastatic adrenal cancer in whom complete resection with negative margins was achieved. The median survival time after open adrenalectomy was 23 months, with an operative mortality of 3.9% [42]. A longer disease-free interval from the time of primary cancer therapy to adrenal metastasis was associated with a longer postoperative survival after adrenalectomy. A longer disease-free interval presumably reflects less aggressive tumor biology.

The primary tumor site appears to significantly affect survival as well. A significantly longer survival has been observed for patients with primary kidney, colon, lung carcinoma and melanoma. Poorer results were found for patients with unknown primary cancer, sarcoma, esophageal and hepatocellular carcinoma [42]. The size of the metastases has not been shown to affect survival, and patients with tumors greater than 7 cm fared just as well as patients with smaller metastases [41, 42]. Therefore metastasis size should not preclude an aggressive surgical approach, assuming complete resection is possible.

Most published data support that resection of isolated adrenal metastases clearly benefits carefully selected patients. One should consider overall patient health, tumor aggressiveness and complete resectability in selecting those patients in whom adrenalectomy should be attempted. Medically fit patients, particularly those with a long disease-free interval (greater than 6 months) and resectable tumors, should be offered resection with low operative mortality. It must be kept in mind though that these patients are not cured by this approach and therefore careful extent-of-disease (staging) workup is clearly indicated prior to adrenalectomy.

15.4.1 The Role of Laparoscopic Adrenalectomy

Laparoscopic adrenalectomy has proven to be effective and safe for the treatment of benign functioning and non-functioning adrenal tumors [47–52]. Skepticism exists, however, currently for laparoscopic removal of primary adrenocortical carcinoma [53, 54]. In the patient with isolated adrenal metastases there are, however, several factors that support the minimally invasive approach. The laparoscopic approach offers excellent visualization, early control of the organ's vasculature and the ability to effectively screen for signs of unresectability. Another factor that may support the use of laparoscopy is the fact that most often simple adrenalectomy is sufficient to remove metastatic lesions, because these lesions seldom penetrate the capsule of the gland [37, 55] (Fig. 3). When extraglandular extension is found, extended resection including the involved organs should be performed (Fig. 4). Initiating a laparoscopic exploration does not preclude subsequent conversion to an open, more extensive resection. There are few absolute contraindications for laparoscopic adrenalectomy: (1) the presence of a locally invasive adrenal or metastatic carcinoma, because of the possible extent and complexity of the operation required; (2) the identification of widespread systemic disease. Other relative contraindications include previous trauma or surgery in the area that may create dense adhesions, and an adrenal size of 10 cm or larger, which would require extensive laparoscopic and probable open adrenal surgical expertise.

The role of laparoscopy for metastatic adrenal tumors remains unclear, since rare and limited outcome

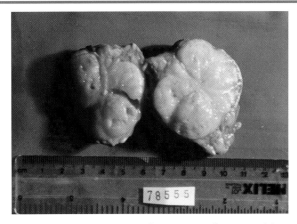

Fig. 3. Metastatic carcinoma laparoscopically removed in a patient treated for cervical cancer several years previously. The capsule of the adrenal remained intact

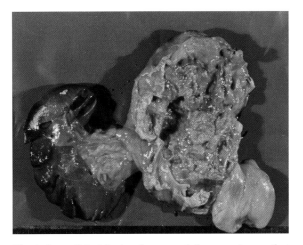

Fig. 4. Large (13×9.5×4 cm) metastatic lung carcinoma that was removed en bloc with the spleen, kidney and tail of the pancreas

data exist in the literature. These reports have been limited to case reports and small cohort studies with short follow-up. In a search of the English literature 11 authors have reported 46 cases of synchronous or metachronous adrenal metastases treated laparoscopically [10, 37, 50, 56–64]. Heniford et al. in a two-institution review of ten patients with metastatic adrenal tumors and one patient with primary adrenal cancer, which were all removed laparoscopically, reported no port-site or local recurrence at a mean follow-up time of 8.3 months [37]. Kebebew et al. retrospectively studied 23 patients who underwent laparoscopic adrenalectomy for metastatic adrenal cancer (13 patients) and adrenocortical carcinoma (10 patients). There were no locoregional or port-site recurrences in any of the 13 patients who underwent laparoscopic adrenal metastasectomy at a mean follow-up time of 3.3 years. Their overall disease-free survival was 65%. Four of the 13 patients who were thought to have solitary adrenal metastasis at the time of their laparoscopic adrenalectomy later had distant recurrences [61]. Feliciotti et al. reported their experience of six patients with isolated adrenal metastasis managed laparoscopically. No postoperative complications occurred, tumor free margins were achieved in every case and no port-site metastasis or local recurrence was observed at follow-up to 24 months [63].

The current available literature is too sparse to allow any treatment management recommendations for metastatic adrenal neoplasms. Unlike for colon cancer, a prospective randomized study comparing open with laparoscopic adrenalectomy is impractical because of the rarity of isolated metastatic adrenal tumors. However, this limited experience has shown that resection of metastatic adrenal lesions is laparoscopically feasible. Because of the many known advantages of the laparoscopic as compared to the open approach, we believe that laparoscopic adrenalectomy for solitary adrenal metastasis should be preferred when technically and oncologically feasible in a highly selective group of patients.

References

1. Lam KY (1994) The pathology of adrenal tumors. Cancer J 7:181–187
2. Glomset DA (1938) The incidence of metastases of malignant tumors of the adrenal. Am J Cancer 32:57–61
3. Abrams HL, Spiro R, Goldstein N (1950) Metastases in carcinoma: analysis of 1000 autopsied cases. Cancer 3:74–85
4. Otabe S, Muto S, Asano Y, et al. (1991) Hyperreninemic hypoaldosteronism due to hepatocellular carcinoma metastatic to the adrenal gland. Clin Nephrol 35:66–71
5. Okuda K, Arakawa M, Kubo Y, et al. (1998) Right-sided pedunculated hepatocellular carcinoma: A form of adrenal metastasis. Hepatology 27:81–85
6. Kennedy RL, Ball RY, Dixon AK, ApSimon AT (1987) Metastatic transitional cell carcinoma of the bladder causing Addison's disease. J Urol 137:986–988
7. Feinmann C, Gillett R, Irving MH (1976) Hodgkin's disease presenting with hypoadrenalism. BMJ 2:455–456
8. Carey RW, Harris N, Kliman B (1987) Addison's disease secondary to lymphomatous infiltration of the adrenal glands. Cancer 59:1087–1090
9. Potepan P, Danesini GM, Spagnoli I, et al. (1992) Adrenal gland metastasis in osteogenic osteosarcoma. A radiological case report. Tumori 78:417–420
10. Einat S, Amir S, Silvia M, et al. (2002) Successful laparoscopic removal of a solitary adrenal metastasis: a case report. Gynecol Oncol 85:201–3
11. Yunta PJ, Ponce JL, Prieto M, et al. (2001) Solitary adrenal gland metastasis of a follicular thyroid carcinoma presenting with hyperthyroidism. Ann Endocrinol (Paris) 62:226–9
12. Allard P, Yanaskas BC, Fletcher RH, et al. (1990) Sensitivity and specificity of computed tomography for the detection of adrenal metastatic lesions among 91 autopsied lung cancer patients. Cancer 66:457–462
13. Salvatierra A, Baamonde C, Llamas JM, et al. (1990) Extra thoracic staging of bronchogenic carcinoma. Chest 97:1052–1058
14. Ettinghausen SE, Burt ME (1991) Prospective evaluation of unilateral adrenal masses in patients with operable non small-cell lung cancer. J Clin Oncol 9:1462–1466
15. Lam KY, Lo CY (2002) Metastatic tumors of the adrenal glands: a 30-year experience in a teaching hospital. Clin Endocrinol 56:95–101
16. Mesurrole B, Mignon F, Travagli JP, et al. (1997) Late presentation of solitary contralateral adrenal metastasis of renal cell carcinoma. Radiology 7:557–558
17. Sagalowski AL, Molberg K (1999) Solitary metastasis of renal cell carcinoma to the contralateral adrenal gland 22 years after nephrectomy. Urology Online 54:162
18. Lo CY, van Heerden JA, Soreide JA, et al. (1996) Adrenalectomy for metastatic disease to the adrenal glands. Br J Surg 83:528–531
19. Kong MF, Jeffcoate W (1994) Eighty-six cases of Addison's disease. Clin Endocrinol 41:757–761
20. Soule S (1999) Addison's disease in Africa – a teaching hospital experience. Clin Endocrinol 50:115–120
21. Trincado T, Playan J, Acha J, et al. (1996) Adrenal failure due to metastasis both to the hypothalamic-pituitary area and the adrenals. Tumori 82:401–404
22. Kinoshita A, Nakano M, Suyama N, et al. (1997) Massive adrenal hemorrhage secondary to metastasis from lung cancer. Int Med 36:815–818
23. Berney CR, Roth AD, Allal A, et al. (1997) Spontaneous retroperitoneal hemorrhage due to adrenal metastasis for non-small cell lung cancer treated by radiation therapy. Acta Oncol 36:91–93
24. Linos DA (2000) Management approaches to adrenal incidentalomas (adrenalomas). A view from Athens, Greece. Endocr Metabol Clin North Am 29:141–157
25. Linos DA, Stylopoulos N (1997) How accurate is computed tomography in predicting the real size of adrenal tumors? Arch Surg 132:740–743
26. Porte HL, Ernst OJ, Delebecq T, et al. (1999) Is computed tomography guided biopsy still necessary for the diagnosis of adrenal masses in patients with resectable non-small cell lung cancer? Eur J Cardiothorac Surg 15:597–601
27. Burt M, Heelan RT, Coit D, et al. (1994) Prospective evaluation of unilateral adrenal masses in patients with operable non-small cell lung cancer. Impact of magnetic resonance imaging. J Thorac Cardiovasc Surg 107:584–589

28. Quraishi MA, Costanzi JJ, Balachandran S (1981) Iodocholesterol adrenal scanning for the detection of adrenal metastases in lung cancer and its clinical significance. Cancer 48:714–716

29. Coleman RF (2001) PET in lung cancer staging. Q J Nucl Med 45:231–4

30. Yun M, Kim W, Alnafisi N, et al. (2001) 18F-FDG Pet in characterizing adrenal lesions detected on CT or MRI. J Nucl Med 42:1795–9

31. Harrison J, Ali A, Bonomi P, et al. (2000) The role of positron emission tomography in selecting patients with metastatic cancer for adrenalectomy. Am Surg 66:432–7

32. Gregoire A, Drahmoune R (2000) Clinical case of the month. Case report of adrenal metastases from lung adenocarcinoma. Rev Med Liege 55:8–10

33. Maurea S, Mainolfi C, Wang H, et al. (1996) Positron emission tomography (PET) with fludexoglucose F18 in the study of adrenal masses: comparison of benign and malignant lesions. Radiol Med (Torino) 92:782–7

34. Luciani L, Scappini P, Pusiol T, et al. (1985) Aspiration cytology of simultaneous bilateral adrenal metastases from renal cell carcinoma. A case report and review of the literature. J Urol 134:315–318

35. Berkman WA, Bernardino ME, Sewell CW, et al. (1984) The computed tomography-guided adrenal biopsy. An alternative to surgery in adrenal mass diagnosis. Cancer 53:2098–2103

36. Pagani JJ (1984) Non-small cell lung carcinoma adrenal metastases. Computed tomography and percutaneous needle biopsy in their diagnosis. Cancer 53:1058–1060

37. Heniford BT, Arca MJ, Walsh RM, et al. (1999) Laparoscopic adrenalectomy for cancer. Semin Surg Oncol 16:293–306

38. Beitler AL, Urschel JD, Verlagapudi SRC, et al. (1998) Surgical management of adrenal metastases from lung cancer. J Surg Oncol 69:54–57

39. Wade TP, Longo WE, Virgo KS, et al. (1998) A comparison of adrenalectomy to other resections for metastatic cancers. Am J Surg 175:183–186

40. Kim SH, Brennan MF, Russo P, et al. (1998) The role of surgery in the treatment of clinically isolated adrenal metastasis. Cancer 82:389–394

41. Paul CA, Virgo KS, Wade TP, et al. (2000) Adrenalectomy for isolated adrenal metastases from non-adrenal cancer. Int J Oncol 17:181–187

42. Porte H, Siat J, Guibert B, et al. (2001) Resection of adrenal metastases from non-small cell lung cancer: a multicenter study. Ann Thorac Surg 71:981–5

43. Luketish JD, Burt ME (1996) Does resection of adrenal metastases from NSCLC improve survival? Ann Thorac Surg 62:1614–6

44. Higashiyama H, Doi O, Kodama K, et al. (1994) Surgical treatment of adrenal metastasis following pulmonary resection for lung cancer: comparison of adrenalectomy with palliative therapy. Int J Surg 79:124–9

45. Soffen EM, Solin LJ, Rubenstein JH, et al. (1990) Palliative radiotherapy for symptomatic adrenal metastases. Cancer 65:1318–20

46. Gagner M, Lacroix A, Bolte E (1992) Laparoscopic adrenalectomy in Cushing's syndrome and pheochromocytoma. N Engl J Med 327:1033

47. Smith CD, Weber CJ, Amerson JR (1999) Laparoscopic adrenalectomy: new gold standard. World J Surg 23:389–396

48. Thompson GB, Grant CS, van Heerden JA, et al. (1997) Laparoscopic versus open posterior adrenalectomy: a case control study of 100 patients. Surgery 122:132–138

49. Zeh HJ, Udelsman R (2003) One hundred laparoscopic adrenalectomies: a single surgeon's experience. Ann Surg Oncol 10:1012–1017

50. Linos DA, Stylopoulos N, Boukis M, et al. (1997) Anterior, posterior or laparoscopic approach for the management of adrenal diseases? Am J Surg 173:120–125

51. Fowler DL (2003) Laparoscopic adrenalectomy: there can be no doubt. Ann Surg Oncol 10:997–8

52. Wells SA, Merke DP, Cutler GB, et al. Therapeutic controversy: the role of laparoscopic surgery in adrenal disease. J Clin Endocrinol Metab 83:3041–49

53. Suzuki K, Ushiyama T, Mugiya S, et al. (1997) Hazards of laparoscopic adrenalectomy in patients with adrenal malignancy. J Urol 158:2227

54. Ayabe H, Tsuji H, Hara S, et al. (1995) Surgical management of adrenal metastasis from bronchogenic carcinoma. J Surg Oncol 58:149–154

55. Elashry OM, Clayman RV, Soble JJ, et al. (1997) Laparoscopic adrenalectomy for solitary metachronous adrenal metastasis from renal cell carcinoma. J Urol 157:1217–1222

56. Bendinelli C, Lucchi M, Buccianti P, et al. (1998) Adrenal masses in non-small cell lung carcinoma patients: is there any role for laparoscopic procedures? J Laparoendosc Adv Surg Tech 8:119–124

57. Tsuji Y, Yashuku M, Haryu T, et al. (1999) Laparoscopic adrenalectomy for solitary metachronous adrenal metastasis from lung cancer: report of a case. Surg Today 29:1277–1279

58. Valeri A, Borrelli A, Presenti L, et al. (2001) Adrenal masses in neoplastic patients. The role of laparoscopic procedure. Surg Endosc 15:90–93

59. Chen B, Zhou M, Cappelli MC, et al. (2002) Port site, retroperitoneal and intra-abdominal recurrence after laparoscopic adrenalectomy for apparently isolated metastasis. J Urol 168:2528–2529

60. Kebebew E, Siperstein AE, Clark OH, et al. (2002) Results of laparoscopic adrenalectomy for suspected and unsuspected malignant adrenal neoplasms. Arch Surg 137:948–953

61. Linos DA, Avlonitis V, Iliadis K (1998) Laparoscopic resection of solitary adrenal metastasis from lung carcinoma: Case report. JSLS 2:291–293

62. Feliciotti F, Paganinin AM, Guerrieri M, et al. (2003) Laparoscopic anterior adrenalectomy for the treatment of adrenal metastases. Surg Laparosc Endosc Percutan Tech 13:328–33

16 Virilizing and Feminizing Adrenal Tumors

Michael Brauckhoff, Oliver Gimm, Henning Dralle

CONTENTS

16.1 Introduction

Androgen- and estrogen-producing adrenal neoplasms are very rare. They may occur at all ages but two peaks of incidence exist: younger than 10 years and between the fourth and fifth decade. The overall annual incidence of adrenocortical tumors is reported to be about 2/1,000,000 [32]. During childhood, the incidence of adrenocortical tumors is about 0.3 per 1,000,000 per year. Adrenocortical tumors constitute 0.2–0.5% of all pediatric tumors [20, 80, 133, 135]. In previous studies, more than 50% of adrenocortical tumors were assumed to be malignant [53]. In more recent studies, a frequency of malignant tumors of about 35% without any difference between children and adults was observed [18, 93].

Less than 60% of symptomatic adrenocortical neoplasms produce hormones. Hyperandrogenism can be found in about 10–15% of adult patients, and a combined production of cortisol and androgens occurs in about 30–35% [32]. In contrast to adults, pure androgen-producing tumors are the predominant entity within endocrine active adrenocortical tumors during childhood [21, 37, 62, 76, 93, 103, 105].

The pathogenesis of adrenal tumors is basically unclear. However, since family members of patients with adrenal carcinoma have a higher than expected incidence of other tumors, a genetic origin can be assumed [105]. Furthermore, adrenocortical tumors occur more frequently in syndromic patients such as those with the Beckwith-Wiedemann syndrome, anomalies of the kidneys, multiple endocrine neoplasia type 1 (MEN 1), Li-Fraumeni syndrome, and McCune-Albright syndrome when compared to healthy subjects [37, 74, 105, 106, 117, 126]. In patients with congenital adrenal hyperplasia, an increased incidence of adrenocortical tumors was observed, suggesting a direct oncogenic effect of chronic adrenocorticotropic hormone (ACTH) stimulation [20, 74, 105].

Because of the rarity of sex hormone-producing adrenocortical tumors, evidence based data regarding diagnosis, classification, therapy, and prognostic factors are barely available. The best therapy and prognostic factor is complete surgical removal of the tumor. Theoretically, two different clinical forms have to be distinguished concerning adrenal neoplasms producing androgens or estrogens: (a) the clinically symptomatic tumor with virilization or feminization, and (b) the clinically asymptomatic incidentaloma producing subclinical amounts of adrenocortical hormones and potentially suppressing the hypothalamic-pituitary-adrenal axis (secondary or tertiary adrenal insufficiency). However, the latter has not been reported in tumors secreting sex hormones to date.

16.2   Physiology of Adrenal Androgens and Estrogens

Androgens [testosterone, dihydrotestosterone, dehydroepiandrosterone (DHEA), DHEA sulfate (DHEA-S), and androstenedione] are C19 steroids (androstane derivates) derived from the conversion of cholesterol. Estrogens [estrone (E1), estriol, and estradiol (E2)] are C18 steroids (estrane derivates) arising from androgens by aromatization. Androgens and estrogens are mainly produced under the control of hypothalamic and pituitary hormones (GnRH, CRH, LH, FSH, and ACTH) in a sex- and age-related pattern by the gonads (testes/ovaries) and the adrenal glands. The most effective androgens biologically are testosterone and dihydrotestosterone; the most effective estrogen is estradiol.

The most frequent adrenal androgens DHEA and DHEA-S (and in smaller amounts androstenedione) are produced mainly in the zona reticularis of the adrenal cortex [limiting enzyme: 17-hydroxylase/17,20-lyase (CYP17)]. In normal subjects, the biologically active androgens and estrogens result from DHEA by extraadrenal enzymatic transformation [involved enzymes: 3β-hydroxysteroid dehydrogenase/isomerase (3β-HSD), 17β-hydroxysteroid dehydrogenase (17β-HSD), 5α-reductase, CYP19] (Fig. 1).

DHEA is mainly produced under the control of ACTH. Adrenal androgen secretion increases at the end of the first decade, plateaus at the end of the second decade and decreases after the fifth decade. During all periods, cortisol levels remain constant. However, the control mechanisms are still unclear [81, 83].

In normal premenopausal females, the ovaries and adrenals both produce about 25% of the circulating testosterone (Table 1). The rest is transformed by peripheral conversion of androstenedione. DHEA and DHEA-S are almost exclusively products of the adrenal glands [44].

Inactivation of androgens and estrogens into several metabolites occurs mainly in the liver [androgens: 17-ketosteroids (epiandrosterone, androsterone, etiocholanolone); estrogens: several estriol derivates]. Almost all of the metabolites are excreted by the kidneys.

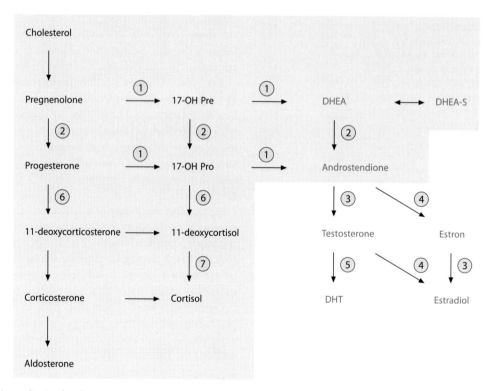

Fig. 1. Biosynthesis of androgens and estrogens (*red*, adrenal androgens; *blue*, extra-adrenal androgens – gonads, peripheral transformation; *17OHPre*, 17-hydroxypregnenolone; *17OHPro*, 17-hydroxyprogesterone; *DHEA*, dehydroepiandrosterone; *DHEA-S*, dehydroepiandrosterone sulfate; *DHT*, dihydrotestosterone; *1*, 17α-hydroxylase/17,20-lyase (P450$_{C17}$, CYP17); *2*, 3β-hydroxysteroid dehydrogenase (3β-HSD); *3*, 17β-hydroxysteroid dehydrogenase (17β-HSD); *4*, P450-aromatase (P450aro); *5*, 5α-reductase; *6*, 21-hydroxylase (P450$_{C21}$, CYP21A2); *7*, 11β-hydroxylase (P450$_{C11}$, CYP11B1)

Table 1. Source of circulating androgens in premenopausal females [44]

	Adrenal glands (zona fasciculata and zona reticularis)	Ovaries (theca cells)
DHEA-S	100%	–
DHEA	90%	10%
Androstenedione	50%	50%
Testosterone[a]	25%	25%

[a] Fifty percent of the circulating testosterone in premenopausal women is produced by peripheral metabolization of DHEA and androstenedione.

16.3 Pathology of Adrenal Androgens and Estrogens

16.3.1 Pathophysiology

Disturbances of the sex and age specific androgen and estrogen levels may lead to a very broad spectrum of masculinization (hyperandrogenism) or feminization (hyperestrogenism). In general, in prepubertal subjects, increased amounts of androgens, but also estrogens, initially accelerate growth and bone aging. However, growth is eventually terminated earlier in these patients compared to normal subjects because of the premature closure of the bone growth centers. Thus, after an increased growth rate during the prepubertal period, the patients do not reach the height of normal adults. In males, androgens result in an isosexual precocious pseudopuberty (which is defined as premature puberty not caused by activation of the hypothalamic-pituitary system) and in females in a contrasexual precocious pseudopuberty (pseudohermaphroditism femininus). Estrogens lead to isosexual precocious pseudopuberty in females and to contrasexual precocious pseudopuberty in males (pseudohermaphroditism masculinus). In adults, hyperandrogenism in males and hyperestrogenism in females are usually oligosymptomatic (Table 2).

Since androgens and estrogens are formed in the gonads and the adrenals, but also by peripheral transformation, an increased effect of androgens or estrogens can be the result of several pathological pathways (autonomic or stimulated overproduction of the hormones, increased transforming activity of peripheral enzymes, increased expression of hormone receptors in sex hormone-producing cells or effector cells, increased fraction of free circulating hormones, reduced inactivation). Thus, symptoms of hyperandrogenism or hyperestrogenism require subtle endocrine investigations (Tables 3, 4).

In general, endocrine symptoms of sex hormone-producing tumors (neoplastic hyperandrogenism/hyperestrogenism) are usually more severe and develop usually more rapidly when compared to non-tumorous causes of sex hormone excess (functional and idiopathic hyperandrogenism/hyperestrogenism).

Adrenal overproduction of androgens or estrogens can be caused by three different pathophysiological processes also influencing therapeutic strategies (Table 5):

1. Several forms of congenital adrenal hyperplasia (CAH) caused by deficiency of glucocorticoid hormone synthesizing enzymes resulting in hypocortisolism and compensatory increased plasma ACTH levels (see Chap. 10, "Classic Congenital Adrenal Hyperplasia")
2. Adrenal hyperplasia without enzyme deficiency probably caused by increased expression of stimulating cell receptors, and
3. Adrenal neoplasms with specific pattern (increased or decreased enzyme activity) of the steroid hormone cascade

16.3.2 Pathology

Macroscopically, sex hormone-producing tumors are usually found as dark red-brown tumors with a gray-red-brown cut-surface which is in sharp contrast to cortisol-producing adrenal tumors. Histologically, androgen- or estrogen-producing tumors present either as typical adrenocortical tumors imitating zonae reticularis and fasciculata (alveolar or solid texture) or as gonadal-like tumors containing Reinke's crystals typically to be found in ovarian hilus cells or testicular Leydig cells [1, 46, 55, 71, 80, 120, 122]. In a few cases, ganglioneuroma containing Leydig cells [1, 46] have been reported, leading to the hypotheses of: (1) the proximity of adrenocortical gland and gonadal tissue

Table 2. Clinical symptoms of hyperandrogenism and hyperestrogenism in males and females with respect to patient age

	Hyperandrogenism	Hyperestrogenism
Prepubertal females	Advanced growth and bone age followed by premature termination of growth Contrasexual precocious pseudopuberty Premature pubarche No thelarche Primary amenorrhea Hirsutism Virilism Clitoris hypertrophy Deep voice Female pseudohermaphroditism	Advanced growth and bone age followed by premature termination of growth Isosexual precocious pseudopuberty Premature thelarche Premature menarche
Prepubertal males	Advanced growth and bone age followed by premature termination of growth Isosexual precocious pseudopuberty Premature pubarche Macrogenitosomia Infantile testes	Advanced growth and bone age followed by premature termination of growth Contrasexual precocious pseudopuberty Gynecomastia Delayed or absent pubic hair and penis growth Azoospermia Male pseudohermaphroditism
Premenopausal female adults	Hirsutism Virilism Secondary amenorrhea Deep voice Clitoris hypertrophy	Disturbance of menstruation
Postmenopausal female adults	Oligosymptomatic hirsutism Virilism Deep voice Clitoris hypertrophy	Vaginal bleeding
Male adults	Oligosymptomatic	Gynecomastia Azoospermia Loss of pubic hair Testes and penis atrophy

Table 3. Causes of masculinization

	Females	Males
Neoplastic forms	Androgen-producing ovarian tumors (Sertoli stromal cell tumors, Leydig cell tumors) Androgen-producing adrenal tumors/hyperplasia Cortisol-producing adrenal tumors/hyperplasia Growth hormone-producing tumors	Androgen-producing testicular tumors (Leydig cell tumors) Gonadotropic tumors (teratoma, germinoma, optic glioma, hypothalamic astrocytoma or hamartoma, choriocarcinoma, hepatoma) Androgen-producing adrenal tumors/hyperplasia Cortisol-producing adrenal tumors/hyperplasia Growth hormone-producing tumors
Functional forms	"Polycystic ovary syndrome" Hyperthecosis CAH	CAH
Idiopathic forms	Increased androgen receptor activity	Not known
Iatrogenic forms	Testosterone, glucocorticoids, danazol	

Table 4. Causes of feminization

	Females	Males
Neoplastic forms	Estrogen-producing ovarian tumors (granulosa cell tumors, theca cell tumors, granulosa-theca cell tumors)	Estrogen-producing testicular tumors (Sertoli cell tumors)
	Estrogen-producing adrenal tumors/hyperplasia	Estrogen-producing adrenal tumors/hyperplasia
	Gonadotropic tumors (teratoma, germinoma, optic glioma, hypothalamic astrocytoma or hamartoma, choriocarcinoma, hepatoma)	Prolactinoma
Functional forms	Familial CYP19 overexpression	Familial CYP19 overexpression 5a-reductase deficiency (Imperato-McGinley syndrome) Androgen receptor deficiency ("hairless women") After castration Hepatic cirrhosis Uremia
Idiopathic forms	Not known	Increased estrogen receptor activity
Iatrogenic forms		Estrogens, antiandrogens, digitalis, spironolactone

Table 5. Causes of adrenal hyperandrogenism/hyperestrogenism and consequences for surgery

Entity	Pathogenesis and clinical presentation	Indication for adrenalectomy
Congenital adrenal hyperplasia	Several forms of hypocortisolism with hyperandrogenism caused by inherited adrenal steroid hormone enzyme deficiency (autosomal recessive) resulting in increased ACTH release and C19 steroid synthesis (see Chap. 10, "Classic Congenital Adrenal Hyperplasia")	Usually not given; only in patients with adrenal tumors (increased frequency in patients with CAH) or in patients with adverse side effects/inefficacy of steroid substitution [14, 89, 128, 131]
Acquired adrenal hyperplasia	Probably related to an increased expression of LH receptors (or others) resulting in symmetric or asymmetric adrenal hyperplasia and increased release of adrenal androgens	In general probably not given; indicated in patients without options/effects of medical treatment or unknown etiology
Androgen- or estrogen-producing adrenocortical adenomas or carcinomas	Caused by overexpression of androgen-producing enzymes	Given in all patients

during early embryogenesis, (2) the common origin of the gonad and the adrenal cortex, (3) thecal metaplasia, and (4) the development of Leydig cells from Schwann cells [46].

The histological pattern of an adrenocortical tumor allows no conclusions to be drawn about its endocrine feature nor about its biological behavior [71, 74]. However, the expression of inhibin α (probably involved in the regulation of FSH) has recently been found to be limited on normal or neoplastic androgen-producing adrenocortical cells when compared to other adrenocortical cells [3, 70].

The nature of androgen- or estrogen-producing tumors is difficult to determine when pathohistological criteria are used [5, 29, 103]. So far, the best predictor for malignancy is the occurrence of metastases or tumor recurrence, and tumor weight [18, 103, 132]. The weight of adrenocortical carcinomas is usually >100 g. In contrast, tumors weighing <30 g are generally considered to be benign [32, 41]. However, benign tumors presenting with a diameter of about 13–16 cm weighing more than 1,500 g have also been reported [41]. Recently, a correlation between patient outcome and several proliferation indices was reported [5, 16].

The majority of pure androgen-producing adrenal tumors have been assumed to be benign [18], whereas in estrogen-producing tumors and tumors with a mixed pattern of hormones produced an adrenocortical carcinoma has to be expected [35, 39].

16.3.3   Enzyme and Cell Receptor Pattern

In adrenal neoplasms, an isolated increase of androgens or estrogens may be the result of:
1. Tumor specific steroidogenesis enzyme pattern: low activity of cortisol-producing enzymes [11β-hydroxylase (CYP11B1), 21-hydroxylase (CYP21A2), 3β-HSD)] and/or high activity of DHEA-producing enzymes (CYP17), testosterone-producing enzymes (3β-HSD, 7β-HSD) (Fig. 2), and estrone-producing enzymes (CYP19), and/or

normal pathway

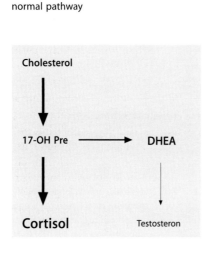

DHEA producing tumor:
increased activity of DHEA producing enzymes (CYP17)

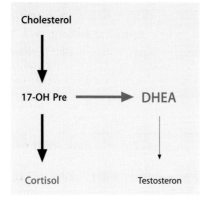

DHEA producing tumor:
reduced activity of cortisol producing enzymes (3β-HSD, CYP11B1, CYP21A2)

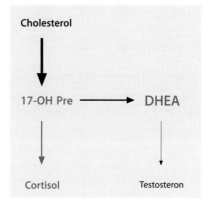

Testosteron producing tumor:
increased activity of testosteron producing enzymes (CYP17, 17β-HSD); reinforced by reduced activity of cortisol producing enzymes (CYP11B1, CYP21A2)

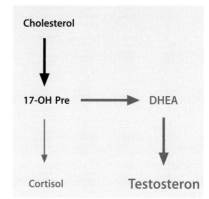

Fig. 2. Principle of normal and impaired enzymatic activities via alternative enzymatic pathways within adrenocortical tumor cells

2. Expression of stimulating receptors in tumor cells, and/or

3. Large tumor volume.

It must be noted that indirect effects by involving extra-adrenal endocrine organs (e.g. inhibition of ACTH or gonadotropins) may modulate the clinical picture.

16.3.3.1   Virilizing Adrenal Tumors

Two distinct types of virilizing adrenal tumors may be distinguished: tumors with high production rates of DHEA/DHEA-S usually presenting as typical adrenocortical tumors and tumors with secretion of testosterone. It has been suggested that testosterone-producing adrenal tumors could somehow be derived from gonadal tissue because gonadal type histology and gonadotropin receptors can be frequently found [57, 108]. However, testosterone-producing tumors with the typical feature of adrenal architecture were found in several patients either with or without gonadotropin responsiveness [7, 107].

DHEA, DHEA-S and Androstenedione-Producing Adrenal Tumors

Low activity of CYP11B1, CYP21A2, and/or 3β-HSD in adrenocortical tumor cells has been reported in several studies [10, 15, 23, 30, 77, 113, 119]. As a consequence of the absent enzyme activity, tumor cells may secrete large amounts of cortisol precursors and as a consequence DHEA, DHEA-S, and/or androstenedione [10]. Virilizing symptoms occur as a result of peripheral conversion from DHEA and/or androstenedione into testosterone and dihydrostosterone. Since the remaining adrenocortical tissue expresses normal enzyme activities leaving the total adrenal production of cortisol unaffected, generally no changes regarding ACTH and cortisol levels have been found causing pure virilization without Cushing symptoms in those patients [10, 119].

The nature of the low enzyme activity is unknown. Since fetal adrenocortical cells exhibit only low levels of CYP11B1, it has been hypothesized that tumor cells with CYP11B1 deficiency arise from undifferentiated fetal adrenal cells or from a cell that regressed to a stage of fetal adrenal cells [10]. However, low CYP11B1 is also found in normal cells of the zona reticularis [87].

Testosterone-Producing Adrenal Tumors

In tumor cells which express testosterone synthesizing enzymes (3β-HSD, 17β-HSD), testosterone can be produced by the tumor cells itself [30, 57, 65, 77, 107, 113]. This pathway seems to be reinforced in patients with tumor cells presenting with CYP11B1 deficiency [30] or CYP21A2 deficiency [77, 113].

16.3.3.2   Feminizing Adrenal Tumors

Adrenocortical tumor cells with testosterone production *and* overexpression of the CYP19 gene, which has low activity in normal adrenocortical cells [9, 68, 129], are able to produce estrone or estradiol by aromatization of androstenedione or testosterone [9, 48, 68, 70, 94, 129, 134].

The CYP19 gene is located on chromosome 15 and contains at least ten exons. Under the control of several distinct promotor regions, alternate splicing of exon 1 and a part of exon 2 seems to be the basis of tissue-specific expression of several aromatase splicing variants [50, 109]. In estrogen-producing adrenal tumors, the CYP19 gene seems to utilize those promoters typically expressed in the gonads but not in the normal adrenals. Since a similar spontaneous, tissue-specific transcription-factor related switch of the alternative exons was found in several tumors (breast cancer, tumors of the liver, colorectal cancer [50, 52]), a similar pathogenetic mechanism has recently been suggested in adrenal tumors [9, 129].

The amount of secreted estrogens depends on the volume of the tumor but also on the activity of the expressed P450-aromatase, which has been reported in a relatively wide range between 0.0125 pmol/min/g protein and 104.4 pmol/min/mg protein [9, 48, 68, 94, 129, 134] (Table 6). It is conceivable that the estrone production would be reinforced by low activity of the 11β-hydroxylase, which was also reported in feminizing tumors [15]. In adrenal tumors secreting both androgens and estrogens, peripheral aromatization of androgens may reinforce the clinical feature of feminization [136].

16.3.3.3   Adrenal Tumors with Mixed Hormone Pattern

Estrogens, androgens, and cortisol-producing tumors may lead to simultaneous feminization and masculinization [4, 8, 50, 82]. Co-secretion of several adrenocortical hormones is probably the result of large tu-

Table 6. Activity of CYP19 in patients with estrogen-producing adrenal tumors

Sex and age (years)	Symptoms	CYP19 activity (v_{max} in pmol/min/mg protein)	CYP19 splicing variant	Reference
Male, 19	Gynecomastia	3.6	nd	[68]
Female, 65	Vaginal bleeding	2.0	nd	[48]
Male, 29	Gynecomastia	~4.0	Gonadal	[134]
Male, 18 1/2	Gynecomastia	71–104.4	Gonadal	[129]
Female, 7	Premature menarche, isosexual precocious pseudopuberty	0.43	Gonadal	[94]
Male, 20	Gynecomastia	0.0125	Gonadal	[9]
Normal adrenocortical tissue		0.0047[a] 0.0054[b] 0.016[c]		

[a] Given by [94].
[b] Given by [9].
[c] Given by [68].

mors (volume effect) with autonomic production of hormones without a preference for any steroid hormone pathway.

The switch of predominately secreted hormones has been considered to be a sign of malignancy [8,50].

In patients with hypercortisolism and hyperandrogenism, cytochrome b_5 has been identified as the determining factor regulating the activity of CYP18, constituting the control enzyme between the cortisol- and androgen hormone-producing pathway [101]. High expression of cytochrome b_5 was found to be associated with a high secretion of adrenal androgens in patients with Cushing's syndrome [100].

16.3.3.4 Gonadotropin-Dependent Androgen and Estrogen-Producing Adrenal Tumors and Adrenal Hyperplasia (Acquired Adrenal Hyperplasia)

Gonadotropin receptors have been detected in cells in both the zona reticularis and fasciculata of the adrenal cortex [92] but without a physiological impact on steroidogenesis [95]. In some cases of testosterone and estrogen-producing adrenal tumors, however, an increased expression of human chorionic gonadotropin (hCG) receptors has been suggested [7, 12, 28, 36, 38, 45, 47, 49, 58, 73, 77, 88, 97, 112, 115, 116, 130]. An early hypothesis of how gonadotropins could stimulate adrenal androgen or estrogen secretion focussed on the presence of gonadal tissue within the adrenals (embryological translocation of gonadal cells). However,

none of the reported gonadotropin responsive virilizing adrenal tumors presented with features of gonadal tissue but with typically adrenocortical features [7, 12, 28, 36, 38, 45, 47, 49, 58, 73, 77, 88, 112, 115, 116, 130]. Thus, overexpression of gonadotropin receptors has been hypothesized as an independent pathogenetic factor concerning the evolution of adrenocortical tumors [47]. The expression of gonadotropin receptors may be the reason for masculinization during pregnancy in women with gonadotropin-dependent androgen-producing adrenal adenoma [26, 38]. On the other hand, the majority of gonadotropin responsive virilizing adrenal tumors occurred in postmenopausal women, suggesting a long history of the tumors achieving clinical significance after permanent elevation of gonadotropins during the menopause [47]. Furthermore, overexpression of gonadotropin receptors or other ectopic receptors (gastric inhibitory peptide, β-adrenergic receptors, vasopressin receptors, serotonin receptors) in adrenocortical cells (Table 7)

Table 7. Potential options of medical therapy for adrenocortical tumors and hyperplasia expressing illicit cell receptors. (Modified from [72])

Illicit receptor	Potential therapy
GIP receptor	Somatostatin
β-Adrenergic receptors	β-Blockers
LH-R	GnRH analogs
5-HT$_4$ receptors	5-HT$_4$ receptor antagonists

seems to be the cause of polyclonal adrenocortical adenoma or bilateral adrenal hyperplasia presenting with hypercortisolism [72] or hyperandrogenism [6, 47, 72, 121].

16.4   Clinical Features

16.4.1   Androgen-Producing Adrenal Tumors

16.4.1.1   *Prepubertal Females*

Hyperandrogenism caused by adrenal tumors leads to contrasexual precocious pseudopuberty. Usually hirsutism, especially with marked pubic hair growth (premature pubarche), clitoris hypertrophy, and voice deepening can be observed. Furthermore, patients are typically above the 90th percentile in growth and weight and present with advanced bone age [17]. In a recent report, growth was accelerated in about 75% of children with virilizing adrenal tumors, and bone age was advanced by at least 1.5 years in 60% of them [132]. The advance in linear growth is in marked contrast to children with hypercortisolism, in whom usually a reduced growth occurs [104]. However, in patients with androgens and cortisol co-secreting tumors, usually the effect of cortisol predominates that of androgens [104]. However, some reports have been published reporting an advanced growth and bone age in children with cortisol- and androgen-producing tumors [4]. In female infants with tumor development before the 4 months of gestation, clitoris hypertrophy may be combined with labial fusion, leading to confusion in sex determination [17, 24].

16.4.1.2   *Prepubertal Males*

In boys with androgen-producing adrenal tumors, an isosexual precocious puberty can be found. Typically, they have significant penile enlargement and advanced growth of pubic hair. As in females, an advanced growth and bone age as well as an advanced development of the musculature has to be considered [17]. Despite the macrogenitosomia praecox, the patients have often small and infantile testes [17], which is in contrast to true pituitary-mediated precocious puberty [34]. However, testicular enlargement with hypertrophy of spermatic tubules does not exclude an adrenal origin of hyperandrogenism probably because of a direct androgen effect in some patients [34, 75].

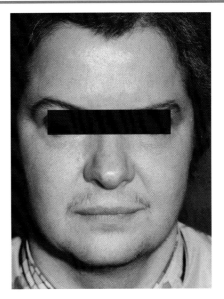

Fig. 3. Hirsutism in a postmenopausal woman with a beard on the upper lips caused by an androgen-producing adrenal tumor on the left side. (Picture kindly provided by U. Schneyer, MD, Halle)

16.4.1.3   *Adult Females*

In females, hirsutism with excessive hair growth on the face (Fig. 3), chest, areola, liena alba, inner thighs and external genitalia, and clitoris hypertrophy is present in almost all patients. In premenopausal women with androgen-producing adrenal tumors, menstrual abnormalities (amenorrhea, oligomenorrhea, irregular cycles) can usually be observed. Deepening of the voice occurs in about 50% of patients. Less frequent symptoms are loss of libido, acne, seborrhea, male type of baldness, and breast atrophy [32, 41, 80, 81]. The clinical features of virilizing adenomas do not differ from those of adrenocortical carcinoma [41]. Typically, symptoms of androgen-producing adrenal tumors develop rapidly when compared to functional hyperandrogenism. However, a long history of symptoms does not exclude a virilizing adrenal tumor [32].

Remarkably, in a few cases, virilization during gravidity has been reported [26, 38, 69, 88], probably related to gonadotropin-responsive androgen-producing adrenal adenoma [38, 26, 88]. In all female newborns, disturbances of sex determination were found. In one girl who presented with severe female pseudohermaphroditism, an apparent feminization occurred during puberty with respect to her female karyotype [69].

16.4.1.4   Adult Males

In men, androgen-producing adrenal tumors may cause infertility by suppression of gonadotropin secretion [81], but usually only slight endocrine symptoms can be observed.

16.4.2   Estrogen-Producing Adrenal Tumors

16.4.2.1   Male Subjects

The extent of feminization in males depends on the ratio of testosterone and estrogens [80]. In adult males, bilateral gynecomastia is the main symptom occurring in almost all patients. As a result of the estrogen induced inhibition of gonadotropins, testicular atrophy, azoospermia related to tubular fibrosis and loss of Leydig cells, and decreased libido can be observed in about 50% of patients [70]. Less than 25% of patients present with feminizing hair changes or penile atrophy [39, 61].

In prepubertal males, bilateral gynecomastia and advanced height and weight (usually above the 90th percentile) are typically found [33].

16.4.2.2   Female Subjects

In adult females, only atypical endocrine symptoms can usually be found. Increased vaginal bleeding but also amenorrhea were most often reported [48, 82, 111]. In prepubertal females, isosexual precocious pseudopuberty with premature thelarche, pubarche [usually classified using the Tanner stages (I–V)], and menarche, with estrogenized pink vaginal mucosa but without clitoris hypertrophy combined with advanced growth and weight can be observed [23].

16.5   Diagnostic Procedures

16.5.1   Clinical Signs

Since hyperandrogenism is caused by several pathogenetic processes, hirsutism and virilism require a complex endocrinological diagnosis. Initially, it is most important to distinguish between neoplastic, functional, or idiopathic hyperandrogenism. The main clinical symptoms suggesting neoplastic hyperandrogenism are rapid development of severe virilizing symptoms. Very careful clinical assessment should include examination of the breast and the vagina (clitoris hypertrophy, estrogenization of the vaginal mucosa, palpation of the adnexae). Severity of hirsutism can be classified using the Ferriman-Gallwey score. Cushing symptoms and medical treatment with androgens or its factitial intake should also be noted [81]. Elevated estrogen levels leading to bilateral gynecomastia and testicular atrophy described by several authors [40] may be the result of non-tumoral activation of the peripheral aromatase [40, 76, 79, 114]. Many causes of hyperestrogenism must be considered (see above).

16.5.2   Laboratory Findings

Laboratory investigations should include analysis of serum testosterone, serum DHEA-S, and urinary excretion of the 17-ketosteroids over 24 h. Dependent on clinical signs (severe masculinization, Cushing feature) and laboratory results, analysis of other hormones and metabolites of the hypothalamus-pituitary-adrenal axis and the hypothalamus-pituitary-gonadal axis such as serum cortisol, aldosterone, 11-hydroxyprogesterone (11-OHPro), 11-OHP-Pre, plasma ACTH, gonadotropins and, in patients with feminization, estrone and estradiol may be required.

Typically, testosterone levels are only slightly elevated in women with functional or idiopathic hirsutism (normal values <2.1 nmol/l). High levels of testosterone (>5–7 nmol/l) and urinary 17-ketosteroids >50 mg/24 h (normal <15 mg) are suggestive for organic hyperandrogenism caused by ovarian or adrenal tumors [32, 44]. DHEA-S levels >18.5 μmol/l (normal <7.5 nmol/l) indicate an androgen-producing adrenal tumor with a high sensitivity. However, normal levels of testosterone, DHEA-S, and urinary 17-ketosteroids can be found even in patients with virilizing adrenocortical carcinoma [32]. Urinary 17-ketosteroids are usually within the normal range in testosterone-producing tumors [45, 81, 130].

In patients with organic hyperandrogenism, dexamethasone usually does not suppress elevated serum levels of testosterone or DHEA-S, or reduce urinary excretion of 17-ketosteroids [32, 64]. Due to the existence of gonadotropin dependent adrenocortical adenoma, the ACTH test and the hCG test are not suitable to distinguish between ovarian and adrenal androgen-producing tumors [32, 73, 81]. Moreover, numerous adrenocortical adenomas are unresponsive for ACTH [57]. However, an ACTH test should be performed to exclude a late onset or non-classical CAH [44]. On the other hand, genetic testing should be performed when CAH is expected. In infants with severe virilism due to an androgen-producing tumor during gestation (child or mother), an analysis of the karyotype may be required to determine the true sex [69].

16.5.3   Localization Techniques

Abdominal and vaginal ultrasonography can reveal adrenal and ovarian tumors in more than 70% of cases. Other localizing imaging techniques are computed tomography (Fig. 4), magnetic resonance imaging, and norcholesterol scintigraphy. However, the positive prediction of all imaging techniques does not reach 90% [32].

In patients with suspected adrenal and ovarian tumors, selective venous catheterization of the adrenal and the ovarian veins for selective measurement of androgens is helpful and should be performed in every case with uncertain localization [10, 13, 31, 41, 81, 86, 98]. However, since the suprarenal and the testicular/ovarian vein on the left side drain into the renal vein, false results might be produced unless superselective catheterization is performed. In this case, intraoperative blood sampling for testosterone measurement may be superior [96]. Laparoscopy might be suitable for minimal-invasive intra-abdominal diagnosis in selected patients with unclear origin of organic hyperandrogenism [113]. The possibility of extra-adrenal localization of adrenocortical adenoma

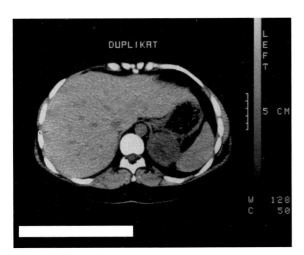

Fig. 4. CT scan of a testosterone-producing adrenal adenoma on the left side in a premenopausal woman with hirsutism and virilism. (Picture kindly provided by U. Schneyer, MD, Halle)

should be considered in patients with high elevation of androgens but a negative imaging examination [66, 84].

16.6   Treatment

Surgery is the only therapeutic option with curative intention for patients with sex hormone-producing tumors. Only complete removal of the tumor tissue offers definitive cure. However, in advanced tumor stages, surgery cannot influence long-term survival [126]. In patients with metastastases or non-resectable tumors, medical treatment combining adrenolysis, chemotherapy, and hormonal treatment is required. However, tumor debulking should be taken into account in all patients with metastases of adrenocortical tumors. However, recent data suggest a benefit of surgical tumor debulking only in those patients who had responded to a prior "neoadjuvant" chemotherapy [126]. In patients with acquired adrenal hyperplasia, medical treatment could be an alternative to surgical treatment on condition that the expression of illicit cell receptors is known [72].

16.6.1   Surgical Strategies

The surgical approach to the adrenal glands in patients with sex hormone-producing adrenal tumors does not differ from that in patients with other adrenal diseases. Laparoscopic or retroperitoneoscopic adrenalectomy is the preferred approach [11, 42, 43, 127] and is also feasible in children [19, 85, 110, 118].

However, the high frequency of malignant adrenal tumors producing androgens or estrogens has to be considered [35, 39]. Although recently an increasing number of studies reporting the endoscopic approach in patients with malignant adrenal tumors have been published [54], open adrenalectomy should be the preferred approach to all patients with suspected malignancy. In patients with advanced tumors spreading into the lower cava vein and the right cardiac atrium, a heart-lung machine may be required. With respect to the potential malignancy of all adrenal tumors secreting androgens or estrogens, regional lymphadenectomy should be considered, and, furthermore, in contrast to cortisol-producing adenomas or aldosterone-producing adenomas [11, 56, 60], subtotal adrenalectomy should only be considered in patients with benign tumors.

In patients with acquired adrenal hyperplasia, total bilateral adrenalectomy has to be considered when medical therapy is ineffective. The effect of bilateral subtotal adrenalectomy should be investigated further before this procedure may be recommended [63, 125].

16.6.2   Perioperative Treatment

Systematic investigations of androgen mediated inhibition of the hypothalamus-pituitary-adrenal axis and its recovery after adrenalectomy have not yet been performed. A direct and indirect inhibitory effect of androgens on the release of corticotropin-releasing hormone (CRH) has been demonstrated in animals by numerous studies [123, 124]. Thus, perioperative administration of exogenous glucocorticoids seems to be required in patients with hyperandrogenism and hyperestrogenism [17, 75]. However, more recently, successful operations without hydrocortisone replacement were reported in patients with an unaffected hypothalamus-pituitary-adrenal axis [11, 57].

To determine function of the hypothalamic-pituitary-adrenal axis, an appropriate test should be performed preoperatively. In patients with an unaffected system, exogenous steroids are not necessary. In those patients with a depression of the hypothalamic-pituitary-adrenal axis, perioperative and postoperative administration of hydrocortisone is required.

In general, patients with sex hormone-producing adrenal tumors and depression of the hypothalamic-pituitary-adrenal axis should receive 100 mg hydrocortisone during operation and 200 mg hydrocortisone during the subsequent 24 h continuously. During the subsequent days, the dosis of hydrocortisone should be continuously decreased.

Duration of hydrocortisone administration in patients with sex hormone-producing tumors depends on the time of secondary/tertiary adrenal insufficiency following tumor resection. No data are available allowing general recommendations. In patients with tumors secreting sex hormones and cortisol, restitution of the hypothalamic-pituitary-adrenal axis usually requires more than 6–12 months. These patients should be treated like patients with Cushing's syndrome. Before termination of exogenous steroid supplementation, a functional test should be performed. For exclusion of a secondary adrenal insufficiency a metyrapone test or an insulin-hypoglycemia test is recommended [91]. Patients with adrenal hyperandrogenism or hyperestrogenism should receive a single shot antibiosis.

16.6.3   Adjuvant and Palliative Treatment Options

Patients with advanced sex hormone-producing adrenocortical neoplasms (perhaps adrenocortical carcinomas) may benefit from a preoperative treatment using mitotane or ketaconazole [32, 90, 99].

In patients with complete removal of adrenal tumors associated with increased levels of androgens or estrogens, no special postoperative treatment is required even in the case of malignancy. However, although controlled studies have not been performed, mitotane may be given in advanced tumor stages to increase the length of time between recurrences [2, 25, 67, 74, 126].

Postoperatively, several drugs may be administered in patients with metastases or non-resectable tumors

Table 8. Options in adjuvant and palliative medical treatment for sex hormone-producing adrenal tumors

Substance	Action	Dose	Side effects
Mitotane	Inhibition of CYP11A1 and CYP11B1, adrenolysis (zona reticularis and zona fasciculata	4–12 g daily	Vomiting, vertigo, somnolence, weakness, confusion
Ketoconazole	Inhibition of CYP21A2 and CYP11B1	400–1,200 mg daily	Vomiting, hepatitis, gynecomastia
Aminoglutethimide	Inhibition of CYP19	500–2,000 mg daily	Headache, exanthema, tiredness
Letrozole	Inhibition of CYP19	1 mg daily	
Tamoxifen	Estrogen receptor antagonism	30 mg daily	
Flutamide	Androgen receptor antagonism	500 mg daily	Hepatotoxicity

(Table 8) to control tumor growth but predominantly endocrine symptoms. Mitotane (o.p'-DDD, 1, 1-dichlorodiphenyldichloroethane) is considered to be the drug of choice in patients with adrenocortical carcinoma. It inhibits steroidogenesis by interfering with cholesterol side-chain-cleavage enzyme (CYP11A1) and CYP11B1. Furthermore, it has a cytotoxic effect on cells of the zonae fasciculata and reticularis. The remission rates depend on the administered dose; however, in patients with metastastic disease, the effect of mitotane is limited [32, 74, 126]. Due to the adrenolytic effect, exogenous steroid substitution must be considered [126]. Ketoconazole has been demonstrated to control tumor symptoms preoperatively [90, 99]. It acts by inhibition of CYP21A2 and CYP11B1. However, long-term survival cannot be influenced. Other adrenolytic drugs or chemotherapeutic regimens used in several protocols included suramin and gossipol or cisplatin, etoposide, doxorubicin, 5-fluorouracil, melphalan, and vincristine [21, 26]. The combination of mitotane and cytotoxic chemotherapy may be of limited success. In general, despite significant remission rates, long-term outcome was not improved [74]. Antiandrogens (cyproterone acetate, flutamide, spironolactone) or antiestrogens (tamoxifen) may control endocrine symptoms like hirsutism or gynecomastia [27, 44, 73, 78].

Radiotherapy does not result in improved patient survival and should be limited as palliative treatment for metastases or non-resectable local recurrences [32].

16.6.4   Prognosis

After complete removal of tumor tissue, virilizing or feminizing symptoms usually disappear within a few months [10, 30, 41, 57, 73]. In prepubertal patients, complete regression of all symptoms may be observed when the patients are operated on before closure of the bone growth centers. The majority of patients will grow along the centile line achieved at presentation [102, 104]. In an univariate analysis, small tumor size, complete surgical removal, and benign behavior were identified to be favorable prognostic factors [117].

Patients with metastatic disease have a poor prognosis. Median survival without treatment is 3 months and with treatment 14 months. The long-term survival rate (5 years) is below 20% [32, 74, 126].

References

1. Aguirre P, Scully RE (1983) Testosterone-secreting adrenal ganglioneuroma containing Leydig cells. Am J Surg Pathol 7:699–705
2. Ahlman H, Khorram-Manesh A, Jansson S, Wangberg B, Nilsson O, Jacobsson CE, Lindstedt S (2001) Cytotoxic treatment of adrenocortical carcinoma. World J Surg 25:927–33
3. Arola J, Liu J, Heikkilä P, Ilvesmäki V, Salmenkivi K, Voutilainen R, Kahri AI (2000) Expression of inhibin a in andrenocortical tumours reflects the hormonal status of the neoplasm. J Endocrinol 165:223–9
4. Balakumar T, Perry LA, Savage MO (1997) Adrenocortical adenoma – an unusual presentation with hypersecretion of oestradiol, androgens and cortisol. J Pediatr Endocrinol Metab 10:227–9
5. Bergada I, Venara M, Maglio S, Ciaccio M, Diez B, Bergada C, Chemes H (1996) Functional adrenal cortical tumors in pediatric patients: a clinicopathologic and immunohistochemical study of a long term follow-up series. Cancer 77:771–7
6. Bertherat J, Gicquel C, Le Bouc Y, Bertagna X (2002) Molecular genetics of adrenal tumors. In: Wass JAH, Shalet SM (eds) Oxford textbook of endocrinology and diabetes. Oxford University Press, Oxford, pp 831–6
7. Blichert-Toft M, Vejlsted H, Hehlet H, Albrechtsen R (1975) Virilizing adrenocortical adenoma responsive to gonadotrophin. Acta Endocrinol (Copenh) 78:77–85
8. Bondy PK (1985) Disorders of the adrenal cortex. In: Wilson JD, Foster DW (eds) William's textbook of endcrinology, 7th edn. WB Saunders Co., Philadelphia, pp 816–890
9. Bouraima H, Lireux B, Mittre H, Benhaim A, Hrrou M, Mahoudeau J, Guillon-Metz F, Kottler ML, Reznik Y (2003) Major hyperestrogenism in a feminizing adrenocortical adenoma despite a moderate overexpression of the aromatase enzyme. Eur J Endocrinol 148:457–461
10. Bradshaw KD, Milewich L, Mason JI, Parker CR Jr, MacDonald PC, Carr BR (1994) Steroid secretory characteristics of a virilizing adrenal adenoma in a woman. J Endocrinol 140:297–307
11. Brauckhoff M, Nguyen Thanh P, Gimm O, Bär A, Dralle H (2003) Functional results after endoscopic subtotal cortical sparing adrenalectomy. Surg Today 33:342–8
12. Breustedt HJ, Nolde S, Tamm J (1997) A feminizing adrenal cortex adenoma with Cushing's syndrome which can be stimulated by HCG. Verh Dtsch Ges Inn Med 83:1340–3
13. Bricaire C, Raynaud A, Benotmane A, Clair F, Paniel B, Mowszowicz I, Wright F, Moreau JF, Kuttenn F, Mauvais-Jarvis P (1991) Selective venous catheterization in the evaluation of hyperandrogenism. J Endocrinol Invest 14:949–56
14. Bruining H, Bootsma AH, Koper JW, Bonjer J, de Jong FH, Lamberts SWJ (2001) Fertility and body composition after laparoscopic bilateral adrenalectomy in a

30-year-old female with congenital adrenal hyperplasia. J Clin Endocrinol Metab 86:482–4

15. Bryson MJ, Young RB, Reynolds WA, Sweat ML (1968) Biosynthesis of steroid hormones in a human feminizing adrenal carcinoma. Cancer 21:501–7

16. Bugg MF, Ribeiro RC, Roberson PK, Lloyd RV, Sandrini R, Silva JB, Epelman S, Shapiro DN, Parham DM (1994) Correlation of pathologic features with clinical outcome in pediatric adrenocortical neoplasia. A study of a Brazilian population. Brazilian Group for Treatment of Childhood Adrenocortical Tumors. Am J Clin Pathol 101:625–9

17. Burrington JD, Stephens CA (1969) Virilizing tumors of the adrenal gland in childhood: report of eight cases. J Pediatr Surg 4:291–302

18. Cagle PT, Hough AJ, Pysher TJ, Page DL, Johnson EH, Kirkland RT, Holcombe JH, Hawkins EP (1986) Comparison of adrenal cortical tumors in children and adults. Cancer 57:2235–7

19. Castilho LN, Castillo OA, Denes FT, Mitre AI, Arap S (2002) Laparoscopic adrenal surgery in children. J Urol 168:221–4

20. Chudler RM, Kay R (1989) Adrenocortical carcinoma in children. Urol Clin North Am 16:469–79

21. Ciftci AO, Senocak ME, Tanyel FC, Buyukpamukcu N (2001) Adrenocortical tumors in children. J Pediatr Surg 36:549–54

22. Clouston WM, Cannell GC, Fryar BG, Searle JW, Martin NI, Mortimer RH (1989) Virilizing adrenal adenoma in an adult with the Beckwith-Wiedemann syndrome: paradoxical response to dexamethasone. Clin Endocrinol (Oxf) 31:467–73

23. Comite F, Schiebinger RJ, Albertson BD, Cassorla FG, Vander Ven K, Cullen TF, Loriaux DL, Cutler GB Jr (1984) Isosexual precocious pseudopuberty secondary to a feminizing adrenal tumor. J Clin Endocrinol Metab 58:435–40

24. Coslovsky R, Ashkenazy M, Lancet M, Barash A, Borenstein R (1985) Female pseudohermaphroditism with adrenal cortical tumor in adulthood. J Endocinol Invest 8:63–5

25. Dackiw AP, Lee JE, Gagel RF, Evans DB (2001) Adrenal cortical carcinoma. World J Surg 25:914–26

26. Danilowicz K, Albiger N, Vanegas M, Gomez RM, Cross G, Bruno OD (2002) Androgen-secreting adrenal adenomas. Obstet Gynecol 100:1099–102

27. Dawber RP (2002) Hirsuties. J Gend Specif Med 5: 34–42

28. De Lange WE, Pratt JJ, Doorenbos H (1980) A gonadotrophin responsive testosterone producing adrenocortical adenoma and high gonadotrophin levels in an elderly woman. Clin Endocrinol (Oxf) 12: 21–8

29. Del Gaudio AD, Del Gaudio GA (1993) Virilizing adrenocortical tumors in adult women. Report of 10 patients, 2 of whom each had a tumor secreting only testosterone. Cancer 72:1997–2003

30. Deng Y, Osamura Y, Tanaka M, Katsuoka Y, Kawamura N, Murakoshi M (1990) A case of testosterone-secreting adrenal cortical adenoma with spironolactone body-like inclusion. Acta Pathol Jpn 40:67–72

31. Derksen J, Nagesser SK, Meinders AE, Haak HR, van de Velde CJ (1994) Identification of virilizing adrenal tumors in hirsute women. N Engl J Med 331:968–973

32. Derksen J (1997) Androgen secreting adrenal neoplasms. In: Azziz R, Nestler JE, Dewailly D (eds) Androgen excess disorders in women. Lippincott-Raven, Philadelphia, pp 545–53

33. Desai MB, Kapadia SN (1988) Feminizing adrenocortical tumors in male patients: adenoma versus carcinoma. J Urol 139:101–3

34. Drago JR, Sheiholislam B, Olstein JS, Palmer JM, Tesluk H, Link D (1979) Virilizing adrenal cortical carcinoma with hypertrophy of spermatic tubules in childhood. Urology 14:70–5

35. Dudley N (2002) Adrenal surgery. In: Wass JAH, Shalet SM (eds) Oxford textbook of endocrinology and diabetes. Oxford University Press, Philadelphia, pp 758–64

36. Faggiano M, Crisuolo T, Sinisi AA, Scialdone A, Bellastella A, Cuccurullo L (1984) Virilization syndrome in a young woman due to an androgen-secreting adenoma. J Endocrinol Invest 7:41–5

37. Federici S, Galli G, Ceccarelli PL, Ferrari M, Cicognani A, Cacciari E, Domini R (1994) Adrenocortical tumors in children: a report of 12 cases. Eur J Pediatr Surg 4: 21–5

38. Fuller PJ, Pettigrew IG, Pike JW, Stockigt JR (1983) An adrenal adenoma causing virilization of mother and infant. Clin Endocrinol (Oxf) 18:143–53

39. Gabrilove JL, Sharma DC, Wotiz HH, Dorfman RI (1965) Feminizing adrenocortical tumors in the male. A review of 52 cases including a case report. Medicine 44:37–96

40. Gabrilove JL, Nicolis GL, Sohval AR (1973) Non-tumorous feminizing adrenogenital syndrome in the male subject. J Urol 110:710–3

41. Gabrilove JL, Seman AT, Sabet R, Mitty HA, Nicolis GL (1981) Virilizing adrenal adenoma with studies on the steroid content of the adrenal venous effluent and a review of the literature. Endocr Rev 2:462–70

42. Gagner M, Lacroix A, Bolte E, Pómp A (1994) Laparoscopic adrenalectomy. The importance of a flank approach in the lateral decubitus position. Surg Endosc 8:135–8

43. Gagner M, Lacroix A, Bolte E (1992) Laparoscopic adrenalectomy in Cushing's syndrome and pheochromocytoma. N Engl J Med 327:1033

44. Gilling-Smith C, Franks S (2002) Hirsutism. In: Wass JAH, Shalet SM (eds) Oxford textbook of endocrinology and diabetes. Oxford University Press, Oxford, pp 1148–59

45. Givens JR, Andersen RN, Wiser WL, Coleman SA, Fish SA (1974) A gonadotropin-responsive adrenocortical adenoma. J Clin Endocrinol Metab 38:126–33

46. Godlewski G, Nguyen Trong AH, Tang J, Semler-Collery R, Joujoux JM, Gaujoux AF (1993) Virilizing adrenal ganglioneuroma containing Leydig cells. Acta Chir Belg 93:181–4

47. Goodarzi MO, Dawson DW, Li X, Lei Z, Shintaku P, Rao CV, Van Herle AJ (2003) Virilization in bilateral macronodular adrenal hyperplasia controlled by luteinizing hormone. J Clin Endocrinol Metab 88:73–77

48. Goto T, Murakami O, Sato F, Haraguchi M, Yokoyama K, Sasano H (1996) Oestrogen producing adrenocortical adenoma: clinical, biochemical and immunohistochemical studies. Clin Endocrinol (Oxf) 45:643–8

49. Guillausseau PJ, Boitard C, Le Charpentier Y, Cedard L, Nahoul K, Blacker C, Kaloustian E, Courtalhac-Kaloustian F, Dubost C, Lubetzki J (1987) Androgen producing adrenal adenoma. Report on a case associated with hyperparathyroidism. J Endocrinol Invest 10: 593–9

50. Halmi KA, Lascari AD (1971) Conversion of virilization to feminization in a young girl with adrenal cortical carcinoma. Cancer 27:931–5

51. Harada N, Utsumi T, Takagi Y (1993) Tissue-specific expression of the human aromatase cytochrome P-450 gene by alternative use of multiple exons 1 and promoters, and switching of tissue-specific exons 1 in carcinogenesis. Proc Natl Acad Sci U S A 90:11312–6

52. Harada N, Ota H, Yoshimura N, Katsuyama T, Takagi Y (1998) Localized aberrant expression of cytochrome P450 aromatase in primary and metastatic malignant tumors of human liver. J Clin Endocrinol Metab 83: 697–702

53. Hayles AB, Hahn HB Jr, Sprague RG, Bahn RC, Priestley JT (1966) Hormone-secreting tumors of the adrenal cortex in children. Pediatrics 37:19–25

54. Henry JF, Sebag F, Icabone M, Mirallie E (2002) Results of laparoscopic adrenalectomy for large and potentially malignant tumors. World J Surg 26:1043–7

55. Hilton CW, Pollock WJ (1988) Virilization due to a Leydig cell adrenal adenoma. South Med J 81:924–5

56. Imai T, Tanaka Y, Kikumori T, Ohiwa M, Matsuura N, Mase T, Funahashi H (1999) Laparoscopic partial adrenalectomy. Surg Endosc 13:343–5

57. Imai T, Tobinaga J, Morita-Matsuyama T, Kikumori T, Sasano H, Seo H, Funahashi H (1999) Virilizing adrenocortical adenoma: in vitro steroidogenesis, immunohistochemical studies of stereogenic enzymes, and gene expression of corticotropin receptor. Surgery 125:396–402

58. Imperato-McGinley J, Young IS, Huang T, Dreyfus JC, Reckler JM, Peterson RE (1981) Testosterone secreting adrenal cortical adenomas. Int J Gynaecol Obstet 19: 421–8

59. Itami RM, Amunsdosn GM, Kaplan SA, Lippe BM (1982) Prepubertal gynecomastia caused by an adrenal tumor. Diagnostic value of ultrasonography. Am J Dis Child 136:584–6

60. Janetschek G, Lhotta K, Gasser R, Finkenstedt G, Jaschke W, Bartsch G (1997) Adrenal-sparing laparoscopic surgery for aldosterone-producing adenoma. J Endourol 11:145–8

61. Jones KL (1974) Feminization, virilization, and precocious sexual development that results from neoplastic processes. Ann N Y Acad Sci 230:195–203

62. Kaddah NM, Dessouky NM (2003) Functioning adrenal tumors in children: A report of 17 cases. Saudi Med J 24:S46–7

63. Kageyama Y, Ishizaka K, Iwashina M, Sasano H, Kihara K (2002) A case of ACTH-independent bilateral macronodular adrenal hyperplasia successfully treated by subtotal resection of the adrenal glands: four-year follow-up. Endocr J 49:227–9

64. Kaltsas GA, Isidori AM, Kola BP, Skelly RH, Chew SL, Jenkins PJ, Monson JP, Grossman AB, Besser GM (2003) The value of the low-dose dexamethasone suppression test in the differential diagnosis of hyperandrogenism in women. J Clin Endocrinol Metab 88: 2634–43

65. Kelly TR, Mayors DJ, Boutsicaris PS (1982) Adrenal adenoma: isolated testosterone secretion. Am Surg 48: 604–6

66. Kepes JJ, O'Boynick P, Jones S, Baum D, McMillan J, Adams ME (1990) Adrenal cortical adenoma in the spinal canal of an 8-year-old girl. Am J Surg Pathol 14:481–4

67. Khorram-Manesh A, Ahlman H, Jansson S, Wangberg B, Nilsson O, Jakobsson CE, Eliasson B, Lindstedt S, Tisell LE (1998) Adrenocortical carcinoma: surgery and mitotane for treatment and steroid profiles for follow-up. World J Surg 22:605–11

68. Kimura M, Itoh N, Tsukamoto T, Kumamoto Y, Takagi Y, Mori Y (1995) Aromatase activity in an estrogen-producing adrenocortical carcinoma in a young man. J Urol 153:1039–40

69. Kirk JM, Perry LA, Shand WS, Kirby RS, Besser GM, Savage MO (1990) Female pseudohermaphroditism due to a maternal adrenocortical tumor. J Clin Endocrinol Metab 70:1280–1284

70. Kuhn JM, Lefebvre H, Duparc C, Pellerin A, Luton JP, Strauch G (2002) Cosecretion of estrogen and inhibin B by a feminizing adrenocortical adenoma: impact on gonadotropin secretion. J Clin Endocrinol Metab 87: 2367–75

71. Lack EE (1997) Tumors of the adrenal gland and extraadrenal paraganglia. Atlas of tumor pathology, 3rd series, fascicle 19. Armed Forces Institute of Pathology, Washington DC, pp 1–468

72. Lacroix A, Ndiaye N, Tremblay J, Hamet P (2001) Ectopic and abnormal hormone receptors in adrenal Cushing's syndrome. Endocr Rev 22:75–110

73. László FA, Tóth S, Kocsis J, Pávó I, Szécsi M (2001) Testosterone-secreting gonadotropin-responsive adrenal adenoma and its treatment with the antiandrogen flutamide. J Endocrinol Invest 24:622–7

74. Latronico AC, Chrousos GP (1997) Extensive personal experience: adrenocortical tumors. J Clin Endocrinol Metab 82:1317–24

75. Lee PD, Winter RJ, Green OC (1985) Virilizing adrenocortical tumors in childhood: eight cases and a review of the literature. Pediatrics 76:437–44

76. Leiberman E, Zachmann M (1992) Familial adrenal feminization probably due to increased steroid aromatization. Horm Res 37:96–102

77. Leinonen P, Ranta T, Siegberg R, Pelkonen R, Heikkila P, Kahri A (1991) Testosterone-secreting virilizing adrenal adenoma with human chorionic gonadotrophin receptors and 21-hydroxylase deficiency. Clin Endocrinol (Oxf) 34:31–5

78. Loszio FA, Toth S, Kocsis J, Pavo, Szecsi M (2001) Testosterone-secreting gonadotrophin-responsive adrenal adenoma and its treatment with the antiandrogen flutamide. J Endocrinol Invest 24:622–7

79. Martin RM, Lin CJ, Nishi MY, Billerbeck AEC, Latronico AC, Russell DW, Mendonca BB (2003) Familial hyperestrogenism in both sexes: clinical, hormonal, and molecular studies of two siblings. J Clin Endocrinol Metab 88:3027–34

80. Masiakos PT, Flynn CE, Donahoe PK (1997) Masculinizing and feminizing syndromes caused by functioning tumors. Semin Pediatr Surg 6:147–55

81. McKenna TJ, Cunningham SK, Loughlin T (1985) The adrenal cortex and virilization. Clin Endocrinol Metab 14:997–1020

82. McKenna TJ, O'Connell Y, Cunningham S, McCabe M, Culliton M (1990) Steroidogenesis in an estrogen-producing adrenal tumor in a young woman: comparison with steroid profiles associated with cortisol- and androgen-producing tumors. J Clin Endocrinol Metab 70: 28–34

83. McKenna TJ, Cunningham SK (1993) The pathogenesis of adrenal and extraadrenal hyperandrogenism. J Steroid Biochem Mol Biol 45:117–121

84. Medeiros LJ, Anasti J, Gardner KL, Pass HI, Nieman LK (1992) Virilizing adrenal cortical neoplasm arising ectopically in the thorax. J Clin Endocrinol Metab 75: 1522–5

85. Mirallie E, Leclair MD, de Lagausie P, Weil D, Plattner V, Duverne C, DeWint A, Podevin G, Heloury Y (2001) Laparoscopic adrenalectomy in children. Surg Endosc 15:156–60

86. Moltz L, Pickartz H, Sorensen R, Schwartz U, Hammerstein J (1984) Ovarian and adrenal vein steroids in seven patients with androgen-secreting ovarian neoplasms: selective catheterization findings. Fertil Steril 42:585–93

87. Munro-Neville A, O'Hare MJ (1982) The human adrenal cortex – pathology and biology – an integrated approach. Springer, New York, pp 16–34

88. Murset G, Zachmann M, Prader A, Fischer J, Labhart A (1970) Male external genitalia of a girl caused by a virilizing adrenal tumour in the mother. Case report and steroid studies. Acta Endocrinol (Copenh) 65: 627–38

89. Nasir J, Royston C, Walton C, White MC (1996) 11 beta-hydroxylase deficiency: management of a difficult case by laparoscopic bilateral adrenalectomy. Clin Endocrinol (Oxf) 45:225–8

90. Neto LS, Filho AG, Bustorff-Silva JM, Koler H, Epelman S, Marini SH, Junior GG (2000) Pre-operative control of arterial hypertension using ketoconazole in pediatric patients with adrenocortical tumors. J Pediatr Endocrinol Metab 13:201–4

91. Oelkers W (1996) Adrenal insufficiency. N Engl J Med 335:1206–12

92. Pabon JE, Li X, Lei ZM, Sanfilippo JS, Yussman MA, Rao CV (1996) Novel presence of luteinizing hormone/chorionic gonadotropin receptors in human adrenal glands. J Clin Endocrinol Metab 81:2397–400

93. Patil KK, Ransley PG, McCullagh M, Malone M, Spitz L (2002) Functioning adrenocortical neoplasms in children. BJU Int 89:562–5

94. Phornphuktul C, Okubo T, Wu K, Harel Z, Tracy TF Jr, Pinar H, Chen S, Gruppuso PA, Goodwin G (2001) Aromatase P450 expression in a feminizing adrenal adenoma presenting as isosexual precocious puberty. J Clin Endocrinol Metab 86:649–52

95. Piltonen T, Koivunen R, Morin-Papunen L, Ruokonen A, Huhtaniemi IT, Tapanainen JS (2002) Ovarian and adrenal steroid production: regulatory role of LH/HCG. Hum Reprod 17:620–4

96. Regnier C, Bennet A, Malet D, Guez T, Plantavid M, Rochaix P, Monrozies X, Louvet JP, Caron P (2002) Intraoperative testosterone assay for virilizing ovarian tumor topographic assessment: report of a Leydig cell tumor of the ovary in a premenopausal woman with an adrenal incidentaloma. J Clin Endocrinol Metab 87:3074–7

97. Rose LI, Williams GH, Jagger PI, Lauler DP (1968) Feminizing tumor of the adrenal gland with positive "chorionic-like" gonadotropin test. J Clin Endocrinol Metab 28:903–8

98. Ruutiainen K, Satokari K, Anttila L, Erkkola R (1992) Adrenal- and ovarian-vein steroids and LH response to GnRH in two patients with adrenocortical adenoma studied by selective catheterizations. Horm Res 37: 49–53

99. Saadi HF, Bravo EL, Aron DC (1990) Feminizing adrenocortical tumor: steroid hormone response to ketoconazole. J Clin Endocrinol Metab 70:540–3

100. Sakai Y, Yanase T, Takayanagi R, Nakao R, Nishi Y, Haji M, Nawata H (1993) High expression of cytochrome b5 in adrenocortical adenomas from patients with Cushing's syndrome associated with high secretion of adrenal androgens. J Clin Endocrinol Metab 76:1286–90

101. Sakai Y, Yanase T, Hara T, Takayanagi R, Haji M, Nawata H (1994) Mechanism of abnormal production of adrenal androgens in patients with adrenocortical adenomas and carcinomas. J Clin Endocrinol Metab 78:36–40

102. Salt AT, Savage MO, Grant DB (1992) Growth patterns after surgery for virilising adrenocortical adenoma. Arch Dis Child 67:234–6

103. Sandrini R, Ribeiro RC, DeLcerda L (1997) Extensive personal experience: childhood adrenocortical tumors. J Clin Endocrinol Metab 82:2027–31

104. Savage MO, Scommegna S, Carroll PV, Ho JT, Monson JP, Besser GM, Grossman AB (2002) Growth in disorders of adrenal hyperfunction. Horm Res 58 Suppl 1:39–43

105. Sawin RS (1997) Functioning adrenal neoplasms. Semin Pediatr Surg 6:156–63

106. Sbragia-Neto L, Melo-Filho AA, Guerra-Junior G, deLemos Marini SHV, Baptista MTM, deMatos PS, deOliveira-Filho AC, Bustorff-Silva JM (2000) Beckwith-

Wiedemann syndrome and virilizing cortical adrenal tumor in a child. J Pediatr Surg 35:1269–71

107. Schteingart DE, Woodbury MC, Tsao HS, McKenzie AK (1979) Virilizing syndrome associated with an adrenal cortical adenoma secreting predominantly testosterone. Am J Med 67:140–6

108. Sciarra F, Tosti-Croce C, Toscano V (1995) Androgen-secreting adrenal tumors. Minerva Endocrinol 20: 63–8

109. Sebastian S, Bulun SE (2001) A highly complexed organization of the regulatory region of the human CYP19 (aromatase) gene revealed by the human genome project. J Clin Endocrinol Metab 86:4600–2

110. Shanberg AM, Sanderson K, Rajpoot D, Duel B (2001) Laparoscopic retroperitoneal renal and adrenal surgery in children. BJU Int 87:521–4

111. Singer F (1991) Adrenal carcinoma presenting with postmenopausal vaginal bleeding. Obstet Gynecol 78: 569–70

112. Smith HC, Posen S, Clifton-Nligh P, Casey J (1978) A testosterone-secreting adrenal cortical adenoma. Aust N Z J Med 8:171–4

113. Spaulding SW, Masuda T, Osawa Y (1980) Increased 17 beta-hydroxysteroid dehydrogenase activity in a masculinizing adrenal adenoma in a patient with isolated testosterone overproduction. J Clin Endocrinol Metab 50:537–40

114. Stratakis CA, Vottero A, Brodie A, Kirschner LS, DeAtkine D, Li Q, Yue W, Mitsiades CS, Flor AW, Chrousos GP (1998) The aromatase excess syndrome is associated with feminization of both sexes and autosomal dominant transmission of aberrant p450 aromatase gene transcription. J Clin Endocrinol Metab 83: 1348–57

115. Takahashi H, Yoshizaki K, Kato H, Masuda T, Matsuka G, Mimura T, Inui Y, Takeuchi S, Adachi H, Matsumoto K (1978) A gonadotrophin-responsive virilizing adrenal tumour identified as a mixed ganglioneuroma and adrenocortical adenoma. Acta Endocrinol (Copenh) 89:701–9

116. Taylor L, Ayers JW, Gross MD, Peterson EP, Menon KM (1986) Diagnostic considerations in virilization: iodo-methyl-norcholesterol scanning in the localization of androgen secreting tumors. Fertil Steril 289:1005–10

117. Teinturier C, Pauchard MS, Brugieres L, Landais P, Chaussain JL, Bougneres PF (1999) Clinical and prognostic aspects of adrenocortical neoplasms in childhood. Med Pediatr Oncol 32:106–11

118. Tobias-Machado M, Cartum J, Santos-Machado TM, Gaspar HA, Simoes AS, Cruz R, Rodrigues R, Juliano RV, Wroclawski ER (2002) Retroperitoneoscopic adrenalectomy in an infant with adrenocortical virilizing tumor. Sao Paulo Med J 120:87–9

119. Touitou Y, Lecomte P, Auzeby A, Bogdan A, Besnier Y (1989) Evidence of 11β-hydroxylase deficiency in a patient with cortical adrenal adenoma. Horm Metab Res 21:272–4

120. Trost BN, Koenig MP, Zimmermann A, Zachmann M, Muller J (1981) Virilization of a post-menopausal woman by a testosterone-secreting Leydig cell type adrenal adenoma. Acta Endocrinol (Copenh) 98:274–82

121. Tsagarakis S, Tsigos C, Vassiliou V, Tsiotra P, Pratsinis H, Kletsas D, Trivizas P, Nikou A, Mavromatis T, Sotsiou F, Raptis S, Thalassinos N (2001) Food-dependent androgen and cortisol secretion by a gastric inhibitory polypeptide-receptor expressive adrenocortical adenoma leading to hirsutism and subclinical Cushing's syndrome: in vivo and in vitro studies. J Clin Endocrinol Metab 86:583–9

122. Vasiloff J, Chideckel EW, Boyd CB, Foshag LJ (1985) Testosterone-secreting adrenal adenoma containing crystalloids characteristic of Leydig cells. Am J Med 79: 772–6

123. Viau V, Chu A, Soriano L, Dallman MF (1999) Independent and overlapping effects of corticosterone and testosterone on corticotropin-releasing hormone and arginine vasopressin mRNA expression in the paraventricular nucleus of the hypothalamus and stress-induced adrenocorticotropic hormone release. J Neurosci 19: 6684–6693

124. Viau V, Soriano L, Dallman MF (2001) Androgens alter corticotropin releasing hormone and arginine vasopressin mRNA within forebrain sites known to regulate activity in the hypothalamic-pituitary-adrenal axis. J Neuroendocrinol 13:442–452

125. Wada N, Kubo M, Kijima H, Ishizuka T, Saeki T, Koike T, Sasano H (1996) Adrenocorticotropin-independent bilateral macronodular adrenocortical hyperplasia: immunohistochemical studies of steroidogenic enzymes and post-operative course in two men. Eur J Endocrinol 134:583–7

126. Wajchenberg BL, Albergaria Pereira MA, Mendonca BB, Latronico AC, Carneiro PC, Ferreira Alves VA, Zerbini MAC, Liberman B, Gomes GC, Kirschner MA (2000) Adrenocortical carcinoma. Cancer 88:711–36

127. Walz MK, Peitgen K, Krause U, Eigler FW (1995) Dorsal retroperitoneoscopic adrenalectomy – a new surgical technique. Zentralbl Chir 120:53–8

128. Warinner SA, Zimmermann D, Thompson GB, Grant CS (2000) Study of three patients with congenital adrenal hyperplasia treated by bilateral adrenalectomy. World J Surg 24:1347–52

129. Watanabe T, Yasuda T, Noda H, Wada K, Kazukawa I, Someya T, Minamitani K, Minagawa M, Wataki K, Matsunaga T, Ohnuma N, Kohno Y, Harada N (2000) Estrogen secreting adrenal adenocarcinoma in an 18-month-old boy: aromatase activity, protein expression, mRNA and utilization of gonadal type promotor. Endocr J 47:723–30

130. Werk EE Jr, Sholiton LE, Kalejis L (1973) Testosterone-secreting adrenal adenoma under gonadotropin control. N Engl J Med 289:767–70

131. White PC, Speiser PW (2002) Congenital adrenal hyperplasia. In: Wass JAH, Shalet SM (eds) Oxford textbook of endocrinology and diabetes. Oxford University Press, Oxford, New York, pp 733–45

132. Wolthers OD, Cameron FJ, Scheimberg I, Honour JW, Hindmarsh PC, Savage MO, Stanhope RG, Brook CG (1999) Androgen secreting adrenocortical tumours. Arch Dis Child 80:46–50

133. Young DL, Miller RW (1975) Incidence of malignant tumors in U.S. children. J Pediatr 86:254–8

134. Young J, Bulun SE, Agarwal V, Couzinet B, Mendelson CR, Simpson ER, Schaison G (1996) Aromatase expression in a feminizing adrenocortical tumor. J Clin Endocrinol Metab 81:3173–6

135. Young JL Jr, Ries LG, Silverberg E, Horm JW, Miller RW (1986) Cancer incidence, survival, and mortality for children younger than age 15 years. Cancer 58 (Suppl 2): 598–602

136. Zayed A, Stock JL, Liepman MK, Wollin M, Longcope C (1994) Feminization as a result of both peripheral conversion of androgens and direct estrogen production from an adrenocortical carcinoma. J Endocrinol Invest 17:275–8

17 Pheochromocytoma

Cord Sturgeon, Quan-Yang Duh

CONTENTS

17.1 Introduction

Pheochromocytomas are neoplasms of the neural crest derived chromaffin cells. Synthesis and secretion of catecholamines in an unregulated and often life-threatening manner is the hallmark of this rare tumor. Chromaffin cells are most frequently found in the adrenal medulla, where they normally function to secrete catecholamines, which modulate stress response, metabolism, and blood pressure. When catecholamine-producing chromaffin cell tumors arise in an extra-adrenal location they are referred to as paragangliomas, or extra-adrenal pheochromocytomas. Although apparently similar in ontogeny, subtle differences exist in the biology of disease between adrenal and extra-adrenal pheochromocytomas, which impact clinical decision making. A thorough understanding of the natural history of the various manifestations of chromaffin cell tumors guides the clinician in the most appropriate and efficacious treatment.

Although considered rare, the importance of screening for and treating pheochromocytomas is underscored by the fact that it is one of the few curable causes of hypertension, with a prevalence in hypertensive patients of 0.1–1% [36]. In autopsy series, a prevalence between 0.3% and 0.95% has been found [46]. In biochemical screening series the prevalence has been reported to be as high as 1.9% [44]. Undiagnosed and untreated pheochromocytomas lead to significant cardiovascular and oncologic morbidity and mortality.

17.2 Epidemiology

Pheochromocytomas can occur sporadically or in association with a number of syndromes. Approximately 90% are believed to be sporadic. Familial syndromes associated with the development of pheochromocytomas include multiple endocrine neoplasia (MEN) types 2A and 2B, von Recklinghausen's neurofibromatosis (NF1), and von Hippel-Lindau disease (VHL). Pheochromocytomas may also accompany nonfamilial syndromes such as Sturge-Weber syndrome, tuberous sclerosis, and Carney's triad. Pheochromocytomas in patients with familial syndromes are unlikely to be malignant [5, 23]. The one exception is patients with a family history of malignant pheochromocytomas; these individuals are felt to be at a higher risk for malignancy.

MEN 2A and 2B are autosomal dominant syndromes caused by mutations in the RET proto-oncogene. Common to MEN2 syndromes are medullary thyroid cancer (MTC; nearly 100% penetrance) and pheochromocytoma (approximately 40%). Pheochromocytomas in MEN 2 are bilateral in approximately 70% and are usually multicentric. Bilateral medullary hyperplasia is almost always present in these patients. Pheochromocytomas are rarely extra-adrenal or malignant in MEN2.

NF1 is an autosomal dominant disorder associated with widespread neurofibromatosis, café au lait spots, and the rare (1%) development of pheochromocytomas. Inheritance of VHL is autosomal dominant, and is characterized by retinal hemangiomatosis, cerebellar hemangioblastoma, pancreatic tumors, kidney cysts or tumors, pancreatic cysts, epididymal cystadenoma, and pheochromocytoma. The incidence of pheochromocytoma in VHL is between 10% and 20% and they are often bilateral. Other neuroectodermal disorders that may be associated with pheochromocytoma include Sturge-Weber syndrome, tuberous sclerosis, and Carney's triad. Carney's triad is a syndrome of gastric leiomyosarcoma, pulmonary chondroma, and functional extra-adrenal pheochromocytoma.

17.3   Untreated Pheochromocytoma

Undiagnosed and untreated pheochromocytoma may lead to profound morbidity due to the unregulated oversecretion of catecholamines. Most complications are cardiovascular. Hypertensive or hypotensive crises, myocardial infarction, dysrhythmias, congestive heart failure, and cerebral vascular accidents account for 75% of mortalities in undiagnosed or untreated pheochromocytomas [33, 46]. Patients may present with seizures, hyperglycemia, hypercalcemia, retinopathy, a palpable flank mass, left ventricular hypertrophy or cardiomegaly, shock, and lactic acidosis. Symptoms are commonly misdiagnosed as panic attacks or anxiety. Other rare manifestations that have been reported include acute pancreatitis, retroperitoneal tumor hemorrhage, renal artery stenosis secondary to mass effect, renal infarction, rhabdomyolysis, renal failure, disseminated intravascular coagulopathy, and vasculitis [33, 46].

17.4   Anatomy, Embryology, Physiology, and Oncogenesis

The adrenal glands are paired retroperitoneal organs located superomedial to each kidney. They are surrounded by loose areolar tissue and fat, and can be identified by their characteristic dark "sulfur yellow" appearance and firm texture. Arterial blood is delivered to the gland through a plexus derived from numerous unnamed branches of three main vessels: the superior, middle, and inferior adrenal arteries. These vessels originate from the inferior phrenic artery, aorta, and renal artery respectively. In contrast to the arterial supply, venous drainage is through a single adrenal vein, either into the renal vein on the left, or directly into the vena cava on the right. Occasionally the right adrenal has an accessory vein that drains into the right renal vein or the right hepatic vein. Lymphatic drainage of the gland is to the periaortic and renal nodes.

The adrenal gland consists of cortex and medulla with distinct functions and embryologic heritages. The medulla normally comprises only 10% of the weight of the gland. Chromaffin cells (also known as pheochromocytes) comprise the majority of the adrenal medulla, and function to synthesize, store, and, under controlled conditions, secrete catecholamines. There are two subtypes of chromaffin cells, the most populous of which produces epinephrine. Norepinephrine is made by a smaller subpopulation of chromaffin cells. Normally, epinephrine accounts for 80% of the catecholamine production of the adrenal medulla. Interestingly, most pheochromocytomas produce an abundance of norepinephrine.

Chromaffin cells are neural crest derivatives, and belong to the amine precursor uptake and decarboxylation (APUD) system. Precursor neural crest cells, known as pheochromoblasts, give rise to other structures along the sympathetic chain (the paraganglia) where pheochromocytomas may be encountered. The most common extra-adrenal site is the organ of Zuckerkandl, which resides within the retroperitoneum between the inferior mesenteric artery and the aortic bifurcation. Extra-adrenal pheochromocytomas are also encountered between the aorta and inferior vena cava (IVC) at the level of the left renal vein, or near the origin of the superior mesenteric artery (SMA). Numerous other sites have been reported along the path of neural crest cell migration from the skull base to the spermatic cord [14].

Catecholamines (epinephrine, norepinephrine, and dopamine) are synthesized in the adrenal medulla from L-tyrosine. The rate-limiting step in catecholamine synthesis is the production of L-DOPA by the enzyme tyrosine hydroxylase. Subsequently, decarboxylation of L-DOPA yields dopamine. Dopamine β-hydroxylase then converts dopamine to norepinephrine. In a reaction linked to the presence of cortisol from the adrenal cortex, norepinephrine is converted to epinephrine in the adrenal medulla by phenylethanolamine-*N*-methyltransferase (PNMT). Norepinephrine can be converted to epinephrine only in tissues that contain PNMT: primarily the adrenal medulla and the organ of Zuckerkandl [20]. The clinical consequence of this is that epinephrine-producing pheochromocytomas are almost always found in one of these two locations [21]. Pheochromocytomas frequently secrete norepinephrine. Epinephrine or dopamine secreting pheochromocytomas are less common [51]. They also frequently secrete chromogranin A. This substance has not been adopted as a tumor marker because it may be falsely elevated with any pertubation in renal function. Numerous other rare secretory products of pheochromocytomas have been described including adrenocorticotropic hormone (ACTH), calcitonin gene-related protein, PTH related protein, atrial natriuretic peptide, and vasoactive intestinal peptide [10]. Pheochromocytomas can also be nonfunctional [51].

The overproduction of catecholamines by pheochromocytomas may be related to loss of feedback inhibition. Normally, norepinephrine production leads to compensatory inhibition of medullary catecholamine production by stimulating inhibitory α_2-receptors, and by inhibiting the rate-limiting enzyme, tyrosine hydroxylase. Catecholamine secretion by the adrenal medulla is normally mediated by calcium-dependent exocytosis, which follows depolarization of the chromaffin cells. Pheochromocytomas are believed to leak catecholamines by simple diffusion, because catecholamines are produced in excess of the vesicular storage capacity [20].

Once released, catecholamines are rapidly metabolized. Neuronal tissue metabolizes catecholamines through monoamine oxidase (MAO) into vanillylmandelic acid (VMA) and homovanillic acid (from dopamine). Circulating catecholamines are metabolized by carboxy-O-methyl transferase (COMT). This enzyme converts norepinephrine into normetanephrine, and epinephrine into metanephrine. The products of catecholamine metabolism are excreted in the urine and can be measured as metanephrines, VMA and conjugated catecholamines.

17.5   Clinical Presentation

The clinical manifestations of pheochromocytoma are primarily due to the elaboration of excess catecholamines. The hallmark is hypertension. Patients may present anywhere along the spectrum from occult disease (incidentaloma) to florid hypertensive crisis. The classic triad of symptoms is relatively non specific and consists of headache, palpitations and diaphoresis. Symptoms are often paroxysmal and last no longer than 15 min. Episodes have been found to increase in severity and frequency as the disease progresses [39]. Hypertension may occur in paroxysms against a backdrop of normal blood pressure, or the patient may have baseline hypertension with or without paroxysms of more extreme hypertension. When the classic triad of symptoms accompanies paroxysms of hypertension the diagnosis is likely, and workup must be initiated. Other symptoms that frequently accompany paroxysms include anxiety or a sense of impending doom, nausea, and abdominal pain. Other nonspecific symptoms include chest pain, diarrhea, dyspnea, paresthesias, flushing, tachycardia, mydriasis, Raynaud's phenomenon, and fever. The natural history of untreated pheochromocytoma, as discussed above, is the high likelihood of the eventual development of cardiovascular morbidity.

Hypertensive paroxysms can occur spontaneously, or may be induced. Mechanical pressure on the tumor itself is an often invoked explanation, but many triggers have been documented including exercise, micturition, defecation, sexual intercourse, pregnancy and parturition, alcohol consumption, smoking, anesthesia induction, invasive procedures (interventional radiology and surgery), and the administration of various medications.

17.6   Diagnosis

The differential diagnosis of pheochromocytoma includes a litany of physiologic and psychologic disorders. Common misdiagnoses include anxiety, panic attacks, migraines, menopause, drug abuse, and essential hypertension. Most of these disorders will be excluded by a careful history and physical examination. Biochemical testing should establish the diagnosis without difficulty, and should always precede localization studies. Clearly, biochemical testing should be performed on all patients who display the classic paroxysmal triad. Incidentally found adrenal tumors also mandate a workup for pheochromocytoma and other functioning neoplasms. Screening should be considered for those patients who have a history of extraordinarily labile hypertension, new-onset hypertension during pregnancy, childhood hypertension, hypertension unresponsive to medical therapy, or a family history of pheochromocytoma or syndromes associated with pheochromocytoma (discussed earlier). One exception to performing localization studies only following biochemical confirmation is in the case of screening for familial syndromes such as MEN2. These persons are at high risk for developing pheochromocytomas. Small tumors may have negative biochemical studies, but may still be found on screening localization studies. Early identification may allow earlier resection or partial adrenalectomy.

There is no consensus on the best test for screening and diagnosis. Measurement of 24-h urine collection specimens for metanephrines is 98% sensitive for the diagnosis [32, 40]. We recommend this as an initial test, followed by confirmation with fractionated 24-h urinary catecholamines by high pressure liquid chromatography (HPLC) [10, 13, 21, 40]. Urinary VMA is slightly less sensitive and specific [12,32], but the combination of 24-h urinary metanephrines and VMA has historically been used in many institutions [28]. When either test is abnormal, the addition of confirmatory 24-h fractionated urinary catecholamines by HPLC should also yield an accuracy of approximately 98% [13, 28].

Despite the episodic nature of symptoms from pheochromocytoma, catecholamines and metabolite levels are usually elevated between attacks, especially when the attacks are frequent. In the face of equivocal test results, some have advocated the clonidine suppression test or the use of provocative testing with glucagon [13]. Provocative tests, however, are obsolete because they have a poor diagnostic accuracy, and may have significant and potentially life-threatening side effects [14]. The need for provocative testing is obviated by ensuring that there are no interfering dietary or pharmacologic substances present (see below), and by obtaining timed urinary and plasma samples during symptomatic episodes and assaying for catecholamines and their metabolites by the very sensitive HPLC method.

Some dietary and pharmacologic substances are known to interfere with catecholamine and metabolite measurement. Fortunately, the newer HPLC methods are less frequently confounded than the older fluorometric and spectrophotometric assays. One of the most important interfering substances to be aware of is methylglucamine (found in some radiographic iodine contrast media), which falsely lowers metanephrine measurements for up to 72 h after administration. This interaction further underscores the importance of establishing biochemical diagnosis prior to embarking upon radiographic localization. Labetalol, α-methyldopa, caffeine, nicotine, and foods such as coffee, bananas, and some peppers are also known to alter catecholamine and metanephrine assays [10].

Many physiologic states affect the levels of catecholamines. Hypertension, noise, stress, and pain increase the plasma catecholamine levels [10]. Elevated catecholamine levels are most diagnostic when measured during a symptomatic episode in the absence of these confounding factors.

Once pheochromocytoma is suspected, biochemical tests are used to establish the diagnosis. Fine needle aspiration (FNA) biopsy has no role in the diagnosis of pheochromocytoma, and should not be attempted for adrenal neoplasms unless pheochromocytoma has been ruled out. In a recent review from the University of California, San Francisco, approximately one-half of patients referred for pheochromocytomas who did not present with classic signs underwent unnecessary FNA biopsy of the tumor prior to any biochemical screening to exclude pheochromocytoma [8]. This practice is very hazardous and should be strongly discouraged because it may precipitate a potentially fatal hypertensive crisis [26]. The proper sequence of tests should be history and physical examination followed by biochemical confirmatory testing, pharmacologic adrenergic blockade, and subsequent localization.

17.7   Tumor Localization

Once the diagnosis of pheochromocytoma is confirmed by biochemical testing, the tumor should be localized and the extent of disease evaluated. Computed tomography (CT), magnetic resonance imaging (MRI), and meta-iodo-benzylguanidine (MIBG) scans are complementary studies and each has utility in localizing these tumors. The approach to tumor localization begins with the knowledge of probable locations based on history, physical, and biochemical testing.

In adults 90% of pheochromocytomas are found in the adrenal medulla, and 97% are located below the diaphragm [21,49,52]. Approximately 70% of pheochromocytomas arising in children are found in the adrenal glands [6]. Right-sided adrenal pheochromocytomas are slightly more common than the left [10]. As discussed earlier, epinephrine-secreting tumors are usually confined to the adrenal medulla or organ of Zuckerkandl due to the tissue specific presence of PNMT, which converts norepinephrine to epinephrine. Bilateral pheochromocytomas are more common in the context of familial syndromes (approximately 70%), but overall 10% of adult and 35% of childhood pheochromocytomas are bilateral [10].

Approximately 10% of pheochromocytomas can be categorized as either bilateral, multifocal, extra-adrenal, familial, or malignant; thus pheochromocytomas are often remembered by medical students as the 10% tumor. Newer reports, however, suggest that pheochromocytomas may be extra-adrenal in up to 30% of cases [45, 52]. Eighty-five percent of extra-adrenal pheochromocytomas are located below the diaphragm [52]. Although most frequently found in the organ of Zuckerkandl, numerous other sites from skull base to spermatic cord have been reported.

In cases where the risk of multifocality or extra-adrenal disease is low, we start with a thin-cut adrenal CT scan or MRI. If the pheochromocytoma is found by one of these studies, no further localization studies are obtained. We use MIBG scanning selectively to screen for and to localize extra-adrenal, multiple, or recurrent pheochromocytomas. If necessary, MRI or CT can then be used to generate more detailed images of the region with MIBG uptake. If this approach fails to localize the tumor, PET scanning or the use of selective venous catheterization (rarely necessary) has been useful.

17.7.1   MRI

The sensitivity and specificity of MRI for adrenal pheochromocytomas is approximately 95% and 100% respectively. Pheochromocytomas are characteristically bright on T2-weighted images (Fig. 1). The major advantage of MRI is the lack of exposure to radiation and IV contrast. Thus, it is the procedure of choice in pregnancy and childhood. Possible limitations to MRI include claustrophobia, cost, and availability. Small metastases, extra-adrenal pheochromocytomas, and

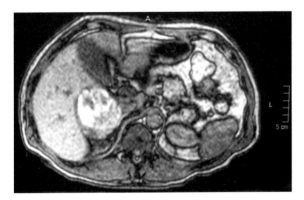

Fig. 1. This is a characteristic image of a T2-weighted MRI demonstrating an enhancing pheochromocytoma in the right adrenal. (Used with permission from Fitzgerald [10])

recurrent disease are not reliably localized by MRI. The only findings consistent with malignancy on MRI (or CT) are local invasion of the tumor into adjacent organs or the presence of metastases. MRI can also identify tumor thrombus in the IVC or renal vein, and help plan extent of resection [14].

17.7.2   CT

CT scanning has greater than 95% sensitivity for adrenal pheochromocytomas. Since the majority of pheochromocytomas are larger than 2 cm and are located in the adrenal gland, CT scanning is an accurate and sensitive study for tumor localization (Fig. 2). CT scans provide excellent anatomic information, including the presence of metastatic disease in the liver, and for this reason CT is preferred by some surgeons. CT scans should be performed in thin section (3 mm) from the diaphragm to the aortic bifurcation. The limitations of CT scanning are that it may miss small metastases, extra-adrenal pheochromocytomas, and recurrent disease. The disadvantages of CT scanning are radiation exposure, need for intravenous contrast (which has been associated with the precipitation of hypertensive crises in unblocked patients), and lack of tissue characterization such as is found with T2 weighted MRI. Characteristics of malignancy are local invasion and metastases.

17.7.3   MIBG

With an overall sensitivity of approximately 80–85% [38], MIBG scanning with iodine-131 (^{131}I) or iodine-123 (^{123}I) can be used to scan the entire body for APUD tumors (Fig. 3). MIBG selectively accumulates in tissues that store catecholamines. Normal adrenal medulla, fortunately, does not take up sufficient MIBG to produce an image. Specificity is reported to range from 88% to 100% [21, 50]. MIBG is most useful for localizing extra-adrenal or recurrent pheochromocytoma. MIBG is the only widely used localizing study that provides functional data about the tumor; uptake is proportional to the quantity of catecholamine containing vesicles in the tumor. Disadvantages of MIBG scanning include radiation exposure, high cost, poor anatomic resolution, and the requirement to pretreat with iodine to prevent ablation of the thyroid. Lugol's solution or saturated solution of potassium iodide (SSKI) must be administered prior to the study in order to prevent the uptake of radioactive iodine by the

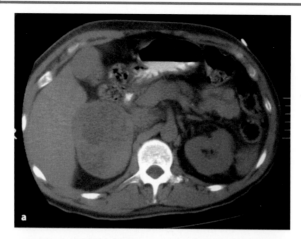

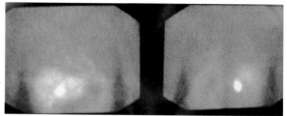

Fig. 3. This ^{123}I-MIBG study demonstrates selective uptake in the right adrenal gland which corresponds to the pheochromocytoma at that location. (Courtesy of Paul Fitzgerald, MD. Used with permission from Fitzgerald [10])

age through single-photon emission computed tomography (SPECT).

17.7.4   Other Imaging Modalities

Although not yet validated for the detection of pheochromocytoma, the PET scan has been shown to be useful in the detection of malignant pheochromocytomas [41]. [^{18}F]-Fluorodeoxyglucose positron emission tomography ([^{18}F]-FDG-PET) scanning detects tissues with a high metabolic rate. Consequently, it is less specific than MIBG scanning. 6-[^{18}F]-Fluorodopamine ([^{18}F]-DA) PET is being studied, and some investigators predict that it may be superior to other nuclear imaging techniques [16, 17, 29–31]. The perceived advantages of PET scanning over MIBG are that pretreatment with iodine to protect the thyroid is unnecessary, and images can be obtained without a 1–2 day delay. PET scanning is costly and less available than the other imaging modalities. [^{18}F]-DA PET is currently only available at the National Institutes of Health.

Somatostatin receptor scintigraphy is another investigational modality for the detection of pheochromocytoma. It appears to have a sensitivity of only approximately 25% for adrenal pheochromocytomas [48]. Conversely, this modality detects 87% of metastases. It may be useful when metastases are not revealed on MIBG scanning, but the index of suspicion is high [24, 48].

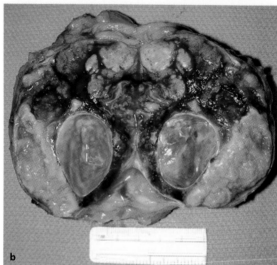

Fig. 2. a This noncontrast CT scan demonstrates a 9-cm right-sided adrenal pheochromocytoma. This is the same tumor as shown in Fig. 1. Areas of inhomogeneity are visible which probably correspond to areas of tumor necrosis and cyst formation seen in **b**. There is no evidence of local or vascular invasion on this study. **b** The 9-cm right pheochromocytoma from Figs. 1 and 2a is shown here in bivalve section. Common to large tumors are areas of cyst formation and tumor necrosis which are demonstrated here. The sulfur-yellow adrenal cortex is displaced inferolaterally to the periphery of the tumor. (Used with permission from Fitzgerald [10])

thyroid. In addition, a delay of 1–2 days is required before imaging after administration of ^{131}I-MIBG, because of excessive background noise preventing the acquisition of good resolution images. Although not widely available, ^{123}I-MIBG scanning is reported to have a sensitivity of approximately 90%, superior to that of ^{131}I-MIBG. It also yields a higher quality image and can be used to generate a three-dimensional im-

17.8   Preoperative Management

Surgical removal is the only effective treatment for pheochromocytoma. The likelihood of complication-free surgery is correlated to the adequacy of the preoperative medical management. The goals of medical management are to correct hypertension, restore vascular volume, and control dysrhythmias. This is achieved primarily through alpha-adrenergic blockade and fluid administration. The most commonly used agent for alpha blockade is phenoxybenzamine. Blockade is usually initiated 1–3 weeks prior to surgery, with a starting dose of 10 mg per day and increased gradually until blood pressure is controlled. Doses as high as 400 mg per day may be required to control blood pressure. Endpoints of alpha blockade are: controlled blood pressure (<160/90) or the development of significant side effects including reflex tachycardia, orthostatic hypotension (<80/45), nasal congestion, nausea, or abdominal pain. A shorter acting alpha antagonist, prazosin, has also been shown to be beneficial and is preferred by some investigators due to its shorter half-life, and lower frequency of reflex tachycardia [4]. Doxazosin and terazosin have also been used.

Beta blockers may be required for patients who develop persistent tachycardia from alpha blockade. This class of drugs should not be used for pheochromocytoma without adequate alpha blockade because of the possibility of precipitating hypertensive crisis from unopposed alpha adrenergic effect.

Calcium channel blockers such as nicardipine and nifedipine are successfully used for preoperative preparation in some centers [9], and can be used to treat hypertensive paroxysms. Calcium channel blockers have been shown to cause less orthostatic hypotension than alpha blockers [51], and may prevent coronary vasospasm [4]. The combination of calcium channel blockers and selective alpha-1 blockers is gaining favor in the recent literature for these reasons and because their use may obviate overshoot hypotension following ligation of the adrenal vein [4]. Other pharmacologic agents used for management of hypertension associated with pheochromocytomas include angiotensin converting enzyme (ACE) inhibitors [40], clonidine, and labetalol. Labetalol competitively blocks alpha-1 and beta adrenergic receptors and has been used with success as an antihypertensive and antidysrhythmic drug. Metyrosine inhibits the rate limiting enzyme in catecholamine synthesis, tyrosine hydroxylase, but because of its side effects is a second line drug [51].

Patients with pheochromocytoma are in a persistently vasoconstricted state. Volume repletion should accompany adequate pharmacologic management. Patients are encouraged to increase oral salt and fluid intake. Preoperative volume repletion is considered essential in order to avoid hypotension following the ligation of the adrenal vein. We continue pharmacologic blockade until the time of operation.

17.9 Surgical Options

The principles of surgery for pheochromocytoma are complete tumor extirpation, avoidance of tumor spillage, minimal manipulation, control of venous drainage and arterial supply, and hemostasis. Adrenalectomy can be performed open or laparoscopically. The choice of approach is dictated by tumor size, signs of local invasion, and surgeon experience. Historically, the open anterior approach has been the standard because it allowed en-bloc tumor resection with exploration of the contralateral adrenal and possible metastatic sites (Fig. 4a, b). Due to the accuracy of contemporary localization studies, contralateral adrenal exploration is usually unnecessary. Furthermore, a thorough evaluation of the liver and peritoneum for metastases is possible with the laparoscopic transabdominal approach. The only absolute contraindications to the laparoscopic approach for pheochromocytoma are findings consistent with malignancy such as invasion into adjacent organs or blood vessels. Laparoscopic adrenalectomy for amenable lesions (Fig. 5) has been shown to be superior to the open approach in terms of pain medicine requirements, hospital stay, return to normal activities, and late incisional complications [25, 35, 47]. With surgeon experience, the operative time is decreased, and large tumors (greater than 6 cm) can be resected [15, 27]. Tumors larger than 15 cm are being resected laparoscopically at some centers. Hand-assist devices may also facilitate laparoscopic resection [3].

Regardless of the approach, communication between surgeon and anesthesiologist is critical to the performance of a safe operation. Tumor manipulation precipitates severe hypertension, even in adequately blocked patients, which can be anticipated and treated with short-acting vasodilating agents (e.g. nitroprusside or nitroglycerin). Often there is a drop in blood pressure following ligation of the adrenal vein. Prior to this maneuver, notifying the anesthesiologist allows them time to cease the administration of vasodilators, or prepare vasopressors.

17.9.1 Principles of Open Adrenalectomy

Several open operations have been described including the anterior, lateral, thoracoabdominal, and poste-

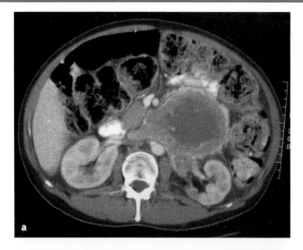

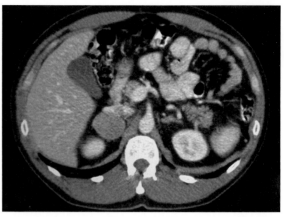

Fig. 5. This contrast CT scan demonstrates a pheochromocytoma of the right adrenal gland. There is no evidence of local invasion or distant disease. The tumor appears well encapsulated, and there is no regional lymphadenopathy. This lesion was removed laparoscopically

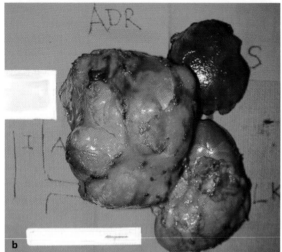

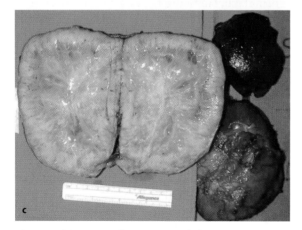

Fig. 4. **a** This CT scan demonstrates a left adrenal pheochromocytoma with features suggestive of local invasion. The lack of discrete tumor margins, and the suggestion of local invasion into the left renal vein, prompted an open en-bloc resection of the left adrenal, kidney, and spleen. **b** Gross specimen with orientation. **c** Bivalved specimen

rior approaches. The thoracoabdominal approach may be useful for large or malignant tumors, but will not be described here. The posterior open approach has been completely replaced by the laparoscopic approach, and is not used in institutions that perform laparoscopic adrenalectomy. Our preferred open approach is through a subcostal incision with the patient in 15–30 degrees of lateral decubitus. A surgical headlight is helpful to illuminate the dissection field. The abdomen is opened and explored briefly. For a right adrenalectomy the right lobe of the liver is mobilized from its lateral peritoneal attachments and retracted anteromedially. Mobilization of the hepatic flexure of the colon provides additional exposure, and is followed by a Kocher maneuver to reveal the inferior vena cava. The peritoneum overlying the vena cava is opened, and the lateral border of the supraduodenal vena cava identified. Dissection is then carried cephalad towards the adrenal. The retroperitoneum is opened over the superolateral aspect of the adrenal, and the incision carried medially towards the vena cava. Small arterial branches will be encountered. Branches from the caudate lobe to the IVC may require division. The right adrenal vein originates from the medial aspect of the adrenal and after traversing a short distance enters the vena cava, often along its posterolateral aspect. The adrenal vein is then ligated and divided. Be aware that there are occasionally accessory veins that drain into the right renal vein, or the right hepatic vein. The arterial branches are divided beginning on the superolateral aspect of the gland and progressing medially. Care is taken to avoid manipulation of the tumor, and violation of the surrounding fat and capsule.

The left adrenal gland is approached in a similar manner. The splenic flexure is mobilized and retracted inferomedially. The spleen is then mobilized from the left upper quadrant, and, along with the stomach and tail of the pancreas, retracted medially. The left adrenal gland is then exposed. The left adrenal vein originates inferomedially and drains into the left renal vein after being joined by the inferior phrenic vein. The adrenal and inferior phrenic veins are ligated and divided when they are encountered. Following control of the small arterial branches, the gland is removed en-bloc.

17.9.2 Principles of Laparoscopic Adrenalectomy

With the development of reliable imaging studies for pheochromocytomas, extensive exploration is no longer necessary and a more focused adrenalectomy is possible. Laparoscopic adrenalectomy has become the standard operative approach for the management of benign adrenal tumors because it allows a safe focused adrenalectomy with less postoperative pain, a shorter hospital stay, shorter time to convalescence, less blood loss and transfusion, and fewer incisional complications [18, 22, 43]. The surgeon must be prepared for open adrenalectomy, if necessary for hemorrhage or to resect invasive malignancies. In addition, patients must be consented for, and physiologically able to tolerate, the open procedure.

Numerous laparoscopic approaches have been described that mimic the open approaches including supine and lateral transabdominal, and posterior and lateral retroperitoneal operations. We prefer the laparoscopic lateral transabdominal approach originally described in 1992 by Gagner [11]. The patient is placed in the lateral decubitus position. The beanbag, and kidney rests are essential to proper positioning. The table is flexed to open the space inferior to the costal margin. We use four 10 mm trocars spaced evenly along the costal margin from the midaxillary line to the midclavicular line. Pneumoperitoneum is established with the Veress needle at Palmer's point [7], and the first trocar is then placed percutaneously at this location. The remaining three trocars are placed under direct vision. The abdominal contents are inspected for evidence of liver or peritoneal metastases. For a laparoscopic right adrenalectomy, the right lobe of the liver is mobilized from the diaphragm by dividing the triangular ligament, and retracted anteriorly with a fan retractor. It is rarely necessary to mobilize the hepatic flexure. Gerota's fascia is incised, and the adrenal gland is identified superomedial to the kidney. Dissection is begun at the cephalad aspect of the gland, and continued inferomedially. Small arterial branches and fatty tissue around the adrenal are divided hemostatically. We continue to mobilize the gland by dissecting in a clockwise fashion, and ligate the vein when it is exposed by the medial dissection. The right adrenal vein is identified as it traverses the short distance between the medial aspect of the gland and the vena cava. The vein is double clipped and divided sharply. The remaining soft tissue attachments and small arterial branches are divided hemostatically, and the specimen is placed into an impervious retrieval bag. The incision can be enlarged to allow intact retrieval of the tumor, or it may be retrieved through the 10 mm trocar incision by morcellation within the specimen bag.

For the left adrenalectomy the abdominal cavity is entered in a similar manner. The retroperitoneum is opened by dividing the splenocolic ligament. Occasionally, it is necessary to mobilize the splenic flexure of the colon as well. The spleen is mobilized from its retroperitoneal attachments and allowed to fall medially by gravity. Just as is done on the right side, dissection is begun at the superior pole of the gland, and continued inferomedially. Small arterial branches contained within the connective tissue surrounding the adrenal are divided hemostatically. The left adrenal vein is identified as it emerges from the inferomedial aspect of the gland and empties into the left renal vein. The adrenal vein is double clipped and divided sharply. The inferior phrenic vein joins the left adrenal vein medially, and also needs to be dissected, clipped and divided. The remaining attachments and small arterial branches are divided hemostatically, and the specimen is placed into the retrieval bag.

Hand-assisted laparoscopic adrenalectomy can be used in cases of large tumors that are difficult to dissect. Retraction, blunt dissection, and control of blood vessels can be performed manually through a 7–8 cm incision [3].

17.10 Postoperative Care

The average postoperative stay in our institution is less than 2 days [8]. Three months following the operation a 24-h urine collection can be obtained for metanephrines to establish the patient's new baseline and ensure that there has been complete tumor removal.

Quarterly screening for urinary catecholamine metabolites can be performed for the first year, and then screening is done annually for at least 5 years. Weekly home blood pressure measurements should be taken for the first year and then monthly thereafter. Metastases can manifest as late as 20 years from surgery, supporting the practice of indefinite follow-up for these patients [34]. Changes in blood pressure or urinary measurements should prompt a workup for metastases or contralateral primary pheochromocytoma.

17.11   Pathology/Malignancy

There are no agreed upon histologic characteristics for malignancy. The presence of metastases or local invasion into surrounding tissues is the most reliable indicator. Approximately 10–20% of pheochromocytomas ultimately prove to be malignant. Malignancy is identified in 10% at the time of diagnosis, and approximately 5% more are identified in the ensuing 5 years [10]. Malignancy is more likely in extra-adrenal pheochromocytomas (30–40%), larger tumors (>6 cm), dopamine-only secreting tumors, and with postoperative persistent hypertension [1, 10, 19]. The diagnosis of malignancy is best made by an imaging study showing metastases or local invasion, or these findings at operation.

The most common sites of metastases are bone (spine, skull, ribs), liver, retroperitoneal or regional lymph nodes, lungs, and peritoneum. The median time to recurrence is between 5 and 6 years [14]. The main treatment for recurrent or metastatic disease is resection and adrenergic blockade. If the tumor or metastases are not completely resectable, chemotherapy, external-beam radiotherapy, or high dose ^{131}I-MIBG are options. Based on data from the Surveillance, Epidemiology and End Results (SEER; 1973–2000) study, the mean survival for malignant pheochromocytoma is approximately 80 months.

The combination of cyclophosphamide, vincristine, and dacarbazine has been used with variable success. One large series showed a 57% overall response, 79% hormonal response, and 21% tumor response. There were no cases of complete response [2]. It remains the regimen of choice in the absence of more effective chemotherapy.

MIBG is used to localized recurrent or residual disease, and it also identifies neoplastic tissue that can potentially be treated with high dose ^{131}I-MIBG [42]. Treatment requires 5–7 days of hospitalization. Patients must be pretreated with iodine in order to prevent thyroid ablation. Prior to ^{131}I-MIBG ablation, some patients are required to undergo leukapheresis and stem cell cryopreservation in the event that they suffer total hematopoietic ablation. Risks of ^{131}I-MIBG ablation include bone marrow suppression, infertility, increased risk of malignancy (lifelong), and possible need for retreatment. External beam radiation has been used for symptomatic metastases to the spine or long bones, or CNS metastases. Five-year survival is between 30% and 50% [10, 13, 37].

17.12   Conclusion

Biochemical testing should be performed on all patients with the classic paroxysmal triad of headache, palpitations and diaphoresis. Incidentalomas also mandate a workup for pheochromocytoma and other functioning neoplasms. Screening should be considered for those patients who have a history of extraordinarily labile hypertension, new-onset hypertension during pregnancy, childhood hypertension, hypertension unresponsive to medical therapy, or a family history of syndromes associated with pheochromocytoma. We recommend 24-h urine metanephrines as the initial test, followed by confirmation with fractionated 24-h urinary catecholamines. We usually start with a thin-cut adrenal CT scan or MRI for localization. We use MIBG scanning selectively to screen for and localize extra-adrenal, multiple, or recurrent pheochromocytomas. The likelihood of complication-free adrenalectomy is dependent upon the adequacy of the preoperative medical management. The goals of medical management are to correct hypertension, restore vascular volume, and control dysrhythmias, usually through alpha adrenergic blockade and fluid administration. The choice of approach for adrenalectomy is dictated by tumor size, signs of local invasion, and surgeon experience. Laparoscopic adrenalectomy has been shown to be superior to the open approach in terms of pain medicine requirements, hospital stay, return to normal activities, and late incisional complications. We have found conversion to hand-assisted laparoscopy to be beneficial in some instances. Patients with pheochromocytoma should have nearly lifelong follow-up. Changes in blood pressure or urinary measurements should prompt a workup for metastases or contralateral primary pheochromocytoma.

References

1. Al-Fehaily M, Duh QY (2003) Malignant adrenal neoplasms. Probl Gen Surg 20:92–102
2. Averbuch SD, Steakley CS, Young RC, Gelmann EP, Goldstein DS, Stull R, Keiser HR (1988) Malignant pheochromocytoma: effective treatment with a combination of cyclophosphamide, vincristine, and dacarbazine. Ann Intern Med 109:267–73
3. Bennett IC, Ray M (2002) Hand-assisted laparoscopic adrenalectomy: an alternative minimal invasive surgical technique for the adrenal gland. ANZ J Surg 72:801–5
4. Bravo EL, Tagle R (2003) Pheochromocytoma: state-of-the-art and future prospects. Endocr Rev 24:539–53
5. Casanova S, Rosenberg-Bourgin M, Farkas D, Calmettes C, Feingold N, Heshmati HM, Cohen R, Conte-Devolx B, Guillausseau PJ, Houdent C, et al. (1993) Phaeochromocytoma in multiple endocrine neoplasia type 2 A: survey of 100 cases. Clin Endocrinol (Oxf) 38:531–7
6. Caty MG, Coran AG, Geagen M, Thompson NW (1990) Current diagnosis and treatment of pheochromocytoma in children. Experience with 22 consecutive tumors in 14 patients. Arch Surg 125:978–81
7. Chang FH, Lee CL, Soong YK (1994) Use of Palmer's point for insertion of the operative laparoscope in patients with severe pelvic adhesions: experience of seventeen cases. J Am Assoc Gynecol Laparosc 1:S7
8. Cheah WK, Clark OH, Horn JK, Siperstein AE, Duh QY (2002) Laparoscopic adrenalectomy for pheochromocytoma. World J Surg 26:1048–51
9. Combemale F, Carnaille B, Tavernier B, Hautier MB, Thevenot A, Scherpereel P, Proye C (1998) Exclusive use of calcium channel blockers and cardioselective beta-blockers in the pre- and per-operative management of pheochromocytomas. 70 Cases. Ann Chir 52:341–5
10. Fitzgerald PA (2003) Pheochromocytoma and paraganglioma. In: Clark OH, Duh QY, Jahan TM (eds) Endocrine tumors. BC Decker, Hamilton, ON, pp 100–122
11. Gagner M, Lacroix A, Bolte E (1992) Laparoscopic adrenalectomy in Cushing's syndrome and pheochromocytoma. N Engl J Med 327:1033
12. Graham PE, Smythe GA, Edwards GA, Lazarus L (1993) Laboratory diagnosis of phaeochromocytoma: which analytes should we measure? Ann Clin Biochem 30:129–34
13. Grant C (1997) Pheochromocytoma. In: Clark OH, Duh QY (eds) Textbook of endocrine surgery. Saunders, Philadelphia, pp 513–522
14. Gray DK, Thompson NW (2001) Pheochromocytoma. In: Doherty G, Skogseid B (eds) Surgical endocrinology. Lippincott Williams & Wilkins, Philadelphia, pp 247–262
15. Henry JF, Sebag F, Iacobone M, Mirallie E (2002) Results of laparoscopic adrenalectomy for large and potentially malignant tumors. World J Surg 26:1043–7
16. Hoegerle S, Nitzsche E, Altehoefer C, Ghanem N, Manz T, Brink I, Reincke M, Moser E, Neumann HP (2002) Pheochromocytomas: detection with 18f dopa whole body PET – initial results. Radiology 222:507–12
17. Ilias I, Yu J, Carrasquillo JA, Chen CC, Eisenhofer G, Whatley M, McElroy B, Pacak K (2003) Superiority of 6-[18f]-fluorodopamine positron emission tomography versus [131i]-metaiodobenzylguanidine scintigraphy in the localization of metastatic pheochromocytoma. J Clin Endocrinol Metab 88:4083–7
18. Jacobs JK, Goldstein RE, Geer RJ (1997) Laparoscopic adrenalectomy. A new standard of care. Ann Surg 225:495–501; discussion 501–2
19. John H, Ziegler WH, Hauri D, Jaeger P (1999) Pheochromocytomas: can malignant potential be predicted? Urology 53:679–83
20. Kacsoh B (2000) The adrenal gland. In: Dolan J (ed) Endocrine physiology. McGraw-Hill, New York, pp 360–447
21. Kebebew E, Duh QY (1998) Benign and malignant pheochromocytoma: diagnosis, treatment, and follow-up. Surg Oncol Clin N Am 7:765–89
22. Kebebew E, Siperstein AE, Duh QY (2001) Laparoscopic adrenalectomy: the optimal surgical approach. J Laparoendosc Adv Surg Tech A 11:409–13
23. Lairmore TC, Ball DW, Baylin SB, Wells SA Jr (1993) Management of pheochromocytomas in patients with multiple endocrine neoplasia type 2 syndromes. Ann Surg 217:595–601; discussion 601–3
24. Lin JC, Palafox BA, Jackson HA, Cohen AJ, Gazzaniga AB (1999) Cardiac pheochromocytoma: resection after diagnosis by 111-indium octreotide scan. Ann Thorac Surg 67:555–8
25. Matsuda T, Murota T, Oguchi N, Kawa G, Muguruma K (2002) Laparoscopic adrenalectomy for pheochromocytoma: a literature review. Biomed Pharmacother 56 Suppl 1:132s–138s
26. McCorkell SJ, Niles NL (1985) Fine-needle aspiration of catecholamine-producing adrenal masses: a possibly fatal mistake. AJR Am J Roentgenol 145:113–4
27. Novitsky YW, Czerniach DR, Kercher KW, Perugini RA, Kelly JJ, Litwin DE (2003) Feasibility of laparoscopic adrenalectomy for large adrenal masses. Surg Laparosc Endosc Percutan Tech 13:106–10
28. Orchard T, Grant CS, van Heerden JA, Weaver A (1993) Pheochromocytoma – continuing evolution of surgical therapy. Surgery 114:1153–8; discussion 1158–9
29. Pacak K, Goldstein DS, Doppman JL, Shulkin BL, Udelsman R, Eisenhofer G (2001) A "pheo" lurks: novel approaches for locating occult pheochromocytoma. J Clin Endocrinol Metab 86:3641–6
30. Pacak K, Eisenhofer G, Carrasquillo JA, Chen CC, Li ST, Goldstein DS (2001) 6-[18f]Fluorodopamine positron emission tomographic (PET) scanning for diagnostic localization of pheochromocytoma. Hypertension 38:6–8
31. Pacak K, Eisenhofer G, Carrasquillo JA, Chen CC, Whatley M, Goldstein DS (2002) Diagnostic localization of pheochromocytoma: the coming of age of positron emission tomography. Ann N Y Acad Sci 970:170–6
32. Peplinski GR, Norton JA (1994) The predictive value of diagnostic tests for pheochromocytoma. Surgery 116:1101–9; discussion 1109–10

33. Platts JK, Drew PJ, Harvey JN (1995) Death from phaeochromocytoma: lessons from a post-mortem survey. J R Coll Phys Lond 29:299–306

34. Plouin PF, Chatellier G, Fofol I, Corvol P (1997) Tumor recurrence and hypertension persistence after successful pheochromocytoma operation. Hypertension 29: 1133–9

35. Prinz RA (1995) A comparison of laparoscopic and open adrenalectomies. Arch Surg 130:489–92; discussion 492–4

36. Samaan NA, Hickey RC, Shutts PE (1988) Diagnosis, localization, and management of pheochromocytoma. Pitfalls and follow-up in 41 patients. Cancer 62:2451–60

37. Shapiro B, Sisson JC, Lloyd R, Nakajo M, Satterlee W, Beierwaltes WH (1984) Malignant phaeochromocytoma: clinical, biochemical and scintigraphic characterization. Clin Endocrinol (Oxf) 20:189–203

38. Shapiro B, Sisson JC, Shulkin BL, Gross MD, Zempel S (1995) The current status of meta-iodobenzylguanidine and related agents for the diagnosis of neuro-endocrine tumors. Q J Nucl Med 39:3–8

39. Sheps SG, Jiang NS, Klee GG (1988) Diagnostic evaluation of pheochromocytoma. Endocrinol Metab Clin North Am 17:397–414

40. Sheps SG, Jiang NS, Klee GG, van Heerden JA (1990) Recent developments in the diagnosis and treatment of pheochromocytoma. Mayo Clin Proc 65:88–95

41. Shulkin BL, Thompson NW, Shapiro B, Francis IR, Sisson JC (1999) Pheochromocytomas: imaging with 2-[fluorine-18]fluoro-2-deoxy-D-glucose PET. Radiology 212: 35–41

42. Sisson JC, Shapiro B, Beierwaltes WH, Glowniak JV, Nakajo M, Mangner TJ, Carey JE, Swanson DP, Copp JE, Satterlee WG, et al. (1984) Radiopharmaceutical treatment of malignant pheochromocytoma. J Nucl Med 25: 197–206

43. Smith CD, Weber CJ, Amerson JR (1999) Laparoscopic adrenalectomy: new gold standard. World J Surg 23: 389–96

44. Smythe GA, Edwards G, Graham P, Lazarus L (1992) Biochemical diagnosis of pheochromocytoma by simultaneous measurement of urinary excretion of epinephrine and norepinephrine. Clin Chem 38:486–92

45. Stenstrom G, Svardsudd K (1986) Pheochromocytoma in Sweden 1958–1981. An analysis of the National Cancer Registry data. Acta Med Scand 220:225–32

46. Sutton MG, Sheps SG, Lie JT (1981) Prevalence of clinically unsuspected pheochromocytoma. Review of a 50-year autopsy series. Mayo Clin Proc 56:354–60

47. Thompson GB, Grant CS, van Heerden JA, Schlinkert RT, Young WF Jr, Farley DR, Ilstrup DM (1997) Laparoscopic versus open posterior adrenalectomy: a case-control study of 100 patients. Surgery 122:1132–6

48. van der Harst E, de Herder WW, Bruining HA, Bonjer HJ, de Krijger RR, Lamberts SW, van de Meiracker AH, Boomsma F, Stijnen T, Krenning EP, Bosman FT, Kwekkeboom DJ (2001) [(123)I]Metaiodobenzylguanidine and [(111)In]octreotide uptake in benign and malignant pheochromocytomas. J Clin Endocrinol Metab 86:685–93

49. van Heerden JA, Roland CF, Carney JA, Sheps SG, Grant CS (1990) Long-term evaluation following resection of apparently benign pheochromocytoma(s)/paraganglioma(s). World J Surg 14:325–9

50. Velchik MG, Alavi A, Kressel HY, Engelman K (1989) Localization of pheochromocytoma: MIGB, CT, and MRI correlation. J Nucl Med 30:328–36

51. Werbel SS, Ober KP (1995) Pheochromocytoma. Update on diagnosis, localization, and management. Med Clin North Am 79:131–53

52. Whalen RK, Althausen AF, Daniels GH (1992) Extra-adrenal pheochromocytoma. J Urol 147:1–10

18 Extra-adrenal and Malignant Pheochromocytoma

Gerard M. Doherty

18.1 Introduction

Pheochromocytomas are rare tumors that are usually benign lesions within the adrenal gland. However, primary tumors can occur outside of the adrenal gland, and tumors that arise either within the adrenal gland or outside of it can be malignant. This tumor is often described by the "rule of 10's," that is, 10% familial, bilateral, extra-adrenal, malignant, and occurring in children. However, this memory tool underestimates the incidence of both malignancy and extra-adrenal primary tumors, each of which probably occur in closer to 20% of patients with pheochromocytoma [15].

18.2 Extra-adrenal Primary Pheochromocytoma

18.2.1 Frequency and Patterns of Extra-adrenal Disease

Extra-adrenal tumors occur along the sympathetic chain, at any site from the base of the skull to the pelvis. The most common site for extra-adrenal pheochro-

mocytomas, which are also sometimes, and probably more correctly, called paragangliomas particularly when they do not make appreciable amounts of catecholamines, is the organ of Zuckerkandl. They have been localized in the neck, posterior chest, atrium, renal hilum and bladder (Fig. 1). A common location of extra-adrenal tumors is between the aorta and vena cava at the level of the left renal vein, cephalad to the organ of Zuckerkandl tumors arising on either side of the superior mesenteric artery or more distally to the aortic bifurcation, where it can also be mistaken for a lymph node metastasis. Middle mediastinal tumors, which may involve the heart, occur more frequently than was previously recognized. Extra-adrenal tumors have a higher reported malignancy rate of 25–40%, although not all reports agree on the differential aggressiveness of the extra-adrenal sites [7, 10].

18.2.2 Diagnosis of Ectopic Sites

The increased recognition of ectopic sites of primary pheochromocytomas is due to a variety of changes in the diagnostic options. First, there is the improved accuracy of biochemical testing for pheochromocytoma. With the current testing, particularly with the widespread availability of plasma metanephrine testing, the diagnosis of excess catecholamine synthesis and secretion can be more certain. With that increased level of certainty, our improved imaging can be selectively and diligently applied. Current imaging, including high-resolution computerized tomographic (CT) and magnetic resonance scanning (MRI), and nuclear imaging with ^{123}I-MIBG or somatostatin receptor scintigraphy can localize tumors in many sites that were simply not practical in the past, particularly if the biochemical diagnosis was equivocal [5, 18].

Patients with disease at ectopic sites typically present with the same symptoms as those with adrenal pheochromocytoma. Most patients have hyperten-

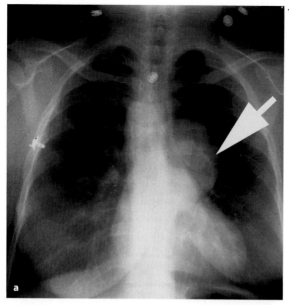

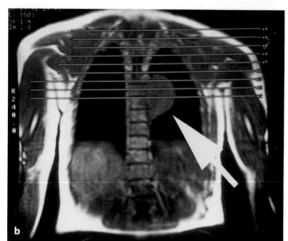

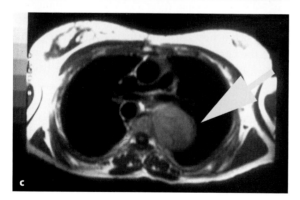

◀ **Fig. 1a–c.** Studies from a woman with ectopic pheochromocytoma during pregnancy. This patient's worsening hypertension led to a biochemical evaluation that diagnosed her pheochromocytoma. Initial imaging of her adrenal glands with ultrasound and an abdominal MRI showed no evidence of the source of her disease. When a chest X-ray (**a**) showed this left thoracic mass (*arrow*), the localization was clear. A subsequent MRI of the chest (**b, c**) provided improved anatomic delineation before resection in the second trimester of the pregnancy (tumor at *arrows*). Mother and daughter have subsequently done well

sion, and describe "spells," which classically include hypertension, but which also may have a variety of symptoms that are consistent within each patient for their episodes. These spells may include paroxysmal headache, dizziness, anxiety, tachycardia, nausea or visual changes. The spells may occur seemingly spontaneously, or may predictably follow some activities. This can be particularly true for some of the ectopic sites, where spells can be caused by local mechanical changes, such as micturition, sexual intercourse, or defecation causing spells from tumors adjacent to the bladder [17]. Patients may occasionally present with severe systemic illness or death from hormone release from a previously occult tumor.

Pheochromocytomas can also produce hormones other than catecholamines, including adrenocorticotropin (ACTH), calcitonin, somatostatin, vasoactive intestinal peptide (VIP) or serotonin. The production of these unusual hormones and their syndromes can lead to an extensive work-up to identify the responsible tumor.

18.2.3   Localization of Tumor

Once the biochemical diagnosis of pheochromocytoma has been made, the tumor must be localized. Since most pheochromocytomas are located in the adrenal gland, the initial localizing test should be a cross-sectional study of the adrenals, either a high-resolution CT scan or an MRI. If that study shows a unilateral adrenal mass, without suggestion of malignancy or other extra-adrenal findings, then no further testing is necessary. In a consecutive series from the University of Michigan, 48 patients with a biochemical diagnosis of pheochromocytoma and a unilateral adrenal mass on CT or MRI, none had additional disease defined by the ^{123}I-MIBG scan. Forty-seven of the 48 patients had a single unilateral focus of uptake defined on MIBG scan, and the remaining patient had a false-negative MIBG scan [8]. Thus, we now reserve the MIBG scan for patients whose disease is either not apparent on the cross-sectional imaging, or who have additional abnormalities (bilateral adrenal masses or extra-adrenal lesions). In these patients, ^{123}I-MIBG scans or somatostatin receptor scintigraphy can identify the site(s) of disease to allow treatment planning [5].

18.2.4 Therapy

The best therapy for extra-adrenal pheochromocytoma is resection, as this is the only potentially curative option. Careful attention to the preoperative localization allows operative planning to include all sites of disease. Once the diagnosis of pheochromocytoma has been firmly established with biochemical testing, and localization studies have been completed, preparations can be made for the operative treatment of the tumor(s). Regardless of the site or number of tumors, all patients should be prepared with an alpha-adrenergic antagonist for 1–2 weeks preoperatively. One proven method is phenoxybenzamine (Dibenzyline), which can be administered three times a day. Starting with a total dose of 30 mg per day, we increase the dose every 3rd day by 30 mg. The endpoint of therapy is orthostatic hypotension, although a clinical sign that the dose is adequate is the development of nasal congestion. This may be achieved with the starting dose, although some patients have required as much as 360 mg per day. An experienced and prepared anesthesiologist should be considered as an essential member of the team. Central venous and arterial pressure lines are placed for monitoring during induction of anesthesia and throughout the operative procedure.

The operative approach should be planned to resect the evident disease. As with most adrenal pheochromocytomas, many extra-adrenal pheochromocytomas can now be resected using minimally invasive techniques (laparoscopy or thoracoscopy). This technology must be applied judiciously by a surgeon familiar with both the disease and the techniques, in order to achieve optimal outcome for the patient.

18.3 Malignant Pheochromocytoma

18.3.1 Incidence and Prevalence

Malignant pheochromocytomas currently account for 10–15% of all cases, although various authors have reported an incidence ranging from 5% to as high as 46%. Extra-adrenal pheochromocytomas have been associated with a higher incidence of malignancy in most series reported ranging from 20% to 40%, but this is not uniform [10]. When collected series of pheochromocytomas are evaluated, and trying to account for selective referral bias, an overall incidence of 15% appears to be a reliable estimate [15].

18.3.2 Diagnosis

There are no certain histologic criteria that distinguish benign from malignant tumors. Even upon retrospective review, the distinction is often impossible since vascular and capsular invasion as well as mitotic figures can be readily identified in both benign and malignant pheochromocytomas. Tumors without evidence of capsular or vascular invasion have metastasized to distant sites while some tumors with local capsular or even major venous invasion have apparently been cured by surgical excision. Malignancy can be positively diagnosed only when there is local invasion of tumor into surrounding soft tissue, or when the presence of tumor in non-chromaffin-bearing tissue outside the region of the sympathetic chain is identified. Tumors that are at increased risk for malignancy are those that are extra-adrenal (30–40% risk vs. 10% adrenal), and those pheochromocytomas that secrete only dopamine.

The median time of recurrence or identification of metastases is 5–6 years. Long-term follow-up is therefore advised which should include regular blood pressure monitoring as well as annual biochemical studies for catecholamine and their metabolites. Our current approach is to evaluate using plasma metanephrine measurements at least annually, except in those tumors that make only dopamine or ACTH, in which case specific biochemical follow-up plans must be made depending upon the initial biochemical presentation [2–4, 13].

The most common site for metastatic lesions is bone, where they commonly present as lytic lesions of the spine, skull or ribs. Other sites include liver, lung, and retroperitoneal or mediastinal lymph nodes. Malignant pheochromocytomas usually are slow growing tumors and long-term survival has been reported (although rare) provided that control of symptoms caused by increased catecholamines is possible.

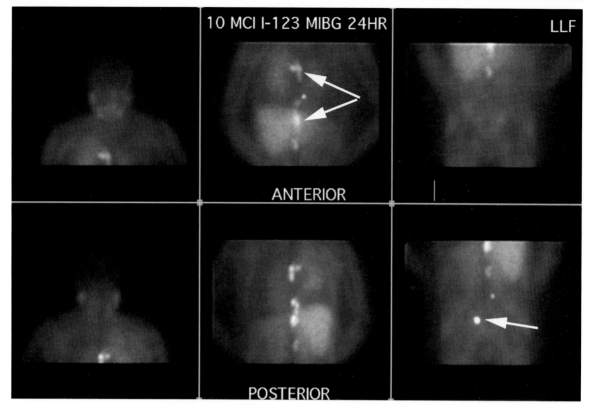

Fig. 2. MIBG scan can demonstrate the sites of systemic disease, as in this patient with diffuse intra-abdominal and intra-tho-racic nodal disease (*double arrows*) and bone metastasis (*single arrow*). (Images courtesy of Dr. Barry Shulkin, University of Michigan)

18.3.3   Localization and Treatment Planning

Once the diagnosis of malignant pheochromocytoma is established or suspected, ^{123}I-MIBG scintiscanning has proven effective in detecting the extent of the disease in most patients (Fig. 2). In some centers, MIBG is used routinely in all pheochromocytoma patients before any operative procedure to rule out occult metastases, although a recent study from our institution shows that in most pheochromocytoma patients, this is not necessary [8]. CT and MRI may give additional anatomic information that may be helpful in determining resectability in patients whose disease is limited to soft tissue. Octreotide scanning and technetium bone scans have also proved useful in some cases [5]. Bone metastases, in vertebral bodies, skull or ribs are the most common location for spread of the disease. They can be identified by any of the scintiscanning techniques.

18.3.4   Therapy

18.3.4.1   Medical Blockade of End-Organ Effects

All patients with malignant pheochromocytomas should initially be treated with an alpha-adrenergic blocking drug with the exception of those rare tumors secreting only dopamine. We prefer phenoxybenzamine, gradually increasing the dose to control hypertension. Starting with a total dose of 30 mg per day, we increase the dose every third day by 30 mg. The endpoint of therapy is orthostatic hypotension, although a clinical sign that the dose is adequate is the development of nasal congestion. Small doses of a beta-blocking drug, even when epinephrine levels are not excessively high, may also prove beneficial. In patients whose symptoms or blood pressure cannot be readily controlled with an alpha-blockade, additional antihypertensive therapy may be required. For patients with unresectable metastatic disease, alpha-methyltyrosine should be considered. This drug inhibits the synthesis of catecholamines and may, in conjunction with an adrenergic blockade, offer long-term control of cate-

Fig. 3a–c. Preoperative imaging can be critical to appropriate ▶ operative planning. This woman with a large right adrenal pheochromocytoma with necrosis (**a**) had a significant thrombus in the inferior vena cava demonstrated on preoperative ultrasound (**b**, *arrow*). Exploration with extensive mobilization and control of the IVC, and intraoperative ultrasound allowed resection of the tumor en bloc with the involved IVC (**c**, with the Satinsky clamp enclosing the region of IVC to be resected)

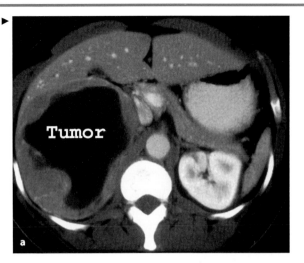

cholamine-related symptoms. Some patients with unresectable disease may live for a number of years, providing their catecholamine secretion is controlled.

18.3.4.2   Extirpative Therapy

After appropriate blockade, management of recurrences includes wide local excision of surgically resectable disease as a first line of treatment (Fig. 3). Unfortunately, this may only be palliative because of the presence of bone metastases. However, when tumor is limited to soft tissue, surgical excision may offer long-term palliation and even cure. Complete resection may require retroperitoneal lymph node dissection, liver resection, or soft tissue resection that includes other intra-abdominal organs (kidney, bowel, distal pancreas). Careful preoperative planning and imaging can help to "draw the dotted lines" sufficiently widely around the tumor to give the best opportunity for cure [10].

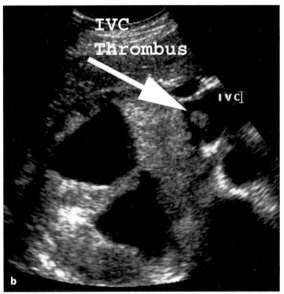

18.3.4.3   Systemic Therapy

Until the past decade, no effective chemotherapeutic regimen had been reported. No single agent such as Adriamycin or streptozotocin has ever been shown to be beneficial. However, a combination of cyclophosphamide, vincristine and dacarbazine has resulted in a high incidence of both biochemical improvement (decrease in catecholamines) and tumor growth inhibition [1, 12, 14, 16]. This combination is currently considered the drug regimen of choice when chemotherapy is indicated (Table 1).

18.3.4.4   Palliative Care

External beam radiation treatment is effective for the palliation of bone pain. Cytotoxic therapy including cyclophosphamide, vincristine and dacarbazine offers

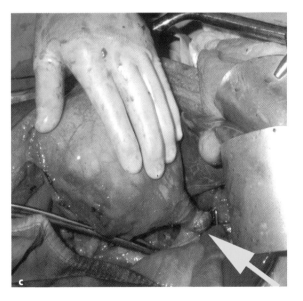

Table 1. Clinical reports of therapy with cyclophosphamide, dacarbazine and vincristine

Authors	Year	Patients (N)	Biochemical response (CR+PR)	Tumor responses (CR+PR)
Averbuch [1]	1988	14	11	8
Tada [15]	1998	3	3	NR
Sisson [13]	1999	6	3	3

only limited improvement in survival rates [1, 12, 14, 16]. Therapeutic ^{131}I-MIBG has been used to treat patients with functioning metastases with encouraging results in selected patients with respect to decrease in both tumor size and circulating catecholamines [6, 9, 11, 14]. Less than a third of patients are candidates for treatment, which is based on the tumor's ability to concentrate sufficient ^{131}I-MIBG to be irradiated effectively. Although regression of tumor has been well documented in some cases, the duration of effect has been limited to approximately 2 years and no patient has been cured.

References

1. Averbuch SD, et al. (1988) Malignant pheochromocytoma: effective treatment with a combination of cyclophosphamide, vincristine, and dacarbazine. Ann Int Med 109:267–73
2. Eisenhofer G (2003) Editorial: biochemical diagnosis of pheochromocytoma – is it time to switch to plasma-free metanephrines? [comment]. J Clin Endocrinol Metab 88:550–2
3. Eisenhofer G, et al. (1999) Plasma normetanephrine and metanephrine for detecting pheochromocytoma in von Hippel-Lindau disease and multiple endocrine neoplasia type 2. N Engl J Med 340:1872–9
4. Eisenhofer G, et al. (1998) Plasma metanephrines are markers of pheochromocytoma produced by catechol-O-methyltransferase within tumors. J Clin Endocrinol Metab 83:2175–85
5. Kaltsas G, et al. (2001) Comparison of somatostatin analog and meta-iodobenzylguanidine radionuclides in the diagnosis and localization of advanced neuroendocrine tumors. J Clin Endocrinol Metabol 86:895–902
6. Loh KC, et al. (1997) The treatment of malignant pheochromocytoma with iodine-131 metaiodobenzylguanidine (131I-MIBG): a comprehensive review of 116 reported patients. J Endocrinol Invest 20:648–58
7. Lumachi F, et al. (1998) Extraadrenal and multiple pheochromocytomas. Are there really any differences in pathophysiology and outcome? J Exp Clin Cancer Res 17:303–5
8. Miskulin J, et al. (2003) Is preoperative iodine 123 metaiodobenzyl guanidine scintigraphy routinely necessary before initial adrenalectomy for pheochromocytoma? Surgery 134:918–22
9. Nakabeppu Y, Nakajo M (1994) Radionuclide therapy of malignant pheochromocytoma with 131I-MIBG. Ann Nucl Med 8:259–268
10. Pommier RF, et al. (1993) Comparison of adrenal and extraadrenal pheochromocytomas. Surgery 114:1160–5; discussion 1165–6
11. Pujol P, et al. (1995) Metastatic pheochromocytoma with a long-term response after iodine-131 metarodobenzylguanidine therapy. Eur J Nucl Med 22:382–384
12. Rao F, Keiser HR, O'Connor DT (2002) Malignant and benign pheochromocytoma: chromaffin granule transmitters and the response to medical and surgical treatment. Ann N Y Acad Sci 971:530–2
13. Sawka AM, et al. (2003) A comparison of biochemical tests for pheochromocytoma: measurement of fractionated plasma metanephrines compared with the combination of 24-hour urinary metanephrines and catecholamines [comment]. J Clin Endocrinol Metab 88:553–8
14. Sisson JC, et al. (1999) Treatment of malignant pheochromocytomas with 131-I metaiodobenzylguanidine and chemotherapy. Am J Clin Oncol 22:364–70
15. Stenstrom G, Svardsudd K (1986) Pheochromocytoma in Sweden 1958–1981. An analysis of the National Cancer Registry Data. Acta Medica Scand 220:225–32
16. Tada K, Okuda Y, Yamashita K (1998) Three cases of malignant pheochromocytoma treated with cyclophosphamide, vincristine, and dacarbazine combination chemotherapy and alpha-methyl-p-tyrosine to control hypercatecholaminemia. Horm Res 49:295–7
17. Thrasher JB, et al. (1993) Pheochromocytoma of urinary bladder: contemporary methods of diagnosis and treatment options. Urology 41:435–439
18. Velchik MG, et al. (1989) Localization of pheochromocytoma: MIBG, CT and MRI correlation. J Nucl Med 30:328–336

19 Pheochromocytoma in MEN-2A, MEN-2B, and von Hippel-Lindau Disease

Geoffrey B. Thompson

CONTENTS

19.1 Introduction

Pheochromocytomas in MEN-2A, MEN-2B, and von Hippel-Lindau disease (VHL) may be bilateral and, less often, extra-adrenal (paragangliomas) [8, 30]. Historically, such patients were explored via an open anterior, transperitoneal approach to provide ready access to both adrenal glands and the paraganglia. Bilateral total adrenalectomy was the preferred operation, to avoid future recurrence in residual adreno-medullary tissue. Pheochromocytomas can be associated with sudden, life-threatening events, especially in the perioperative and peripartum periods [2, 8]. With the likely need for multiple operative procedures, in these familial disorders, over the course of a patient's lifetime, missing a small or occult pheochromocytoma could have disastrous perioperative consequences.

The downside of bilateral total adrenalectomy (BTA) is the lifelong commitment to exogenous steroid dependence. More recent follow-up studies have documented the true incidence of acute adrenal insufficiency following bilateral total adrenalectomy. The numbers are not inconsequential, and morbidity is significant [4, 9, 20].

The risk of malignancy [2, 8, 33] in patients with familial pheochromocytoma is so low that concerns regarding malignancy should be, at best, a very weak argument supporting routine bilateral total adrenalectomy.

With a better understanding of the genetics and natural history of these disorders, coupled with improved methods of diagnosis, localization, and resection, more conservative operations can now be made available to patients with MEN2 and VHL, so as to avoid lifelong steroid dependence.

19.2 MEN-2A, MEN-2B

Multiple endocrine neoplasia type 2 (MEN-2) is an autosomal dominant genetic syndrome characterized by multiple endocrine tumors, including medullary thyroid carcinoma (seen in 100% of patients), parathyroid neoplasia, and pheochromocytoma. In MEN-2A, pheochromocytomas are seen in approximately 50% of affected kindred members. The same is true of MEN-2B patients. In MEN-2B, the marfanoid habitus is seen in virtually all patients, along with mucosal neuromas and occasional intestinal ganglioneuromas. Parathyroid disease is seen in 10–20% of MEN-2A patients, and is not seen in MEN-2B kindreds [15].

Germline mutations in the RET proto-oncogene have been found to be responsible for both inherited syndromes. The causative gene was mapped to the centromeric chromosome 10 in 1987 [22, 35]. The RET proto-oncogene is a tumor-suppressor gene and encodes a tyrosine kinase receptor. In more than 95% of patients with MEN-2A, a germline mutation affects one of five codons specifying a conserved cysteine residue within the extracellular ligand-binding domain of RET. All MEN-2A patients exhibit allelic heterogeneity. Ninety-eight percent of patients with MEN-2B syndrome harbor a single point mutation located within the tyrosine kinase catalytic domain of RET [5, 12, 24, 34]. Through direct mutational analysis, it is now possible to determine the genetic status of patients at risk for the development of MEN-2 in most cases.

The reported incidence of pheochromocytomas in affected MEN-2 patients ranges from 30% to 55% [30]. Pheochromocytoma is the first presenting feature in only 10–25% of MEN-2 patients. Medullary thyroid carcinoma is diagnosed before or simultaneously in 75–90% of cases. The average age at diagnosis for pheochromocytoma in MEN-2 patients is approximately 37 years. When medullary thyroid carcinoma is diagnosed first, there is an average interval of at least 10 years before a pheochromocytoma becomes evident either clinically or biochemically. Pheochromocytomas in MEN-2 are rarely malignant and paragangliomas occur in less than 1% of MEN-2 patients [25].

It is absolutely necessary to exclude the presence of pheochromocytoma in any patient in whom thyroidectomy is planned for medullary thyroid carcinoma, particularly when a family history of MEN-2 is suspected or known.

The diagnosis of pheochromocytoma in MEN-2 patients is made by a combination of history, biochemical screening, and imaging. Today, because of genetic screening and surveillance, 50–80% of patients with adrenomedullary tumors are asymptomatic. When symptomatic, headache (69%), palpitations (62%), hypertension (57%), and diaphoresis (50%) are the most common signs and symptoms [25]. Combined measurement of 24-h fractionated urinary catecholamines and total metanephrines is diagnostic in over 90% of patients with (familial) pheochromocytomas [8, 28]. Measurement of plasma metanephrines and normetanephrines may be more sensitive, resulting in more false positive studies [13]. We find plasma levels helpful when the clinical and radiographic suspicion is high, but the 24-h urinary levels are repeatedly normal.

Computed tomography (CT), magnetic resonance imaging (MRI), and nuclear scintigraphy (MIBG) are all very accurate at localizing pheochromocytomas (85–90%) [25]. Somatostatin receptor scintigraphy has also been used with some success. Because of the low rate of malignancy and extra-adrenal tumors, there is little role for meta-iodobenzyl guanidine (MIBG) imaging in early screening. In addition, MIBG will light up hyperplastic glands in MEN 2, thereby creating both diagnostic and management dilemmas [11].

Lairmore et al. [20] have published the most important study with regard to the operative management of MEN-2 pheochromocytomas. In 23 patients undergoing unilateral adrenalectomy alone, 48% had not developed a contralateral tumor with a mean follow-up time of 5.2 years. In those that did develop a contralateral pheochromocytoma (52%), the mean follow-up was 11.9 years. In addition, of their patients undergoing bilateral total adrenalectomy, 25% had at least one episode of acute adrenal insufficiency requiring hospital admission and intravenous corticosteroid infusion.

19.3   von Hippel-Lindau Disease

VHL is an autosomal dominant tumor predisposition syndrome characterized by multiple benign and malignant tumors of the central nervous system, kidneys, pancreas, adrenal medulla, and paraganglia (Table 1) [2, 8]. Renal cell carcinomas are the most lethal tumors seen in over 50% of VHL patients [2, 8]. Retinal angiomas and central nervous system hemangioblastomas are the hallmarks of this disease [2, 8]. Approximately 7–20% of VHL patients develop pheochromocytomas [2, 8].

The incidence of VHL is roughly 1 per 40,000, and it has been observed across all ethnic groups and both sexes [2, 8]. Genetic testing is available and can be used to determine whether an individual carries a mutation of the VHL gene. VHL is due to germline mutations in a tumor suppressor gene mapped to the chromosomal region 3p25–26 [8]. Deleterious mutations in the VHL gene can be identified in 80% or more of the VHL families [8]. In kindreds where a mutation has been identified, genetic testing can rule out VHL in family members lacking that specific mutation, thus avoiding the

Table 1. von Hippel-Lindau tumor types seen in 109 patients, January 1975 to June 2000

Tumor type	No. (%)
Renal cell carcinoma	50 (46)
Cerebellar/cerebral hemangioblastomas	83 (76)
Retinal angiomas	69 (63)
Pheochromocytomas (adrenal masses)	17 (16)
Paragangliomas	3 (3)
Benign renal cysts	66 (61)
Spinal cord hemangioblastoma	33 (30)
Pancreatic lesions	47 (43)
Ovarian cysts	7 (6)
Epididymal cysts	10 (9)
Endolymphatic sac tumors	5 (5)
Hepatic hemangiomas	7 (6)

expense, anxiety, and inconvenience of lifelong surveillance. There appears to be a strong correlation between the type of mutation and the clinical phenotype in VHL. In VHL type 2 (with pheochromocytomas), 96% of families have missense mutations. However, not all missense mutations are associated with pheochromocytoma [8].

Minimal clinical diagnostic criteria for VHL of known family members require documentation of at least one major lesion (retinal angioma, central nervous system hemangioblastoma, renal cell cancer, or pheochromocytoma) [8]. In a suspected proband, the individual must demonstrate two or more retinal or CNS vascular tumors or one vascular tumor and one characteristic visceral lesion [8].

Pheochromocytomas in VHL tend to occur in younger patients and are more frequently smaller, multiple, bilateral, and extra-adrenal, compared to their sporadic counterparts [8]. Similar to MEN-2 patients, metastasis is rare. Clustering of pheochromocytomas in a subset of VHL families is well recognized in VHL, VHL 2A (pheochromocytomas but no renal call carcinoma), and VHL 2B (pheochromocytomas and renal cell carcinoma) [8].

In our most recent review of 109 VHL patients at Mayo Clinic [2], the mean age at VHL diagnosis was 29 years (range, 7–66 years). One-third of patients had no first-degree relatives with VHL. Seventeen (16%) patients had an adrenal mass, and three (3%) had paragangliomas. In six patients (6%), pheochromocytoma or paraganglioma was the first documented VHL tumor. Forty-one percent of patients were asymptomatic, but 29% presented with significant cardiac manifestations (arrhythmia and/or cardiomyopathy). The urinary excretion of fractionated catecholamines and total metanephrines was elevated in only two-thirds of VHL patients with pheochromocytomas. CT scanning detected 83% of the known tumors. ^{123}I-MIBC scintigraphy detected the remaining lesions. Sixteen patients underwent surgical resection during this 25-year period at our institution. Fifty percent of the patients underwent concurrent abdominal surgery for renal and/or pancreatic tumors. In only two cases were bilateral total adrenalectomies performed. Mean tumor size was 2.7 cm (range, 1.5–6.5 cm). No malignant tumors were identified. There were no deaths, and only two transient perioperative complications (atrial fibrillation and pancreatitis; each in one patient). Of the three excised paragangliomas, two were located in the inner ear, and one was in the juxtarenal, para-aortic position. Of the adrenalectomies performed, nine were unilateral procedures (three laparoscopic; of which

one was partial), four were bilateral (two bilateral total adrenalectomies; two were cortical-sparing – one of which was laparoscopic). Only the two patients who underwent bilateral total adrenalectomy remain steroid dependent. No metastases or recurrences have developed with a mean follow-up of 6.8 years (range, 3 months to 37 years) in the entire group and 1 year (range, 11–47 months) in the cortical-sparing group.

19.4 Screening MEN-2 and VHL Patients for Pheochromocytoma

Biochemical screening for pheochromocytoma in affected kindred members should begin during early adolescence in MEN-2 patients and childhood in VHL patients, seeing that the earliest reports of pheochromocytoma in these patients appear to be approximately 10 years later [8, 25]. Screening should consist of 24-h urinary catecholamines and metanephrines and CT scanning on a yearly basis for both MEN-2 and VHL patients. Elevated urinary studies in the face of a negative CT scan should prompt an MRI examination in MEN-2 patients and an MRI or MIBG scan in VHL patients. Normal urinary studies in the face of an adrenal mass on CT should prompt the measurement of plasma metanephrines and normetanephrines. If normal, MIBG scanning or MRI should be considered. Lack of symptoms or normotension is not an indication for continued observation in a patient with a documented pheochromocytoma. The quiescent nature of these smaller familial tumors makes screening and early detection essential to avoid life-threatening crises during surgery, trauma, or childbirth.

19.5 Preoperative Preparation

Once the diagnosis of pheochromocytoma is established, preoperative pharmacologic blockade with the α-blocker dibenzyline is our preferred agent of choice. The drug is titrated for 7–10 days to orthostatic hypotension and nasal congestion. Replenishment of the patient's effective circulating volume with added salt and fluid intake is imperative for safe perioperative management. β-Blockers are added 2–3 days prior to surgery if tachyarrhythmias are present. Alternative, effective regimens utilizing calcium channel blockers or labetalol have been described.

19.6   Surgical Management

Anesthetic management is similar to that described for sporadic cases and is presented elsewhere in this text. Surgical management in MEN-2 and VHL has evolved as a result of a better understanding of the natural history of these disease processes. Given the low incidence of malignancy and the low risk of (early) recurrence, adrenal-sparing procedures [2, 8, 30] have become increasingly popular and are proving to be both safe and efficacious. Autotransplantation of devascularized cortical tissue is fraught with unacceptably high failure rates [16, 27], but the preservation of a vascularized remnant (as little as one-third of one gland) of adrenal cortex can provide sufficient cortisol secretion at rest and during times of stress [2, 3, 7]. We and others have demonstrated the safety and success of the laparoscopic approach for pheochromocytomas both unilateral and bilateral, total and cortical-sparing (Table 2) [1, 2, 4, 10, 14, 17, 18, 21, 23, 26, 29, 31, 32, 38, 39]. The availability of ultrasound and harmonic ultrasonic dissectors for both open and laparoscopic procedures has made cortical-sparing surgery an appropriate alternative to bilateral total adrenalectomy in most patients with bilateral pheochromocytomas (Fig. 1). Although minimal steroid supplementation may be necessary for short periods of time after cortical-sparing surgery, most can be weaned based on the results of cortrosyn stimulation testing.

Cortical-sparing surgery (either unilateral or bilateral) is easier with smaller tumors (<1.5–2.0 cm) and tumors at either pole (away from the central hilum)

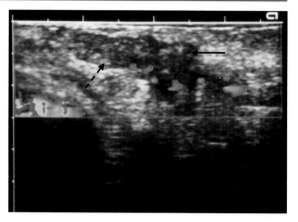

Fig. 1. Laparoscopic ultrasound demonstrating non-visible tumor in lower pole

but is possible under a variety of situations (see Chap. 36). Contraindications to cortical-sparing surgery include large, centrally located, invasive or malignant tumors and multiple tumors throughout the gland. Open anterior procedures are still utilized when concomitant intra-abdominal operations are planned in VHL patients, such as nephron-sparing surgery and pancreatic surgery for islet cell tumors, or in many cases requiring a completion adrenalectomy.

When performing laparoscopic or open adrenalectomy in MEN-2 patients, the liver should be carefully inspected for evidence of metastatic medullary thyroid carcinoma. Open posterior adrenalectomy remains an option for patients with extensive intra-abdominal adhesions, but the morbidity (musculoskeletal) is not insignificant [36]. An extraperitoneal

Table 2. Laparoscopic and cortical-sparing adrenalectomy for MEN 2 and VHL pheochromocytomas (recent literature review)

Author	Patients (no.)	VHL or MEN 2	Cortical sparing	Laparoscopic	Mean FU (months)	Recurrence	Steroid independence
Lee et al. 1996 [21]	15	Both	15	0	138	3	93%
Janetschek et al. 1998 [18]	4	VHL	4	4	13.5	0	All
de Graaf et al. 1999 [10]	6	MEN 2	6	0	40	1	All
Mugiya et al. 1999 [23]	1	MEN 2	1	1	3	0	All
Neumann et al. 1999 [26]	4	VHL	4	4	2–24	0	All
Walther et al. 1999 [38]	14	VHL	12	0	18	2	92%
Inabnet et al. 2000 [16]	5	Both	5	0	84	3	40%
Radmayr et al. 2000 [32]	1	VHL	1	1	24	0	All
Walther et al. 2000 [39]	3	VHL	3	3	13	0	All
Al-Sobhi et al. 2002 [1]	1	VHL	1	1	3	0	All
Baghai et al. 2002 [2]	5	VHL	3/5	4/5	12	0	All
Brunt et al. 2002 [4]	18	Both	0	18	57	4/12 MEN 2	N/A
Porpiglia et al. 2002 [31]	1	MEN 2	1	1	12	0	All

endoscopic approach is another option in this situation, but is technically quite demanding [23].

One remaining controversy focuses on the appropriateness of cortical-sparing surgery in MEN-2 patients. Virtually all MEN-2 patients have nodular or diffuse adrenomedullary hyperplasia [6, 19, 37]. These hyperplastic and neoplastic cells are the precursor cells for MEN-2 pheochromocytomas. Adrenomedullary hyperplasia is not found in other cases of familial pheochromocytoma. Is it then appropriate to transect an adrenal gland with adrenomedullary hyperplasia, assuming that some neoplastic precursor cells will be spilled into the retroperitoneum? No definitive answer is available. Numerous cortical-sparing adrenalectomies have been performed on MEN-2 patients without any reported cases of pheochromocytomatosis. Remnant recurrences are reportedly low, but follow-up in most cases is short. Definitive answers regarding this question may not be available for another 15–20 years.

19.7   Paragangliomas

Paragangliomas can occur anywhere from the base of the skull to the bladder along the sympathetic paraganglia. Because of their location and the reactive tissue that often surrounds these tumors, open surgical excision is our procedure of choice, but laparoscopic resection of such tumors has been performed [18]. Unlike their sporadic counterparts, paragangliomas in MEN-2 (exceedingly rare) and VHL tend to behave in a benign fashion.

19.8   Summary

Fifty percent of MEN-2 patients develop pheochromocytomas, and 10–20% of affected members of VHL families will do the same. Familial pheochromocytomas are more often bilateral, multiple, small, and asymptomatic compared to their sporadic counterparts. Genetic testing is available for both disorders, and when mutations are present, patients should be screened regularly for pheochromocytoma with biochemical and imaging studies. After preoperative pharmacologic blockade, resection of all pheochromocytomas should be performed either in an open or laparoscopic fashion. Adrenal-sparing surgery and cortical-sparing surgery seem appropriate in most cases, given the low risk of malignancy, the acceptable rate of contralateral or remnant recurrence, and the

clear advantage for avoidance of prolonged exogenous steroid dependence. Concerns (at least theoretic) regarding gland transection remain in MEN-2 patients with adrenomedullary hyperplasia, and further study is warranted.

References

1. Al-Sobhi S, Peschel R, Zihak C, Bartsch G, Neumann H, Janetschek G (2002) Laparoscopic partial adrenalectomy for recurrent pheochromocytoma after open partial adrenalectomy in von Hippel-Lindau disease. J Endourol 16:171–174
2. Baghai M, Thompson GB, Young WF Jr, Grant CS, Michels VV, van Heerden JA (2002) Pheochromocytomas and paragangliomas in von Hippel-Lindau disease. Arch Surg 137:682–689
3. Barker NW (1929) The pathologic anatomy in twenty-eight cases of Addison's disease. Arch Pathol 8:432–450
4. Brunt LM, Lairmore TC, Doherty GM, Quasebarth MA, DeBenedetti M, Moley JF (2002) Adrenalectomy for familial pheochromocytoma in the laparoscopic era. Ann Surg 235:713–721
5. Carlson KM, Dou S, Chi D, et al. (1994) Single missense mutation in the tyrosine kinase catalytic domain of the *RET* protooncogene is associated with multiple endocrine neoplasia type 2B. Proc Natl Acad Sci USA 91:1579–1583
6. Carney JA, Sizemore GW, Sheps SG (1976) Adrenal medullary disease in multiple endocrine neoplasia, type 2: pheochromocytoma and its precursors. Am J Clin Pathol 66:279–290
7. Cedemark BJ, Sjoberg HE (1981) The clinical significance of metastases to the adrenal glands. Surg Gynecol Obstet 152:607–610
8. Couch VMS, Lindor NM, Karnes PS, Michels VV (2000) von-Hippel-Lindau disease. Mayo Clin Proc 75:265–272
9. de Graaf JS, Dullaart RPF, Swierstra RP (1999) Complications after bilateral adrenalectomy for phaeochromocytoma in multiple endocrine neoplasia type 2 – a plea to conserve adrenal function. Eur J Surg 165:843–846
10. de Graaf JS, Lips CJM, Rütter JE, van Vroonhoven TJMV (1999) Subtotal adrenalectomy for phaeochromocytoma in multiple endocrine neoplasia type 2A. Eur J Surg 165:535–538
11. de Graaf JS, Dullaart RPF, Kok T, Piers DA, Swierstra RP (2000) Limited role of meta-iodobenzylguanidine scintigraphy in imaging phaeochromocytoma in patients with multiple endocrine neoplasia type II. Eur J Surg 166:289–292
12. Donis-Keller H, Dou S, Chi D, et al. (1993) Mutations in the *RET* proto-oncogene are associated with MEN 2A and FMTC. Hum Mol Genet 2:851–856
13. Eisenhofer G, Lenders JW, Linehan WM, Walther MM, Goldstein DS, Keiser HR (1999) Plasma normetanephrine and metanephrine for detecting pheochromocytoma in

von Hippel-Lindau disease and multiple endocrine neoplasia type 2. N Engl J Med 340:1872–1879

14. Gagner M, Breton G, Pharand D, Pomp A (1996) Is laparoscopic adrenalectomy indicated for pheochromocytomas? Surgery 120:1076–1080

15. Howe JR, Norton JA, Wells SA Jr (1993) Prevalence of pheochromocytoma and hyperparathyroidism in multiple endocrine neoplasia type 2A: results of long-term follow-up. Surgery 114:1070–1077

16. Inabnet WB, Caragliano P, Pertsemlidis D (2000) Pheochromocytoma: inherited associations, bilaterality, and cortex preservation. Surgery 128:1007–1012

17. Janetschek G, Neumann HP (2001) Laparoscopic surgery for pheochromocytoma. Urol Clin North Am 28:97–105

18. Janetschek G, Finkenstedt G, Gasser R, Waibel UG, Peschel R, Bartsch G, Neumann HPH (1998) Laparoscopic surgery for pheochromocytoma: adrenalectomy, partial resection, excision of paragangliomas. J Urol 160:330–334

19. Koch CA, Mauro D, Walther MM, Linehan M, Vortmeyer AO, Jaffe R, Pacak K, Chrousos GP, Zhuang Z, Lubensky IA (2002) Pheochromocytoma in von Hippel-Lindau disease: distinct histopathologic phenotype compared to pheochromocytoma in multiple endocrine neoplasia type 2. Endocr Pathol 13:17–27

20. Lairmore TC, Ball DW, Baylin SB, et al. (1993) Management of pheochromocytomas in patients with multiple endocrine neoplasia type 2 syndromes. Ann Surg 217:595–603

21. Lee JE, Curley SA, Gagel RE, Evans DB, Hickey RC (1996) Cortical-sparing adrenalectomy for patients with bilateral pheochromocytoma. Surgery 120:1064–1071

22. Mathew CG, Chin KS, et al. (1987) A linked genetic marker for multiple endocrine neoplasia type 2A on chromosome 10. Nature 6130:527–528

23. Mugiya S, Suzuki K, Saisu K, Fujita K (1999) Unilateral laparoscopic adrenalectomy followed by contralateral retroperitoneoscopic partial adrenalectomy in a patient with multiple endocrine neoplasia type 2a syndrome. J Endourol 13:99–104

24. Mulligan LM, Kwok JBJ, Healey CS, et al. (1993) Germ-line mutations of the RET proto-oncogene in multiple endocrine neoplasia type 2A. Nature 363:458--460

25. Mutch MG, Lairmore TC (2001) Pheochromocytoma and hyperparathyroidism in multiple endocrine neoplasia type 2. In: Doherty GM, Skogseid B (eds) Clinical endocrinology. Lippincott Williams & Wilkins, Philadelphia, p 569

26. Neumann HPH, Reincke M, Bender BU, Elsner R, Janetschek G (1999) Preserved adrenocortical function after laparoscopic bilateral adrenal sparing surgery for hereditary pheochromocytoma. J Clin Endocrinol Metab 84:2608–2610

27. Okamoto T, Obara T, Ito Y, Yamashita T, Kanbe M, Iihara M, Hirose K, Yamazaki K (1996) Bilateral adrenalectomy with autotransplantation of adrenocortical tissue or unilateral adrenalectomy: treatment options for pheochromocytomas in multiple endocrine neoplasia type 2A. Endocr J 43:169–175

28. Orchard T, Grant CS, van Heerden JA, Weaver A (1993) Pheochromocytoma – continuing evolution of surgical therapy. Surgery 114:1153–1158

29. Pautler SE, Choyke PL, Pavlovich CP, Caryanani K, Walther MM (2002) Intraoperative ultrasound aids in dissection during laparoscopic partial adrenalectomy. J Urol 168:1352–1355

30. Pomares FJ, Canas R, Rodriguez JM, Hernandez AM, Parrilla P, Tebar FJ (1998) Differences between sporadic and multiple endocrine neoplasia type 2A phaeochromocytoma. Clin Endocrinol 48:195–200

31. Porpiglia F, Destefanis P, Bovio S, Allasino B, Orlandi F, Fontana D, Angeli A, Terzolo M (2002) Cortical-sparing laparoscopic adrenalectomy in a patient with multiple endocrine neoplasia type IIA. Horm Res 57:197–199

32. Radmayr C, Neumann H, Bartsch G, Elsner R, Janetschek G (2000) Laparoscopic partial adrenalectomy for bilateral pheochromocytomas in a boy with von Hippel-Lindau disease. Eur Urol 38:344–348

33. Scopsi L, Castellani MR, Gullo M, Cusumano F, Camerini E, Pasini B, Orefice S (1996) Malignant pheochromocytoma in multiple endocrine neoplasia type 2B syndrome: case report and review of the literature. Tumori 82: 480–484

34. Seizinger BR, Rouleau GA, Ozelius LJ, et al. (1988) von Hippel-Lindau disease maps to the region of chromosome 3 associated with renal cell carcinoma. Nature 332: 268–269

35. Simpson NE, Kidd KK, et al. (1987) Assignment of multiple endocrine neoplasia type 2A to chromosome 10 by linkage. Nature 6130:528–530

36. Thompson GB, Grant CS, van Heerden JA, et al. (1997) Laparoscopic versus open posterior adrenalectomy: a case-control study of 100 patients. Surgery 122:1132–1136

37. van Heerden JA, Sizemore GW, Carney JA, et al. (1984) Surgical management of the adrenal glands in the multiple endocrine neoplasia type II syndrome. World J Surg 8:612–621

38. Walther M, Keiser HR, Choyke PL, Rayford W, Lyne JC, Linehan WM (1999) Management of hereditary pheochromocytoma in von Hippel-Lindau disease kindreds with partial adrenalectomy. J Urol 161:395–398

39. Walther MM, Herring J, Choyke PL, Linehan WM (2000) Laparoscopic partial adrenalectomy in patients with hereditary forms of pheochromocytoma. J Urol 164: 14–17

20 Benign Paragangliomas

Abbie L. Young, William F. Young, Jr.

Paraganglia are specialized neural crest-derived cells (chromaffin cells) that are divided into sympathoadrenal and parasympathetic paraganglia [14, 22]. The sympathoadrenal paraganglia are symmetrically distributed along the paravertebral axis from high in the neck near the superior cervical ganglion to the abdomen and pelvis. Small sympathoadrenal paraganglia can also be associated with organs such as the urinary bladder and prostate gland. The parasympathetic paraganglia are primarily localized to the skull base and neck. Paragangliomas are rare tumors that arise from extra-adrenal paraganglia; they represent 10–18% of all chromaffin tissue-related tumors [5, 40], which are reported at a rate of 2–8 cases per million per year [5, 34]. The diagnosis, localization, and treatment of paragangliomas offers potential cure of symptoms associated with functional tumors, prevention of a lethal hypertensive paroxysm, prevention of morbidity from mass effects, and the early diagnosis of malignant tumors [41].

20.1   Presentation

Benign paragangliomas are diagnosed in the following clinical settings: signs and symptoms related to catecholamine hypersecretion, mass effect symptoms, incidental finding on imaging, or family screening for hereditary paraganglioma. We recently reported our experience with benign paragangliomas diagnosed over a 20-year period at Mayo Clinic [13]. The patient population consisted of 141 females (60%) and 95 males (40%). The mean age at the time of diagnosis was 47±16 years (range, 14–93). Most of the patients presented with mass effect symptoms or an incidental imaging finding; only 19.8% had documented catecholamine hypersecretion. In the patients with catecholamine hypersecretion, most tumors were localized to the abdomen and pelvis. Only 3.6% of the head and neck paragangliomas were documented to have catecholamine hypersecretion [13].

The majority of paragangliomas are non-functioning; for the minority of tumors that are hormone-producing, the diagnosis and treatment is complex. Symptomatic catecholamine-hypersecretion results in signs and symptoms identical to those in patients with hyperfunctioning adrenal pheochromocytoma. Episodic symptoms or spells include abrupt onset of throbbing headaches, generalized diaphoresis, palpitations, anxiety, chest pain, and abdominal pain. These spells can be extremely variable in their presentation and may be spontaneous or precipitated by postural changes, anxiety, exercise, or maneuvers that increase intra-abdominal pressure. The catecholamine-hypersecretion spell may last 10–60 min and may occur daily to monthly. The clinical signs include hypertension (paroxysmal in half of the patients and sustained in the other half), orthostatic hypotension, pallor, grade I–IV retinopathy, tremor, and fever. Catecholamine-secreting urinary bladder paragangliomas may be associated with painless hematuria and paroxysmal attacks induced by micturition or bladder distension.

20.2   Diagnosis

When a catecholamine-secreting tumor is suspected in a patient because of paroxysmal symptoms, biochemical documentation of catecholamine hypersecretion should precede any form of imaging study. Most laboratories measure catecholamines and metanephrines by high-pressure liquid chromatography with electrochemical detection or by gas-chromatographic/mass-spectrometric methods. Refined laboratory techniques have overcome the problems associated with fluorometric analysis (e.g., false-positive results caused by α-methyldopa and other drugs with high native fluorescence). Catecholamines and metanephrines can be measured in the blood or the urine.

The 24-h urinary excretion rates of metanephrines and catecholamines are the tests of choice to screen for symptomatic catecholamine-secreting tumors [21, 38]. For a patient with episodic hypertension, the 24-h urine collection should start with the onset of a spell. When collected in this manner, patients with catecholamine-secreting paraganglioma have more than a twofold increase above the upper normal limit in the 24-h urinary levels of catecholamines or increased total metanephrine values. Measurements of fractionated plasma free metanephrines are highly sensitive [23] but lack specificity when compared to the combination of 24-h urinary total metanephrines and catecholamines [32]. Normal fractionated plasma free metanephrine measurement effectively rules out the diagnosis of a catecholamine-secreting tumor, even in high-risk individuals, with the possible exception of a dopamine-secreting tumor [32]. Thus, measurement of fractionated plasma free metanephrines may be the biochemical test of choice in high-risk patients (those with familial paraganglioma or a vascular mass consistent with paraganglioma discovered incidentally on imaging). However, in the more common clinical setting when a sporadic catecholamine-secreting tumor is suspected, particularly in older hypertensive patients, measurement of 24-h urinary metanephrines and catecholamines may provide adequate sensitivity, with a lower rate of false-positive tests.

Although it is best to evaluate patients who are not receiving any medication, treatment with most medications may be continued, with some exceptions (Table 1). Tricyclic antidepressants are the agents that interfere most frequently with the interpretation of 24-h urine catecholamines and metabolites. To effectively screen for catecholamine-secreting tumors, treatment with tricyclic antidepressants and other psychoactive agents listed in Table 1 should be tapered

Table 1. Medications that may alter measured levels of catecholamines and metabolites

Increase the values
   Tricyclic antidepressants
   Levodopa
   Amphetamines, buspirone, and most psychoactive agents
   Labetalol, sotalol, and methyldopa (in spectrophotometric metanephrine assays)
   Withdrawal from clonidine hydrochloride (Catapres) and other drugs
   Ethanol

Decrease the values
   Metyrosine
   Methylglucamine[a]

[a] A component of iodinated contrast media that may cause metanephrine values to be falsely normal for as long as 72 h when measured with Pisano's spectrophotometric method.

and discontinued at least 2 weeks before any hormonal assessments.

20.3   Localization

Localization studies should not be initiated until biochemical studies have confirmed the diagnosis of a catecholamine-secreting tumor. Computer-assisted imaging (magnetic resonance imaging [MRI] or computed tomography [CT]) of the adrenal glands, abdomen, and pelvis should be the first localization test (sensitivity, >95%; specificity, >65%) [17, 18, 24]. Approximately 90% of catecholamine-secreting tumors are found in the adrenal glands and 98% in the abdomen and pelvis [25, 38]. Catecholamine-secreting paragangliomas are found where chromaffin tissue is located, e.g., along the para-aortic sympathetic chain, or within the organ of Zuckerkandl at the origin of the inferior mesenteric artery [6], the wall of the urinary bladder, and the sympathetic chain in the neck or mediastinum [13, 30, 40] (Fig. 1). The imaging characteristics on MRI scanning are quite typical for paraganglioma (Fig. 2). If the results of abdominal imaging are negative, scintigraphic localization with ^{123}I-metaiodobenzylguanidine is indicated (Fig. 3). This radiopharmaceutical agent accumulates preferentially in catecholamine-producing tumors; however, this procedure is not as sensitive as initially hoped (sensi-

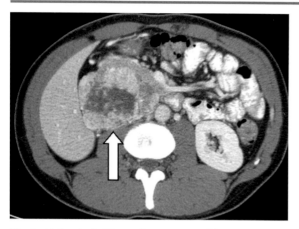

Fig. 1. Abdominal CT scan in a 39-year-old man with biochemically silent familial paraganglioma (*SDHB*, mutation). The large (9.6×6.0×5.3 cm) abdominal paraganglioma is shown (*arrow*)

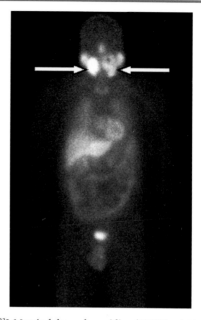

Fig. 3. ^{123}I-Metaiodobenzylguanidine (MIBG) scintigraphy in a 48-year-old man with familial paraganglioma (*SDHD*, mutation). The MIBG scan shows large areas of intense uptake in the neck (*arrows*) consistent with bilateral carotid body tumors

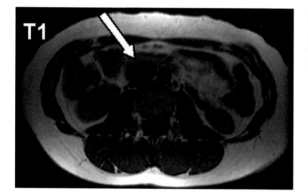

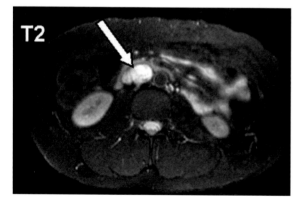

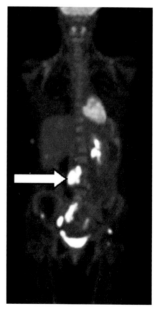

Fig. 2. MRI of the abdomen in a 32-year-old woman with labile hypertension, documented catecholamine excess, and family history of paraganglioma (sister of the patient shown in Fig. 1). The 3.9×3.4×2.0-cm paraganglioma (*arrow*) is seen in the typical location between the aorta and inferior vena cava. Increased signal on T2-weighted imaging is also demonstrated

Fig. 4. ^{18}F-Fluorodeoxyglucose (FDG) PET scan in a 14-year-old girl who presented with spells and hypertension and biochemical documentation of catecholamine hypersecretion. The PET scan was obtained because of inconclusive findings on MRI and no tumoral uptake on ^{123}I-MIBG scintigraphy. This scan shows a 5.0×3.0×2.8-cm paraganglioma along the inferior vena cava (*arrow*) and metastatic disease to the right ovary, the right external iliac lymph nodes, posterior pelvic lymph nodes bilaterally, right lobe of liver, distal right humeral diaphysis, 10th and 11th thoracic vertebral bodies, and right iliac crest. Normal FDG uptake is seen over her heart, solitary left kidney, and urinary bladder

tivity, 88%; specificity, 99%) [10, 33]. In certain cases, 6-[(18)F]-fluorodopamine or ^{18}F-fluorodeoxyglucose positron emission tomography may be indicated to investigate metastatic disease [16] (Fig. 4).

In the Mayo Clinic series, multicentric tumors (99 total with 2 to 6 paragangliomas per patient) were present in 39 patients: 26 (67%) had disease in the head and neck, 7 (18%) below the neck, and 6 (15%) had disease both within the head and neck and below the neck [13]. Twenty-four patients with multiple paragangliomas presented with 66 synchronous tumors and 15 patients presented with 33 metachronous tumors. The mean time from diagnosis of the first tumor to diagnosis of a metachronous tumor was 80.8±62.8 months (range, 6–180).

20.4   Syndromic Paraganglioma and Role for Genetic Testing

Overall, 10–50% of paragangliomas are thought to be hereditary [26]. Approximately 10–20% of patients with catecholamine-secreting tumors have associated germline mutations (inherited mutations present in all cells of the body) in genes known to cause genetic disease [8, 28]. Catecholamine-secreting paragangliomas may be associated with familial paraganglioma, neurofibromatosis type 1, von Hippel-Lindau disease, Carney triad, and rarely multiple endocrine neoplasia (MEN) type 2. From the Mayo Clinic series of 236 paraganglioma patients, 29 patients (12.3%) had a documented family history of paragangliomas; 19 of these had familial paraganglioma, five had von Hippel-Lindau disease (retinal hemangiomatosis, cerebellar hemangioblastoma, renal cell carcinoma, pheochromocytoma/paraganglioma), and one had MEN type 2B (Erickson et al. 2001). Four patients presented with the Carney triad (paraganglioma, gastric stromal sarcoma, and pulmonary chondroma) [9, 13]. Genetic testing is available for nearly all of these disorders; genetic counseling should be considered prior to performing genetic testing.

20.4.1   Familial Paraganglioma

Familial paraganglioma is an autosomal dominant condition characterized by paragangliomas that are most often located in the head and neck, but have also been found to occur in the thorax, abdomen, pelvis, and urinary bladder. The occurrence of catecholamine

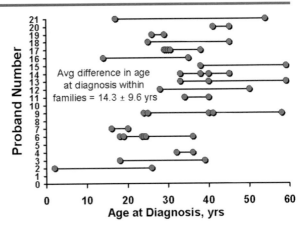

Fig. 5. Age at diagnosis of familial benign paraganglioma and distribution within kindreds. Data were collected retrospectively on 21 Mayo Clinic patients who presented during the years 1978–1998. The family members were first and second degree relatives of the proband. The average age at diagnosis was 32.5 years in patients with head and neck paragangliomas and 28.5 years in patients with abdominal paragangliomas. Within families, the average age difference between members at diagnosis was 14.3±9.6 years (range, 0–37 years)

hypersecretion in familial paraganglioma depends on tumor location; approximately 5% of head and neck paragangliomas and 50% of abdominal paragangliomas are hormone-producing [13]. The average age at diagnosis is approximately 30–35 years, and it can vary greatly within a family (average of 14.3±9.6 years difference, range 0–37 years) (Fig. 5). Familial paraganglioma is caused by mutations in the succinate dehydrogenase (SDH; succinate:ubiquinone oxidoreductase) subunit genes *SDHB*, *SDHC*, *SDHD*, which compose portions of mitochondrial complex II [3]. Most germline mutations in *SDHD*, located on chromosome 11q23, have been identified in multi-generational families with head and neck paragangliomas [4, 35] (Fig. 3). In families with *SDHD* mutations, penetrance is dependent upon parent of origin such that the disease is not manifest when the mutation is inherited from the mother but is highly penetrant when inherited from the father [3]. *SDHB*, located on chromosome 1p35–36, and *SDHC*, located on chromosome 1q21, mutations have been associated with families that have abdominal as well as head and neck familial paraganglioma [1, 29, 41] (Figs. 1, 2). In families with *SDHB* and *SDHC* mutations, no imprinting effects have been observed in inheritance pattern. The *SDH* gene mutation detection rate for individuals with familial paraganglioma is currently unknown. *SDHD* and *SDHB* germline mutation screening are commercially available and should be considered in all patients with paraganglioma. In the near future, commercial testing for mutations in *SDHC* should be available [29].

20.4.2 Neurofibromatosis Type 1

Approximately 1–2% of patients with neurofibromatosis type 1 (NF1) develop a catecholamine-secreting neoplasm (typically an adrenal pheochromocytoma). The prevalence of NF1, an autosomal dominant condition, is approximately 1 in 3,000 individuals. NF1 is caused by mutations in a tumor-suppressor gene (*NF1*) located on chromosome 17q11.2. Utilizing a multi-step testing protocol, greater than 95% of mutations within the *NF1* gene can be identified. However, unless a patient with abdominal paraganglioma presents with additional clinical characteristics consistent with a diagnosis of NF1 (e.g., multiple café au lait spots, axillary and inguinal freckling, subcutaneous fibromas, macrocephaly), molecular genetic testing of the *NF1* gene is currently not recommended.

20.4.3 von Hippel-Lindau Disease

von Hippel-Lindau (VHL) disease is an autosomal dominant syndrome [2]. The VHL phenotype includes pheochromocytoma (usually bilateral adrenal neoplasms), retinal angiomas, cerebellar hemangioblastoma, epididymal cystadenoma, renal and pancreatic cysts, and renal cell carcinoma [15]. Rarely, these patients may have an extra-adrenal paraganglioma [13, 36]. The prevalence of VHL is approximately 1 in 35,000 individuals. Pheochromocytoma is reported to occur in approximately 50% of VHL patients. The *VHL* tumor suppressor gene is located on chromosome 3p25–26. More than 300 *VHL* germline mutations have been identified. In up to 97% of cases, pheochromocytoma is associated with missense mutations (rather than truncating or null mutations) within the *VHL* gene. Nearly 100% of patients with VHL will have an identifiable mutation in the *VHL* gene. VHL germline mutation analysis is commercially available and should be considered in patients with bilateral pheochromocytoma, or patients with co-phenotype disorders.

20.4.4 Carney Triad or Syndrome

The Carney triad or syndrome is a rare disorder that affects primarily young women and includes gastric stromal sarcoma, pulmonary chondroma, paraganglioma, adrenal cortical adenoma, and esophageal leiomyomas [9]. The longest reported interval between detection of the first and second components of the syndrome is 26 years (mean, 8.4 years; median, 6 years) [9]. The Carney triad is a chronic, persistent, and indolent disease. Although the disorder may be familial, the responsible gene has yet to be identified.

20.4.5 Multiple Endocrine Neoplasia Type 2

MEN type 2A is an autosomal dominant disorder [12, 19]. The MEN 2A phenotype includes pheochromocytoma (usually bilateral adrenal neoplasms), medullary carcinoma of the thyroid (MTC), and hyperparathyroidism. MTC is almost always detected before pheochromocytoma. Very rarely the patient with MEN 2A may have an extra-adrenal paraganglioma. The prevalence of MEN 2A is approximately 1 in 35,000 individuals. Numerous mutations throughout the *RET* proto-oncogene have been documented in individuals with MEN 2A. The *RET* proto-oncogene, located on chromosome 10q11.2, encodes a receptor tyrosine kinase. Pheochromocytoma is most frequently associated with mutations in codon 634 (exon 11) of the *RET* proto-oncogene.

MEN type 2B is also an autosomal dominant disorder, and it represents approximately 5% of all MEN 2 cases. This genetic condition is also very rarely associated with extra-adrenal paraganglioma. The MEN 2B phenotype includes pheochromocytoma (usually bilateral adrenal neoplasms), MTC, mucosal neuromas, thickened corneal nerves, intestinal ganglioneuromatosis, and marfanoid body habitus. Like MEN 2A, MEN 2B is caused by mutations in the *RET* proto-oncogene. MEN 2B is primarily associated with mutations in codon 918 (exon 16).

Overall, pheochromocytoma occurs in approximately 50% of patients with MEN 2. More than 95% of patients with MEN 2A and more than 98% of patients with MEN 2B will have an identifiable mutation in the *RET* proto-oncogene. *RET* proto-oncogene germline mutation analysis is commercially available and should be considered in patients with bilateral pheochromocytoma, or patients with co-phenotype disorders.

20.5   Treatment

The treatment of choice for paraganglioma is surgical resection; most are benign and can be excised totally. From the Mayo Clinic series, of the 246 resected benign paragangliomas, the average volume was 17.1 cm³ for head and neck tumors and 94.1 cm³ for tumors below the neck.

If the tumor is catecholamine-secreting, the chronic and acute effects of excess circulating catecholamines should be reversed prior to the operation.

20.5.1   Preoperative Management

Combined α- and β-adrenergic blockade are required preoperatively to control blood pressure and to prevent intraoperative hypertensive crises. α-Adrenergic blockade should be started at least 7 days preoperatively to allow for expansion of the contracted blood volume. A liberal salt diet is advised during the preoperative period. Once adequate α-adrenergic blockade is achieved, β-adrenergic blockade is initiated (e.g., 3 days preoperatively). With this approach, only 7% of patients undergoing catecholamine-secretion tumor resection at Mayo Clinic have needed postoperative hemodynamic management [20].

20.5.1.1   α-Adrenergic Blockade

Phenoxybenzamine is an irreversible, long-acting, α-adrenergic blocking agent. Approximately 25% of an oral dose of phenoxybenzamine is absorbed. Phenoxybenzamine is available in 10-mg capsules. The initial dosage is 10 mg orally once or twice daily; the dosage is increased by 10–20 mg every 2–3 days as needed to control the blood pressure and spells. The effects of daily administration are cumulative for nearly a week. The average dosage is 20–100 mg per day. Side-effects include postural hypotension, tachycardia, miosis, nasal congestion, inhibition of ejaculation, diarrhea, and fatigue. Prazosin, terazosin, and doxazosin are selective α₁-adrenergic blocking agents; the more favorable side-effect profiles of these agents may be preferable to phenoxybenzamine when long-term pharmacologic treatment is indicated (e.g., for metastatic pheochromocytoma). However, phenoxybenzamine is the preferred drug for preoperative preparation because it provides α-adrenergic blockade of long duration. Effective α-adrenergic blockade permits expansion of blood volume, which usually is severely decreased as a result of excessive adrenergic vasoconstriction.

20.5.1.2   β-Adrenergic Blockade

The β-adrenergic antagonist should be administered only after α-adrenergic blockade is effective because β-adrenergic blockade alone may result in more severe hypertension due to the unopposed α-adrenergic stimulation. Preoperative β-adrenergic blockade is indicated to control the tachycardia associated with both the high circulating catecholamine concentrations and the α-adrenergic blockade. Caution is indicated if the patient is asthmatic or has congestive heart failure. Chronic catecholamine excess can produce a myocardiopathy, and β-adrenergic blockade can result in acute pulmonary edema. Noncardioselective β-adrenergic blockers such as propranolol and nadolol or cardioselective β-adrenergic blockers such as atenolol and metoprolol may be used. When administration of the β-adrenergic blocker is begun, the drug should be used cautiously and at a low dose. For example, propranolol is usually started at 10 mg orally every 6 h at least 5–7 days after the initiation of α-adrenergic blockade. The dose is then increased and converted to a long-acting preparation as necessary to control the tachycardia.

20.5.1.3   Catecholamine Synthesis Inhibitor

A catecholamine synthesis inhibitor may be used in the rare patient where α-adrenergic blockade cannot be used or in patients with large invasive tumors and a prolonged resection is anticipated. α-Methyl-L-tyrosine (metyrosine) inhibits the synthesis of catecholamines by blocking the enzyme tyrosine hydroxylase. It is rapidly absorbed from the gastrointestinal tract and most of it is excreted in the urine unchanged. Metyrosine is available as 250-mg capsules. The initial dosage is 250 mg orally four times daily. The dosage may be increased by 500 mg per day every day to a maximum of 4 g per day (1 g four times per day) as needed for blood pressure control. Side effects include sedation, depression, diarrhea, anxiety, nightmares, crystalluria and urolithiasis, galactorrhea, and extrapyramidal manifestations. Therefore, this agent should be used with caution and only when other agents have been ineffective or are contraindicated. The extrapyramidal effects of phenothiazines or haloperidol may be potentiated, and the use of these agents concomitant with metyrosine should be avoided. High fluid intake to avoid crystalluria is suggested for any patient taking more than 2 g daily. Although some centers have used this agent preoperatively, most clinicians have reserved it primarily for those patients who, for cardiopulmonary reasons, cannot be treated with combined α- and β-adrenergic blockade.

20.5.1.4 Calcium Channel Blockade

Calcium channel blockers, which block norepinephrine-mediated calcium transport into vascular smooth muscle, have been used successfully at several medical centers for the preoperative preparation of pheochromocytoma patients [7, 11, 37]. Nicardipine is the most commonly used calcium channel blocker. It is given orally to control blood pressure preoperatively and then as an intravenous infusion intraoperatively. In a study from France, 70 pheochromocytoma patients were operated on between 1988 and 1996 and managed with calcium channel blockers [11]. Nicardipine was used in 61 patients and other calcium channel blockers in the remaining patients. The duration of preoperative treatment ranged from 24 h to several weeks depending on plasma volume and blood pressure control. Intraoperatively, nicardipine infusion was started after intubation, adjusted according to systolic blood pressure and stopped before ligation of the tumor venous drainage. Increases in SBP greater than 200 mmHg were observed in ten patients and were effectively controlled by nicardipine in all cases. Heart rate greater than 100 bpm occurred in 51 patients and was easily controlled with esmolol. Arrhythmias were infrequent (n=4) and required treatment in only one case [11]. A review of the perioperative management of 113 pheochromocytoma patients operated at Cleveland Clinic showed no surgical mortalities [37]. Although this study suggested that that preoperative α-adrenergic blockade is not essential in pheochromocytoma patients, most centers continue to use α- and β-adrenergic blockade because of the excellent outcomes associated with this approach. Calcium channel blockers serve as a good option for patients that are intolerant of α- and β-adrenergic blockade.

20.5.1.5 Acute Hypertensive Crises

Acute hypertensive crises may occur before or during operation and should be treated with nitroprusside or phentolamine administered intravenously. Phentolamine is a short-acting, nonselective, α-adrenergic blocker. It is available in lyophilized form in vials containing 5 mg. An initial test dose of 1 mg is administered and, if necessary, this is followed by repeat 5-mg boluses or a continuous infusion. The response to phentolamine is maximal in 2–3 min after a bolus injection and lasts 10–15 min. A solution of 100 mg of phentolamine in 500 ml of 5% dextrose and water can be infused at a rate titrated for blood pressure control. The use of nitroprusside is discussed below.

20.5.2 Anesthesia and Surgery

Extirpating a paraganglioma is a high-risk surgical procedure, and an experienced surgeon/anesthesiologist team is required [31]. The last oral doses of α- and β-adrenergic blockers can be administered early in the morning on the day of operation. Cardiovascular and hemodynamic variables must be monitored closely. Continuous measurement of intra-arterial pressure and heart rhythm is required. In the setting of congestive heart failure or decreased cardiac reserve, monitoring of pulmonary capillary wedge pressure is indicated. Premedication includes minor tranquilizers and barbiturates. Fentanyl and morphine should not be used because of the potential for stimulating catecholamine release from the pheochromocytoma. In addition, parasympathetic nervous system blockade with atropine should be avoided because of the associated tachycardia. Induction usually is accomplished with thiopental, and general anesthesia is maintained with a halogenated ether such as enflurane or isofluorane. Hypertensive episodes should be treated with phentolamine (2–5 mg intravenously) or nitroprusside intravenous infusion (0.5–5.0 µg/kg per minute; maximum dose should not exceed 800 µg per minute). Lidocaine (50–100 mg intravenously) or esmolol (50–200 µg/kg per minute intravenously) is used for cardiac arrhythmia. Adverse perioperative events or complications occurred in 32% of 143 patients operated at Mayo Clinic from 1983 to 1996 [20]. The most common adverse event was sustained hypertension (36 patients). There were no perioperative deaths, myocardial infarctions, or cerebrovascular events. Preoperative factors univariately associated with adverse perioperative events included larger tumor size (P=0.007), prolonged duration of anesthesia (P=0.015), and increased levels of preoperative urinary catecholamines and catecholamine metabolites: total metanephrines (P=0.004), norepinephrine (P=0.014), and epinephrine (P=0.004). Despite premedication of most patients with phenoxybenzamine and a beta-adrenergic blocker, varying degrees of intraoperative hemodynamic lability occurred [20].

20.5.3   Postoperative Management

Hypotension may occur after surgical resection of the pheochromocytoma and should be treated with fluids and colloids. Postoperative hypotension is less frequent in patients who have had adequate α-adrenergic blockade preoperatively. Hypoglycemia can occur in the immediate postoperative period, and therefore blood glucose levels should be monitored and the fluid given intravenously should contain 5% dextrose. Blood pressure usually is normal by the time of dismissal from the hospital. Some patients remain hypertensive for up to 8 weeks postoperatively. Long-standing, persistent hypertension does occur and may be related to accidental ligation of a polar renal artery, resetting of baroreceptors, established hemodynamic changes, structural changes of the blood vessels, altered sensitivity of the vessels to pressor substances, renal functional or structural changes, or coincident primary hypertension.

Approximately 2 weeks postoperatively, either fractionated plasma free metanephrines or a 24-h urine sample should be obtained for measurement of catecholamines and metanephrines. If the levels are normal, the resection of the catecholamine-secreting tumor can be considered to have been complete. Increased levels of metanephrines or catecholamines postoperatively indicate the probable presence of residual tumor, a second primary lesion, or occult metastases. Lifelong biochemical testing should be performed annually as surveillance for tumor recurrence, metastatic disease, or delayed appearance of multiple primary tumors [39].

References

1. Astuti D, Latif F, Dallol A, Dahia PL, Douglas F, George E, Skoldberg F, Husebye E, Eng C, Maher ER (2001) Gene mutation in the succinate dehydrogenase subunit SDHB causes susceptibility to familial pheochromocytoma and to familial paraganglioma. Am J Hum Genet 69:49–54
2. Atuk NO, Stolle C, Owen JA Jr, Carpenter JT, Vance ML (1998) Pheochromocytoma in von Hippel-Lindau disease: clinical presentation and mutation analysis in a large multigenerational kindred. J Clin Endocrinol Metab 83: 117–120
3. Baysal BE, Ferrell RE, Willett-Brozick JE, Lawrence EC, Myssiorek D, Bosch A, van der Mey A, Taschner PEM, Rubinstein WS, Myers EN, Richard CW 3rd, Cornelisse CJ, Devilee P, Devlin B (2000) Mutations in SDHD, a mitochondrial complex II gene, in hereditary paraganglioma. Science 287:848–851
4. Baysal BE, Willett-Brozick JE, Lawrence EC, Drovdlic CM, Savul SA, McLeod DR, Yee HA, Brackmann DE, Slattery WH 3rd, Myers EN, Ferrell RE, Rubinstein WS (2002) Prevalence of SDHB, SDHC and SDHD germline mutations in clinic patients with head and neck paragangliomas. J Med Genet 39:178–183
5. Beard CM, Sheps SG, Kurland LT, Carney JA, Lie JT (1983) Occurrence of pheochromocytoma in Rochester, Minnesota, 1950 through 1979. Mayo Clin Proc 58:802–804
6. Brantigan CO, Katase RY (1969) Clinical and pathologic features of paragangliomas of the organ of Zuckerkandl. Surgery 65:898–905
7. Bravo EL (2002) Pheochromocytoma: an approach to antihypertensive management. Ann N Y Acad Sci 970:1–10
8. Bryant J, Farmer J, Kessler LJ, Townsend RR, Nathanson KL (2003) Pheochromocytoma: the expanding genetic differential diagnosis. J Natl Cancer Inst 95:1196–1204
9. Carney JA (1999) Gastric stromal sarcoma, pulmonary chondroma, and extra-adrenal paraganglioma (Carney triad): natural history, adrenocortical component, and possible familial occurrence. Mayo Clin Proc 74:543–552
10. Chatal JF, Charbonnel B (1985) Comparison of iodobenzylguanidine imaging with computed tomography in locating pheochromocytoma. J Clin Endocrinol Metab 61: 796–772
11. Combemale F, Carnaille B, Tavernier B, Hautier MB, Thevenot A, Scherpereel P, Proye C (1998) Exclusive use of calcium channel blockers and cardioselective beta-blockers in the pre- and per-operative management of pheochromocytomas. 70 cases. Ann Chir 52:341–345
12. Eng C, Clayton D, Schuffenecker I, Lenoir G, Cote G, Gagel RF, van Amstel HK, Lips CJ, Nishisho I, Takai SI, Marsh DJ, Robinson BG, Frank-Raue K, Raue F, Xue F, Noll WW, Romei C, Pacini F, Fink M, Niederle B, Zedenius J, Nordenskjold M, Komminoth P, Hendy GN, Mulligan LM, et al. (1996) The relationship between specific RET proto-oncogene mutations and disease phenotype in multiple endocrine neoplasia type 2: International RET mutation consortium analysis. JAMA 276:1575–1579
13. Erickson D, Kudva YC, Ebersold MJ, Thompson GB, Grant CS, van Heerden JA, Young WF Jr (2001) Benign paragangliomas: clinical presentation and treatment outcomes in 236 patients. J Clin Endocrinol Metab 86:5210–5216
14. Fries JG, Chamberlin JA (1968) Extra-adrenal pheochromocytoma: literature review and report of a cervical pheochromocytoma. Surgery 63:268–279
15. Hes FJ, Hoppener JW, Lips CJ (2003) Clinical review 155: Pheochromocytoma in Von Hippel-Lindau disease. J Clin Endocrinol Metab 88:969–974
16. Ilias I, Yu J, Carrasquillo JA, Chen CC, Eisenhofer G, Whatley M, McElroy B, Pacak K (2003) Superiority of 6-[(18)F]-fluorodopamine positron emission tomography versus

[(131)I]-metaiodobenzylguanidine scintigraphy in the localization of metastatic pheochromocytoma. J Clin Endocrinol Metab 88:4083–4087

17. Jackson JA, Kleerekoper M, Mendlovic D (1993) Endocrine grand rounds: A 51-year-old man with accelerated hypertension, hypercalcemia, and right adrenal and paratracheal masses. Endocrinologist 3:5

18. Jalil ND, Pattou FN, Combemale F, Chapuis Y, Henry JF, Peix JL, Proye CA (1998) Effectiveness and limits of preoperative imaging studies for the localisation of pheochromocytomas and paragangliomas: a review of 282 cases. Eur J Surg 164:23–28

19. Januszewicz A, Neumann HP, Lon I, Szmigielski C, Symonides B, Kabat M, Apel TW, Wocial B, Lapinski M, Januszewicz W (2000) Incidence and clinical relevance of RET proto-oncogene germline mutations in pheochromocytoma patients. J Hypertens 18:1019–1023

20. Kinney MA, Warner ME, van Heerden JA, Horlocker TT, Young WF Jr, Schroeder DR, Maxson PM, Warner MA (2000) Perianesthetic risks and outcomes of pheochromocytoma and paraganglioma resection. Anesth Analgesia 91:1118–1123

21. Kudva YC, Sawka AM, Young WF Jr (2003) The laboratory diagnosis of adrenal pheochromocytoma: the Mayo Clinic experience. J Clin Endocrinol Metab (in press)

22. Lack EE (2000) Tumours of adrenal and extra-adrenal paraganglia. In: Solae E, Kloppel G, Sobin LH (eds) Histological typing of endocrine tumors, 2nd edn. Springer, Berlin, pp 38–48

23. Lenders JW, Pacak K, Walther MM, Linehan WM, Mannelli M, Friberg P, Keiser HR, Goldstein DS, Eisenhofer G (2002) Biochemical diagnosis of pheochromocytoma: which test is best? JAMA 287:1427–1434

24. Maurea S, Coucolo A, Reynolds JC, Neumann RD, Salvatore M (1996) Diagnostic imaging in patients with paragangliomas. Computed tomography, magnetic resonance and MIGB scintigraphy comparison. Q J Nucl Med 40:365–371

25. Melicow MM (1977) One hundred cases of pheochromocytoma (107 tumors) at the Columbia-Presbyterian Medical Center, 1926–1976: a clinicopathological analysis. Cancer 40:1987–2004

26. Milunsky JM, Maher TA, Michels VV, Milunsky A (2001) Novel mutations and the emergence of a common mutation in the SDHD chain causing familial paraganglioma. Am J Med Genet 100:311–314

27. Modlin IM, Farndon JR, Shepherd A, Johnston ID, Kennedy TL, Montgomery DA, Welbourn RB (1979) Phaeochromocytomas in 72 patients: clinical and diagnostic features, treatment and long term results. Br J Surg 66:456–465

28. Neumann HP, Bausch B, McWhinney SR, Bender BU, Gimm O, Franke G, Schipper J, Klisch J, Altehoefer C, Zerres K, Januszewicz A, Eng C, Smith WM, Munk R, Manz T, Glaesker S, Apel TW, Treier M, Reineke M, Walz MK, Hoang-Vu C, Brauckhoff M, Klein-Franke A, Klose P, Schmidt H, Maier-Woelfle M, Peczkowska M, Szmigielski C, Eng C; Freiburg-Warsaw-Columbus Pheochromocytoma Study Group (2002) Germ-line mutations in nonsyndromic pheochromocytoma. N Engl J Med 346: 1459–1466

29. Niemann S, Muller U (2000) Mutations in SDHC cause autosomal dominant paraganglioma, type 3. Nat Genet 26:268–270

30. O'Riordain DS, Young WF Jr, Grant CS, Carney JA, van Heerden JA (1996) Clinical spectrum and outcome of functional extraadrenal paraganglioma. World J Surg 20:916–921

31. O'Riordan JA (1997) Pheochromocytomas and anesthesia. Int Anesthesiol Clin 25:99–127

32. Sawka AM, Jaeschke R, Singh RJ, Young WF Jr (2003) A comparison of biochemical tests for pheochromocytoma: measurement of fractionated plasma metanephrines compared with the combination of 24-hour urinary metanephrines and catecholamines. J Clin Endocrinol Metab 88:553–558

33. Shapiro B, Gross MD, Fig L, et al. (1990) In: Endocrine hypertension. Raven Press, New York, p 235

34. Stenstrom G, Svardsudd K (1986) Pheochromocytoma in Sweden 1958–1981. An analysis of the National Cancer Registry Data. Acta Med Scand 220:225–232

35. Taschner PE, Jansen JC, Baysal BE, Bosch A, Rosenberg EH, Brocker-Vriends AH, van Der Mey AG, van Ommen GJ, Cornelisse CJ, Devilee P (2001) Nearly all hereditary paragangliomas in the Netherlands are caused by two founder mutations in the SDHD gene. Genes Chromosomes Cancer 31:274–281

36. Trobs RB, Reichardt P, Friedrich T, Kloppel R, Bennek J (2002) Pheochromocytoma and multifocal functioning paraganglioma in a 9-year-old boy with von Hippel-Lindau disease. Urol Int 68:299–301

37. Ulchaker JC, Goldfarb DA, Bravo EL, Novick AC (1999) Successful outcomes in pheochromocytoma surgery in the modern era. J Urol 161:764–767

38. van Gils AP, Falke TH, van Erkel AR, Arndt JW, Sandler MP, van der Mey AG, Hoogma RP (1991) MR imaging and MIBG scintigraphy of pheochromocytomas and extraadrenal functioning paragangliomas. Radiographics 11: 37–57

39. van Heerden JA, Roland CF, Carney JA, Sheps SG, Grant CS (1990) Long-term evaluation following resection of apparently benign pheochromocytoma(s)/paraganglioma(s). World J Surg 14:325–329

40. Whalen RK, Althausen AF, Daniels GH (1992) Extraadrenal pheochromocytoma. J Urol 147:1–10

41. Young AL, Baysal BE, Deb A, Young WF Jr (2002) Familial malignant catecholamine-secreting paraganglioma with prolonged survival associated with mutation in the succinate dehydrogenase B gene. J Clin Endocrinol Metab 87:4101–4105

21 Neuroblastoma

Jed G. Nuchtern, Heidi V. Russell, Jason M. Shohet

CONTENTS

21.1   Introduction

Neuroblastoma is the third most common childhood cancer following leukemia and brain tumors. With more than 600 cases diagnosed in the United States each year, this disease accounts for more than 15% of all pediatric cancer fatalities. It is primarily a tumor of young children with a median age at diagnosis of 17.3 months; approximately one-third of patients are less than 1 year of age [3].

The term neuroblastoma actually represents a spectrum of tumors that arise from primitive ganglion cells throughout the sympathetic nervous system including neuroblastoma, ganglioneuroblastoma, and ganglioneuromas. Outcome varies along this spectrum from almost certain survival with ganglioneuroma to a 30–50% 3-year survival with advanced-stage neuroblastoma.

21.2   Clinical Presentation

Neuroblastoma tumors can arise from anywhere along the sympathetic chain. The most common sites are the adrenal glands, the abdominal and pelvic retroperitoneum, and the thorax (see Figs. 1, 2). These tumors can metastasize to lymph nodes, bone marrow, cortical bone, dura, orbits, liver and skin (see Figs. 3, 4) [13]. Symptoms depend on the location of the tumor and metastases, if present. Because of the frequency of abdominal tumors, abdominal pain, fullness, and a palpable mass are not uncommon. Orbital tumors can cause periorbital ecchymosis (raccoon eyes), ptosis and proptosis and are commonly unilateral. Metastatic spread to the bones and bone marrow can cause pain, especially with ambulation, and blood count abnormalities such as anemia or thrombocytopenia.

Because the tumor cells arise from paravertebral ganglia, they are able to invade the spinal canal

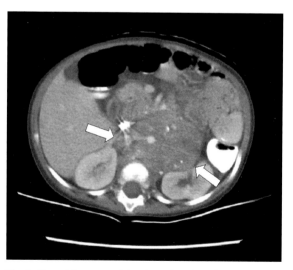

Fig. 1. Neuroblastoma arising from the adrenal gland. The tumor is heterogeneous in appearance, containing calcifications. Note how it surrounds and displaces the aorta

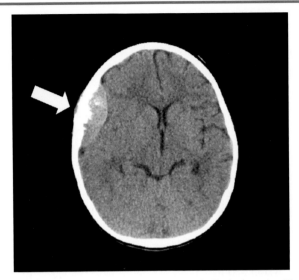

Fig. 2. Neuroblastoma metastatic to the skull. The bone itself has developed an osteoclastic reaction. There is an intracranial component of the metastasis, putting pressure on the brain and causing a midline shift

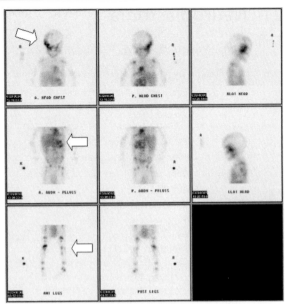

Fig. 4. MIBG scan of a newly diagnosed patient with multiple metastases. *Arrows* specifically demonstrate cranial and leg bone metastases as well as the primary adrenal tumor

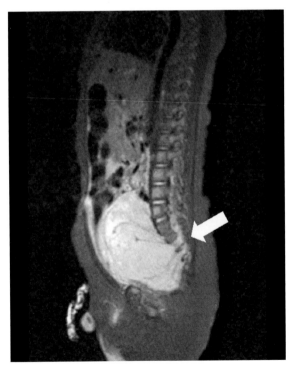

Fig. 3. MRI of a large pelvic neuroblastoma with extension into the spine

through the neural foramina, creating a so-called dumbbell tumor (see Fig. 2). The subsequent spinal cord compression can cause motor deficits, pain, loss of bowel or bladder control, or sensory loss. Subtle and gradual onset of neurologic symptoms may present diagnostic challenges in young children. These dumbbell tumors are normally well localized, and rapid treatment can halt, and in many cases reverse, neurologic deficits; the overall outlook for these children is quite good [12].

Two well-known paraneoplastic syndromes are associated with the presentation of neuroblastoma. Opsoclonus-myoclonus-ataxia syndrome (OMA) occurs in approximately 2–3% of cases [40]. Children develop rapid, dancing, eye movements, rhythmic jerking and/or ataxia. Substantial clinical and experimental evidence suggests that OMA is caused by tumor-reactive anti-neuronal antibodies, although absolute proof of this hypothesis is lacking [41]. Neuroblastoma tumors associated with OMA are likely to be of lower stage and their outcome is favorable. However, approximately 63% of children with OMA will have delays in speech, motor, or cognitive abilities [44]. Vasoactive intestinal peptide (VIP) can be secreted by some neuroblastoma tumors causing abdominal distension and intractable secretory diarrhea with associated hypokalemia [24]. VIP releasing tumors also tend to be less aggressive ganglioneuroblastomas and ganglioneuromas [11] and symptoms resolve following removal of the tumor [17].

21.2.1 Risk Factors and Familial Neuroblastoma

There are several case reports of neuroblastoma occurring in siblings and the incidence of familial neuroblastoma is estimated at less than 6% of all cases [28]. These children usually present at an early age (mean around 9 months of age) and a large percentage have bilateral adrenal or multifocal disease. No constitutional predisposition syndrome or associated congenital anomalies have been identified which correlate with the disease. A recent genetic linkage study suggests that disruption of a locus at 16p12–13 may confer an increased familial predisposition [35]. In families without a history of multiple affected individuals, it is unlikely that a sibling of a neuroblastoma patient will also be affected. The risk for children of survivors of neuroblastoma is difficult to assess due to small numbers and treatment-related infertility.

21.3 Diagnosis

A complete evaluation of the primary tumor and possible metastatic sites requires multiple imaging studies, laboratory assays, and biopsies. All of these studies are best completed at a major pediatric center. Pediatric oncologists and radiologists familiar with the diagnosis and treatment of neuroblastoma should be closely involved in the planning and coordination of these studies. Computerized tomography (CT) or magnetic resonance imaging (MRI) of the primary tumor may reveal an inhomogeneous mass, possibly containing calcifications. When the mass is adjacent to the spine, an MRI is particularly helpful for evaluation of spinal canal invasion. Ultrasound may be helpful for finding a mass and usually can be obtained quickly, but should be followed by either CT or MRI [4].

Technetium bone scan is a sensitive tool for evaluating metastatic spread to cortical bone. The primary mass is sometimes seen as well. In small children less than 1 year of age, a skeletal survey may be needed because the bone scan may be difficult to interpret. Plain radiographs, however, are not as sensitive because of the degree of cortical bone destruction needed to visualize a lesion.

Metaiodobenzylguanidine (MIBG) is a chemical analogue of norepinephrine that is selectively concentrated in sympathetic nervous tissues such as neuroblastoma. It can be labeled with radioactive iodine and imaged by scintigraphy. This type of scan is both sensitive and specific for neuroblastoma in this age group and is recommended at diagnosis and repeat evaluations of the tumor [39, 52]. Because radioactive iodine is used, the thyroid must be protected with non-radioactive iodine administered simultaneously. Despite prophylaxis, thyroid dysfunction becomes a potential complication in around 50% of patients [57].

Neuroblastoma tumor cells have defective synthesis of catecholamines resulting in the accumulation and excretion of the intermediates homovanillic acid (HVA), vanillylmandelic acid (VMA), and dopamine. HVA and VMA tumor markers can be measured in the urine and are useful in both diagnosis and follow-up. Screening programs for neuroblastoma using urine catecholamines are discussed below.

A biopsy is required for definitive diagnosis of neuroblastoma. The most common methods include incisional biopsy of the primary tumor or bone marrow aspirate/biopsy in those patients with a high suspicion of bone marrow metastasis. Because bone marrow biopsy does not give information about the histologic grade of the primary tumor, it may not be sufficient to guide therapy in a subset of cases. For tumors that appear to be localized and resectable without substantial morbidity, a complete or 95% resection of the primary tumor can be performed as the initial diagnostic procedure, along with sampling of non-adherent ipsilateral and contralateral lymph nodes.

As a general rule, the initial procedure should not include resection of vital structures such as kidney or spleen or major motor or sensory nerves whose section would lead to permanent disability. The nature and extent of the initial diagnostic procedure for a child with suspected neuroblastoma should be decided in consultation between a pediatric surgeon and oncologist who are familiar with current treatment of this disease. Tumor tissue or bone marrow, if positive for tumor, is evaluated for MYCN status (see below) and DNA ploidy at a centralized laboratory. Because treatment hinges on proper handling of tissues after biopsy, whenever possible biopsy of the tumor should be undertaken with the guidance of a pediatric oncologist.

Bone marrow disease is evaluated by aspiration and biopsy of the marrow, usually at the iliac crests. Two separate sites are assayed, resulting in four samples (two aspirations, two biopsies). If any of the four assays demonstrate tumor cells, the bone marrow is considered positive for disease [4]. All four assays must be without evidence of tumor for the bone marrow to be considered clear.

The differential diagnosis of primary tumors in children varies with the location. When the tumor arises in a suprarenal location, Wilms' tumor and hepatoblastoma should be entertained as possibilities. In other retroperitoneal and thoracic locations lymphoma, germ cell tumors and infection should also be considered. Definitive diagnosis of neuroblastoma must be made by either histologic review of the tumor or evidence of metastases to bone marrow with concomitant elevation of catecholamines in the urine [4].

21.4   Risk Categories for Treatment

As understanding of neuroblastoma tumors has increased, it is apparent that tumors behave differently both in aggressiveness and in response to treatment. This has allowed treatment to be tailored based on factors associated with the tumor and the child. The Children's Oncology Group (COG) divides neuroblastoma patients into low, intermediate, and high risk categories based on the age of the patient, the stage of the disease when first diagnosed, the histologic appearance of the tumor, the quantitative DNA content of the tumor (ploidy), and the presence or absence of the amplification of the MYCN oncogene (see Table 1). The

clinical heterogeneity of neuroblastoma suggests that further insights into the biology of this tumor will permit the refinement of these risk categories, and hopefully reveal new biologically specific therapeutic targets in the future.

21.4.1   Staging

The most important factor in determining outcome for patients with neuroblastoma is the degree of metastatic spread at presentation [8, 16, 22]. Neuroblastoma tumors can spread to lymph nodes either attached to the tumor or in the close area without significantly affecting the outcome. However, distant metastatic disease (e.g. bone marrow involvement) confers a much worse prognosis as detailed below. One exception to the generally dismal prognosis of children with widespread metastases is a special category of disease in infants, described as 4S, who have resectable primary tumors and metastases limited to the liver, skin and bone marrow, but not cortical bone. The tumor cells in infants with 4S neuroblastoma can undergo spontaneous apoptosis without treatment [10] and overall survival is greater than 85% [25].

Historically, different pediatric cancer cooperative groups used different staging systems based on the clinical presentation and extent of metastatic spread of

Table 1. Children's Oncology Group Risk Assignment Schema

INSS stage	Age	MYCN status	Pathology classification	DNA ploidy	Risk group assignment
1	0–21y	Any	Any	Any	Low
2	<365d	Any	Any	Any	Low
	>365d–21y	Non-amp.	Any	–	Low
	>365d–21y	Amp	Fav.	–	Low
	>365d–21y	Amp	Unfav.	–	High
3	<365d	Non-amp.	Any	Any	Intermediate
	<365d	Amp	Any	Any	High
	>365d–21y	Non-amp.	Fav.	–	Intermediate
	>365d–21y	Non-amp.	Unfav.	–	High
	>365d–21y	Amp	Any	–	High
4	<365d	Non-amp.	Any	Any	Intermediate
	<365d	Amp	Any	Any	High
	>365d–21y	Any	Any	–	High
4S	<365d	Non-amp.	Fav.	>1	Low
	<365d	Non-amp.	Any	=1	Intermediate
	<365d	Non-amp.	Unfav.	Any	Intermediate
	<365d	Amp	Any	Any	High

y, Year; *d*, day; *Amp.*, amplified; *Fav.*, favorable; *Unfav.*, unfavorable.

Table 2. International Neuroblastoma Staging System [12]

Stage	Definition
1	Localized tumor with complete gross excision, with or without microscopic residual disease; representative ipsilateral lymph nodes negative for tumor microscopically (nodes attached to and removed with the primary tumor may be positive)
2A	Localized tumor with incomplete gross excision; representative ipsilateral nonadherent lymph nodes negative for tumor microscopically
2B	Localized tumor with or without complete gross excision, with ipsilateral nonadherent lymph nodes positive for tumor. Enlarged contralateral lymph nodes must be negative microscopically
3	Unresectable unilateral tumor infiltrating across the midline, with or without regional lymph node involvement; or localized unilateral tumor with contralateral regional lymph node involvement; or midline tumor with bilateral extension by infiltration (unresectable) or by lymph node involvement
4	Any primary tumor with dissemination to distant lymph nodes, bone, bone marrow, liver, skin and/or other organs (except as defined for stage 4S)
4S	Localized primary tumor (as defined for stage 1, 2A or 2B), with dissemination limited to skin, liver, and/or bone marrow (limited to infants <1 year of age)

the tumor. This posed difficulty in comparing treatments and outcomes among the research groups. In the early 1990s a single staging system, the International Neuroblastoma Staging System (INSS), was adopted and is currently in use (see Table 2) [4]. It is based on the resectability of the tumor and the spread to local lymph nodes and distant sites. Uniformity of staging has advanced the understanding and treatment of this disease.

21.4.2 Age at Diagnosis

The age at presentation has a profound impact on the overall outcome of children with neuroblastoma. Infants, younger than 1 year of age, have a considerably better survival rate than children over 1 year. Differences in metastatic potential and tumor biology between infants and older children are primarily responsible for these divergent clinical outcomes. Children under 1 year of age are more likely than older children to have localized tumors [13], and only infants have the favorable stage 4S disease. However, even within the same staging category, infants generally have more favorable outcomes than older children of comparable stages [36, 53].

One exception in infants is the newborn, under 4–6 weeks, diagnosed with stage 4S neuroblastoma. In this small subset of infants, there is often rapid growth of the neuroblastoma in the liver resulting in pulmonary compromise and renal failure in approximately 30% [15, 56]. These children should be monitored closely even after the initiation of treatment.

Age also modulates the impact of tumor histology (more completely described below). In the studies leading to the development of the International Neuroblastoma Classification System, less aggressive-appearing neuroblastomas faired worse in older children [48]. Therefore, age is taken into account when defining a neuroblastoma tumor as favorable or unfavorable (see Table 3).

21.4.3 Histology

Neuroblastoma tumors are thought to arise from a pluripotent neural crest cell and, as such, can appear in various degrees of differentiation. The balance between neural-type cells (neuroblasts, maturing neuroblasts, and ganglion cells) and Schwann-type cells (schwannian blasts and mature Schwann cells) helps to categorize the tumor into neuroblastoma, ganglioneuroblastoma, and ganglioneuroma. It should be stressed that central review of neuroblastoma histology through the Children's Oncology Group (COG) is vital to ensure accurate risk category assignment.

Neuroblastoma, the most undifferentiated-appearing and aggressive of this family of tumors, is composed almost entirely of neuroblasts with very few schwannian or stromal cells. Because of the lack of schwannian cells, these tumors are called "stroma-poor". Primitive neuroblasts are 10 μm in diameter, have hyperchromatic nuclei and scanty cytoplasm and

Table 3. International Neuroblastoma Pathology Classification [25] (*MKI*, mitosis karyorrhexis index)

Tumor type	Histology	Prognostic group
Neuroblastoma	(Schwannian stroma-poor)	
Favorable		Favorable
<1.5 years	Poorly differentiated or differentiating and low or intermediate MKI tumor	
1.5–5 years	Differentiating and low MKI tumor	
Unfavorable		Unfavorable
<1.5 years	a) Undifferentiated tumor b) High MKI tumor c) Undifferentiated or poorly differentiated tumor	
1.5–5 years	a) Undifferentiated or poorly differentiated tumor b) Intermediate or high MKI tumor	
>5 years	All tumors	
Ganglioneuroblastoma	(Schwannian stroma-rich)	Favorable

Ganglioneuroma
  Maturing
  Mature
	(Schwannian stroma-dominant)	Favorable

Ganglioneuroblastoma, nodular	(Composite schwannian stroma-rich/stroma-dominant and stroma-poor)	Unfavorable

may form Homer-Wright rosettes. The density of the neuroblasts, rate of mitosis or mitosis-karyorrhexis index (MKI) and neuroblastic differentiation can vary between neuroblastomas and even within the tumor itself. Ganglioneuroblastoma are called "intermediate stroma-rich" or "stroma-rich" tumors because of the increased proportion of schwannian cells. The neuroblasts, which generally have a more mature appearance, are clustered together in foci or nests surrounded by schwannian cells. Ganglioneuroma is predominantly composed of schwannian cells studded with fully mature ganglion cells [48].

Because neuroblastoma in its undifferentiated or immature forms can be difficult to distinguish from other malignancies such as rhabdomyosarcoma or lymphoma, panels of antibodies have been employed to help make a diagnosis. Neuroblastoma tumors generally react to antibodies that distinguish neural tissue such as neuron-specific enolase (NSE), synaptophysin, chromogranin, and S-100.

The degree of differentiation and stromal component of neuroblastoma tumors can be predictive of outcome and is used to determine treatment based on the COG risk. Tumors are classified as having favorable or unfavorable histology after taking into account the appearance of the tumor as described above, the frequency of cell division or the mitosis-karyorrhexis in-

dex (MKI) and the age of the patient (see Table 3). This classification scheme was first described by Shimada et al. in the mid 1980s [49] and is the basis for the current International Neuroblastoma Pathology Classification system [50]. Its prognostic significance was evaluated prospectively on 746 tumors on various risk-based treatment plans of the Children's Cancer Group. This analysis showed a distinct difference in outcome between favorable histology tumors (90% event free survival, EFS) and unfavorable histology tumors (27% EFS) ($p<0.0001$) [51].

21.4.4 Molecular Genetics

Neuroblastoma is a remarkably heterogeneous disease and to date no single pathomnemonic chromosomal alteration or gene has been identified. However, molecular and cytogenetic characterization of neuroblastoma aids in risk classification and, as described above, therapy is tailored according to risk category [2].

Cytogenetic analysis reveals multiple characteristic changes correlating with prognosis and may ultimately reveal clues to the pathogenesis of neuroblastoma. Overall chromosome content as measured by DNA content, or ploidy, has prognostic impact in young children where hyperdiploidy confers a better prognosis [31]. Chromosomal deletions suggesting deficiencies of tumor suppressor genes have been located to the short arm of chromosome1 (1p-) and the long arms of chromosomes 11 and 14 (11q-, 14q-) [59]. Gains of chromosome 17 (17q+) are also found in a significant subset of patients. Increased *MYCN* copy number is associated with 1p- loss and possibly 17q gain and identifies a particularly high risk for treatment failure [34]. The search for specific oncogenes and tumor suppressor genes within these and other less commonly altered chromosomal regions is an active field of research.

The *MYCN* oncogene is clearly associated with altered biologic behavior and a poor clinical outcome. A close relative of the *MYCC* oncogene, *MYCN* copy number is amplified 50–400 fold in about 25% of neuroblastomas with consequent persistently high protein levels [46]. The MYCN protein is a DNA binding transcription factor known to cause malignant transformation in both in vitro and in vivo tumor models [9, 33]. A recent study of infants with stage 4S neuroblastoma demonstrated <50% survival for children with *MYCN*-amplified tumors and >90% survival for a similar population without *MYCN* amplification [25]. Outcome is also dramatically worse for older children with *MYCN*-amplified compared to non-amplified metastatic disease [37]. Despite these clinical and genetic observations, the transcriptional targets of MYCN accounting for this particularly malignant phenotype remain unidentified [2].

The Trk family of tyrosine kinase receptors for neurotrophic factors (TrkA, TrkB and TrkC) are also associated with prognosis. The primary ligands for these receptors are nerve growth factor (NGF), brain derived neurotrophic factor (BDNF) and neurotrophin-3, respectively. Elevated expression of TrkA appears to confer an increased apoptotic response to stimulation and a favorable clinical response to therapy while the converse applies to TrkB and TrkC expression (less favorable clinical group [5, 14].

Much work is still needed to better understand the molecular pathogenesis of neuroblastoma; the importance of obtaining additional materials for research should be stressed. Current molecular studies including methodologies such as gene expression profiling and array-based comparative genomic hybridization coupled with the recently available complete human genome sequence will accelerate the elucidation of molecular pathways essential for neuroblastoma tumorigenesis and metastasis. This critical information will facilitate the development of novel molecular targeted therapies with the promise of decreased treatment-related toxicity and increased long-term survival.

21.5 Treatment

21.5.1 Surgical Aspects of Treatment

Surgical resection is a key component in treatment of all patients with neuroblastoma. The vast majority of patients with localized tumors are cured by complete or subtotal resection alone [23, 29]. In this sense neuroblastoma is unique among cancers because children with less than complete resections or local nodal metastases can often be cured without chemotherapy or radiation. The exceptions to this rule are those with extensive or locally invasive masses with unfavorable histology or *MYCN* amplification.

Patients with large, infiltrating masses, especially those with distant metastases, are normally approached with an initial incisional biopsy of the tumor. This biopsy should include sufficient tissue for definitive histology and molecular studies for risk group assignment. Because most neuroblastoma tumors are responsive to chemotherapy, patients with extensive disease are treated with four or five cycles of chemotherapy prior to attempting a complete resection of the mass. This delayed approach is associated with fewer surgical complications and a decreased rate of incidental nephrectomy [47]. Numerous studies suggest that surgical resection of the primary tumor is associated with better outcome even in patients with distant metastases [18, 21, 30, 55, 58]. Only a pediatric surgeon with training and experience in resecting these extensive, infiltrating tumors should perform these arduous and lengthy procedures.

21.5.1.1 Operative Procedure

Adrenal neuroblastomas range from small, localized masses to extensive tumors that encase the major abdominal blood vessels. The surgical plan should be adapted to the individual patient's position on this spectrum of disease.

Smaller tumors are normally approached via a transverse upper abdominal incision. On the right side, the ascending colon and duodenum are mobilized, followed by exposure of the vena cava above and below the level of the tumor. The right renal artery and vein are identified and preserved. Working from the vena cava toward the tumor, the adrenal vessels are controlled and divided and the mass is excised. For small left adrenal masses, the descending colon is mobilized. The surgeon must decide whether visceral medial rotation of the spleen, pancreas and stomach are required, based on the size and location of the primary tumor. After visualizing the aorta above and below the level of the mass, the left renal vessels are identified and protected. It may be helpful to mobilize the left kidney to aide in this maneuver. Working from the aorta toward the mass, the adrenal vessels are ligated in continuity and divided. There may be several adrenal veins draining into the left renal vein that must be controlled without injuring the larger vessel. After the blood supply is divided, the tumor is removed. Ipsilateral and contralateral non-adherent lymph nodes should be sought and sampled to adequately stage the disease.

Resection of larger, infiltrating tumors can often be approached better through a thoracoabdominal incision. This exposure facilitates proximal vascular control and is usually well tolerated in young children. In addition to division of the lateral attachments of the colon, the dissection is normally aided by mobilization of the ipsilateral kidney. For right-sided lesions, the triangular ligament of the right lobe of the liver is divided to help with exposure. The adventitia overlying the vena cava is incised longitudinally caudad to the tumor. Working in the subadventitial plane, the anterior wall of the vena cava is cleared of tumor, dividing the mass anterior to the plane of dissection if needed. On the lateral side of the cava, the right renal vein is freed from the tumor. With the kidney reflected anteriorly, the renal artery is dissected away from the tumor from where it emerges from behind the vena cava to the renal hilum. As the dissection proceeds proximally on the lateral aspect of the vena cava, the adrenal veins are encountered and divided. When the vena cava has been completely cleared, the remaining attachments of the tumor are readily sectioned.

Large left adrenal masses often encase the aorta and its major abdominal branches, including the celiac axis, superior and inferior mesenteric arteries (SMA and IMA), and the renal vessels. Kiely and La Quaglia have contributed substantially to a coherent and organized approach to these challenging cases [26, 30]. Medial visceral rotation of the spleen, stomach and pancreas is very helpful in providing access to the aorta at the hiatus. The aorta is surrounded with a tape either below the hiatus or by dividing the diaphragm and encircling the vessel in the thorax. The dissection can be initiated either proximal or distal to the mass on the anterior aspect of the aorta, although the distal approach is often more straightforward. In the first stage, the subadventitial plane is developed and the tumor is divided over the aorta for a length of 2–5 cm. The origin of the IMA is identified and protected. Next the left renal vein, which is often encased in tumor in the plane anterior to the aorta, is dissected out for a distance of 5–7 cm. The right and left renal arteries are identified, and just proximal to these the SMA and celiac axis. After exposing each major artery, the subadventitial plane is followed along the axis of the vessel, dividing tumor as the dissection proceeds. As each vessel is mobilized circumferentially, the tumor is removed piecemeal. After the SMA and celiac are freed, the renal vessels are exposed completely (into the hilum if necessary) and branches directly feeding the tumor are divided. The IMA and aorta below the renal hilum are then cleared of tumor. The remainder of the dissection is concerned with resecting tumor posterior to the aorta and separating the mass from its attachments to the kidney, ureter, diaphragm and retroperitoneum.

On some occasions left sided masses will infiltrate around the splenic, superior mesenteric and portal veins. When dissecting tumor in the region between the SMA and celiac axis, extra caution should be used to follow the course of the splenic vein proximally from the hilum of the spleen to its junction with the superior mesenteric vein. If there is substantial involvement of the portal vein, it is better approached from the right side after the bulk of the tumor on the left side is removed.

21.5.1.2   Postoperative Care and Complications

The postoperative course is typical of infants and children after a major laparotomy. In major series the operative mortality is between 0% and 2%, almost exclusively due to severe hemorrhage or the sequelae of massive transfusions. Persistent postoperative diarrhea occurs in approximately one-third of these patients. The extensive dissection around the SMA and celiac axis is the likely cause of this problem. Although there is some improvement over time, many children have permanent symptoms that are often resistant to treatment with antimotility agents [42].

21.5.2 Treatment by Risk Group

21.5.2.1 Low Risk

Patients in the low risk category have low stage disease, stage 1, 2A or 2B. They generally have favorable MYCN status, DNA index and histology. Surgery is the primary treatment for these tumors and is effective for most patients. Disease free survival at 2 years is between 85% and 100% and is dependent on the degree of resection [29, 38, 54]. Chemotherapy with a combination of agents including platinums, etoposide, Adriamycin, and cyclophosphamide is employed if there are symptoms such as spinal cord compression, respiratory or bowel compromise, or if less than half of the tumor can be resected. Radiation therapy is used only for emergency symptom management.

21.5.2.2 Intermediate Risk

Intermediate risk patients include those children less than 1 year of age with stage 3 disease regardless of *MYCN* status or histology, or over 1 year with favorable features. Also included are infants with stage 4 and some 4S disease that are not *MYCN*-amplified. Complete surgical resection is an important part of these children's treatment plans, but is not adequate by itself to completely eradicate this disease [53, 54]. For children with widespread disease, surgical resection may not be possible at diagnosis. Children felt to have intermediate risk disease, therefore, receive surgery to biopsy or resect their primary tumor if possible. Chemotherapy is recommended for these children using a combination of known agents: carboplatin, etoposide, Adriamycin and cyclophosphamide. The chemotherapy will usually allow an unresectable tumor to become resectable as well as eliminate tumor cells remaining in the local and metastatic sites. Radiation therapy is used if tumor remains after surgery and chemotherapy.

Despite the need for chemotherapy in these children, the outcome remains excellent. Three-year event-free survival is predicted to be 70–98%, with a good chance for salvage in the face of recurrent disease [36, 53, 54].

21.5.2.3 High Risk

Patients at the highest risk for disease progression and mortality are those over 1 year of age with disseminated disease at diagnosis, or localized disease with unfavorable biologic and histologic markers such as MYCN amplification. Because of their particularly poor outcome, treatment is aggressive and employs a multi-modality approach. Intensive chemotherapy with a combination of agents is used to shrink the tumor, both at the site of the primary tumor and at metastatic sites. Surgery is used to biopsy the tumor for diagnosis as well as for resection of the primary tumor after chemotherapy when the tumor is smaller and less invasive locally. When the bulk of the tumor has been decreased by chemotherapy and surgery, the patient receives higher dose chemotherapy followed by autologous stem cell rescue. Radiation therapy to a dose of 24–30 Gy is added for control of the primary tumor bed. Biologic differentiation therapy with *cis*-retinoic acid (Accutane) has recently been added to the regimen after completion of the more intensive components.

This intensive treatment regimen is the result of multiple clinical trials over the last several decades. In the 1990s, high dose chemotherapy with autologous stem cell rescue followed by *cis*-retinoic acid provided a survival advantage to children with high-risk neuroblastoma in a randomized clinical trial [37]. However, the results of this best treatment remain poor with only approximately 30% of children remaining disease free at 2 years. A somewhat better preliminary outcome has been achieved with tandem transplants, i.e. more than one autologous stem cell rescue cycle. Both two [19, 20] and three cycles [27] have been piloted with 3-year survival rates of >55%.

The most frequent long-term outcome of high-risk neuroblastoma is recurrence of disease followed by death, despite intensification of therapy over time. Developing new methods to treat this disease is an active area of research in pediatric oncology. Although new chemotherapeutics are being developed and tested in clinical trials, more hope is placed on novel types of treatment based on better understanding of the molecular basis of the tumors. Immunotherapies such as antibodies targeted at GD2 [6], a disialoganglioside on the surface of neuroblastoma, and neuroblastoma vaccines [1, 43] have shown some promise and are vigorously being tested. Generalized targeting of tumor cells with drugs that induce apoptosis [32] or angiogenesis is increasingly desired. Several institutions are evaluating submyeloablative allogenic bone marrow transplant to induce a donor vs tumor effect that has shown promise in some adult tumors such as renal cell carcinoma [7]. Studies into the molecular workings of neuroblastoma will hopefully also yield tumor specific targets for the development of new agents.

21.6   Prevention of Neuroblastoma

Because many neuroblastoma tumors secrete catecholamines that are excreted in the urine, several groups have attempted urine-screening programs in infancy. The aim of these studies was to detect tumors when they were in lower stages, thus decreasing the incidence of high-risk tumors.

Three large studies from Japan, Canada, and Europe have screened approximately 3.6 million children at either 6 months or 1 year of life. The incidence of neuroblastoma diagnosis was compared with either historic controls [61] or unscreened populations in other cities [45, 60].

All study results were similar – there was an increase in diagnosis of neuroblastoma in the screened populations. However, the additional tumors were low stage. There was not a decrease in incidence of high-risk tumors in children beyond the screening age. Nor was there a decrease of mortality in the screened populations. In the study from Canada, two of the 43 patients whose tumors were detected by screening had significant adverse affects because of treatment for their favorable prognosis neuroblastoma [60]. The conclusions of these studies have been that screening for neuroblastoma with urine catecholamines does not reduce mortality of this disease and is not recommended of the population as a whole.

References

1. Bowman L, Grossmann M, Rill D, Brown M, et al. (1998) IL-2 adenovector-transduced autologous tumor cells induce antitumor immune responses in patients with neuroblastoma. Blood 92:1941–1949
2. Brodeur GM (2003) Neuroblastoma: biological insights into a clinical enigma. Nat Rev Cancer 3:203–216
3. Brodeur GM, Maris JM (2002) Neuroblastoma. In: Pizzo PA, Poplack DG (eds) Principles and practice of pediatric oncology. Lippincott Williams & Wilkins, Philadelphia, p 895
4. Brodeur GM, Pritchard J, Berthold F, Carlsen NL, et al. (1993) Revisions of the international criteria for neuroblastoma diagnosis, staging, and response to treatment. J Clin Oncol 11:1466–1477
5. Brodeur GM, Nakagawara A, Yamashiro DJ, Ikegaki N, et al. (1997) Expression of TrkA, TrkB and TrkC in human neuroblastomas. J Neurooncol 31:49–55
6. Cheung NK, Kushner BH, Cheung IY, Kramer K, et al. (1998) Anti-G(D2) antibody treatment of minimal residual stage 4 neuroblastoma diagnosed at more than 1 year of age. J Clin Oncol 16:3053–3060
7. Childs R, Chernoff A, Contentin N, Bahceci E, et al. (2000) Regression of metastatic renal-cell carcinoma after nonmyeloablative allogeneic peripheral-blood stem-cell transplantation. N Engl J Med 343:750–758
8. Coldman AJ, Fryer CJ, Elwood JM, Sonley MJ (1980) Neuroblastoma: influence of age at diagnosis, stage, tumor site, and sex on prognosis. Cancer 46:1896–1901
9. Cole MD, McMahon SB (1999) The Myc oncoprotein: a critical evaluation of transactivation and target gene regulation. Oncogene 18:2916–2924
10. D'Angio GJ, Evans AE, Koop CE (1971) Special pattern of widespread neuroblastoma with a favourable prognosis. Lancet 1:1046–1049
11. Davies RP, Slavotinek JP, Dorney SF (1990) VIP secreting tumours in infancy. A review of radiological appearances. Pediatr Radiol 20:504–508
12. De Bernardi B, Pianca C, Pistamiglio P, Veneselli E, et al. (2001) Neuroblastoma with symptomatic spinal cord compression at diagnosis: treatment and results with 76 cases. J Clin Oncol 19:183–190
13. DuBois SG, Kalika Y, Lukens JN, Brodeur GM, et al. (1999) Metastatic sites in stage IV and IVS neuroblastoma correlate with age, tumor biology, and survival. J Pediatr Hematol Oncol 21:181–189
14. Eggert, A, Grotzer MA, Ikegaki N, Liu XG, et al. (2000) Expression of neurotrophin receptor TrkA inhibits angiogenesis in neuroblastoma. Med Pediatr Oncol 35: 569–572
15. Evans AE, Chatten J, D'Angio GJ, Gerson JM, et al. (1980) A review of 17 IV-S neuroblastoma patients at the Children's Hospital of Philadelphia. Cancer 45:833–839
16. Evans AE, D'Angio GJ, Propert K, Anderson J, et al. (1987) Prognostic factor in neuroblastoma. Cancer 59:1853–1859
17. Funato M, Fujimura M, Shimada S, Takeuchi T, et al. (1982) Rapid changes of serum vasoactive intestinal peptide after removal of ganglioneuroblastoma with watery-diarrhea-hypokalemia-achlorhydria syndrome in a child. J Pediatr Gastroenterol Nutr 1:131–135
18. Garaventa A, De Bernardi B, Pianca C, Donfrancesco A, et al. (1993) Localized but unresectable neuroblastoma: treatment and outcome of 145 cases. Italian Cooperative Group for Neuroblastoma. J Clin Oncol 11:1770–9
19. Grupp SA, Stern JW, Bunin N, Nancarrow C, et al. (2000) Tandem high-dose therapy in rapid sequence for children with high-risk neuroblastoma. J Clin Oncol 18:2567–2575
20. Grupp SA, Bowman LC, von Allmen D, Guzikowski V, et al. (2002) Rapid sequence tandem transplant for advanced neuroblastoma: update and patterns of relapse. Adv Neuroblastoma Res 2002:120
21. Haase GM, O'Leary MC, Ramsay NK, Romansky SG (1991) Aggressive surgery combined with intensive chemotherapy improves survival in poor-risk neuroblastoma. J Pediatr Surg 26:1119–24

22. Jereb B, Bretsky SS, Vogel R, Helson L (1984) Age and prognosis in neuroblastoma. Review of 112 patients younger than 2 years. Am J Pediatr Hematol Oncol 6: 233–243

23. Kaneko M, Iwakawa M, Ikebukuro K, Ohkawa H (1998) Complete resection is not required in patients with neuroblastoma under 1 year of age. J Pediatr Surg 33:1690–4

24. Kaplan SJ, Holbrook CT, McDaniel HG, Buntain WL, et al. (1980) Vasoactive intestinal peptide secreting tumors of childhood. Am J Dis Child 134:21–24

25. Katzenstein HM, Bowman LC, Brodeur GM, Thorner PS, et al. (1998) Prognostic significance of age, MYCN oncogene amplification, tumor cell ploidy, and histology in 110 infants with stage D(S) neuroblastoma: the pediatric oncology group experience – a pediatric oncology group study. J Clin Oncol 16:2007–2017

26. Kiely EM (1993) Radical surgery for abdominal neuroblastoma. Semin Surg Oncol 9:489–92

27. Kletzel M, Katzenstein HM, Haut PR, Yu AL, et al. (2002) Treatment of high-risk neuroblastoma with triple-tandem high-dose therapy and stem-cell rescue: results of the Chicago Pilot II Study. J Clin Oncol 20:2284–2292

28. Kushner BH, Gilbert F, Helson L (1986) Familial neuroblastoma. Case reports, literature review, and etiologic considerations. Cancer 57:1887–1893

29. Kushner BH, Cheung NK, LaQuaglia MP, Ambros PF, et al. (1996) Survival from locally invasive or widespread neuroblastoma without cytotoxic therapy. J Clin Oncol 14: 373–381

30. La Quaglia MP, Kushner BH, Heller G, Bonilla MA, et al. (1994) Stage 4 neuroblastoma diagnosed at more than 1 year of age: gross total resection and clinical outcome. J Pediatr Surg 29:1162–6

31. Look AT, Hayes FA, Shuster JJ, Douglass EC, et al. (1991) Clinical relevance of tumor cell ploidy and N-myc gene amplification in childhood neuroblastoma: a Pediatric Oncology Group study. J Clin Oncol 9:581–591

32. Lovat PE, Ranalli M, Annichiarrico-Petruzzelli M, Bernassola F, et al. (2000) Effector mechanisms of fenretinide-induced apoptosis in neuroblastoma. Exp Cell Res 260: 50–60

33. Lutz W, Schurmann J, Wenzel A, et al. (1996) Conditional expression of N-myc in human neuroblastoma cells increases expression of alpha-prothymosin and ornithine decarboxylase and accelerates progression into S-phase early after mitogenic stimulation of quiescent cells. Oncogene 13:803–812

34. Maris JM, Weiss MJ, Guo C, Gerbing RB, et al. (2000) Loss of heterozygosity at 1p36 independently predicts for disease progression but not decreased overall survival probability in neuroblastoma patients: a Children's Cancer Group study. J Clin Oncol 18:1888–1899

35. Maris JM, Weiss MJ, Mosse Y, Hii G, et al. (2002) Evidence for a hereditary neuroblastoma predisposition locus at chromosome 16p12–13. Cancer Res 62:6651–6658

36. Matthay KK, Perez C, Seeger RC, Brodeur GM, et al. (1998) Successful treatment of stage III neuroblastoma based on prospective biologic staging: a Children's Cancer Group study. J Clin Oncol 16:1256–1264

37. Matthay KK, Villablanca JG, Seeger RC, Stram DO, et al. (1999) Treatment of high-risk neuroblastoma with intensive chemotherapy, radiotherapy, autologous bone marrow transplantation, and 13-cis-retinoic acid. Children's Cancer Group. N Engl J Med 341:1165–1173

38. Nitschke R, Smith EI, Shochat S, Altshuler G, et al. (1988) Localized neuroblastoma treated by surgery: a Pediatric Oncology Group Study. J Clin Oncol 6:1271–1279

39. Perel Y, Conway J, Kletzel M, Goldman J, et al. (1999) Clinical impact and prognostic value of metaiodobenzylguanidine imaging in children with metastatic neuroblastoma. J Pediatr Hematol Oncol 21:13–18

40. Pranzatelli MR (1992) The neurobiology of the opsoclonus-myoclonus syndrome. Clin Neuropharmacol 15: 186–228

41. Pranzatelli MR, Tate ED, Wheeler A, Bass N, et al. (2002) Screening for autoantibodies in children with opsoclonus-myoclonus-ataxia. Pediatr Neurol 27:384–387

42. Rees H, Markley MA, Kiely EM, Pierro A, Pritchard J (1998) Diarrhea after resection of advanced abdominal neuroblastoma: a common management problem. Surgery 123:568–72

43. Rousseau RF, Haight AE, Hirschmann-Jax C, Yvon ES, et al. (2003) Local and systemic effects of an allogeneic tumor cell vaccine combining transgenic human lymphotactin with interleukin-2 in patients with advanced or refractory neuroblastoma. Blood 101:1718–1726

44. Rudnick E, Khakoo Y, Antunes NL, Seeger RC, et al. (2001) Opsoclonus-myoclonus-ataxia syndrome in neuroblastoma: clinical outcome and antineuronal antibodies – a report from the Children's Cancer Group Study. Med Pediatr Oncol 36:612–622

45. Schilling FH, Spix C, Berthold F, Erttmann R, et al. (2002) Neuroblastoma screening at one year of age. N Engl J Med 346:1047–1053

46. Schwab M (1999) Oncogene amplification in solid tumors. Semin Cancer Biol 9:319–325

47. Shamberger RC, Allarde-Segundo A, Kozakewich HP, Grier HE (1991) Surgical management of stage III and IV neuroblastoma: resection before or after chemotherapy? J Pediatr Surg 26:1113–8

48. Shimada H (1992) Neuroblastoma. Pathology and biology. Acta Pathol Jpn 42:229–241

49. Shimada H, Chatten J, Newton WA Jr, Sachs N, et al. (1984) Histopathologic prognostic factors in neuroblastic tumors: definition of subtypes of ganglioneuroblastoma and an age-linked classification of neuroblastomas. J Natl Cancer Inst 73:405–416

50. Shimada H, Ambros IM, Dehner LP, Hata J, et al. (1999) The International Neuroblastoma Pathology Classification (the Shimada system). Cancer 86:364–372

51. Shimada H, Umehara S, Monobe Y, Hachitanda Y, et al. (2001) International neuroblastoma pathology classification for prognostic evaluation of patients with peripheral neuroblastic tumors: a report from the Children's Cancer Group. Cancer 92:2451–2461

52. Shulkin BL, Shapiro B (1998) Current concepts on the diagnostic use of MIBG in children. J Nucl Med 39: 679–688

53. Strother D, Shuster JJ, McWilliams N, Nitschke R, et al. (1995) Results of pediatric oncology group protocol 8104 for infants with stages D and DS neuroblastoma. J Pediatr Hematol Oncol 17:254–259

54. Strother D, van Hoff J, Rao PV, Smith EI, et al. (1997) Event-free survival of children with biologically favourable neuroblastoma based on the degree of initial tumour resection: results from the Pediatric Oncology Group. Eur J Cancer 33:2121–2125

55. Tsuchida Y, Yokoyama J, Kaneko M, Uchino J, Iwafuchi M, Makino S, Matsuyama S, Takahashi H, Okabe I, Hashizume K, et al. (1992) Therapeutic significance of surgery in advanced neuroblastoma: a report from the study group of Japan. J Pediatr Surg 27:616–22

56. van Noesel MM, Hahlen K, Hakvoort-Cammel FG, Egeler RM (1997) Neuroblastoma 4S: a heterogeneous disease with variable risk factors and treatment strategies. Cancer 80:834–843

57. van Santen HM, de Kraker J, van Eck BL, de Vijlder JJ, et al. (2002) High incidence of thyroid dysfunction despite prophylaxis with potassium iodide during (131)I-meta-iodobenzylguanidine treatment in children with neuroblastoma. Cancer 94:2081–2089

58. von Schweinitz D, Hero B, Berthold F (2002) The impact of surgical radicality on outcome in childhood neuroblastoma. Eur J Pediatr Surg 12:402–9

59. Westermann F, Schwab M (2002) Genetic parameters of neuroblastomas. Cancer Lett 184:127–47

60. Woods WG, Gao RN, Shuster JJ, Robison LL, et al. (2002) Screening of infants and mortality due to neuroblastoma. N Engl J Med 346:1041–1046

61. Yamamoto K, Ohta S, Ito E, Hayashi Y, et al. (2002) Marginal decrease in mortality and marked increase in incidence as a result of neuroblastoma screening at 6 months of age: cohort study in seven prefectures in Japan. J Clin Oncol 20:1209–1214

22 Miscellaneous Adrenal Neoplasms (Cysts, Myelolipoma, Hemangioma, Lymphangioma)

Melanie L. Richards

Adrenal neoplasms that are non-functional and have benign characteristics on imaging studies may pose a management dilemma. This is particularly true of the uncommon neoplasms that have an uncertain natural history. These tumors usually present as adrenal incidentalomas, with an incidence of 1–4% on imaging studies. With liberal computed tomography (CT) scanning and advanced imaging techniques, they are becoming a more frequent entity. While the majority of adrenal incidentalomas are adenomas or metastases [14], this chapter will focus on the diagnosis and management of the less common adrenal neoplasms.

The best studies to obtain to aid in the diagnosis of these neoplasms are CT scanning and magnetic resonance imaging (MRI). A non-enhanced CT scan is the most common modality used in adrenal imaging. Density criteria are used to assist in characterizing the adrenal pathology. The helical scanning techniques using smaller slices (3 mm) have improved the accuracy in assessing density. MRI with chemical shift imaging has excellent contrast resolution, allowing imaging of tumors as small as 0.5 cm. The T1-weighted images are the best for assessing anatomic detail. Accurate imaging and interpretation of these neoplasms is critical because the majority are clinically benign and do not require an operation.

If an operation is recommended; the patient can usually undergo a laparoscopic adrenalectomy. An open adrenalectomy should be performed if there is any suspicion for a primary malignancy. The role of fine-needle aspiration for cytology is limited secondary to sparse cellularity. Prior to any surgical or other invasive procedure (aspiration), the lesion must be evaluated for function. Functional studies should include a 24-h urine for cortisol, metanephrines, catecholamines and vanillylmandelic acid to assess for either a cortisol-producing neoplasm or a pheochromocytoma. A serum potassium level and possibly an aldosterone level should be obtained to screen for an aldosterone-producing tumor.

22.1 Adrenal Cysts

The first adrenal cyst of record was described in 1670 by Greiselius, a Viennese anatomist [4]. Since that time, adrenal cysts have been rare, with an incidence of less than 0.1% [1]. They account for 4–22% of adrenal incidentalomas [14]. Occurring more commonly in women, they are equally distributed bilaterally. They can occur at any age, but children may actually have a cystic neuroblastoma. Overall, adrenal cysts are most accurately identified and evaluated with CT scanning.

The most common presentation is as an incidentaloma. In a review of 286 cases, they were found incidentally in 34% of patients (Table 1) [16]. Other presentations included: abdominal pain in 19%, abdominal mass in 10%, pain and a mass in 10% and hypertension in 9% [16]. Patients with hypertension may also have a cystic pheochromocytoma, which supports the importance of functional studies.

In 1966, Foster classically divided adrenal cysts into four categories: endothelial cysts, pseudocysts, epithelial cysts and parasitic cysts (Table 2) [3,6]. The largest review was reported in 1999 by Neri and Nance, which included 515 patients with adrenal cysts (Table 3) [16]. They found that most adrenal cysts were pseudocysts (56%), followed by endothelial (24%), unspecified be-

Table 1. Clinical presentation of 286 patients with adrenal cysts [16]

Presentation	Number of patients (%)
Incidental	97 (34%)
Abdominal pain	53 (19%)
Abdominal mass	30 (10%)
Abdominal pain and mass	30 (10%)
Hypertension	26 (9%)
Flank pain	17 (6%)
Hypertension and a symptom or sign	13 (5%)
Back pain	7 (2%)
Trauma	7 (2%)
Loin pain	2 (1%)
Shock (ruptured angiomatous cysts)	2 (1%)
Vague	2 (1%)

Table 2. Foster's 1966 classification of adrenal cysts [6]

Histologic type	Frequency
Parasitic cysts (hydatid cysts)	7%
Epithelial cysts	9%
Embryonal cysts	
Cystic adenomas	
True glandular (mesothelial)	
Endothelial cysts	45%
Lymphangiomatous	42%
Angiomatous	3%
Pseudocysts	39%

of small benign-appearing asymptomatic adrenal cysts [3]. Surgical excision or enucleation of benign cysts can safely be performed laparoscopically.

nign (12%), epithelial (6%) and parasitic (2%). Many simply classify adrenal cysts as either a true cyst or a pseudocyst.

There are varying opinions regarding the management of adrenal cysts. Some authors have recommended aspiration of asymptomatic small non-functioning cysts and surgical excision of cysts greater than 5 cm diameter [13]. Tung recommended attempts at aspiration in all symptomatic benign cysts, reserving surgery for recurrence after aspiration [21]. The current recommendation is for continued observation

22.1.1   True Cyst

A *true cyst* may be a benign or malignant lesion containing *epithelial* or *endothelial* cells. The endothelial cysts include lymphangiomatous (lymphangiectatic or serous) (Fig. 1) and angiomatous (hemangioma) cysts. These cysts are typically small and multiple. The epithelial cysts are also referred to as "glandular" cysts. Since normal adrenal contains no glandular or ductal structures, it has been proposed that these epithelial

Table 3. Classification of adrenal cysts in 515 patients [16]

Classification (%)	Subtype	Case number (%)
Parasitic (2%)	Echinococcus	12 (2%)
Epithelial (6%)	Congenital glandular/retention	6 (1%)
	Cystic adenoma	14 (3%)
	Epithelial unspecified	8 (2%)
Endothelial (24%)	Lymphangiomatous	83 (16%)
	Angiomatous	13 (3%)
	Unspecified or mixed angio and lymph	23 (5%)
Pseudocyst (56%)	Hemorrhagic	188 (37%)
	In adenoma	7 (1%)
	Pheochromocytoma	21 (4%)
	Malignant tumor	
	– Neuroblastoma	11 (2%)
	– Adrenocortical carcinoma	5 (1%)
	– Metastatic	1 (<1%)
	– Unspecified	1 (<1%)
	Pyogenic	3 (<1%)
	Unspecified pseudocyst	55 (11%)
Unspecified benign (12%)		64 (12%)

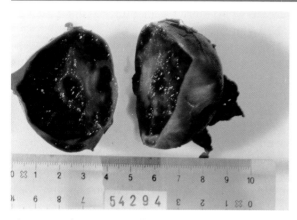

Fig. 1. Lymphangiectatic adrenal cyst 6.5 cm in diameter. (Courtesy of D. Linos, M.D.)

cysts are derived from embryonic rests. This category includes cystic adenomas, glandular retention cysts and embryonal cysts.

22.1.2   Pseudocysts

Pseudocysts are the most common clinically diagnosed adrenal cysts. A pseudocyst lacks an epithelial lining and is often a result of hemorrhage or infarction. Calcification within the wall of a cyst is suspicious for either a pseudocyst or a parasitic cyst. Rarely, a benign or malignant adrenal tumor may undergo cystic degeneration and result in a pseudocyst. Recently, it has been shown that hemorrhagic adrenal pseudocysts often contain thin-walled vascular channels [20]. Immunohistochemical studies of these channels are consistent with a vascular origin, suggesting that many of these hemorrhagic cysts are endothelial cysts. A 47-year literature review by Torres identified 107 patients with 111 vascular adrenal cysts; 79% were hemorrhagic pseudocysts and 21% were endothelial cysts [20]. The differentiation may be difficult because organizing thrombus may form endothelial cells. Histologically, hemorrhagic pseudocysts may also display papillary endothelial hyperplasia [10]. Papillary endothelial hyperplasia may be confused with an angiosarcoma. It is differentiated from an angiosarcoma by the lack of endothelial cell atypia, the presence of a hyaline core and the absence of gross invasion of adjacent tissues.

Most patients may complain of a vague discomfort; others may have severe pain that results from an intracystic hemorrhage or rupture. Adrenal cysts may also become infected. Infected cysts may also present with pain and these patients will often have a leukocytosis. Surgical resection is recommended for symptoms or a suspicion of malignancy.

22.1.3   Parasitic

Parasitic infections, most commonly a hydatid cyst, can also present as adrenal cysts. These cysts are the result of an *Echinococcus* tapeworm infestation. *Echinococcus granulosus* is the most common parasite causing cystic echinococcosis. Echinococcosis is uncommon in northern Europe and North America. It is endemic to areas of South America, the Mediterranean, the Middle East, Africa, Australia and New Zealand. Of all patients with echinococcus, less than 0.5% will have adrenal involvement [6]. These patients may have an eosinophilia or a hypogammaglobinemia. Serology for echinococcus can be obtained to aid in the diagnosis of a hydatid cyst. The enzyme-linked immunosorbent assay (ELISA) and the indirect hemagglutination test are the most sensitive screening tests. Testing for antibodies to echinococcus will confirm the diagnosis. A CT scan is also a highly sensitive and accurate method to aid in the diagnosis because it can identify daughter cysts.

Patients will often remain asymptomatic until the cyst has increased in size to over 5 cm. Aspiration is generally not recommended because there is a risk of cyst disruption and subsequent dissemination of a parasitic infection. There is no adequate medical treatment for cystic echinococcal infections. These patients should be surgically treated with an adrenalectomy. It is critical to avoid spillage of cyst contents, not only to prevent spread of the disease, but to avoid an allergic anaphylaxis.

22.2   Myelolipoma

Adrenal myelolipomas were first described in 1905 by Gierke [7]. These rare tumors are reported in 0.08–2% of the population [5]. They are benign, non-functional and usually asymptomatic (Fig. 2). They are most often found incidentally as solitary lesions on imaging studies or at autopsy. Rarely, they may present with symptoms secondary to hemorrhage, infarction or from compression of adjacent structures. There are a few reports of associated endocrine function, most often a 21-hydroxylase deficiency or Cushing's syndrome [22]. Adrenal insufficiency, primary hyperaldosteronism and pheochro-

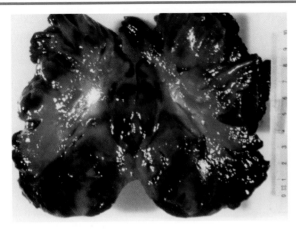

Fig. 2. Gross specimen of a 13-cm right adrenal myelolipoma. (Courtesy of D. Linos, M.D.)

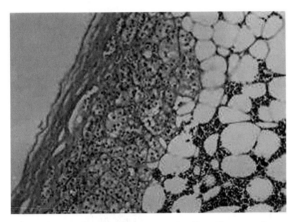

Fig. 3. A thin rim of adrenocortical cells adjacent to bone marrow tissue and mature adipose tissue in a myelolipoma [25]. H&E stain, ×200

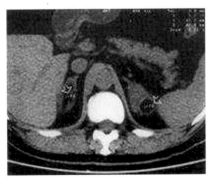

Fig. 4. Non-contrast CT scan showing bilateral adrenal masses with fat densities similar to retroperitoneal or subcutaneous fat consistent with myelolipomas [22]

mocytoma have also been found in association with adrenal myelolipomas.

Histopathology studies show these tumors to consist of both fat and hematopoietic or myeloid tissue (Fig. 3). It is this finding that suggests that these tumors originate from reticuloendothelial cells of the blood capillaries. These cells may undergo adrenocortical cell metaplasia in response to stimuli such as necrosis, hemorrhage, infection or stress [19]. It has also been postulated that these tumors originate from the embolization of hemopoietic stem cells and ectopic myeloid hyperplasia [23]. The association with other functional tumors has led other authors to suggest that adrenal myelolipomas are within the spectrum of a multiple endocrine neoplasia [2].

These benign tumors are easily identified by their well-encapsulated fatty appearance on CT scanning (Fig. 4). They have a low density, typically with negative Hounsfield units (–100 to –200) and may have areas of calcification. The presence of gross fat, with a density below –30 HU confirms the diagnosis [12]. The fatty-appearing adrenal myelolipomas should be differentiated from teratomas, liposarcomas, adenomas, metastatic lesions and primary adrenal malignancy. Retroperitoneal lipomas and renal angiomyolipomas are also in the radiologic differential. If the diagnosis is uncertain, an MRI may be useful to assess tissue planes for invasion or to identify the origin of extra-adrenal tumors.

These tumors are rare and the largest series of adrenal myelolipomas consisted of 21 tumors in 20 patients [8]. Four patients underwent an adrenalectomy; two for abdominal pain, one for Cushing's syndrome and one for a large tumor (10.5 cm). The patient with Cushing's syndrome did have both an adrenal myelolipoma and an adrenal adenoma. Fifteen non-operative patients were evaluated over a mean follow-up period of 3.2 years. Thirteen of these patients remained asymptomatic and two patients had vague abdominal complaints. Serial CT scans were obtained in 12 patients. The mean tumor size increased from 5.1 cm (range 2.2–12 cm) to 5.6 cm (range 2.5–17 cm). Fifty percent of patients had tumors that had increased in size. Tumor size did not appear to correlate with symptoms and no adverse outcomes occurred with non-operative management. These authors felt that routine imaging was unnecessary, but that patients should be followed clinically in order to monitor for clinically significant growth.

Depending on the level of suspicion for malignancy; the patient may be explored or a fine-needle aspiration may be performed in a patient with normal adrenal function. Otherwise, these tumors are benign and do not require surgical intervention unless they are symptomatic.

22.3   Hemangioma

Adrenal hemangiomas are rare and benign. There have been approximately 50 cases reported in the world literature since the first adrenalectomy for a hemangioma by Johnson and Jeppesen in 1955 [11, 15]. They are usually small, non-functional and asymptomatic. Large tumors (25 cm) have been reported and these are at risk for bleeding. Histologically, most have a cavernous appearance with the presence of hypervascularization (Figs. 5, 6). The patients are often in the 5th through 7th decade of life. They are twice as likely to occur in women [18].

The diagnosis can be made on both CT and MRI studies. A CT scan with contrast will show peripheral enhancement and a central area of low attenuation. (Fig. 7). This central area may fill with contrast with delayed imaging. These lesions typically contain calcifications, which may be speckled in appearance. These calcifications may have the appearance similar to a phlebolith. MRI imaging will show a low T1 signal and a moderate to high T2 signal. If there are areas of hemorrhage or necrosis, these will enhance on T1-weighted images [9].

Adrenalectomy has been recommended by some authors [17]. However, most reserve adrenalectomy for symptomatic tumors, tumors that are suspicious for a malignancy such as a hemangiosarcoma and for larger tumors at risk for bleeding. Patients with a symptomatic or large tumor with benign characteristics are candidates for laparoscopic adrenalectomy.

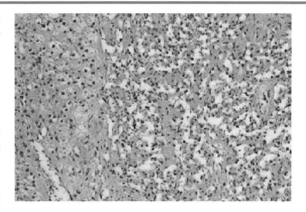

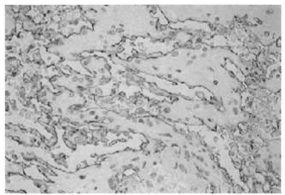

Fig. 6. Hypervascularization and normal adjacent adrenal tissue in an adrenal hemangioma [24]. H&E stain, ×100

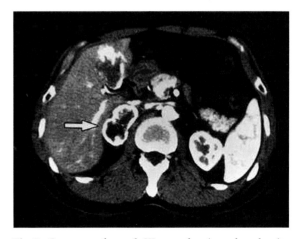

Fig. 7. Contrast-enhanced CT scan showing a low-density mass with peripheral enhancement in the right adrenal gland consistent with a hemangioma [24]

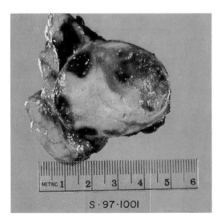

Fig. 5. Gross specimen of a 9.5-cm left adrenal gland containing a cavernous hemangioma. (Thiele 2001 [19a])

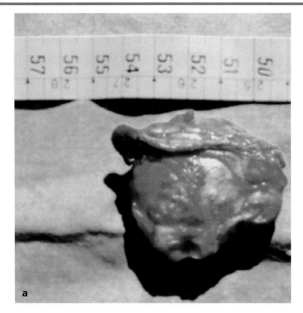

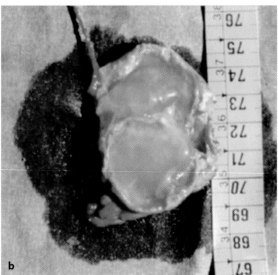

Fig. 8a, b. A 5-cm right adrenal lymphangioma. **a** Outer appearance and **b** clear inner lymphatic content. (Courtesy of D. Linos, M.D.)

22.4   Lymphangioma

The lymphangioma is one of the most common cystic adrenal neoplasms (Fig. 8). Classified as endothelial cysts, they account for 16% of all adrenal cysts (Table 3). Only the hemorrhagic pseudocyst is more prevalent. Lymphangiomas are typically small and most are reported as incidental findings at autopsy. These lesions are multiloculated and many have calcifications present on imaging studies. The cyst contents may range from clear to milky to hemorrhagic. They are difficult to differentiate from organizing hemorrhagic pseudocysts because both lesions may contain endothelial cells. Surgery is rarely indicated in these lesions because they are usually small and asymptomatic.

References

1. Abeshouse GA, Goldstein RB, Abeshouse BS (1959) Adrenal cysts. Review of the literature and report of three cases. J Urol 81:711–719
2. Banik S, Hasleton PS, Lyon RL (1984) An unusual variant of MEN syndrome: A case report. Histopathology 8:134–144
3. de Bree E, Schoretsanitis G, Melissas J, Christodoulakis M, Tsiftsis D (1998) Cysts of the adrenal gland: diagnosis and management. Int Urol Nephrol 30:369–76
4. Doran AHG (1903) Cystic tumor of the suprarenal body successfully removed by operation. BMJ 1:1558–62
5. Enzinger FM, Sharen WW (1995) Benign lipomatous tumors. In: Enzinger FM, Sharen WW (eds) Sort tissue tumors, 3rd edn. Mosby, St. Louis, pp 409–410
6. Foster DG (1966) Adrenal cysts. Review of literature and report of case. Arch Surg 92:131–43
7. Gierke E (1995) Uber Knochenmarksgewebe in der Nebenniere. Bietr Z Pathol Anat Suppl 7, 37:311
8. Han M, Burnett AL, Fishman EK, Marshall FF (1997) The natural history and treatment of adrenal myelolipoma. J Urol 157:1213–1216
9. Honig SC, Klavans MS, Hyde C, Siroky MB (1991) Adrenal hemangioma: an unusual adrenal mass delineated with magnetic resonance imaging. J Urol 146:400–402
10. Jennings TA, Ng B, Boguniewicz A (1998) Adrenal pseudocysts: Evidence of their posthemorrhagic nature. Endocr Pathol 9:353–361
11. Johnson CC, Jeppesen FB (1955) Hemangioma of the adrenal. J Urol 74:573–7
12. Kenney PJ, Wagner BJ, Rao P, Heffess CS (1998) Myelolioma: CT and pathologic features. Radiology 208:87–95
13. Klimopoulos S, Perdikides T, Fratzidou E, Pissiotis CA (1995) Laparoscopic resection of a large right adrenal gland cyst. Surg Endosc 9:1295–7
14. Kloos RT, Gross MD, Francis IR, Korobkin M, Shapiro B (1995) Incidentally discovered adrenal masses. Endocr Rev 16:460–484
15. Llado CC, Arango TO, Vesa LJ, Bielsa GO, Gelabert MA (1996) Adrenal hemangioma: Review of the literature. Prog Urol 6:292–6
16. Neri LM, Nance FC (1999) Management of adrenal cysts. Am Surg 2:151–163
17. Otal P, Escourrou G, Mazerolles C, Janne d'Othee B, Mezghani S, Musso S, Colombier D, Rousseau H, Joffre F (1999) Imaging features of uncommon adrenal masses with histologic correlation. Radiographics 19:569–581
18. Salup R, Finegold R, Borochovitz D, Boehnke M, Posner M (1992) Hemangioma of the adrenal gland. J Urol 147:110–112

19. Sanders R, Bissada N, Curry N, Gordon B (1995) Clinical spectrum of adrenal myelolipoma: analysis of tumors in 7 patients. J Urol 153:1791

20. Torres C, Ro JY, Batt MA, Park YW, Ordonez NG, Ayala AG (1997) Vascular adrenal cysts: a clinicopathologic and immunohistochemical study of six cases and a review of the literature. Mod Pathol 10:530–6

21. Tung GA, Pfister RC, Papanicolaou N, Yoder IC (1989) Adrenal cysts: imaging and percutaneous aspiration. Radiology 173:107–110

22. Umpierrez MB, Fackler S, Umpierrez GE, Rubin J (1997) Adrenal myelolipoma associated with endocrine dysfunction: review of the literature. Am J Med Sci 314: 338–341

23. Vierna J, Laforga JB (1994) Giant adrenal myelolipoma. Scand J Urol Nephrol 28:301–304

24. Yagisawa T, Amano H, Ito F, Horita S, Yamaguchi Y, Toma H (2001) Adrenal hemangioma removed by a retroperitoneoscopic procedure. Int J Urol 8:457–458

25. Yildiz L, Akpolat I, Erzurumlu K, Aydin O, Kandemir B (2001) Giant adrenal myelolipoma: Case report and review of the literature. Pathol Int 50:502–504

23 Adrenal Incidentalomas

Miguel F. Herrera, Juan Pablo Pantoja, Nayví España

CONTENTS

ically unapparent adrenal masses". Since image studies are increasingly available worldwide and they are used more frequently, this finding may become a real public health challenge.

Diagnostic and therapeutic implications of incidentalomas are different in several populations. Such is the case of patients with arterial hypertension, in whom the likelihood of an adrenal tumor to be functioning is higher than in the population with normal blood pressure. Patients with history or concurrent lung, breast, colon and other extra-adrenal malignancies have high potential for developing adrenal metastases. The frequency of adrenal metastases from lung cancer at autopsy ranges from 17% to 38% and patients with adrenal masses in the setting of extra-adrenal malignancy have a frequency of adrenal metastases between 32% and 73% [32]. Based on these facts, to consider an adrenal tumor as truly incidental, patients should not have any clinical condition that may imply a higher risk for an adrenal tumor.

23.1 Definition

Adrenal incidentaloma is a tumor discovered serendipitously in the course of diagnostic evaluation or follow-up of unrelated disorders. Adrenal incidentalomas may represent a variety of entities or diseases. Based on their silent nature, they have also been called "clin-

23.2 Prevalence

The prevalence of adrenal incidentalomas ranges from 1.1% to 32% in autopsy series (Table 1) and from 0.3% to 1.9% in series based on computed tomography (CT) (Table 2). The frequency of adrenal tumors increases with age, being 0.2% in young people and 7% in sub-

Table 1. Prevalence of adrenal incidentalomas in autopsy series

Year of the study	First author	No. of patients	Prevalence (%)
1967	Devenyi [11]	5,120	3.5
1967	Kokko [24]	2,000	1.0
1970	Gragner [17]	2,425	2.5
1972	Russell [46]	35,000	1.9
1985	Abecassis [1]	988	1.9
1996	Reinhard [45]	498	5.0

Table 2. Prevalence of adrenal incidentalomas in CT scan series

Year of the study	First author	No. of patients	Prevalence (%)
1982	Glazer [16]	2,200	0.7
1982	Printz [42]	1,423	0.3
1985	Abecassis [1]	1,459	1.3
1986	Balldegrun [5]	12,000	0.7
1991	Herrera [20]	61,054	0.4
1994	Caplan [8]	1,779	1.9

jects older than 70 years. No sex differences have been reported in autopsy series and no significant geographic or ethnic variability has been reported [4]. Considering the continuous technological improvements, the number of incidental small tumors that can be found in imaging studies may be higher than published figures using old generation CTs. However, tumors smaller than 1 cm rarely represent a clinical problem.

23.3   Clinical Importance

Adrenal incidentalomas are clinically important, with the main concerns relating to hormonal overproduction and the risk of malignancy. In terms of function, clinically silent adrenal masses may subsequently be proven to be pheochromocytomas, aldosteronomas, or cortisol-producing adenomas, which may lead to complications if they remain untreated. In terms of malignancy, since adrenal cortical carcinoma has a dismal prognosis and metastatic tumors cannot be cured, it is particularly important to make the diagnosis at an early stage. In the evaluation of adrenal incidentalomas, diagnostic efforts are therefore directed to investigate hormonal hyperfunction initially and in the presence of a nonfunctioning tumor, to differentiate benign from malignant lesions. The majority of surgically resected adrenal incidentalomas are nonfunctioning cortical adenomas [59]. Among the functioning tumors, pheochromocytoma is the most frequently found [20, 35]. The frequency of pheochromocytoma is particularly higher in the older population. Cortisol secreting adenomas are the second in frequency, followed by aldosteronomas [44,59]. Diagnoses found in 380 surgically treated patients reported in a large multicentric Italian study are shown in Table 3 [35].

23.4   Natural History

The natural course of adrenal incidentalomas is still unknown. In the few follow-up studies published in the literature, it seems that most adrenal incidentalomas diagnosed as benign and non-functioning in the initial evaluation remain unchanged. Up to 20% of non-functioning tumors develop hyperfunction. Tumors 3 cm or larger are more likely to develop hyperfunction than smaller lesions. Tumor enlargement by at least 1 cm has been identified with a frequency between 5% and 25% and reduction in mass size has been documented in few cases [4, 19].

23.5   Biochemical Evaluation

23.5.1   Pheochromocytoma

Many laboratory tests have been used to screen for pheochromocytoma. Considering that tests are laboratory dependent, the optimal screening test is still debatable. Traditionally, the 24-h urinary measurement of total metanephrines has been the suggested method [20]. However, considering the sensitivity and specificity of different tests in certain situations, for patients with vascular or inhomogeneous adrenal masses, in whom the pretest probability of having a

Table 3. Histology of 380 surgically resected adrenal incidentalomas [35]

Diagnosis	No. of patients	%
Cortical adenoma	198	52
Cortical carcinoma	47	12
Pheochromocytoma	42	11
Cyst	20	5.2
Myelolipoma	30	7.8
Metastasis	7	1.8
Ganglioneuroma	15	3.9
Other	21	5.5

pheochromocytoma is high, it has been suggested to screen the patient with both fractionated plasma free metanephrines (normetanephrine and metanephrine) and 24-h urinary measurements of total metanephrines and catecholamines. On the other hand, when the clinical and imaging suspicion is low, 24-h measurement of total metanephrines and catecholamines is sufficient. The reason for not advising the measurement of plasma metanephrines in this group is because their specificity is approximately 89% and false positive elevation of plasma metanephrines may result in needless further laboratory testing, imaging or even surgery [41, 59].

23.5.2   Cortisol-Producing Adenoma

Patients with cortisol-producing adenomas have so-called subclinical Cushing's syndrome, which is characterized by the lack of the usual obvious stigmata of Cushing's syndrome but with the side effects of continuous endogenous cortisol secretion. Cortisol-producing adenomas account for 5–10% of all adrenal incidentalomas [44, 59]. Therefore, evaluation of cortisol overproduction is essential in these patients. The 1 mg dexamethasone suppression test has been the preferred method. After dexamethasone administration, most normal individuals have serum cortisol concentrations suppressed to less than 139.75 nmol/l. There is a consensus that patients with levels above this value need further testing. Some authors have proposed testing of patients with cortisol values ≥149.7 nmol/l in order to increase the detection [44]. Some centers have used a higher dose of dexamethasone (3 mg) to reduce false positive results [3, 4].

23.5.3   Aldosterone-Producing Adenoma

In approximately 1% of patients with adrenal incidentalomas, an aldosterone-producing adenoma (APA) is diagnosed. Initial recommendation was to screen these patients with serum electrolytes [20]. However, many authors have described primary hyperaldosteronism in the absence of hypokalemia. The ratio of plasma aldosterone concentration to plasma renin activity (PAC/PRA) has proven to be the most useful tool for screening [21]. The mean value for the ratio in normal patients and in patients with essential hypertension rages from 4 to 10, whereas most patients with APA have a ratio between 30 and 50 [58, 59]. The combination of a PAC above 20 ng/dl and a PAC/PRA ratio above 30 has a sensitivity of 90% for the diagnosis of an APA [57].

23.5.4   Other Hormonally Producing Adenomas

Sex-hormone secreting adenomas are rare and patients usually present with symptoms; thus routine screening for sex hormone excess in patients with adrenal incidentalomas is not warranted. Nonclassic congenital adrenal hyperplasia can present with adrenal masses. Due to its infrequency and the fact that cosynotropin may give misleading results in some patients with adenomas, cosynotropin stimulation testing is only suggested on the basis of clinical suspicion of the disease [59].

23.6   Radiologic Evaluation

The imaging phenotype characteristic of a pheochromocytoma includes enhancement of the lesion on an intravenous contrasted CT scan and high signal intensity on T2-weighted MR imaging (Fig. 1).

Adrenal cysts appear as homogeneous spherical masses with a density near that of water. The cyst wall is usually thin and does not enhance with intravenous contrast (Fig. 2). A complicated cyst cannot be reliably distinguished from an abscess or a metastatic tumor. A pseudocyst can arise in patients with previous adrenal hemorrhage. These lesions usually have thick walls, calcification, nodularity, septation, and soft-tissue components [54].

Adrenal myelolipomas are benign tumors, composed of mature fat cells and hematopoietic tissue [12]. These tumors have classic fat attenuation values, occasionally with areas of focal calcification. They can be correctly diagnosed by CT scans in most patients. It is highly important to identify these lesions, since they are usually asymptomatic and no further treatment is required [54].

Several radiologic characteristics of adrenal tumors on CT scan may help to differentiate benign from malignant cortical tumors. First of all, tumor size has proven to be an important predictor of malignancy. Adrenal cortical carcinoma accounts for 2% of tumors that are ≤4 cm, 6% of tumors that are 4.1–6 cm and 25% of tumors that are greater than 6 cm [27]. Linos et al. compared CT and histology reports and found that CT scan underestimated true dimensions. Based on this evidence, his group proposed a mathematical calculation to "correct" the tumor size determined by radiology [29].

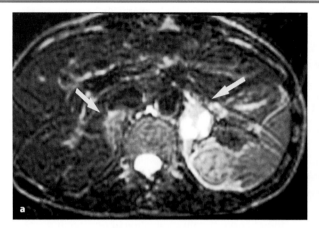
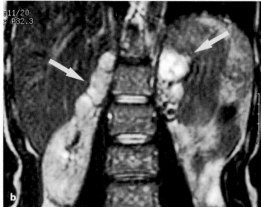

Fig. 1a, b. MRI T2 (2,400/120). **a** Axial image. **b** Coronal image. The *arrows* highlight a bilateral multinodular pheochromocytoma. Note the characteristic hyperintensity of the lesions

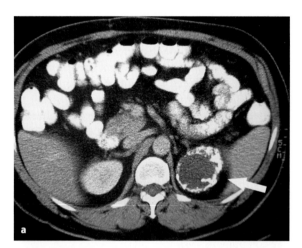

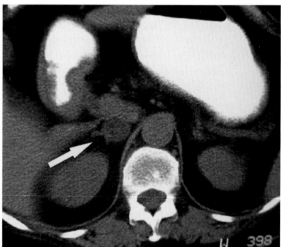

Fig. 3. CT scan shows a small homogeneous round mass with smooth borders in the center of the right adrenal gland (*arrow*). This image is characteristic of a cortical adenoma

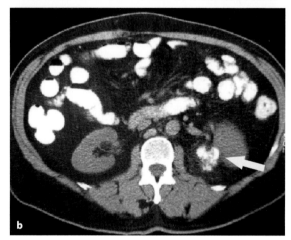

Fig. 2a, b. CT scan showing a left adrenal cyst (*arrows*). **a** The tumor has an evident peripheral calcification and a very low central absorption coefficient (8 UH). **b** A more caudal image showing that the lesion is separate from the left kidney

CT densitometry may help in delineation of the differential diagnosis. An attenuation value expressed in Hounsfield units (HU) of 10 HU has a sensitivity of 71% and a specificity of 98% for the diagnosis of an adrenal adenoma. Intravenous contrast-enhanced CT values on the other hand show too much overlap between benign and malignant tumors. Heterogeneity and border shape are also of importance. A <4 cm homogeneous mass with a smooth border and an attenuation value of less than 10 HU on non-contrasted CT strongly suggests a benign adrenal adenoma [26] (Fig. 3). A big non-homogeneous invasive mass, on the other hand, most frequently represents a carcinoma (Fig. 4).

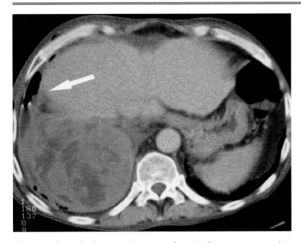

Fig. 4. Adrenal adenocarcinoma. The CT shows an extensive neoplastic solid mass of the right adrenal. The low density in the center represents necrosis. An area of gross invasion to the liver is shown by the *arrow*

Magnetic resonance imaging has similar effectiveness to the CT scan in the differential diagnosis between benign and malignant adrenal tumors. There is evidence suggesting that chemical shift MR could be used to characterize adrenal masses. Characteristics associated with benignity are a signal drop on chemical-shift imaging and a similar intensity to that of the liver on a T2-weighted image [39].

Other studies that have been used to characterize adrenal masses are radioiodocholesterol scanning using NP-59 and positron emission tomography. Unfortunately, both techniques have limited use and there is little published data on their accuracy [18].

23.7 Adrenal Biopsy

Both fine-needle aspiration biopsy (FNAB) and Tru-cut biopsy have a limited role in the evaluation of adrenal incidentalomas. They are useful in the diagnosis of adrenal metastases. In patients with a known extra-adrenal malignancy and a suspicious lesion, they have a sensitivity and specificity of approximately 90% [51]. It is important to rule out the presence of a pheochromocytoma prior to the adrenal biopsy, as biopsy may cause hypertensive crisis that may even lead to death [9]. In patients with adrenal incidentalomas and no history of malignancy, it is generally accepted that adrenal biopsy has no proven efficacy.

The differential diagnosis between an adrenal adenoma and carcinoma is based on the presence of vascular or capsular invasion, which cannot be evaluated by cytology. In a prospective German study, the diagnostic accuracy of adrenal biopsy was evaluated in 231 tumor samples by an ex vivo puncture. Conventional histology and immunohistochemistry (keratin KL1, vimentin, S100 protein, chromogranin A, synaptophysin, neuron-specific enolases, D11, Ki-67, and p53) were used. The overall sensitivity of the core biopsy for malignancy was 99% and the specificity was 96% [47, 48]. From this data, it appears that under optimal conditions, adrenal biopsy may be a valuable method.

23.8 Novel Tumor Markers

It has been demonstrated that major histocompatibility complex class II antigens are absent in adrenal carcinomas whereas normal adrenal glands and most adrenal adenomas express these proteins [37]. There is evidence that cancer cells exhibit uncontrolled growth as a result of a diminished ability to communicate with the surrounding cells. A major route for the cell-cell communication is through gap junction pores composed of connexin [10]. Using immunocytochemical techniques, Murray and colleagues compared α1-connexin 43-gap junction protein levels in normal adrenal tissue, in adrenal adenomas and in a human adrenal cancer cell line (H295). In the normal cell gland, the zona fasciculata showed to have the highest incidence of gap junctions per cell. The number of gap junctions per cell was significantly reduced in benign adrenocortical adenomas when compared to normal tissue and there were few or no α1-connexin 43-gap junctions in the H295 cell line [40].

23.9 Management

If hormonal hyper secretion is identified, surgery is indicated. There is no question that the risk involved with a hypertensive crisis in patients with pheochromocytoma supports early surgical intervention. These patients should receive α and β blockade before surgery to avoid or reduce intraoperative hemodynamic instability. Aldosterone-producing cortical adenomas that present as adrenal incidentalomas should also be removed. Primary aldosteronism is a known cause of curable arterial hypertension and patients are benefited by early adrenalectomy since it has been demonstrated that long lasting arterial hypertension may not resolve after adrenalectomy. Subclinical Cushing's syndrome, on the other hand, is a more controversial indication for surgical treatment. The long-term outcome of the disease is still under evaluation. However, in the absence of non-surgical curative treatment and considering that adrenalectomy has a very low morbidity and almost no mortality, it seems reasonable to treat these patients with surgery.

In terms of the risk of malignancy, all suspicious masses on imaging studies should be removed. For non-suspicious lesions, surgical indications have been based on the likelihood of a tumor being malignant according to tumor size and age of patient. Schteingart, for example, has recommended surgery for masses >6 cm. Considering the low frequency of malignancy in tumors <3 cm, he recommends observation with further imaging for these lesions, and for masses between 3 and 6 cm he suggests surgical intervention if the patient is younger than 50 years [49].

Based on the analysis of a large cohort of patients, we and others have suggested surgical treatment for masses larger than 4 cm and clinical observation for nonsecretory adrenal incidentalomas smaller than 4 cm. Serial radiologic scanning at 3–6 month intervals during the first year after detection and every 1–2 years thereafter seems to be appropriate for these patients, and surgery is indicated for lesions that grow or become functional during follow-up [20, 31, 34].

23.10   Surgical Approaches

Surgical approaches to the adrenal gland include open anterior transabdominal, flank, thoracoabdominal, posterior and, most recently, laparoscopic adrenalectomy that can be performed using a transperitoneal or retroperitoneal approach. Since Gagner and colleagues described laparoscopic adrenalectomy in 1992 [14], laparoscopic adrenalectomy has become the standard technique in most institutions.

Several retrospective case-controlled studies have demonstrated that laparoscopic adrenalectomy is associated with marked decrease in the postoperative length of stay, the amount of pain medication and the total recovery time until resumption of normal activity (Table 4). The indications for laparoscopic adrenalectomy have been extended for virtually all non-malignant adrenal tumors. Most endocrine surgeons agree that large tumors and clearly malignant tumors should be excised using an open technique. Patients with invasive adrenal carcinomas should undergo en bloc excision of the adrenal cancer with Gerota's fascia and surrounding involved organs [7, 15, 50].

Between the two most common laparoscopic approaches, most surgeons have adopted the transperitoneal flank approach. Advantages of this approach are

Table 4. Laparoscopic versus open adrenalectomy

Study		Laparo-scopic	Open anterior
Prinz [43]	n	10	11
	OR time (min)	212	174
	PO Stay (days)	2.1	6.4
Brunt [7]	n	24	25
	OR time	183	142
	PO stay	3.2	8.7
MacGillivray [33]	n	14	9
	OR time	289	201
	PO stay	3	7.9
	Return to activity	8.9	14.6
Vargas [55]	n	20	20
	OR time	193	178
	PO Stay	3.1	7.2
Korman [25]	n	10	10
	OR time	164	124
	PO stay	4.1	5.9
Linos [30]	n	18	86
	OR time	116	155
	PO stay	2.2	8
Shell [50]	n	22	17
	OR time	267	257
	PO stay	1.7	7.8
	Return to activity	1.6	7.9
Acosta [2]	n	17	12
	OR time	180	120
	PO stay	6	6

n, number of patients; *OR*, operative room time; *PO*, postoperative stay.

good anatomic landmarks, the possibility of removing larger adrenal masses and the benefit of gravity to ensure good view of the field in the case of hemorrhage [28]. The posterior retroperitoneal approach although is the preferred technique for some surgeons, having selected advantages in patients with previous intra-abdominal surgery [56].

23.10.1   Surgical Complications

In general, pheochromocytomas involve higher intra-operative risk due to extreme fluctuations in blood pressure and the risk of bleeding. Surgical complications correlate with tumor size. For this reason, some authors choose laparoscopy for pheochromocytomas <6 cm and favor an open approach for larger or extra-adrenal pheochromocytomas [6].

Table 5. Outcomes in laparoscopic adrenalectomy

Study	No. of patients	Converted	Complica tions (%)
Vargas [55]	20	2	10
Duh [13]	23	0	4
Gagner [15]	85	2	15
Marescaux [36]	26	5	12
Miccoli [38]	25	0	0
Smith [52]	28	1	1
Acosta [2]	17	1	11

The most common complications of the open abdominal approach are incidental splenectomy, wound infection, hemorrhage and lung problems. Complications of the open retroperitoneal approach include pleural injury, wound infection, and bleeding [22,53]. Complications of laparoscopic surgery are bleeding, wound infection, subcutaneous emphysema, and pancreatic or splenic injury. However, complications of laparoscopic adrenalectomy are usually mild and unfrequent (Table 5).

23.11 Cost Effectiveness Analysis for the Diagnosis and Treatment

Most adrenal incidentalomas should be left untreated because the majority are either benign adenomas or other disorders that neither affect the patient's health nor warrant the cost and risks of diagnostic or therapeutic interventions. However, some disorders such as cancer or pheochromocytoma may cause serious health risk and deserve treatment. Therefore identifying and curing primary adrenocortical cancer, pheochromocytoma and Conn's syndrome achieve the most cost-effective results. This is guided by the aim of improving life expectancy at acceptable cost. If a 3 cm adrenal incidentaloma is left untreated, quality-adjusted life expectancy is decreased by a mean of one quality-adjusted life year (QALY). By contrast, a pheochromocytoma decreases life expectancy in 4 QALY and the presence of cancer in 15 QALY [23].

Pheochromocytoma screening by urinary metanephrines is warranted in all patients except the most elderly or unfit. Full hormonal analysis is likewise warranted when Conn's syndrome is suspected. In patients with large incidentalomas, screening for adrenocortical cancer is cost-effective. Small non-suspect lesions (<4 cm) may be ignored in elderly and/or unfit patients [23].

23.12 Conclusions

Adrenal incidentalomas require the exclusion of hyperfunction and malignancy. Surgical excision is recommended for patients with hormonally functioning tumors, for masses suspicious of malignancy and for non-suspicious non-functioning tumors equal to or greater than 4 cm. For non-resected tumors, further laboratory and image evaluation for a minimum of 1 year is highly recommended.

References

1. Abecassis M, McLoughlin MJ, Langer B, Kudlow JE (1985) Serendipitous adrenal masses: prevalence, significance, and management. Am J Surg 149:783–8
2. Acosta E, Pantoja JP, Gamino R, Rull JA, Herrera MF (1999) Laparoscopic versus open adrenalectomy in Cushing's syndrome and disease. Surgery 126:1111–6
3. Angeli A, Terzolo M (2002) Adrenal incidentaloma: a modern disease with old complications. J Clin Endocrinol Metab 87:4869–71
4. Barzon L, Scaroni C, Sonino N, Fallo F, Paoletta A, Boscaro M (1999) Risk factors and long-term follow-up of adrenal incidentalomas. J Clin Endocrinol Metab 84:520–6
5. Belldegrun A, Hussain S, Seltzer S (1986) Incidentally discovered mass of the adrenal gland. Surg Gynecol Obstet 163:203–8
6. Bentrem DJ, Pappas SG, Ahuja Y, Murayama KM, Angelos P (2002) Contemporary surgical management of pheochromocytoma. Am J Surg 184:621–5
7. Brunt LM, Doherty GM, Norton JA (1996) Laparoscopic adrenalectomy compared to open adrenalectomy for benign adrenal neoplasms. J Am Coll Surg 183:1–10
8. Caplan RH, Strutt PJ, Wickus GG (1994) Subclinical hormone secretion by incidentally discovered adrenal masses. Arch Surg 129:291–6
9. Casola G, Nicolet V, vanSonnenberg E, Withers C, Bretagnolle M, Saba RM, Bret PM (1986) Unsuspected pheochromocytoma: risk of blood pressure alterations during percutaneous adrenal biopsy. Radiology 159:733–5
10. Cesen-Cummings K, Fernstrom MJ, Malkinson AM, Fuch RJ (1998) Frequent reduction of gap junctional intercellular communication and connexin 43 expression in human and mouse lung carcinoma cells. Carcinogenesis 19:219–31
11. Devenyi I (1967) Possibility of normokalaemic primary aldosteronism as reflected in the frequency of adrenal cortical adenomas. J Clin Pathol 20:49–51
12. Dieckmann KP, Hamm B, Pickartz H (1987) Adrenal myelolipoma: Clinical, radiologic and histologic features. Urology 29:1–8
13. Duh QY, Siperstein AE, Clark OH, Schecter WF, Horn JK, Harrison MR, Hunt TK, Way LW (1996) Laparoscopic adrenalectomy: comparison of the lateral and posterior approaches. Arch Surg 131:870–5

14. Gagner M, Lacroix A, Bolte E (1992) Laparoscopic adrenalectomy in Cushing's syndrome and pheochromocytoma. N Engl J Med 327:1033

15. Gagner M (1996) Laparoscopic adrenalectomy. Surg Clin North Am 76:523–37

16. Glazer HS, Weyman PJ, Sagel SS, Levitt RG, McClennan BL (1982) Nonfunctioning adrenal masses: incidental discovery on computed tomography. Am J Roentgenol 139: 81–5

17. Granger P, Genest J (1970) Autopsy study of adrenals in unselected normotensive and hypertensive patients. Can Med Assoc J 103:34–6

18. Gross MD, Shapiro B, Francis IR (1994) Scintigraphic evaluation of clinically silent adrenal masses. J Nucl Med 35:1145–52

19. Grumbach M, Biller B, Braunstein G, Campbell K, Carney A, Godley P, Harris E, Lee J, Oertel Y, Posner M, Schlechte J, Wieand S (2003) Management of the clinically inapparent adrenal mass ("incidentaloma"). Ann Intern Med 138:424–9

20. Herrera MF, Grant CS, van Heerden JA, Sheedy PF, Ilstrup DM (1991) Incidentally discovered tumors: an institutional perspective. Surgery 110:1014–21

21. Hiramatsu K, Yamada T, Yukimura Y (1981) A screening test to identify aldosterone producing adenoma by measuring plasma renin activity. Arch Intern Med 141: 1589–93

22. Jossart G, Burpee SE, Gagner M (2000) Surgery of the adrenal glands. Endocrinol Metab Clin North Am 29: 57–68

23. Kievit J, Haak HR (2000) Diagnosis and treatment of adrenal incidentaloma. A cost-effectiveness analysis. Endocrinol Metab Clin North Am 29:69–88

24. Kokko JP, Brown TC, Berman MM (1967) Adrenal adenoma and hypertension. Lancet 1:468–70

25. Korman JE, Ho T, Hiatt JR (1997) Comparison of laparoscopic and open adrenalectomy. Am Surg 63:908–12

26. Korobkin M, Brodeur FJ, Francis IR, Quint LE, Dunnick NR, Londy F (1998) CT time-attenuation washout curves of adrenal adenomas and non-adenomas. Am J Roetgenol 170:747–52

27. Korobkin M (2000) CT characterization of adrenal masses: the time has come. Radiology 217:629–32

28. Lezoche E, Guerrieri M, Feliciotti F, Paganini AM, Perretta S, Baldarelli M, Bonjer J, Miccoli P (2002) Anterior, lateral and posterior retroperitoneal approaches in endoscopic adrenalectomy. Surg Endosc 16:96–9

29. Linos DA, Stylopoulos N (1997) How accurate is computed tomography in predicting the real size of adrenal tumors? A retrospective study. Arch Surg 132:740–3

30. Linos DA, Stylopoulos N, Boukis M (1997) Anterior, posterior or laparoscopic approach for the management of adrenal disease? Am J Surg 173:120–5

31. Linos DA (2000) Management approaches to adrenal incidentalomas. A view from Athens, Greece. Endocrinol Metab Clin North Am 29:141–57

32. Linos DA (in press) Management of clinically silent adrenal masses. In: Textbook of endocrine surgery, 2nd edition. WB Saunders, Philadelphia

33. MacGillivray DC, Shichman SJ, Ferrer SJ (1996) A comparison of open vs laparoscopic adrenalectomy. Surg Endosc 10:987–90

34. Mantero F, Arnaldi G (2000) Management approaches to adrenal incidentalomas. A view from Ancona, Italy. Endocrinol Metab Clin North Am 29:107–25

35. Mantero F, Terzolo M, Arnaldi G, Osella G, Masini A, Ali A, Giovagnetti M, Opocher G, Angeli A (2000) A survey on adrenal incidentaloma in Italy. Study Group on Adrenal Tumors of the Italian Society of Endocrinology. J Clin Endocrinol Metab 85:637–44

36. Marescaux J, Mutter D, Wheeler MH (1996) Laparoscopic right and left adrenalectomies: surgical procedures. Surg Endosc 10:912–5

37. Marx C, Wolkersdorfer GW, Brown JW, Scherbaum WA, Bornstein SR (1996) MHC class II expression: a new tool to assess dignity in adrenocortical tumours. J Clin Endocrinol Metab 81:4488–91

38. Miccoli P, Iacconi P, Conte M, Goletti O, Buccianti P (1995) Laparoscopic adrenalectomy. J Laparoendosc Surg 5: 221–6

39. Mitchell DG, Crovello M, Matteucci T, Petersen RO, Miettinen MM (1992) Benign adrenocortical masses: diagnosis with chemical shift MR imaging. Radiology 185:345–51

40. Murray SA, Davis K, Fishman LM, Bornstein SR (2000) Alpha1 connexin 43 gap junctions are decreased in human adrenocortical tumors. J Clin Endocrinol Metab 85:890–5

41. Pacak K, Linehan WM, Eisenhofer G, McClellan MW, Goldstein DS (2001) NIH Conference: Recent advances in genetics, diagnosis, localization and treatment of pheochromocytoma. Ann Intern Med 134:315–29

42. Prinz RA, Brooks MH, Churchill R, Graner JL, Lawrence AM, Paloyan E, Sparagana M (1982) Incidental asymptomatic adrenal masses detected by computed tomographic scanning. Is operation required? JAMA 248:701–4

43. Prinz RA (1995) A comparison of laparoscopic and open adrenalectomies. Arch Surg 130:489–94

44. Reincke M (2000) Subclinical Cushing's syndrome. Endocrinol Metab Clin North Am 29:43–56

45. Reinhard C, Saeger W, Schubert B (1996) Adrenocortical nodules in post-mortem series. Development, functional significance, and differentiation from adenomas. Gen Diagn Pathol 141:203–8

46. Russell RP, Masi AT, Richter ED (1972) Adrenal cortical adenomas and hypertension. A clinical pathologic analysis of 690 cases with matched controls and a review of the literature. Medicine (Baltimore) 51:211–25

47. Saeger W, Beuschlein F, Prager G, Nies C, Lorenz K, Bärlehner E, Simon D, Niederle B, Allolio B, Reincke M (2001) Ex-vivo biopsies of adrenal lesions: Morphology of 231 cases. Exp Clin Endocrinol Diabetes 109 (Suppl 1):S19

48. Saeger W, Fassnacht M, Chita R, Prager G, Nies Clorenz K, Barlehner E, Simon D, Niederle B, Beuschlein F, Allolio B, Reincke M (2003) High diagnostic accuracy of adrenal core biopsy: results of the German and Austrian Adrenal Network Multicenter Trial in 220 Consecutive Patients. Hum Pathol 34:180–6

49. Schteingart DE (2000) Management approaches to adrenal incidentalomas. A view from Ann Arbor, Michigan. Endocrinol Metab Clin North Am 29:127–39

50. Shell SR, Talamini MA, Udelsman R (1998) Laparoscopic adrenalectomy for non-malignant disease: improved safety, morbidity and cost-effectiveness. Surg Endosc 13:30–4

51. Silverman SG, Mueller PR, Pinkney LP, Koenker RM, Seltzer SE (1993) Predictive value of image-guided adrenal biopsy: analysis of results of 101 biopsies. Radiology 187:715–8

52. Smith CD, Weber CJ, Amerson JR (1999) Laparoscopic adrenalectomy: New Gold Standard. World J Surg 23:389–96

53. Thompson GB, Grant CS, van Heerden JA (1997) Laparoscopic versus open posterior adrenalectomy: A case-control study of 100 patients. Surgery 122:1132–6

54. Udelsman R, Fishman EK (2000) Radiology of the adrenal. Endocrinol Metab Clin North Am 29:27–42

55. Vargas HI, Kavoussi LR, Bartlett DK, Wagner JR, Venzon DJ, Fraker DL, Alexander HR (1997) Laparoscopic adrenalectomy: a new standard of care. Urology 49:673–8

56. Walz MK, Peitgen K, Sallaer B (1998) Subtotal adenalectomy by the posterior retroperitoneoscopic approach. World J Surg 22:621–7

57. Weinberger MH, Fineberg NS (1993) The diagnosis of primary aldosteronism and separation or two major subtypes. Arch Intern Med 153:2125–9

58. Wheeler MH, Harris DA (2003) Diagnosis and management of primary aldosteronism. World J Surg 27:627–31

59. Young WF Jr (2000) Management approaches to adrenal incidentalomas: A view from Rochester, Minnesota. Endocrinol Metab Clin North Am 29:159–85

24 Clinically Inapparent Adrenal Mass (Incidentaloma or Adrenaloma)

Dimitrios A. Linos

24.1 Introduction

Historically, the adrenal tumor that was discovered incidentally, usually during an imaging procedure (CT, MRI, ultrasound) for symptoms unrelated to adrenal disease (e.g., back pain), was called an incidentaloma [1].

As more physicians (and patients on their own) ordered these easily available imaging studies for common diseases potentially related to adrenal pathology (and not the known syndromes), such as mild and nonparoxysmal hypertension, diffuse obesity, and diabetes, an increasing number of unsuspected (but hardly incidental) adrenal tumors were found. I have proposed that these tumors be included with the true incidentalomas under the broader term "adrenaloma" because they share the same diagnostic and therapeutic dilemmas [2]. The term adrenaloma implies that the discovered tumor (incidentally or not) arises from the adrenal but is not obviously an aldosteronoma, a Cushing's syndrome adenoma, a pheochromocytoma, a virilizing or feminizing tumor, or a functioning adrenal carcinoma.

Recently, at a State of the Science Conference at the National Institute of Health, the term "clinically inapparent adrenal mass" was coined [3]. The widespread teaching is that most adrenalomas are indolent tumors, nonfunctioning and asymptomatic, causing no harm to the patient [4, 5]. Recent studies, however, have shown that a high percentage of these tumors can be subclinically functioning, causing symptoms milder than those encountered in the well known adrenal hyperfunctioning syndromes but still harmful to the patient [6–14]. Thus, the screening tests of serum potassium, urinary VMA and serum cortisol do not suffice and more detailed and in depth laboratory investigation is necessary. The fear of adrenal carcinoma that dictated the approach to these tumors in the past (with the main emphasis on the size of the tumor) should be changed to the fear of the subtle function of these usually benign adrenal cortical adenomas with coexistent metabolic pathology (e.g., hypertension, obesity, diabetes).

24.2 Frequency

The overall frequency of adrenal adenomas in 87,065 autopsies in 25 studies was 5.9% (range 1.1–32%) [15]. The frequency of adrenal masses discovered by CT, MRI or ultrasonography is somewhat lower. Abecassis et al. [16] in a 2-year period examined 1,459 patients and found 63 (4.3%) with adrenal masses. Of those, 19 patients (1.3% of examined patients and 30% of patients with adrenal masses) had adrenalomas. At the Mayo Clinic [17], in a 5-year period, 61,054 patients underwent CT scanning. In 2,066 (3.4%) patients, an adrenal abnormality was found; among these, 259 patients (12.5%) had an adrenaloma or adrenal lesion larger than 1 cm, without biochemical evidence or symptoms suggestive of cortical or medullary hypersecretion or general constitutional symptoms suggestive of malignant disease. Similar findings have been described in more recent studies [18–20]. Thus, in the era of widespread use of high-resolution ultrasonography, new generation CT scans and MRI, we can anticipate a 5% incidence of adrenalomas.

24.3 Pathology

The majority of surgically removed clinically inapparent adrenal masses have been classified as non-functioning cortical adenomas [21–23]. Benign masses such as nodular hyperplasia, adrenal cysts, myelolipomas, ganglioneuromas, hematomas, hamartomas, hemangiomas, leiomyomas, neurofibromas, teratomas, as well as infections (tuberculosis, fungal, echinococcosis, nocardiosis) are also included in the pathology of these resected tumors. Potentially lethal neoplasms, however, such as pheochromocytomas and primary carcinomas are always first on the list of resected adrenalomas [24–28]. Pheochromocytoma is the most frequently found hormone-producing adrenaloma that occasionally has a normal preoperative laboratory evaluation [29–33]. Few cases of aldosteronomas and androgen-producing adenomas have been described among cases of surgically removed adrenalomas [3–34]. In a large multicenter, retrospective Italian study of 380 surgically treated adrenalomas (out of 1,096 collected), 198 (52%) were cortical adenomas, 47 (12%) were cortical carcinomas, 42 (11%) were pheochromocytomas and 93 were other less frequent tumors [7].

24.4 The Goal of Evaluation

Although by definition the clinically inapparent adrenal masses appear "nonfunctioning", on the basis of clinical and essential laboratory findings more and more investigators have shown that a high percentage may be subclinically functioning and/or associated with other metabolic abnormalities (Fig. 1). In a multicenter, retrospective evaluation of 1,096 patients with adrenal incidentaloma, the work-up revealed that 9.2% had subclinical Cushing's syndrome, 4.2% had

pheochromocytoma and 1.6% had clinically unsuspected aldosteronomas [22].

Rossi et al. [10] prospectively followed 50 consecutive patients with clinically inapparent adrenal masses. Detailed hormonal investigation found 12 of 50 (24%) to have subclinical Cushing's syndrome defined as an abnormal response to at least two standard tests of the hypothalamic-pituitary-adrenal axis function, in the absence of clinical signs of Cushing's syndrome. In the same study, 92% of patients had hypertension, 50% obesity, 42% type 2 diabetes mellitus and 50% abnormal serum lipid concentrations. The clinical and hormonal features improved in all patients treated by adrenalectomy but were unchanged in all who did not undergo surgery (follow-up 9–73 months).

Interestingly, all 13 patients who had resection of truly nonfunctioning adenomas because of large size had improved clinically to such an extent that antihypertensive and antidiabetic therapy was reduced or discontinued. All the improvements persisted during follow-up.

Another multicenter study [12] of 64 consecutive patients with clinically inapparent adrenal masses found a higher than expected prevalence of abnormal glucose tolerance in 39 (61%) patients. The same authors [35] following 62 consecutive patients with clinically inapparent adrenal masses found abnormal glucose tolerance curves in 66%.

Midorikawa et al. [11] studying 15 patients with clinically inapparent adrenal masses (4 with subclinical Cushing and 11 with truly nonfunctioning tumors) found a high prevalence of altered glucose tolerance and insulin resistance. Adrenalectomy reversed insulin resistance in all patients with subclinical functioning and truly nonfunctioning adrenal adenomas.

Terzolo et al. [8] followed 41 patients with clinically inapparent adrenal masses (12 with subclinical Cushing's syndrome) and compared them with 41 controls. He found that the 2-h post-challenge glucose was significantly higher in these patients than in controls. Similarly, both systolic and diastolic blood pressures were higher in studied patients. The calculated whole-body insulin sensitivity index (derived from the oral glucose tolerance test) was significantly reduced in the patients. They concluded that patients with these tumors (subclinically functioning or nonfunctioning) display some features of the metabolic syndrome such as impaired glucose tolerance, increased blood pressure and high triglyceride levels.

Garrapa et al. [3] evaluated body composition and fat distribution, as measured by DEXA (dual-energy X-ray absorptiometry) in women with nonfunction-

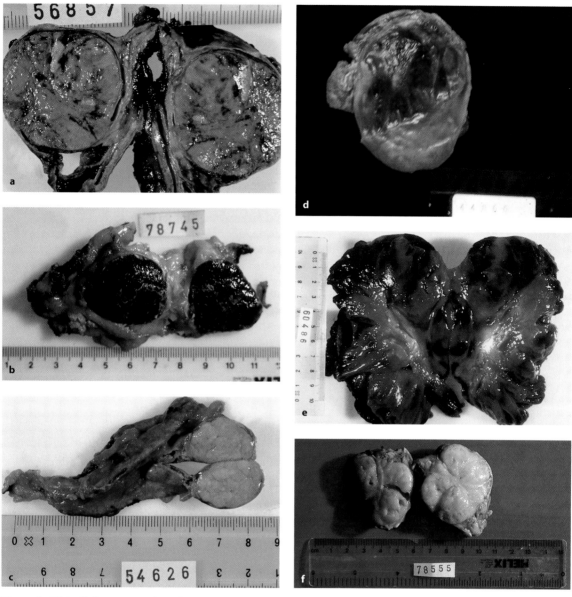

Fig. 1a–f. Clinically inapparent adrenal masses with 'unexpected' clinical behavior. **a** Cortical adenoma on a 37 y.o. female with subclinical Cushing's syndrome and metabolic syndrome significantly improved after surgery. **b** Cortical adenoma on a 40 y.o. male that during a 3 years follow up turned from 'non-functioning' to overt Cushing's syndrome. **c** Aldosteronoma on a 45 y.o. hypertensive but normokalemic male followed for years for this 2.5 cm "incidental" mass. **d** Pheochromocytoma on a 32 y.o. asymptomatic normotensive female. **e** 'Indolent' myelolipoma that ruptured during its follow up causing severe intraabdominal bleeding on a 27 y.o. male. **f** Solitary metastatic adrenal carcinoma, 10 years after hysterectomy for cervical cancer on a 62 y.o. female

ing clinically inapparent adrenal masses and in women with Cushing's syndrome compared with healthy controls matched for age, menopausal status and body mass index. Women with clinically inapparent adrenal masses had larger waist circumference reflecting intra-abdominal fat. The blood pressure was higher in patients with these tumors than in controls

and 50% of patients were hypertensive. High density lipoprotein cholesterol levels and mean triglyceride values were also higher in patients with clinically inapparent adrenal masses than in controls. If central fat deposition, hypertension and low HDL are important risk factors for cardiovascular disease, then patients with clinically inapparent adrenal masses, whether subclinically functioning or nonfunctioning, are at higher risk than the general population for cardiovascular disease.

Chiodin et al. [14] performed a longitudinal study evaluating the rate of spinal and femoral bone loss levels in 24 women with clinically inapparent adrenal masses. They were divided into two groups on the basis of the median value of urinary cortisol excretion. The group with higher cortisol values (subclinical Cushing levels) had more lumbar trabecular bone loss than those with low cortisol secretion (not hypersecreting tumors).

Therefore the cavalier attitude towards clinically inapparent adrenal masses should be changed. These tumors are at an intermediate stage in between normal and pathological. They should be screened to rule out: (a) subclinical Cushing's syndrome, (b) subclinical pheochromocytoma, (c) subclinical primary aldosteronism, (d) adrenal carcinoma (primary or solitary metastasis).

24.5   Screening for Subclinical Cushing's Syndrome

Patients with subclinical Cushing's syndrome have none of the signs and symptoms of typical Cushing's syndrome (plethora, moon face, central obesity, easy bruising, proximal muscle weakness, acne, osteoporosis, etc.).

The frequency of subclinical Cushing's syndrome among patients with adrenaloma ranges from 12% to 24% [10, 36]. Depending on the amount of glucocorticoids secreted, the clinical significance of subclinical Cushing's syndrome ranges from slightly attenuated diurnal cortisol rhythm to atrophy of the contralateral adrenal gland, a dangerous condition after unilateral adrenalectomy if appropriate therapeutic measures are not taken early enough [37].

The best screening test for autonomous cortisol secretion is the short dexamethasone suppression test. A 2- or 3-mg dose is better than the usual 1-mg dose to reduce false-positive results. A suppressed serum cortisol (<3 µg/dl or 80 nmol/l) excludes Cushing's syndrome. A serum cortisol greater than 3 µg/dl requires further investigation, including a confirmatory high-dose dexamethasone suppression test (8 mg), a corticotropin-releasing hormone (CRH) test and analysis of diurnal cortisol rhythm. If serum cortisol concentrations are not suppressible by high-dose dexamethasone, the diagnosis of subclinical Cushing's syndrome is established. Another suggested test is the

growth hormone (GH) response to GHRH. A blunted GH release might prove a sensitive and early sign of subclinical Cushing's syndrome [8]. As already discussed, glucose tolerance is altered in patients with clinically inapparent adrenal masses (with and without subclinical Cushing) and a glucose tolerance test is recommended in patients with clinically inapparent adrenal masses [10, 12, 38]. Finally, bone mineral density of the spine should be performed to detect reduced bone mass in patients with subclinical Cushing's syndrome [14].

Adrenal scintigraphy with ^{131}I-6β-iodomethylnorcholesterol (NP 59) can reveal a "functioning" but not "hypersecretory" tumor when there is an uptake of the nucleotide in the tumor site and no-uptake in the contralateral suppressed gland. Some authors [39, 40] suggested a significant positive correlation between abnormal cortical secretion and NP 59 uptake, making NP 59 scanning a cost effective diagnostic tool for evaluating clinically inapparent adrenal masses.

Others [15] found it cumbersome because it requires several days to obtain the images, and owing to the inability to take up NP 59 when there is hemorrhage or inflammation they do not recommend routine use of NP-59 scanning.

24.6   Screening for "Subclinical Pheochromocytoma"

The typical patient with pheochromocytoma is hypertensive and may have paroxysmal hypertension and related symptoms (headache, hypertensive crisis, sweating and cardiac arrhythmias). The proposed term "subclinical pheochromocytoma" refers to the totally asymptomatic clinically inapparent adrenal masses that histologically prove to be a pheochromocytoma. In several series of clinically inapparent adrenal masses, the frequency of pheochromocytomas range from 10% to 40% [31, 33]. Although the percentage of asymptomatic pheochromocytomas among patients with nonfunctioning adrenal tumors is relatively high, most test positive on hormonal evaluation, which is a measurement of 24-h urinary metanephrines and vanillylmandelic acid (VMA) or fractionated urinary catecholamines. In the National Italian Study Group, 27 patients (3.4% of the total patients with incidentaloma) were found to have pheochromocytoma; 24-h urinary catecholamine and VMA concentrations were elevated in 86% and 4.6% of patients, respectively [22], indicating that a combination of tests is more useful clinically than an individual test. The efficacy of single-voided ("spot") urine metanephrine and normetanephrine assays for diagnosing pheochromocytoma has recently been documented. Such tests may avoid the inconvenience of 24-h urine collection [41].

There is no indication for routine use of ^{131}I-metaiodobenzylguanidine (I-MIBG) scintigraphy in the evaluation of an adrenaloma unless catecholamine and urinary metabolites are elevated.

Because there are cases of clinically inapparent adrenal masses that preoperatively had negative urinary VMA, metanephrines and MIBG scanning but which intraoperatively behaved (with later histologic proof) as pheochromocytomas, prophylactic measures should always be taken (e.g., arterial line, immediate access to intravenous nipride) during surgery.

24.7 Screening for "Subclinical Primary Aldosteronism"

Typical primary aldosteronism is characterized by hypertension with hypokalemia, elevation of plasma aldosterone and suppressed plasma renin activity. Subclinical primary aldosteronism describes the patient with an adrenaloma who is normotensive or hypertensive with normokalemia [42]. More than 40% of patients with primary aldosteronism are normokalemic; therefore, the previously recommended measurement of potassium as the only test to rule out primary aldosteronism in the case of clinically inapparent adrenal masses should be abandoned [42]. Instead, a detailed time-consuming evaluation is necessary, especially in all hypertensive patients, to rule out primary aldosteronism which may be the cause of hypertension in up to 15% of these patients [43, 44]. In a normotensive patient with a serum potassium level greater than 3.9 nmol/l, no further hormonal evaluation is necessary. The screening for subclinical primary aldosteronism should include, in addition to serum potassium, the upright aldosterone level to plasma renin activity (PRA) ratio, since a single value of aldosterone may be normal. Patients with two or more samples positive for aldosterone/PRA ratio (>40) should undergo the fluorocortisone suppression test (0.4 mg every day for 4 days) or the acute saline suppression test (2 l of 0.9% NaCl solution infused intravenously in 4 h) to confirm the diagnosis. Bilateral adrenal venous sampling with measurement of aldosterone and cortisol levels is the necessary next step to lateralize, and determine the subtype of primary aldosteronism in order to identify the patient who will be cured by surgery.

24.8 Screening for Adrenal Carcinoma

The risk of a clinically inapparent adrenal mass harboring a primary carcinoma of the adrenal is very low [45]. The annual incidence of the latter has been estimated to range from 1 case per 600,000 to 1 case per 1.6 million persons. Its prevalence is approximately 0.0012% [46]. In contrast, metastatic carcinoma to the adrenal is a common finding in patients with lung, breast, colon and other extra-adrenal malignancies. In published series of surgically resected adrenalomas, the frequency of histologically confirmed primary adrenal carcinoma ranges from 4.2% to 25% [7]. The frequency of adrenal metastasis from lung cancer at autopsy ranges from 17% to 38%. In patients with an adrenal mass in the setting of extra-adrenal malignancy, the probability of this mass being metastatic ranges from 32% to 73% [5, 33, 47].

24.9 Size of Tumor

The size of a clinically inapparent adrenal mass is frequently used to predict potential malignancy and the need for surgery. Although most clinically treated adrenal malignancies are discovered when they are larger than 6 cm in diameter, several reports have described very large tumors that never metastasized and small adrenal tumors that did (Figs. 2 and 3). In several series, adrenocortical carcinomas with a maximum diameter of 3 cm or less have been described [15, 33, 37, 47].

The size of a clinically inapparent adrenal mass as reported on a CT scan is usually less than the size reported histologically. This underestimation ranges from 16% to 47% [48]. In an analysis of the CT and histology reports of 76 patients with various diseases, we found that the mean estimated diameter of the adrenal tumor was 4.64 cm on the CT report when the real size (pathology report) was 5.96 cm. Further analysis of different CT scans revealed a consistent underestimation in all groups. In the group of adrenal tumors with a maximum diameter of less than 3 cm, the mean diameter reported on CT was 2.32 cm in contrast to the true histological size of 3.63 cm ($P<0.001$). We therefore proposed the formula Histologic Size = 0.85 + (1.09 × CT size) to correct the underestimated CT size and thus to use the size criterion more accurately [48]. A recent study [49] showed that the above "Linos formula" turned out to be significantly more accurate than direct radiologic measurements in predicting the real pathological size of the tumor.

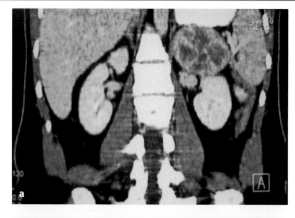

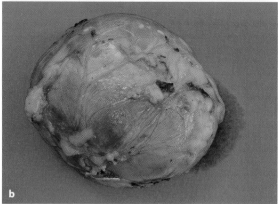

Fig. 2a, b. This larger than 6-cm clinically inapparent adrenal mass was suspicious for malignancy on CT scan (**a**) but histologically was proved a benign cortical tumor (**b**)

24.10   Imaging

In addition to assessing distant metastasis and tumor size, imaging studies may suggest malignancy. On CT, one may see a poorly delineated ragged tumor with stippled calcifications and with areas of necrosis; such lesions are suggestive of malignancy, especially if enlarged lymph nodes or local invasion is also detected.

On MR imaging studies, one should look for heterogeneously increased, early T2-weighted signal, weak and late enhancement after gadolinium injection or an intravascular signal identical to the tumor signal. When NP59 scintigraphy is available, the lack of (or very weak) uptake in the tumor and normal contralateral uptake is suspicious for malignancy. Positron emission tomography (PET) can be used following the administration of 2-deoxy-2[18F]-fluoro-D-glucose. The 18F-FDG-PET scan is a useful tool for confirming isolated metastases and selecting patients for adrenalectomy. It has been used in studies to distinguish be-

tween primary and metastatic adrenal lesions, especially in patients with other primary malignancies [50] (Fig. 3).

24.11   Fine-Needle Aspiration

Fine-needle aspiration (FNA) biopsy of a clinically inapparent adrenal mass has a limited role. It is useful in cases of coexistent extra-adrenal carcinoma (usually lung cancer) to confirm the radiologic evidence of adrenal metastasis. Generally, FNA cannot differentiate cortical adenoma from carcinoma because it cannot detect invasion of the tumor into the capsule.

In a study by Silverman and co-workers [51], 3 of 33 FNA specimens that contained "benign" adrenal tissue were later proved to be malignant. Each malignant lesion was smaller than 3 cm in diameter. In 14 patients in whom the FNA was nondiagnostic, two masses proved to be malignant.

Although it has been suggested that FNA is useful in the differential diagnosis of a cystic adrenal mass, we strongly object to such practice because cystic pheochromocytomas are prevalent. Diagnostic puncture of such a lesion (or of a rare cystic echinococcal parasitic cyst) can be harmful to the patient. The possibility of seeding a malignant adrenal neoplasm in the retroperitoneum is an additional reason that FNA should be discouraged.

24.12   Genetic and Molecular Biology Studies

Currently, the only accepted criteria for determining whether a clinically inapparent adrenal mass is benign or malignant are metastasis (synchronous or metachronous) and local invasion into adjacent structures. The mapping and identification of genes responsible for hereditary syndromes (e.g., multiple endocrine neoplasia type 1, Li-Fraumeni) have increased our understanding of adrenocortical tumorigenesis. Oncogenes and tumor suppressor genes involved in adrenal carcinomas include mutations in the p53 tumor suppressor gene. Amongst these, the Ki67 index (% immunopositive cells) when above 5% can be a useful indicator in the differentiation of adenomas from carcinomas [52]. Adrenal carcinomas are monoclonal, whereas adrenal adenomas may be polyclonal in approximately 25–40% of cases [53]. Although these findings do not have direct clinical application, it is hoped that future research will facilitate

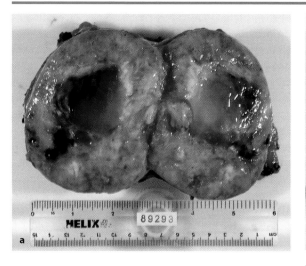

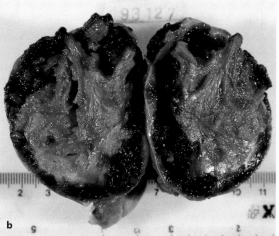

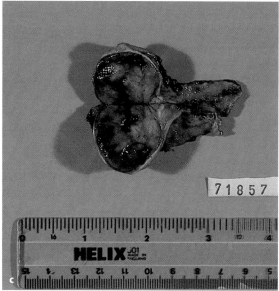

Fig. 3a–c. The size of the clinically inapparent adrenal mass does not necessarily predict the clinical severity of the problem. **a** A 9 cm maximum diameter benign swanoma. **b** A 7 cm maximum diameter benign hemorrhagic cortical adenoma. **c** A 2.9 cm potentially lethal pheochromocytoma

the diagnosis and predict the natural course of these tumors.

24.13 Management of Clinically Inapparent Adrenal Masses: Surgery Versus Follow-Up

Several recent studies that we briefly discussed demonstrated that:

1. A relatively high percentage of clinically inapparent adrenal masses, especially adrenal cortical adenomas, are subclinically functioning.
2. A relatively high percentage of patients with clinically inapparent adrenal mass display pathological features such as: impaired glucose tolerance, insulin resistance, increased blood pressure, high triglyceride levels, low HDL, central fat deposition and reduced trabecular bone mineral density.
3. When adrenalectomy was done in patients who either had proven subclinical hypercortisolism or even truly nonfunctioning tumors, the associated abnormalities and symptoms (such as hypertension, obesity, altered glucose tolerance) were normalized or significantly improved.

In the era of laparoscopic adrenalectomy that carries a minimal mortality and morbidity, it appears logical to advocate surgery in patients with clinically inapparent adrenal mass when:

1. There is laboratory evidence for a subclinically functioning tumor

2. There are associated pathological features such as hypertension, impaired glucose tolerance (or diabetes), pathological triglyceride profile, central fat deposition, reduced bone mineral density
3. There is clinical and radiological evidence for primary or solitary metastatic adrenal carcinoma

The age and the anxiety of the patient should also play a role in the decision to operate or not.

Conservative management is recommended of those patients with clinically inapparent adrenal mass in whom: (a) there is no clinical or laboratory evidence for subclinical function of the tumor; (b) there are no associated symptoms potentially related to the clinically inapparent adrenal mass; (c) there is no suspicion of adrenal carcinoma. In these patients a yearly check-up should be continued for 5–10 years with the main emphasis on the possibility that the silent, nonfunctioning tumor may develop hyperfunction.

Limited, complete follow-up studies (with repeated radiologic and hormonal evaluation) have been performed on patients with clinically inapparent adrenal masses. Barzon and associates [54] followed 75 patients with clinically inapparent adrenal masses [6], observed them for a median of 4 years, and found 9 clinically inapparent adrenal masses to have enlargement. Overt Cushing's syndrome developed in two patients, subclinical Cushing's syndrome in three and clinical pheochromocytoma in one. No patient had a malignancy. The estimated cumulative risks for mass enlargement and hyperfunction were 18% and 9.5% respectively after 5 years, and 22.8% and 9.5% after 10 years. In an other study [55], 53 patients with clinically inapparent adrenal masses were followed for 6–78 months (medium 24 months). During the follow-up, 22 lesions (41.5%) increased in size and 6 lesions (11.3%) decreased in size or disappeared. No clinically inapparent adrenal mass grew or developed hypersecretion. Thus, during follow-up of the truly nonfunctioning clinically inapparent adrenal masses, yearly hormonal evaluation should be emphasized rather than repeating imaging studies.

24.14 What Is the Best Surgical Approach in the Management of Clinically Inapparent Adrenal Masses?

Traditionally, surgical approaches to the adrenals have been anterior transperitoneal, posterior extraperitoneal and thoracoabdominal (for large tumors) [56]. The application of laparoscopic techniques in surgery of the adrenal glands has essentially replaced all traditional open approaches in the same manner that laparoscopic cholecystectomy has replaced traditional open cholecystectomy. Because there are so many benefits associated with the laparoscopic approach, open andrenalectomy should be reserved for very large adrenal carcinomas invading the surrounding tissue. We have compared the anterior, posterior and laparoscopic approach in 165 patients who underwent adrenalectomy between 1984 and 1994 [57]. Although in this study we included our early cases and learning experience, the advantages of the laparoscopic approach were clearly shown in terms of morbidity (12.2% in the anterior approach, 8.1% in the posterior approach and 0% in the laparoscopic approach), mean operating time, mean length of postoperative hospitalization (8.1 days versus 4.5 days versus 2.7 days) and minimal postoperative pain. The lack of long incisions and their immediate and long-term complications (e.g., wound infection, hernia, esthetic dissatisfaction) and the opportunity for an early return to full activity make the laparoscopic approach the procedure of choice for nearly all clinically inapparent adrenal masses, including the laparoscopically removable primary or secondary carcinomas [31,58] (Fig. 3). Although the posterior open adrenalectomy has more advantages than the anterior open andrenalectomy, the advantages of anterior laparoscopic adrenalectomy outweigh the advantages of the posterior laparoscopic approach [59, 60]. The anterior (or lateral) laparoscopic adrenalectomy enables the removal of large tumors, the performance of additional procedures (e.g., cholecystectomy) and the performance of bilateral laparoscopic adrenalectomies when indicated [61,62]. We have simplified [63] the anterior laparoscopic technique, which has become easier and more "friendly" to the surgeon compared to the originally described techniques [58]. Thus, more and more surgeons will switch to the laparoscopic approach for the management of adrenal tumors.

References

1. Copeland PM (1984) The incidentally discovered adrenal mass. Ann Surg 199:116
2. Linos D (1989) Adrenaloma: A better term than incidentaloma. Surgery 105:456
3. Grumbach M, Biller B, Braunstein G, et al. (2003) Management of the clinically inapparent adrenal mass ("incidentaloma"). Ann Intern Med 138:424–429
4. Young AE, Smellie WD (2001) In: Farndon JR (ed) The adrenal glands in endocrine surgery, 2nd edn. WB Saunders, London, pp 123–124

5. Ross NS, Aron DC (1990) Hormonal evaluation of the patient with an incidentally discovered adrenal mass. N Engl J Med 323:1401

6. Barzon L, Boscaro M (2000) Diagnosis and management of adrenal incidentalomas. J Urol 163:398

7. Mantero F, Terzolo M, Arnaldi G, Osella G, Masini AM, et al. (2000) A survey on adrenal incidentaloma in Italy. J Clin Endocrinol Metab 85:637–644

8. Terzolo M, Bossoni S, Ali A, Doga M, Reimondo G, Milani G, Peretti P, Manelli F, Angeli A, Giustina A (2000) Growth hormone (GH) responses to GH-releasing hormone alone or combined with arginine in patients with adrenal incidentaloma: evidence for enhanced somatostatinergic tone. J Clin Endocrinol Metab 85:1310–1315

9. Terzolo M, Pia A, Ali A, Osella G, et al. (2002) Adrenal incidentaloma: a new cause of the metabolic syndrome. J Clin Endocrinol Metab 87:998–1003

10. Rossi R, Tauchmanova L, Luciano A, Di Martino M, Battista C, DelViscovo L, Nuzzo V, Lombardi G (2000) Subclinical Cushing's syndrome in patients with adrenal incidentaloma: clinical and biochemical features. J Clin Endocrinol Metab 85:1440–1448

11. Midorikawa S, Sanada H, Hashimoto S, Suzuki T, Watanabe T (2001) The improvement of insulin resistance in patients with adrenal incidentaloma by surgical resection. Clin Endocrinol 54:797–804

12. Fernadez-Real JM, Engel WR, Simon R, et al. (1998) Study of glucose tolerance in consecutive patients harbouring incidental adrenal tumours: Study Group of Incidental Adrenal Adenoma. Clin Endocrinol (Oxf) 49:53

13. Garrapa GGM, Pantanetti P, Arnaldi G, Mantero F, Faloia E (2001) Body composition and metabolic features in women with adrenal incidentaloma or Cushing's syndrome. J Clin Endocrinol Metab 86:5301–5306

14. Chiodini I, Torlontano M, Carnevale V, Guglielmi G, Cammisa M, Trischitta V, Scillitani A (2001) Bone loss rate in adrenal incidentalomas: a longitudinal study. J Clin Endocrinol Metab 86:5337–5341

15. Young WF (2000) Management approaches to adrenal incidentalomas. A view from Rochester, Minnesota. Endocrinol Metab Clin North Am 29:159–185

16. Abecassis M, McLoughlin MJ, Langer B, et al. (1985) Serendipitous adrenal masses: Prevalence, significance and management. Am J Surg 149:783

17. Herrera MF, Grant CS, van Heerden JA, et al. (1991) Incidentally discovered adrenal tumors: An institutional perspective. Surgery 110:1014

18. Caplan RH, Srutt PJ, Wickus G (1994) Subclinical hormone secretion by incidentally discovered adrenal masses. Arch Surg 129:291

19. Prinz RA, Brooks MH, Churchill R, et al. Incidental asymptomatic adrenal masses detected by computed tomographic scanning: Is operation required? JAMA 248:701

20. Glazer HS, Weyman PJ, Sagel SS, et al. (1982) Nonfunctioning adrenal masses: Incidental discovery on computed tomography. AJR Am J Roentgenol 139:81

21. Belldegrun A, Hussain S, Seltzer SE, et al. (1986) Incidentally discovered mass of the adrenal gland. Surg Gynecol Obstet 163:203

22. Mantero F, Masini AM, Opocher G, et al. (1997) Adrenal incidentaloma: An overview of hormonal data from the National Italian Study Group. Horm Res 47:284

23. Linos DA, Stylopoulos N, Raptis SA (1996) Adrenaloma: A call for more aggressive management. World J Surg 20:788

24. Bitter DA, Ross DS (1989) Incidentally discovered adrenal masses. Am J Surg 158:159

25. Caplan RH, Kisken WA, Huiras CM (1991) Incidentally discovered adrenal masses. Minn Med 74:23

26. Cajraj H, Young AE (1993) Adrenal incidentaloma. Br J Surg 80:422

27. Geelhoed GW, Druy EM (1992) Management of the adrenal "incidentaloma". Surgery 92:866

28. Didolkar MS, Bescher RA, Elias EG, et al. (1984) Natural history of adrenal cortical carcinoma: A clinicopathologic study of 42 patients. Cancer 47:2153

29. Sutton MG, Sheps SG, Lie JT (1981) Prevalence of clinically unsuspected pheochromocytoma: Review of a 50-year autopsy series. Mayo Clin Proc 56:354

30. Proye C, Fossati P, Fontaine P, et al. (1986) Dopamine secreting pheochromocytoma: An unrecognised entity? Classification of pheochromocytomas according to their type of secretion. Surgery 100:1154

31. Kebebew E, Siperstein AE, Clark OH, Duh QY (2002) Results of laparoscopic adrenalectomy for suspected and unsuspected malignant adrenal neoplasms. Arch Surg 137:948–953

32. Aso Y, Homma Y (1992) A survey on incidental adrenal tumors in Japan. J Urol 147:1478

33. Terzolo M, Ali A, Osella G, et al. (1997) Prevalence of adrenal carcinoma among incidentally discovered adrenal masses: A retrospective study from 1989 to 1994. Gruppo Piemontese Incidentalomi Surrenalici. Arch Surg 132:8, 14

34. Yamakita N, Saitoh M, Mercado-Asis LB, et al. (1990) Asymptomatic adrenal tumor: 38 cases in Japan including seven of our own. Endocrinol Jpn 37:671

35. Fernadez-Real JM, Gonzalbez J, Ricart W (2001) Metabolic abnormalities in patients with adrenal incidentaloma [letters to the editor]. J Clin Endocrinol Metab 86:950–951

36. Terzolo M, Osella G, Ali A, et al. (1998) Subclinical Cushing's syndrome in adrenal incidentaloma. Clin Endocrinol (Oxf) 48:89

37. Chidiac RM, Aron DC (1997) Incidentalomas: A disease of modern technology. Endocrinol Metab Clin North Am 26:233

38. Beuschlein F, Borgemeister M, Schirra J, Goke B, Fassnacht M, Arlt W, Allolio B, Reincke M (2000) Oral glucose tolerance testing but not intravenous glucose administration uncovers hyperresponsiveness of hypothalamo-pituitary-adrenal axis in patients with adrenal incidentalomas. Clin Endocrinol 52:617–623

39. Barzon L, Scaroni C, Sonino N, et al. (1998) Incidentally discovered adrenal tumors: Endocrine and scintigraphic correlates. J Clin Endocrinol Metab 83:55

40. Dwamena BA, Kloos RT, Fendrick AM, et al. (1998) Diagnostic evaluation of the adrenal incidentaloma: Decision and cost-effectiveness analysis. J Nucl Med 39:707

41. Ito Y, Obara T, Okamoto T, et al. (1998) Efficacy of single-voided urine metanephrine and normetanephrine assay for diagnosing pheochromocytoma. World J Surg 22:684

42. Linos DA (2000) Management approaches to adrenal incidentalomas (adrenalomas). A view from Athens, Greece. Endocrinol Metab Clin North Am 29:141–157

43. Gordon RD, Ziesak MD, Tunny TJ, et al. (1993) Evidence that primary aldosteronism may not be uncommon: 12% incidence among antihypertensive drug trial volunteers. Clin Exp Pharmacol Physiol 20:296

44. Gordon R, Stowasser M, Rutherford J (2001) Primary aldosteronism: are we diagnosing and operating on too few patients? World J Surgery 25:941–947

45. Proye C, Jafari Manjili M, Combemale F, et al. (1998) Experience gained from operation of 103 adrenal incidentalomas. Langenbecks Arch Surg 338:330

46. Schteingart DE (2000) Management approaches to adrenal incidentalomas. A view from Ann Arbour Michigan. Endocrinol Metab Clin North Am 29:127–139

47. Linos DA, Avlonitis VS, Iliadis K (1998) Laparoscopic resection of solitary adrenal metastasis from lung carcinoma: A case report. J Soc Laparoendoscopic Surg 2:291

48. Linos DA, Stylopoulos N (1997) How accurate is computed tomography in predicting the real size of adrenal tumors? Arch Surg 132:740

49. Fajardo R, Montalvo J, Velazquez D, Arch J, Bezaury P, Gamino R, Herrera MF (2004) Correlation between radiologic and pathologic dimensions of adrenal masses. World J Surg 28(5):494–497

50. Yun M, Kim W, Alnafisi N, Lacorte L, Jang S, Alavi A (2001) 18 F-FDG PET in characterizing adrenal lesions detected on CT or MRI. J Nucl Med 42:1795–9

51. Silverman SG, Mueller PR, Pinkey LP, et al. (1993) Predictive value of image-guided adrenal biopsy: Analysis and results of 101 biopsies. Radiology 187:715

52. Wachenfeld C, Beuschlein F, Swermann O, Mora P, Fassnacht M, Allolio B, Reincke M (2001) Discerning malignancy in adrenocortical tumors: are molecular markers useful? Eur J Endocrinol 145:335–341

53. Reincke M, Beuschlein F, Slawik M, Borm K (2000) Molecular adrenocortical tumourgenesis. Eur J Clin Invest 30:63–68

54. Barzon L, Scaroni C, Sonino, et al. (1999) Risk factors and long-term follow-up of adrenal incidentalomas. J Clin Endocrinol Metab 84:520

55. Grossrubatscher E, Vignati F, Posso M, Lohi P (2001) The natural history of incidentally discovered adrenocortical adenomas: a retrospective evaluation. J Endocrinol Invest 24:846–855

56. Linos DA (1989) Surgical approach to the adrenal gland. In: van Heerden JA (ed) Common problems in endocrine surgery: recommendations of the experts. Year Book Medical, St. Louis, pp 349–355

57. Linos DA, Stylopoulos N, Boukis M, et al. (1997) Anterior, posterior or laparoscopic approach for the management of adrenal diseases? Am J Surg 173:120

58. Gagner M, Pomp A, Heniford BT, et al. (1997) Laparoscopic adrenalectomy: lessons learned from 100 consecutive procedures. Ann Surg 226:238

59. Thompson GB, Grant CS, van Heerden JA, et al. (1997) Laparoscopic versus open posterior adrenalectomy: A case-control study of 100 patients. Surgery 122:1132

60. Ting Ac, Lo CY, Lo CM (1998) Posterior or laparoscopic approach for adrenalectomy. Am J Surg 175:488

61. Lanzi R, Montorsi F, Losa M, et al. (1998) Laparoscopic bilateral adrenalectomy for persistent Cushing's disease after transsphenoidal surgery. Surgery 123:144

62. Miccoli P, Raffaelli M, Berti P, Materazzi G, Massi M, Bernini G (2002) Adrenal surgery before and after the introduction of laparoscopic adrenalectomy. Br J Surg 89:779–782

63. Linos D (2002) Laparoscopic right adrenalectomy in perative techniques in general surgery. In: van Heerden JA, Farley DF (eds) vol 4(4). WB Saunders, Philadelphia, pp 304–308

25 Genetic Syndromes Associated with Adrenal Tumors

Göran Åkerström, Per Hellman

25.1   Introduction

Hereditary genetic syndromes associated with adrenal tumors have become increasingly important to identify in order to appropriately treat not only the adrenal disease but to recognize and manage other syndrome manifestations as well. This association has been recognized in patients with pheochromocytomas, where hereditary disease was recently identified in nearly every fourth patient [64]. Fewer patients with adrenocortical tumors have had a genetic predisposition for hereditary syndromes, all of which have been rare. The identification of genetic syndromes can be expected to become an increasingly important aid in disease classification and prognostic evaluation, and for the treatment of individual patients.

25.2   Hereditary Pheochromocytoma

Classification ▶ Paraganglia are neural ganglionic tissues distributed from the middle ear and the base of the skull, along the great vessels of the thorax and abdomen down to the pelvis. Chromaffin-negative paraganglia belong to the parasympathetic nerve system, and act as chemical sensors involved in pH regulation or oxygen sensing, similar to the carotid body. Chromaffin-positive paraganglia, including the adrenal medulla, are part of the sympathetic nervous system, and can secrete catecholamines in response to stress. The specific function of extra-adrenal sympathetic paraganglia (such as the organ of Zuckerkandel at the aortic bifurcation) has not been clearly elucidated [65].

Pheochromocytomas are uncommon tumors with a characteristic chromaffin tissue reaction originating in the neural crest-derived cells of the adrenal medulla, or in extra-adrenal sympathetic paraganglia, where they may be denoted as *extra-adrenal pheochromocytomas.*

The term "paraganglioma" should refer to neoplasia of the paraganglion system. The nomenclature overlaps, since the name *paraganglioma* is commonly used to depict only the non-functioning tumors originating in parasympathetic ganglia, which occur most often in the head and neck region. The inactive paragangliomas in the head and neck are also called glomus tumors, the most common of which originate in the carotid body and are often called chemodectomas.

Prevalence of Hereditary Disease ▶ It has long been thought that most pheochromocytomas were sporadic and only about 10% were hereditary, constituting part of the familial syndromes, principally multiple endocrine neoplasia type 2 (MEN 2), von Hippel-Lindau (VHL) disease, and rarely neurofibromatosis type 1 (NF 1) [10, 25, 34, 41, 46, 49, 62, 63, 65, 90, 91]. Recently other germ-line mutations in genes encoding succinate dehydrogenase subunits D and B (*SDHD, SDHB*) were identified in familial paraganglioma, and in cases of familial pheochromocytoma [3, 7, 31, 46, 65]. A subsequent molecular study revealed an unexpectedly high incidence of hereditary disease by identifying germ-line mutations in susceptibility genes for pheochromocytoma or paraganglioma, in as many as 24% of patients in a large series of apparently sporadic pheochromocytomas [64]. Of patients with mutations, 45% had VHL mutations, 20% *RET* mutations, 17% *SDHD* and 18% *SDHB* mutations. Young age, multifocal or bilateral, and extra-adrenal tumors were significantly associated with mutations. Of patients presenting at the age of 10 years or younger, 70% had germ-line mutations, and *VHL* mutations in particular were identified in 42% of patients aged 18 years of age or younger. Medullary thyroid carcinoma developed during follow-up in patients with *RET* mutations, while hemangioblastoma, islet-cell pancreatic tumors, or renal cell carcinoma appeared in patients with *VHL* mutations, and glomus tumors in patients with *SDHD* or *SDHB* mutations. This study emphasized that hereditary disease may be more common in patients with apparently sporadic pheochromocytoma and paraganglioma than was previously anticipated. Identification of germ-line mutations is obviously crucially important for appropriate screening and management of syndrome-associated lesions during follow-up in both the proband and the family. Genetic screening to disclose the hereditary tumor syndromes should therefore be recommended routinely in patients with pheochromocytoma, and especially so in young patients with multifocal or extra-adrenal tumors. It should also be routine when diagnostic methods become readily available in patients with paraganglioma, where 50% may have a hereditary predisposition.

25.2.1   Multiple Endocrine Neoplasia Type 2

In multiple endocrine neoplasia type 2 (MEN 2A), which was described by Sipple in 1961 [75], virtually all patients have medullary thyroid carcinoma, 50% have pheochromocytoma, and approximately 15% hyperparathyroidism (HPT) [15, 19, 38]. Variants of MEN 2A include MEN 2A with cutaneous lichen amyloidosis, and MEN 2A with Hirschsprung's disease.

The MEN-2B syndrome is rare, and consists of medullary thyroid carcinoma, pheochromocytoma in approximately 50% of patients, and developmental abnormalities consisting of a marfanoid habitus, tall slender body and long extremities, thick lips, and mucosal neuromas [68]. The characteristic mucosal neuromas often cover the anterior parts of the tongue, lips, buccal mucosa, conjunctiva and eyelids. Gastrointestinal complaints due to intestinal ganglioneuromatosis with obstipation and megacolon are common, but

clearly have a different genesis than the aganglionosis of Hirschsprung's disease.

The medullary thyroid carcinoma is aggressive in patients with MEN 2B, and often develops already during the early years of life, with mean age at diagnosis of approximately 16 years. Due to early development the disease is often advanced at diagnosis, and cure by surgery is rarely possible. Extensive local spread and metastases from the thyroid carcinoma have been the common cause of death. Most patients represent de novo mutations where no other cases in the family can be recognized.

The MEN-2 genetic syndrome also comprises cases of familial medullary thyroid carcinoma, without evidence of other endocrinopathies [26].

Genetics ▶ MEN-2 patients have germ-line mutations in the *RET* proto-oncogene, located on chromosome 10q11.2 [16, 27, 37, 44, 58, 59]. This large gene encodes a tyrosine kinase receptor, with an important role for neural growth differentiation. *RET* consists of 21 exons, and has six "hot-spot" exons in either the extracellular or the intracellular domains, where mutations occur in more than 97% of MEN-2 patients [44, 46] (Table 1). The result of many of these mutations is dimerization at steady stage and constitutive activation of downstream signal transduction. Ligands to *RET* are glial

Table 1. Specific mutations associated with multiple endocrine neoplasia type 2 and pheochromocytoma. This table presents the most common mutations associated with MEN-2 and pheochromocytoma (*FMTC*, familial medullary thyroid carcinoma). (From Kikumori et al. with permission) [44]

Exon	Affected codon	Clinical syndrome	% Of all MEN-2 mutations
Extracellular domain			
10	609	MEN-2A/FMTC	0–1
	611	MEN-2A/FMTC	2–3
	618	MEN-2A/FMTC	3–5
	620	MEN-2A/FMTC	6–8
11	630	MEN-2A/FMTC	0–1
	634	MEN-2A	80–90
Intracellular domain			
13	790	MEN-2A/FMTC	
14	804	MEN-2A/FMTC	
	806	MEN-2A (MEN-2B)	
15	883	MEN-2B	
16	918	MEN-2B	3–5

cell line-derived neurotrophic factor (GDNF), a member of the transforming growth factor (TGF)-B family, and neurturin [46]. Mutations of the ligands do not cause medullary thyroid carcinoma or MEN 2, but GDNF is mutated in 50% of patients with Hirschsprung's disease.

Extracellular Domain Mutations ▸ Mutations in codon 634, exon 10 of *RET* account for 75–85% of all mutations in MEN 2 and hereditary medullary thyroid carcinoma, and are most commonly associated with the classical MEN-2A or Sipple's syndrome [44, 46] (Table 1). MEN 2A and cutaneous lichen amyloidosis have been found only in persons with the 634 mutation. Mutations of codon 609, 611, 618 and 620 constitute an additional ~10% of mutations in MEN 2A [44, 46]. Mutations of these codons and codon 630 will most commonly cause familial medullary thyroid carcinoma, but may also lead to MEN 2A. MEN 2A and Hirschsprung's disease have occurred with 609, 618 and 620 mutations.

Intracellular Domain Mutations ▸ The most common intracellular mutation is codon 918 of exon 16 in the thyrosine kinase domain, which constitutes 3–5% of all mutations, but has been found in more than 95% of patients with MEN 2B [16, 37, 44, 46, 58] (Table 1). This mutation affects the tyrosine kinase catalytic site of the receptor protein. A smaller proportion of MEN-2B patients have codon 883 mutations, whereas mutations at codons 790 and 804 of the intracellular domain have been associated with MEN 2A.

Pheochromocytomas in MEN 2 have been associated with certain RET mutations [44, 46, 58] (Table 1). The risk of development of pheochromocytoma is higher with 634 mutations than with other exon 10 and 11 mutations at codons 609, 611, 618, 620 and 630. Pheochromocytomas occur also with mutations in the intracellular domain, codons 790, 804, 806, 883 and 918 [46].

Genetic testing for the MEN-2 syndrome is well established clinically, and thus makes it possible to advise prophylactic thyroidectomy and a clinical surveillance program for individuals with the diseased gene [44, 46, 58, 64, 65]. Screening of exons 10, 11, 13, 14, 15, and 16 excludes 99% of mutations associated with hereditary disease. Screening is recommended at the age of 6 years in MEN 2A, and immediately after birth in MEN-2B kindred, in order to avoid deaths from thyroid carcinoma. Genetic testing has been included in the clinical management of MEN-2 patients more than in any other genetic malignancy [44, 46, 58, 64, 65].

Characteristics of Pheochromocytomas in MEN 2 ▸ Pheochromocytomas have occurred in 30–55% of MEN-2A and 50% of MEN-2B patients [15, 19, 38, 68]. Medullary thyroid carcinoma has generally been diagnosed before or concomitantly with the pheochromocytoma in MEN 2A and B, and consequently pheochromocytomas have rarely (10–25%) been the first expression of the syndrome [19, 26, 38, 59, 68]. When medullary thyroid carcinoma is diagnosed first, pheochromocytomas have developed after an average duration of 11 years [15, 23, 57, 58]. Mean age at diagnosis of pheochromocytomas in MEN 2A is 37 years, and in MEN 2B 25 years [15, 19, 23, 38, 57, 58]. The pheochromocytomas are frequently bilateral and multifocal in MEN 2 (Fig. 1), but may develop asynchronously [50, 53, 58, 86].

The histological patterns of the adrenal medulla are similar in MEN 2A and B, with single or multiple tumors in a background of micronodular, or diffuse, medullary hyperplasia [18, 23, 53, 58, 70, 86, 87] (Fig. 1). A diameter >1 cm has been used to distinguish pheochromocytomas from nodules of smaller size.

Pheochromocytomas in MEN 2 are rarely extra-adrenal (<1%) [15, 19, 50, 57, 86]. Malignant pheochromocytomas are uncommon (around 10%), but are more likely to be present with large tumors, and in tumors exceeding 5 cm in diameter [15, 18, 19, 50, 53, 57, 86, 87]. Histological features have been uncertain determinants of benign versus malignant tumors, and a diagnosis of malignancy has generally required demonstration of metastases. On occasion the malignant diagnosis has been disclosed only after decades of follow-up [17, 18, 46, 47, 63, 70, 87, 91], and in older series the malignancy rate has reached nearly 25% after ~25 years of follow-up [17, 47].

Diagnosis, Clinical Features ▸ Measurement of the 24-h urinary epinephrine, norepinephrine and metanephrine excretion is usually diagnostic for pheochromocytoma in MEN-2A and B patients [33]. Determination of plasma metanephrines may be even more predictive and has now been introduced at many centers [24]. Pheochromocytomas in MEN-2 patients predominantly excrete epinephrine and metanephrine, and present an *adrenergic biochemical phenotype* [47]. Computed tomography (CT) or magnetic resonance imaging (MRI) can usually efficiently visualize the pheochromocytoma in MEN-2 patients, and may routinely identify lesions larger than 1 cm. Positron emission tomography (PET) can be used with [^{11}C]-hydroxyephedrine as a marker for functional diagnosis of medullary lesions, and [^{11}C]-metomidate as a

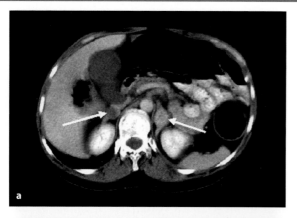

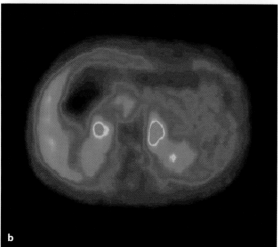

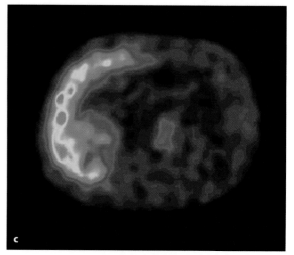

Fig. 1. a CT image of bilateral adrenal tumors in a MEN-2B patient; **b** with bilateral uptake of [11C]-hydroxyephedrine on PET investigation; and **c** no uptake of [11C]-metomidate. Histopathological examination of operative specimens in this patient revealed bilateral pheochromocytomas with concomitant medullary hyperplasia in both adrenals; **d** right adrenal; **e** left adrenal (**d** and **e** represent chromogranin-stained, rearranged operative specimens). Pheochromocytoma with vague demarcation towards concomitant medullary hyperplasia is typical for MEN2

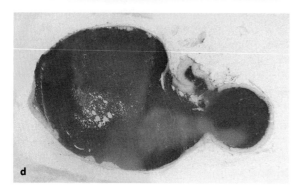

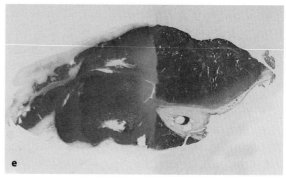

marker for cortical lesions [43, 73] (Fig. 1). Functional diagnosis may sometimes be important since incidental cortical tumors may occur with some prevalence in patients with a presumed pheochromocytoma diagnosis as they do in the normal population (Fig. 2). 131MIBG has been of less value for routine screening of the MEN-2 patients, but may be of special value in extra-adrenal and occult pheochromocytomas, or for the detection of metastases [76, 84]. Pheochromocytomas frequently express somatostatin receptors, but octreoscans have not been specific or sensitive enough to be routinely utilized for pheochromocytoma diagnosis [48, 84].

Annual biochemical screening and CT is done to exclude development of pheochromocytoma in patients with MEN 2. Unrecognized pheochromocytomas may cause significant morbidity and mortality during surgical procedures or pregnancy, and should

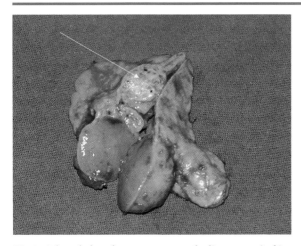

Fig. 2. Adrenal pheochromocytoma and adjacent cortical incidentaloma (*arrow*). The possible presence of incidental cortical tumors emphasizes the need for functional diagnosis of adrenal tumors

always be excluded prior to thyroidectomy for medullary thyroid carcinoma.

Due to increased detection by screening, ~50% or more of MEN-2 patients with pheochromocytoma have been found to be asymptomatic at the time of diagnosis. Patients with symptoms have had the common complaints of headache, palpitations, excessive sweating, and hypertension.

Surgical Treatment ▶ Prior to pheochromocytoma surgery MEN-2 patients need α-receptor blockade as do patients with sporadic disease. Pheochromocytomas in MEN 2 are currently generally removed by laparoscopy, with only the few large tumors needing open surgery [11, 12, 30, 85]. Megacolon in MEN-2B patients may be managed with open insertion of the laparoscope [12]. Bilateral tumors can be removed by bilateral laparoscopy, which is time-consuming because the patient's position has to be changed. This is probably associated with better patient comfort than open surgery via a subcostal incision, which can also be performed.

Since virtually all MEN-2 patients have bilateral nodular hyperplasia with a strong disposition for bilateral tumors, it has been controversial whether patients with unilateral tumors should be treated with routine bilateral adrenalectomy, or if unilateral adrenalectomy might be sufficient [12, 19, 50, 53, 58, 86, 87]. Most surgeons still support excision of the unilateral pheochromocytoma only, and will leave a macroscopically normal gland for careful follow-up [12, 50, 58, 86]. After unilateral adrenalectomy for pheochro-

mocytoma in MEN 2, the risk of recurrent contralateral pheochromocytoma has been 33% after 5 years, and 50% after 11 years, of follow-up [23, 50, 53, 57, 58, 66, 86]. The contralateral tumors have developed especially in patients where the size of the primary tumor exceeded 5 cm [86].

When bilateral adrenalectomy has been required the patients can be managed with glucocorticoid and mineralocorticoid replacement, combined with dehydroepiandrosterone in females, to prevent osteoporosis and improve well-being [1, 94]. The addisonian crisis is reported to develop in 25–33% of patients, and almost half of patients may feel handicapped despite adequate hormonal substitution [12, 50, 58].

In order to avoid adrenal insufficiency, efforts have been made to preserve adrenal function by partial "cortical-sparing" open adrenalectomy for familial pheochromocytomas [4, 51, 63, 66, 88]. In one series with long-term follow-up, recurrence was reported in 21% of patients, and all of these were MEN-2 patients [51]. Recently there has been increased interest in performing unilateral or even bilateral partial adrenalectomies by laparoscopy [4, 40, 51, 63, 92, 95]. These procedures can be aided by intraoperative ultrasound, but are rather time-consuming (average operative time for bilateral procedures 8 h), and more difficult and potentially hazardous with lesions larger than 4 cm [94]. Some authors avoid partial adrenalectomy in MEN-2 patients due to the general presence of medullary hyperplasia, and do this mainly in VHL patients (Fig. 2). Transplantation of adrenal cortex has been successful in isolated patients [39].

25.2.2 Von-Hippel Lindau Disease

Von Hippel-Lindau (VHL) disease is an autosomal dominant disorder where patients have central nervous system hemangioblastoma (cerebellar, cerebral and spinal), retinal angioma, renal cysts and renal carcinoma, endolymphatic sac tumors, neuroendocrine tumors and cysts of the pancreas, epididymal cystadenoma, and pheochromocytoma in varying combinations [21, 28, 29, 74]. The incidence has been estimated to 1/36,000 [54]. Patients have been classified as *VHL type 1 without pheochromocytoma, and VHL type 2 with pheochromocytoma*. Type 2A appears without renal carcinoma (and low frequency of hemangioblastoma and retinal angioma); type 2B patients have renal carcinoma (and high frequency of other manifestations), and type 2C patients have only pheochromocytoma [92]. Deaths have been due to complications of cerebellar hemangioblastoma, or metastatic clear cell renal carcinoma [29]. Retinal lesions may cause blindness due to retinal detachment or hemorrhage, but usually respond to treatment with laser or cryotherapy [29]. Pheochromocytomas have been found in 7–20% of VHL families, with a cumulative occurrence of 15% in VHL patients [4, 29]. VHL germ-line mutations may cause at least 10–20% of all pheochromocytomas, and many cases represent de novo mutations, where the VHL disease has not been recognized [21, 64].

Genetics ▶ The VHL gene located on chromosome 3p25–26 is a tumor suppressor gene. VHL type 1 families most often have larger deletions of the VHL gene, with a resulting non-functioning protein [74]. VHL type 2 families with pheochromocytoma often have missense mutations (92%), with a functioning VHL protein, which may be necessary for the development of pheochromocytoma [21, 46, 92]. Among mutation carriers in type 2 families there is a 60–80% risk of developing a pheochromocytoma. Missense mutations in codon 167 have been found in 33% of VHL patients with type 2 disease and pheochromocytoma [91].

VHL Pheochromocytoma ▶ Pheochromocytomas may be the first manifestation of VHL. The disease often presents in young patients (median age 28 years) and is a common cause of pheochromocytomas in children [29, 46, 72, 74, 91]. The pheochromocytomas are often small, multifocal and bilateral (50%) at the time of diagnosis [4, 29, 46, 72, 94]. Extra-adrenal pheochromocytomas occur in 12%, most of them abdominal, but rare thoracic, neck and middle ear paragangliomas have also been reported [65, 91]. Thus, multifocal tumors can be expected in >60% of VHL patients. Malignant pheochromocytomas have been encountered in 3%, the risk being higher with large tumors (>5 cm). Occasional patients present with metastatic malignant disease (personal observation).

Many VHL pheochromocytomas are small and functionally inactive, and patients are often normotensive and asymptomatic, especially when detected by screening [4, 29, 72, 91, 94]. They still constitute a serious threat because a sudden release of catecholamines may occur during surgery or pregnancy and cause unexpected death [4, 35]. *VHL pheochromocytomas mainly release norepinephrine, indicating a biochemical noradrenergic phenotype* [47].

Recommendations from the National Institute of Health infer that lifelong monitoring of all VHL patients, apart from ophthalmologic examination and MRI of brain and spine, should include screening for pheochromocytoma [29]. This may be done by determination of urinary catecholamines (or plasma metanephrines), and abdominal CT (or ultrasound in young individuals) every 1–2 years. Screening for pheochromocytoma should begin at the earliest reported age of diagnosis, which has been 4 years [91]. A large proportion of VHL patients (35%) with smaller pheochromocytomas initially have normal urinary catecholamines [4, 24]. Plasma metanephrines may be better for screening and have demonstrated a 97% sensitivity [4, 24, 91]. MIBG may be negative in 40% of VHL pheochromocytomas, and functional diagnosis may be efficiently made by [^{11}C]-hydroxyephedrine PET [73].

Surgical Treatment ▶ When evaluating VHL patients for surgery it is important to ensure that other VHL manifestations are correctly treated. VHL patients may have pheochromocytomas and concomitant extra-adrenal paraganglioma, and also renal carcinoma and endocrine pancreatic tumors (most likely non-functioning).

Small, apparently non-functioning and slow growing VHL pheochromocytomas may be followed without surgery, if urinary catecholamines and plasma metanephrines are normal [91, 93]. Surgery is recommended for larger (>2 cm) and symptomatic tumors, but should also be considered when other surgery is indicated or pregnancy planned. Prior to surgery the patients should be treated with α-blockade as in other pheochromocytoma patients.

Laparoscopic removal is recommended for both unilateral and bilateral tumors. After unilateral adrenalectomy new pheochromocytomas have developed in the remaining adrenal gland in 19–33% of patients after a median of 4 years [94]. Laparoscopic partial adrenalectomy has been advocated and half to one-third of one adrenal has appeared sufficient to avoid corticoid replacement therapy [4, 39, 40, 92, 94, 95]. Partial adrenalectomy may be especially well suited for VHL pheochromocytoma, since VHL patients generally lack adrenal medullary hyperplasia [4, 47] (Fig. 3). Ultrasound is of value to help localize a tumor [94]. The right adrenal tail contains little medullary tissue, and the risk of recurrence in a remnant in this location is most likely limited [94]. Partial adrenalectomy is recommended mainly for smaller tumors (2–3 cm in diameter) or those located at one end of the adrenal gland. Larger tumors (>4 cm) may cause distortion and make partial adrenalectomy more difficult, and are associated with increased risk of recur-

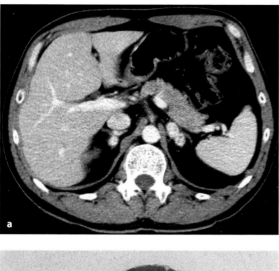
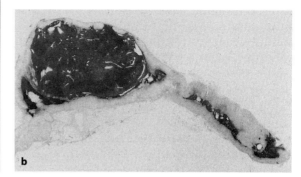
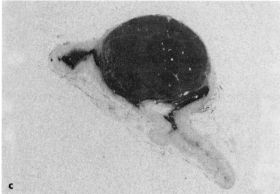
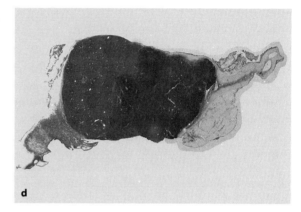

Fig. 3. a CT image of bilateral and multifocal pheochromocytomas in a VHL patient, one tumor in the left and two in the right adrenal. Histopathological examination revealed one left (**b**) and two right-sided pheochromocytomas (**c, d**), without signs of adrenal medullary hyperplasia (**b, c** and **d** represent chromogranin-stained rearranged operative specimens). The adrenal medulla in VHL patients is typically normal or atrophic

rence [94]. Recurrence can be expected after partial resection, but generally with a long delay; repeat surgery is then indicated [4].

25.2.3   Neurofibromatosis

Neurofibromatosis or von Recklinghausen's disease is characterized by multiple café-au-lait spots appearing early in life, multiple subcutaneous or cutaneous neurofibromas, optic gliomata, iris hamartomas (LISCH nodules), and specific dysplastic bone lesions (sphenoid dysplasia, pseudarthrosis, or scoliosis) [27, 46, 93]. The patients may develop sarcomatoid degeneration of neurofibromas (rhabdomyosarcoma), malignant peripheral nerve sheet tumors, and brain tumors.

Neurofibromatosis occurs in families without acoustic neuromas (neurofibromatosis type 1, NF1), and those with acoustic neuromas (neurofibromatosis

type 2, NF2). NF1 affects 1/4,000 individuals, and is the most common familial cancer syndrome with predisposition to pheochromocytoma [46]. However, the risk of pheochromocytoma is low in NF1, about 2% [46, 93]. In autopsy series the prevalence of pheochromocytomas has been 3–13% [93]. Pheochromocytomas are not part of NF2, for which the gene has been located to chromosome 22 [71, 93]. NF1 patients may suffer from macrocephaly, height retardation, and cognitive disorders [32]. They may also present with duodenal carcinoid tumors (often in the papilla of Vater), with positive staining for somatostatin, and they may have combinations of such carcinoid tumors and pheochromocytoma [42, 93, 96]. NF1 patients have also had the occasional co-occurrence with thyroid carcinoma [14, 60, 93].

Genetics ▶ NF1 is an autosomal dominant trait with variable expression, and 50% of patients represent new mutations [46]. The *NF1* gene is a tumor suppressor gene mapped to chromosome 17q11.2 [46]. Because of the large gene size mutation analysis has been difficult, although recent reports have indicated that 70% of NF1 patients have truncation mutations [69]. The gene product, neurofibromin, has homology with guanosine triphosphatase (GTPase)-activating proteins, involved in regulation of *ras* oncoproteins [46]. NF1 accounts for more than 90% of cases with neurofibromatosis. As many as 30–50% of NF1 patients represent new germ-line mutations and have no family history of neurofibromatosis [46,93]. Specific mutations associated with pheochromocytoma have not been identified in NF1.

Pheochromocytomas ▶ Pheochromocytomas in NF1 occur at a later age than in MEN 2 and VHL, with a mean age at diagnosis of around 50 years, and seldom occur before 20 years of age [46]. *The NFI pheochromocytomas are mainly norepinephrine secreting.* Approximately 10% of NF1 patients with pheochromocytoma have multiple or bilateral tumors [93]. Extra-adrenal pheochromocytomas are rare in NF1 (6%). Malignant pheochromocytomas, with metastases to liver, lung, and bone, have been reported in 12%. Mixed pheochromocytoma and ganglioneuroma, ganglioneuroblastoma, and neuroblastoma may also occur [93].

Clinical Features/Treatment ▶ NF1 has been associated with high incidence of spontaneous abortions [93]. Undiagnosed pheochromocytomas in NF1 patients during pregnancy have caused high fetal and maternal mortality, and patients should be evaluated for pheochromocytoma before pregnancy is planned [93]. Neurofibromatosis may be challenging for the anesthesiologist due to facial deformity or presence of neurofibromas obstructing the airway, and possible adverse reactions to neuromuscular blockade. The treatment is surgical as for other pheochromocytomas.

25.3   Hereditary Extra-adrenal Paraganglioma

Paragangliomas are rare tumors of the parasympathetic system composed of neural crest-derived chief cells. Tumors of the head and neck region occur most often in the carotid bodies, which sense hypoxia and may stimulate increase in heart rate and ventilation [5]. Other locations include the jugular, vagal, tym-panic, and mediastinal paraganglia. Both parasympathetic paraganglioma and sympathetic, extra-adrenal pheochromocytomas may occur around the abdominal aorta, mainly in the upper abdomen, and in the organ of Zuckerkandel at the aortic bifurcation. Paragangliomas are thought to be hereditary in 50% of cases, with an autosomal predisposition for the development of tumors mainly in other parasympathetic ganglia [7, 9]. Some families may develop tumors in sympathetic paraganglia, as extra-adrenal pheochromocytoma, and some families have combinations of these two entities, and adrenal pheochromocytomas.

Genetics ▶ The enzyme complex succinate dehydrogenase (SDH) is part of the mitochondrial complex II with an important role in the mitochondrial respiratory chain. Proteins SDHA and SDHB form the catalytic core of the enzyme complex, while SDHD and SDHC form to anchor complex II to the inner mitochondrial membrane [20,65]. The mitochondrial complex is thought to play a role in the oxygen sensing of the carotid body. Germ-line mutations in the mitochondrial complex II genes, *SDHD* at chromosome 11q23, *SDHB* at chromosome 1p36, and *SDHC* at chromosome 1q21–23, are reported to cause hereditary paraganglioma (PGL) [2, 5, 9, 20, 46, 65, 67, 79]. *SDHD* gene mutations (PGL1) are revealed in a majority (50%) of families with hereditary head and neck parasympathetic paraganglioma, and in one family with both parasympathetic and sympathetic paraganglioma. *SDHD* acts as a tumor suppressor gene, and in PGL1 families the disease is expressed only with mutation transmitted by the father, indicating imprinting of the maternal gene. Germ-line *SDHB* mutations (PGL2) are reported in 20% of families with head and neck paragangliomas [5]. *SDHB* mutations are more common in families with adrenal or extra-adrenal sympathetic paragangliomas, with or without parasympathetic paragangliomas (Fig. 4). Both maternal and paternal imprinting has been demonstrated for SDHB mutations [9]. In some families the SDHB positive parent had not presented with disease although the proband had manifested disease at an early age, indicating a variably penetrant gene. It is claimed to be important to test for *SDHB* mutations in patients with pheochromocytoma, with or without associated paragangliomas, especially in families where the proband is young and no parent has evidence of disease [9]. Co-occurrence of head and neck or extra-adrenal paraganglioma or pheochromocytomas, in the same person or other family members, indicates germ-line mutations in mitochondrial complex II genes. Germ-line

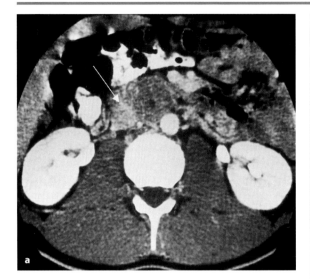

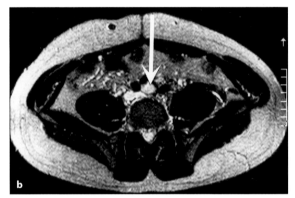

Fig. 4. a CT image of a large pheochromocytoma growing around the abdominal vena cava and aorta (*arrow*) in a 14-year-old boy with severe hypertension and norepinephrine excess. The tumor was removed with the vena cava below the renal veins, without aortic resection. b Recurrence occurred after 7 years with a Zuckerkandel extra-adrenal pheochromocytoma below the aortic bifurcation (again norepinephrine excess) displayed in an MRI image (*arrow*). This tumor was successfully removed. The patient's mother had a history of adrenal pheochromocytoma and pharyngeal paraganglioma. Mutation in the *SDHB* gene was identified in this family [3, 79]

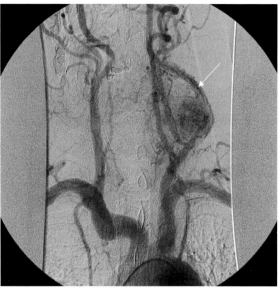

Fig. 5. Angiographic image of carotid body tumor in a patient with a previous operation for pheochromocytoma, with typical vascular supply from the external carotid artery (*arrow*). The patient has high risk for *SDHB* mutation and will be subjected to genetic investigation

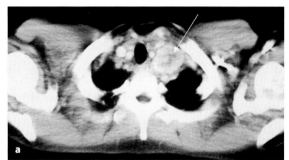

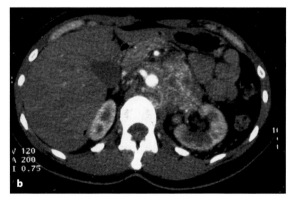

Fig. 6. a Patient with cervical paraganglioma (*arrow*) at the origin of the vertebral artery, which was resected. b The patient had concomitant extra-adrenal paraganglioma involving part of the left kidney and growing around the abdominal aorta. Removal of the tumor required resection of the abdominal aorta and multiple separate grafts to major abdominal arteries

SDHC gene mutations (PGL3) have been revealed in one family [5].

Paragangliomas should be surgically resected if possible. The most common carotid body paraganglioma generally does not involve the internal carotid artery (Fig. 5). Larger paragangliomas, especially in the abdomen, may be locally invasive and require extensive surgery for removal (Fig. 6).

25.4　Hereditary Cortical Tumor Syndromes

25.4.1　Multiple Endocrine Neoplasia Type 1

Adrenocortical lesions are overrepresented in MEN 1 patients (36–41%), and the majority are bilateral, non-functioning adrenal cortical hyperplasia, or adenoma [13, 77, 78]. Adrenocortical carcinoma is exceedingly rare [13, 78]. The adrenocortical lesions in MEN 1 are probably not due to menin gene mutations [78]. They seem to occur especially in patients with endocrine pancreatic tumors, and are hypothetically thought to be due to the influence of locally secreted insulin and insulin-like growth factors [78]. The lesions need to be removed for malignancy prevention if there is obvious growth, or if the tumor diameter exceeds 3 cm.

25.4.2　Carney Complex

The Carney complex (CNC) was first reported in 1985. CNC is described as a form of multiple endocrine hyperplasia, with tumors of two or more endocrine glands, including primary pigmented adrenocortical disease (PPNAD), GH- and prolactin-producing pituitary adenomas, testicular neoplasms, thyroid adenoma or carcinoma, and ovarian cysts [81, 82].

A minority group of CNC patients presents during the first 2–3 years of life, but the majority in the 2nd or 3rd decade. Spotty skin pigmentations are the most common manifestation at the time of presentation, but are not invariably present. Pigmentations include blue nevi and café-au-lait spots, which may be seen on the border of the lips, the conjunctiva, and on the vaginal and penile mucosa. Heart myxomas may occur at a young age; other myxomas with predilection for eyelids, nipple, and external ear canals may also be identified in infancy. Mammary myxoid fibroadenomas may occur together with other myxoid changes. Cushing's syndrome is the most common endocrine manifestation, and is characterized by an atypical, asthenic rather than obese body habitus, and sometimes a periodic Cushing's syndrome. Cushing's syndrome is always caused by PPNAD, which typically consists of multiple, small, pigmented nodules, and typical atrophy between nodules. Acromegaly may occur in 10% of patients, being due to a GH-secreting pituitary adenoma. Testicular tumors can be of different types, and occur in half of affected males; testicular microcalcifications can be visualized by ultrasound in every adult male patient. Thyroid nodules may be seen by ultra-sound in 75% of patients; most represent follicular adenomas, and occasional patients may have follicular thyroid carcinoma.

Genetics ▶ Half of CNC cases are familial [81, 82]. The syndrome is autosomal dominant, but transmission most often occurs with a female affected parent. Two genetic loci have been identified in CNC families. One locus is found at chromosome 2p16, where the gene is not yet identified [83]. Several other CNC families have mapped to another locus at chromosome17q22–24. At this locus the *PRKARIA* gene coding for a regulatory subunit of protein kinase A is identified as a tumor suppressor gene responsible for development of the disease [45].

Clinical and biochemical screening is recommended for the diagnosis of CNC. Testing for *PRKARIA* mutations is not presently recommended for patients with CNC, but is suggested for patients from families with known mutations, to avoid medical surveillance of non-carriers [82].

25.4.3　Beckwith-Wiedemann Syndrome

The Beckwith-Wiedemann syndrome (BWS) is a rare disease characterized by macroglossy, earlobe pits or creases, abdominal wall defects, gigantism, and with increased risk of benign or malignant tumors of multiple organs [8, 36, 97]. Most common is Wilms' tumors of the kidney, rhabdomyosarcoma, hepatoblastoma, and adrenal carcinoma. Most BWS cases are sporadic; families exist with an autosomal dominant trait with incomplete penetrance. BWS maps to chromosome11p15.5, and uniparental paternal isodisomi for this locus including the IGFII gene have been identified in affected individuals [36]. Complete loss of one IGFII allele and a duplication of the remaining allele in association with IGFII overexpression are demonstrated in tumors of the BWS.

25.4.4　Li-Fraumeni Syndrome

The Li-Fraumeni syndrome is a rare, autosomal, dominant familial syndrome with high incidence of multiple malignancies at an early age, including breast cancer, leukemias, soft tissue sarcomas, gliomas, laryngeal carcinoma, lung cancer and adrenocortical carcinoma [52, 55]. Affected patients often develop the first tumor before the age of 30 years, and new neoplasms are often encountered especially in patients treated with chemotherapy or irradiation [55]. The disease is due to germ-line point mutations in the p53 tumor suppressor gene, situated at chromosome 17p13 [80]. The second allele is inactivated in tumors by deletion of the short arm of chromosome 17 (17p). p53 germ-line mutations are found in children with adrenocortical carcinoma without the classical family history of the Li-Fraumeni syndrome [89]. It has been recommended that genetic testing for *p53* mutations should be undertaken in all children with adrenal cancer; and that also the relatives should be tested.

25.4.5   Familial Adenomatous Polyposis

Familial adenomatous polyposis (FAP) is an autosomal dominant disorder with multiple adenomatous polyps of the colon and rectum, which can undergo malignant change [46]. The adenomatous polyposis coli (APC) gene is located at 5q21. Spontaneous germ-line mutations are common. Somatic APC mutations are seen in many other human carcinomas. Patients with FAP develop various extracolonic manifestations, including adrenocortical adenomas and carcinomas and with an apparent higher incidence than in normal individuals [56]. The incidence of adrenal incidentaloma thus appears to be increased, 7.4% compared to 0.6–3.4% reported for a normal population.

References

1. Arlt W, Callies F, van Vlijmen JC, et al. (1999) Dehydroepiandrosterone replacement in women with adrenal insufficiency. N Engl J Med 341:1013–1020
2. Astuti D, Douglas F, Lennard TWJ, et al. (2001) Germline SDHD mutation in familial phaeochromocytoma. Lancet 357:1181–1182
3. Astuti D, Latif F, Dallol A, et al. (2001) Gene mutations in the succinate dehydrogenase subunit SDHB cause susceptibility to familial pheochromocytoma and to familial paraganglioma. Am J Hum Genet 69:49–54
4. Baghai M, Thompson GB, Young WF, et al. (2002) Pheochromocytomas and paragangliomas in von Hippel-Lindau disease. A role for laparoscopic and cortical-sparing surgery. Arch Surg 137:682–689
5. Baysal BE (2002) Hereditary paraganglioma targets diverse paraganglia. J Med Genet 39:617–622
6. Baysal BE, Ferrell RE, Willett-Brozick JE, et al. (2000) Mutations in SDHD, a mitochondrial complex II gene in hereditary paraganglioma. Science 287:848–851
7. Baysal BE, Rubinstein WS, Taschner PEM (2001) Phenotypic dichotomy in mitochondrial complex II genetic disorders. J Mol Med 79:495–503
8. Beckwith JB (1969) Macroglossia, omphalocoele, adrenal cytomegaly, gigantism and hyperplastic visceromegaly. Birth Defects 5:188–196
9. Benn DE, Croxson MS, Tucker K, et al. (2003) Novel succinate dehydrogenase subunit B (SDHB) mutations in familial phaeochromocytomas and paragangliomas, but an absence of somatic SDHB mutations in sporadic phaeochromocytomas. Oncogene 22:1358–1364
10. Brauch H, Hoppner W, Jahnig H, et al. (1997) Sporadic pheochromocytomas are rarely associated with germline mutations in the VHL tumor suppressor gene or the RET protooncogene. J Clin Endocrinol Metab 82:4101–4104
11. Brunt LM, Doherty GM, Norton JA, et al. (1996) Laparoscopic adrenalectomy compared to open adrenalectomy for benign adrenal neoplasms. J Am Coll Surg 183:1–10
12. Brunt LM, Lairmore TC, Doherty GM, et al. (2001) Adrenalectomy for familial pheochromocytoma in the laparoscopic era. Ann Surg 235:713–721
13. Burgess JR, Harle RA, Tucker P, et al. (1996) Adrenal lesions in a large kindred with multiple endocrine neoplasia type 1. Arch Surg 131:699–702
14. Burke AP, Sobin LH, Shekitka KM, et al. (1990) Somatostatin-producing duodenal carcinoids in patients with von Recklinghausen's neurofibromatosis. A predilection for black patients. Cancer 65:1591–1595
15. Cance WG, Wells SA Jr (1985) Multiple endocrine neoplasia type IIa. Curr Probl Surg 22:1–56
16. Carlson KM, Dou S, Chi D, et al. (1994) Single missense mutation in the tyrosine kinase catalytic domain of the RET protooncogene is associated with multiple endocrine neoplasia type 2B. Proc Natl Acad Sci USA 91:1579–1583
17. Carney JA, Sizemore GW, Sheps SG (1976) Adrenal medullary disease in multiple endocrine neoplasia type 2: pheochromocytoma and its precursors. Am J Clin Pathol 66:279–290
18. Carney JA, Sizemore GW, Tyce GM (1975) Bilateral adrenal medullary hyperplasia in multiple endocrine neoplasia, type 2: the precursor of bilateral pheochromocytoma. Mayo Clin Proc 50:3–10
19. Casanova S, Rosenberg-Bourgin M, Farkas D, et al. (1993) Phaeochromocytoma in multiple endocrine neoplasia type 2A: survey of 100 cases. Clin Endocrinol 38:531–537
20. Chew SL (2001) Paraganglioma genes. Clin Endocrinol 54:573–574
21. Couch V, Lindor NM, Karnes PS, et al. (2000) von Hippel-Lindau disease. Mayo Clin Proc 75:265–272
22. Donis-Keller H, Dou S, Chi D, et al. (1993) Mutations in the RET proto-oncogene are associated with MEN 2A and FMTC. Hum Mol Genet 2:851–856
23. Easton DF, Ponder MA, Cummings T, et al. (1989) The clinical and screening age-at-onset distribution for the MEN-2 syndrome. Am J Hum Genet 44:208–215
24. Eisenhofer G, Lenders JW, Linehan WM, et al. (1999) Plasma normetanephrine and metanephrine for detecting pheochromocytoma in von Hippel-Lindau disease and multiple endocrine neoplasia type 2. N Engl J Med 340:1872–1879

25. Eng C, Crossey PA, Mulligan LM, et al. (1995) Mutations in the RET proto-oncogene and the von Hippel-Lindau disease tumor suppressor gene in sporadic and syndromic pheochromocytomas. J Med Genet 32:934–937

26. Farndon JR, Leight GS, Dilley WG, et al. (1986) Familial medullary thyroid carcinoma without associated endocrinopathies: a distinct clinical entity. Br J Surg 73:278–281

27. Friedman JM, Birch PH (1997) Type 1 neurofibromatosis: a descriptive analysis of the disorder in 1,728 patients. Am J Med Genet 70:138–143

28. Friedrich CA (1999) Von Hippel-Lindau syndrome. A pleomorphic condition. Cancer 86:2478–2482

29. Friedrich CA (2001) Genotype-phenotype correlation in von Hippel-Lindau syndrome. Hum Mol Genet 10:763–767

30. Gagner M, Lacroix A, Bolte E (1992) Laparoscopic adrenalectomy in Cushing's syndrome and pheochromocytoma. N Engl J Med 327:1033

31. Gimm O, Armanios M, Dziema H, et al. (2000) Somatic and occult germline mutations in SDHD, a mitochondrial complex II gene, in nonfamilial pheochromocytoma. Cancer Res 60:6822–6825

32. Gutmann DH, Aylsworth A, Carey JC, et al. (1997) The diagnostic evaluation and multidisciplinary management of neurofibromatosis 1 and neurofibromatosis 2. JAMA 278:51–57

33. Hamilton BP, Landsberg L, Levine RJ (1978) Measurement of urinary epinephrine in screening for pheochromocytoma in multiple endocrine neoplasia type II. Am J Med 65:1027–1032

34. Hansford JR, Mulligan LM (2000) Multiple endocrine neoplasia type 2 (MEN 2) and RET: from neoplasia to neurogenesis. J Med Genet 37:817–827

35. Harrington JL, Farley DR, van Heerden JA, et al. (1999) Adrenal tumors and pregnancy. World J Surg 23:182–186

36. Henry I, Bonaiti-Pellie C, Chehensse V, et al. (1991) Uniparental paternal disomy in a genetic cancer-predisposing syndrome. Nature 351:665–667

37. Hofstra RM, Landsvater RM, Ceccherini I, et al. (1994) A mutation in the RET proto-oncogene associated with multiple endocrine neoplasia type 2B and sporadic medullary thyroid carcinoma. Nature 367:375–376

38. Howe JR, Norton JA, Wells SA Jr (1993) Prevalence of pheochromocytoma and hyperparathyroidism in multiple endocrine neoplasia type 2A: results of long-term follow-up. Surgery 114:1070–1077

39. Inabnet W, Caragliano P, Pertsemlidis D (2000) Pheochromocytoma: inherited associations, bilaterality, and cortex preservation. Surgery 128:1007–1012

40. Janetschek G, Finkenstedt G, Gasser R, et al. (1998) Laparoscopic partial adrenalectomy in patients with hereditary forms of pheochromocytoma. J Urol 164:14–17

41. Jhiang SM (2000) The RET protooncogene in human cancers. Oncogene 19:5590–5597

42. Kapur BM, Sarin SK, Anand CS, et al. (1983) Carcinoid tumour of ampulla of Vater associated with viscero-cutaneous neurofibromatosis. Postgrad Med 59:734–735

43. Khan TS, Sundin A, Juhlin C, et al. (2003) 11C-metomidate PET imaging of adrenocortical cancer. Eur J Nucl Med Mol Imaging 30:403–410

44. Kikumori T, Evans D, Lee JE, et al. (2001) Genetic abnormalities in multiple endocrine neoplasia type 2. In: Doherty GM, Skogseid B (eds) Surgical endocrinology. Lippincott Williams & Wilkins, Philadelphia, pp 531–540

45. Kirschner LS, Carney JA, Pack SD, et al. (2000) Mutations of the gene encoding the protein kinase A type I-alpha regulatory subunit in patients with the Carney complex. Nat Genet 26:89–92

46. Koch CA, Vortmeyer AO, Huang SC, et al. (2001) Genetic aspects of pheochromocytoma. Endocr Regul 35:43–52

47. Koch C, Mauro D, McClellan MW, et al. (2002) Pheochromocytoma in von Hippel-Lindau disease: distinct histopathologic phenotype compared to pheochromocytoma in multiple endocrine neoplasia type 2. Endocrine Pathol 13:17–27

48. Kopf D, Bockisch A, Steinert H, et al. (1997) Octreotide scintigraphy and catecholamine response to an octreotide challenge in malignant phaeochromocytoma. Clin Endocrinol 46:39–44

49. Korf BR (2000) Malignancy in neurofibromatosis type 1. The Oncologist 5:477–485

50. Lairmore TC, Ball DW, Baylin SB, et al. (1993) Management of pheochromocytomas in patients with multiple endocrine neoplasia type 2 syndromes. Ann Surg 217:595–603

51. Lee JE, Curley SA, Gagel RF, et al. (1996) Cortical-sparing adrenalectomy for patients with bilateral pheochromocytoma. Surgery 120:1064–1071

52. Li FP, Fraumeni JF (1969) Soft-tissue sarcomas, breast cancer, and other neoplasms: a familial syndrome? Ann Int Med 71:747–752

53. Lips KJ, Van der Sluys Veer J, Struyvenberg A, et al. (1981) Bilateral occurrence of pheochromocytoma in patients with the multiple endocrine neoplasia syndrome type 2A (Sipple's syndrome). Am J Med 70:1051–1060

54. Maher ER, Iselius L, Yates JR, et al. (1991) Von Hippel-Lindau disease: a genetic study. J Med Genet 28:443–447

55. Malkin D, Jolly KW, Barbier N, et al. (1992) Germline mutations of the p53 tumor-suppressor gene in children and young adults with second malignant neoplasms. N Engl J Med 326:1309–1315

56. Marchesa P, Fazio VW, Church JM, et al. (1997) Adrenal masses in patients with familial adenomatous polyposis. Dis Colon Rectum 40:1023–1028

57. Modigliani E, Vasen HM, Raue K, et al. (1995) Pheochromocytoma in multiple endocrine neoplasia type 2: European study. J Internal Med 238:363–367

58. Moley JF, Albinson C (2001) Medullary thyroid carcinoma and the multiple endocrine neoplasia type 2 syndromes. In: Doherty GM, Skogseid B (eds) Surgical endocrinology. Lippincott Williams & Wilkins, Philadelphia, pp 541–557

59. Mulligan LM, Kwok JB, Healey CS, et al. (1993) Germ-line mutations of the RET proto-oncogene in multiple endocrine neoplasia type 2A. Nature 363:458–460

60. Nakamura H, Koga M, Higa S, et al. (1987) A case of von Recklinghausen's disease associated with pheochromocytoma and papillary carcinoma of the thyroid gland. Endocrinol Jpn 34:545–551

61. Neumann HPH, Berger DP, Sigmund G, et al. (1993) Pheochromocytomas, multiple endocrine neoplasia type 2, and von Hippel-Lindau disease. N Engl J Med 329:1531–1538. [Erratum (1994) N Engl J Med 331:1535]

62. Neumann HPH, Eng C, Mulligan LM, et al. (1995) Consequences of direct genetic testing for germline mutations in the clinical management of families with multiple endocrine neoplasia type 2. JAMA 274:1149–1151

63. Neumann HPH, Bender BU, Reincke M, et al. (1999) Adrenal-sparing surgery for phaeochromocytoma. Br J Surg 86:94–97

64. Neumann HPH, Bausch B, McWhinney SR, et al. (2002) Germ-line mutations in nonsyndromic pheochromocytoma. N Engl J Med 346:1459–1466

65. Neumann HPH, Hoegerle S, Manz T, et al. (2002) How many pathways to pheochromocytoma? Semin Nephrol 22:89–99

66. Nguyen L, Niccoli-Sire P, Caron P, et al. (2001) Pheochromocytoma in multiple endocrine neoplasia type 2: a prospective study. Eur J Endocrinol 144:37–44

67. Niemann S, Müller U (2000) Mutations in SDHC cause autosomal dominant paraganglioma, type 3. Nat Genet 26:268–270

68. O'Riordain DS, O'Brien T, Crotty TB, et al. (1995) Multiple endocrine neoplasia type 2B: more than an endocrine disorder. Surgery 118:936–942

69. Park VM, Pivnick EK (1998) Neurofibromatosis type 1 (NF1): A protein truncation assay yielding identification of mutations in 73% of patients. J Med Genet 35:813–820

70. Pomares FJ, Canas R, Rodriguez JM, et al. (1998) Differences between sporadic and multiple endocrine neoplasia type 2A phaeochromocytoma. Clin Endocrinol 48:195–200

71. Ponder BA (1992) Neurofibromatosis: from gene to phenotype. Semin Cancer Biol 3:115–120

72. Richard S, Beigelman C, Duclos JM, et al. (1994) Pheochromocytoma as the first manifestation of von Hippel-Lindau disease. Surgery 116:1076–1081

73. Shulkin BL, Wieland DM, Schwaiger M, et al. (1992) PET scanning with hydroxyephedrine: an approach to the localization of pheochromocytoma. J Nucl Med 33:1125–1131

74. Sims KB (2001) Von Hippel-Lindau disease: gene to bedside. Curr Opin Neurol 14:695–703

75. Sipple JH (1961) The association of pheochromocytoma with carcinoma of the thyroid gland. Am J Med 31:163–166

76. Sisson JC, Frager MS, Valk TW, et al. (1981) Scintigraphic localization of pheochromocytoma. N Engl J Med 305:12–17

77. Skogseid B, Larsson C, Lindgren PG, et al. (1992) Clinical and genetic features of adrenocortical lesions in multiple endocrine neoplasia type 1. J Clin Endocrinol Metab 75:76–81

78. Skogseid B, Rastad J, Gobl A, et al. (1995) Adrenal lesion in multiple endocrine neoplasia type 1. Surgery 118:1077–1082

79. Sköldberg F, Grimelius L, Woodward ER, et al. (1998) A family with hereditary extra-adrenal paragangliomas without evidence for mutations in the von Hippel-Lindau disease or ret genes. Clin Endocrinol 48:11–16

80. Srivastava S, Zou Z, Pirollo K, et al. (1990) Germ-line transmission of a mutated p53 gene in a cancer-prone family with Li-Fraumeni syndrome. Nature 348:747–749

81. Stratakis CA (2001) Clinical genetics of multiple endocrine neoplasias, Carney complex and related syndromes. J Endocrinol Invest 24:370–383

82. Stratakis CA, Kirschner LS, Carney JA (2001) Genetics of endocrine disease. Clinical and molecular features of the Carney complex: diagnostic criteria and recommendations for patient evaluation. J Clin Endocrinol Metab 86:4041–4046

83. Taymans SE, Macrae CA, Casey M, et al. (1997) A refined genetic, radiation hybrid, and physical map of the Carney complex (CNC) locus on chromosome 2p16; evidence for genetic heterogeneity in the syndrome. Am J Hum Genet 61 Suppl:A84

84. Tenenbaum F, Lumbroso J, Schlumberger M, et al. (1995) Comparison of radiolabeled octreotide and meta-iodobenzylguanidine (MIBG) scintigraphy in malignant pheochromocytoma. J Nucl Med 36:1–6

85. Thompson GB, Grant CS, van Heerden JA, et al. (1997) Laparoscopic versus open posterior adrenalectomy: a case-control study of 100 patients. Surgery 122:1132–1136

86. Tibblin S, Dymling JF, Ingemansson S, et al. (1983) Unilateral versus bilateral adrenalectomy in multiple endocrine neoplasia IIA. World J Surg 7:201–208

87. van Heerden JA, Sizemore GW, Carney JA, et al. (1984) Surgical management of the adrenal glands in the multiple endocrine neoplasia type II syndrome. World J Surg 8:612–621

88. van Heerden JA, Sizemore GW, Carney JA, et al. (1985) Bilateral subtotal adrenal resection for bilateral pheochromocytomas in multiple endocrine neoplasia, type IIa: a case report. Surgery 98:363–365

89. Wagner J, Portwine C, Rabin K, et al. (1994) High frequency of germline p53 mutations in childhood adrenocortical cancer. J Natl Cancer Inst 86:1707–1710

90. Walther MM, Herring J, Enquist E, et al. (1999) Von Recklinghausen's disease and pheochromocytomas. J Urol 162:1582–1586

91. Walther MM, Reiter R, Keiser HR, et al. (1999) Clinical and genetic characterization of pheochromocytoma in von Hippel-Lindau families: comparison with sporadic pheochromocytoma gives insight into natural history of pheochromocytoma. J Urol 162:659–664

92. Walther MM, Herring J, Choyke PL, et al. (2000) Laparoscopic partial adrenalectomy in patients with hereditary forms of pheochromocytoma. J Urol 164:14–17

93. Walther MM, Linehan WM, Libutti SK (2001) von Hippel-Lindau disease and von Recklinghausen's disease. In: Doherty GM, Skogseid B (eds) Surgical endocrinology. Lippincott Williams & Wilkins, Philadelphia, pp 581–591

94. Walther MM (2002) New therapeutic and surgical approaches for sporadic and hereditary pheochromocytoma. Ann N Y Acad Sci 970:41–53

95. Walz MK, Peitgen K, Saller B, et al. (1998) Subtotal adrenalectomy by the posterior retroperitoneoscopic approach. World J Surg 22:621–627

96. Wheeler MH, Curley IR, Williams ED (1986) The association of neurofibromatosis, pheochromocytoma, and somatostatin-rich duodenal carcinoid tumor. Surgery 100:1163–1169

97. Wiedemann HR (1964) Complex malformatif familial avec hernie ombilicale et macroglossie – un syndrome nouveau? J Genet Hum 13:223–232

26 Adrenal Tumors and Pregnancy

M. Nicole Lamb, David R. Farley

CONTENTS

26.1 Introduction

Adrenal tumors identified during pregnancy are extraordinarily rare. While incidentalomas (adrenalomas) are commonly identified with abdominal computed tomography (CT) imaging (1–4%) or autopsy (5–17%), pregnant women should undergo neither CT scanning nor autopsy! [8]. Therefore, identifying those rare, functioning adrenal tumors during pregnancy is uncommon. The most widely reported of this unique combination is with pheochromocytomas. Its prevalence in full-term pregnancies is 1/50,000–54,000 [12]. Other adrenal tumors found during pregnancy are even more unusual; in fact, the English medical literature uncovers only 18 pregnant women with aldosteronomas and 97 with cortisol producing tumors [11, 13]. Such rarity should not be surprising: uncovering inherently very rare retroperitoneal tumors that may affect weight gain, swelling, hypertension, headache, malaise, and the like during a 9-month gestational period in young women is difficult (Fig. 1). Clearly, to identify such rare lesions, one must have serendipity, a high index of suspicion, or the adrenal tumor must be "functional" (hormonally active).

At the Mayo Clinic in Rochester, Minnesota, only 4 cases of adrenal tumors were reported in 30,246 pregnant patients between 1975–1996 [5]. These four pa-

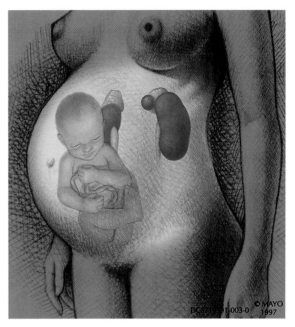

Fig. 1. The retroperitoneal location of the adrenal glands and the hormonal milieu of pregnancy make detection difficult

tients, plus a recent fifth case, showcase, and well represent, the rare patients surgeons may encounter and highlight truisms for their treatment.

Patient 1: A 36-year-old woman at 27 weeks' gestation (gravida 2, para 1) presented to the emergency room with intractable emesis and dyspnea. She suffered a myocardial infarction (Fig. 2) resulting in her death and that of her fetus. At autopsy an unsuspected right-sided pheochromocytoma measuring 13×10×10 cm was found. In retrospect, during her previous pregnancy she had experienced symptoms (palpitations, flushing, headache, and emesis) of catecholamine excess. Unfortunately most adrenal tumors will be masked by the "symptoms" of a normal pregnancy – and most adrenal tumors will, therefore, go undiagnosed.

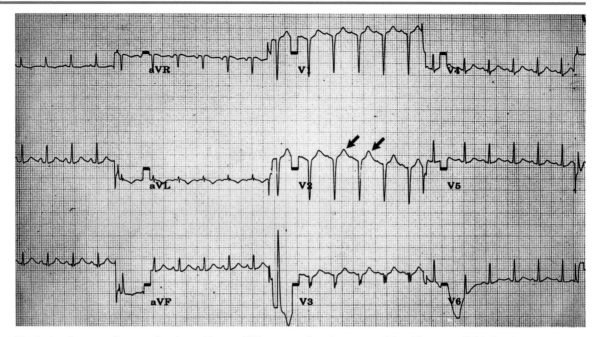

Fig. 2. An electrocardiogram showing evidence of ST segment elevation compatible with myocardial infarction

Truism #1 One needs a high index of suspicion to diagnose adrenal tumors!

Truism #2 Most pregnant women with symptomatic adrenal masses have pheochromocytomas.

Truism #3 Untreated pheochromocytomas are lethal.

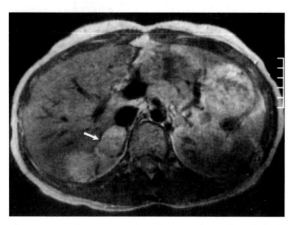

Fig. 3. Magnetic resonance imaging reveals a right-sided adrenal mass in a young woman with von Hippel-Lindau disease. (From Harrington et al. [5]. Reprinted with permission of Springer-Verlag)

Patient 2: A 29-year-old woman (gravida 2, para 1) with a family history of von Hippel-Lindau (vHL) disease was found to have a 3-cm right adrenal mass (Fig. 3), a 6-cm pancreatic mass, and an unsuspected pregnancy while undergoing routine screening for vHL disease. Early in the second trimester (17 weeks), she underwent an open right adrenalectomy, distal pancreatectomy, and an elective suction and curettage with bilateral tubal ligation. She died 3 years later due to metastatic pancreatic islet cell cancer.

Truism #4 Most adrenal tumors – whether in pregnant or non-pregnant patients – are found serendipitously.

Truism #5 Familial endocrine syndromes (multiple endocrine neoplasia [MEN], vHL, etc.) should lower thresholds to evaluate possible adrenal abnormalities.

Truism #6 If surgical intervention is advisable during pregnancy, the second trimester is best.

Patient 3: A 22-year-old woman (gravida 2, para 1) was seen at 12 weeks' gestation with increasing weakness and fatigue. Identification of hypertension and hypokalemia led to documentation of hyperaldosteronism and suppressed renin levels. An abdominal magnetic resonance imaging (MRI) study showed a 3×2×2-cm right-sided adrenal mass (Fig. 4). She had induced labor at 32 weeks' gestation for superimposed preeclampsia. The infant had respiratory distress syndrome for 15 days but eventually recovered. Two months postpartum the mother underwent a right-sided posterior adrenalectomy without complication.

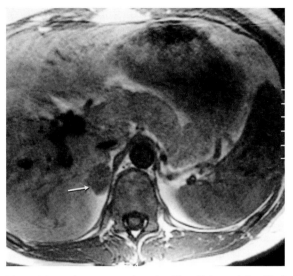

Fig. 4. Magnetic resonance imaging identifying a right-sided aldosteronoma. (From Harrington et al. [5]. Reprinted with permission of Springer-Verlag)

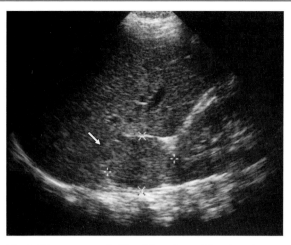

Fig. 6. Ultrasonography identifies a 6-cm right adrenal mass. (From Harrington et al. [5]. Reprinted with permission of Springer-Verlag)

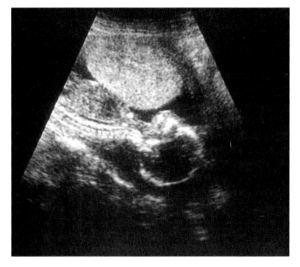

Fig. 5. Ultrasonography depicts a healthy fetus

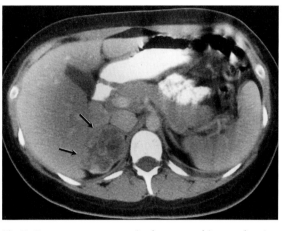

Fig. 7. Postpartum computerized tomographic scan showing a heterogeneous right adrenal mass

Truism #7 MRI is the best imaging modality to visualize adrenal glands during pregnancy.

Truism #8 Most adrenal masses found during pregnancy do not require immediate resection.

Truism #9 Functional adrenal tumors carry morbidity to the mother *and* the fetus.

Patient 4: A 21-year old woman (gravida 2, para 1) presented at 30 weeks' gestation complaining of intermittent right upper quadrant abdominal and back pain. Abdominal ultrasonography (US) revealed a healthy fetus (Fig. 5) and a 6×5×4-cm solid right-sided adrenal mass (Fig. 6). An exhaustive endocrine work-up found no laboratory abnormalities. The patient delivered a healthy baby at 39 weeks' gestation. A postpartum CT scan showed a heterogeneous mass (Fig. 7). The mass was resected laparoscopically and found to be a benign adrenal adenoma with central hemorrhage (Fig. 8).

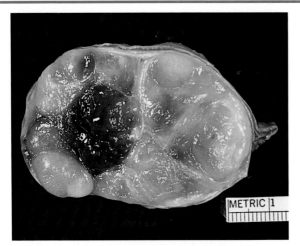

Fig. 8. Benign adrenal adenoma with central hemorrhage

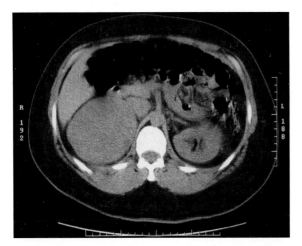

Fig. 9. Preoperative computerized tomographic scan showing what turned out to be an adrenal cortical cancer

Truism #10 Most adrenal masses are benign.
Truism #11 Laparoscopic adrenalectomy is the gold standard procedure for all patients unless hemodynamic instability or tumor size compromise surgical technique.
Truism #12 Laboratory testing during pregnancy is an inexact science.

Patient 5: A previously healthy 38-year-old woman developed difficulties during early pregnancy. Extended work-up led to identification of a large adrenal mass (Fig. 9). Concern for malignancy arose, surgical consultation was obtained, and an open adrenalectomy was performed. Histologic analysis revealed adrenal cortical carcinoma (ACC). The patient is fit and well now 9 months later.

Truism #13 Although rare, physicians must worry about adrenal masses being malignant.
Truism #14 Most adrenal masses occur in women.
Truism #15 Adrenalectomy is the only treatment for ACC.

26.2   Diagnosis and Risk

Early diagnosis and expedient treatment facilitate fetal and maternal survival in most pregnant patients with adrenal tumors. Unfortunately, in the undiagnosed mother with a pheochromocytoma, the mortality rate is 17–48% [12]. When the tumor is diagnosed in the antenatal period, maternal mortality rates are 2–4% [10]. Diagnosis intrapartum or after delivery carries a maternal mortality of 14–25% [10]. Diagnosis before delivery has a fetal mortality of 11–15%. In delayed diagnosis, fetal mortality is a staggering 26–54%. While it is important to diagnose adrenal abnormalities, the accuracy is clearly suboptimal in the pregnant patient. In fact, the sensitivity is 89% and specificity 67% for diagnosing pheochromocytomas in pregnancy [10].

The maternal mortality in undiagnosed pregnant women with cortisol-producing tumors with 5 years of follow-up is 50% [3]. The complications of being hypercortisolemic during pregnancy are hypertension (65%), superimposed preeclampsia (32%), diabetes (32%), congestive heart failure (11%), wound break down (8%), and death (5%). Although no comprehensive data exists for pregnancy and aldosteronomas, diagnosis and treatment of a cortisol- or catecholamine-producing tumor appears crucial to the survival of both the mother and the fetus.

There are several key signs and symptoms that should prompt further investigation of a possible functioning adrenal mass (especially when these features are present in the first trimester). One must remember that pheochromocytomas are, in fact, responsible for 1/200 cases of hypertension in all patients [2]. Even in pregnancy, pheochromocytoma is rarely associated with proteinuria (<20%) or thrombocytopenia as is commonly seen in women with preeclampsia or eclampsia. The primary symptoms of a pheochromocytoma are indeed: hypertension (98%), headaches (80%), hyperhidrosis (65%), and heart palpitations (60%). The symptoms of pregnant women with Cushing's syndrome are the same as in the non-pregnant state: truncal obesity, abdominal striae, moon facies, and glucose intolerance. As such, they are often masked by pregnancy. Signs specific for cortisol-producing tumors include hypertension, hypokalemia, muscle weakness, or paralysis. The diagnosis of an adrenal tumor will therefore only occur if the physician is actively looking for such signs and thinking about them. The presence of such foreshadowing signs raises suspicion for the presence of an adrenal mass; serologic, urine, and imaging studies should then be considered.

26.3   Hormone Levels and Lab Analysis

Laboratory studies can be difficult to interpret due to the biochemical changes that a woman's body undergoes during pregnancy. While pregnancy causes many hormone levels to be elevated, most hormone levels remain the same as when a woman is not pregnant. Importantly, catecholamine levels remain normal in pregnancy, but do become elevated in the presence of a pheochromocytoma. Therefore, changes in catecholamine levels can be measured accurately without considering the effect of pregnancy. In order to diagnose a pheochromocytoma, a 24-h urine specimen should be obtained. Although several groups now tout plasma catecholamine analysis, we prefer the greater accuracy of 24-h urinary studies. Urinary-free catecholamines (epinephrine, norepinephrine, and dopamine) levels should be measured (Table 1). Breakdown products of metanephrines (M) and vanillylmandelic acid (VMA) should also be checked. While the sensitivity for urinary M (67–91%) or VMA (28–56%) is low, the specificity for both M (83–100%) and VMA (98–100%) urinary levels are excellent. If normal levels of urine catecholamines are obtained on two separate occasions, then a diagnosis of pheochromocytoma can be excluded.

In normal pregnancy both aldosterone and renin levels are increased. By 8 weeks' gestation there is a fourfold increase in aldosterone levels, which continues to rise to a maximum of ten times the normal level at delivery. Progesterone is markedly increased in pregnancy and acts as a competitive inhibitor of aldosterone in the distal tubules; therefore, the physiological effects of increased aldosterone are tempered in pregnancy [6]. Consequently, measuring aldosterone is inherently inaccurate during pregnancy. There is sparse literature on the biochemical diagnosis of aldosterone-producing tumors during pregnancy. When attempting to assess aldosterone levels, hypokalemia should be corrected because a low potassium level will suppress aldosterone. Urine potassium levels must be measured to confirm potassium wasting. Plasma renin levels can be checked, but levels are usually higher in pregnancy. While virtually all pregnant women will have "physiologic" hyperaldosteronism, coupling low potassium levels and lower than normal (typically high) renin levels should prompt imaging for an aldosteronoma.

There are no definitive criteria for hypercortisolemia in pregnancy; normally, urinary-free cortisol and plasma cortisol levels are elevated (68–252 µg/dl) at least three times as high as in the non-pregnant state (11–83 µg/dl). Diurnal rhythms are normally maintained in pregnancy but are typically blunted in Cushing's syndrome [9]. Hence the plasma cortisol levels of pregnant women remain elevated but on a normal cycle. Having stated that, making the diagnosis and identifying the source of hypercortisolism in pregnancy is difficult. A dexamethasone suppression test is not accurate in the estrogen excess state of pregnancy because of the elevation of total serum cortisol. In preg-

Table 1. Measurement of urinary-free catecholamine levels

	Normal pregnancy values	Non-pregnancy values
Epinephrine (µg/24 h)	0.5–20	0.5–20
Norepinephrine (µg/24 h)	10–70	10–70
Metanephrine (µg/24 h)	<1.3	<1.3
Vanillylmandelic acid (µg/24 h)	<6.5	<6.5
Dopamine (nmol/24 h)	300–3,900	300–3,900
Aldosterone	4–10× increase	1–21 ng/dl
Renin	Elevated	?
Serum cortisol	?	7–25 µg/dl AM 2–14 µg/dl PM
Urine-free cortisol	68–252 µg/dl	24–108 µg/24 h

nancy there will effectively be a lack of suppression by dexamethasone. It has been suggested that a 24-h urine-free cortisol level in multiple samples and serum cortisol measurements at 0800 and 2300 hours (assessing the diurnal rhythm) be drawn. If these results suggest an unusually elevated cortisol, plasma ACTH levels should be measured in order to differentiate the tumor as ACTH dependent or independent.

26.4   Adrenal Imaging During Pregnancy

Imaging studies should follow a confirmed biochemical diagnosis (especially in the case of a pheochromocytoma). MRI is the preferred modality to use in the pregnant patient because it will produce high quality images but will not expose the fetus to harmful radiation or toxic contrast dye. Pheochromocytomas often appear as bright masses on T2-weighted images, allowing one to distinguish a pheochromocytoma from the asymptomatic or incidental adrenal adenoma found in as many as 5% of such studies [10]. More recent literature suggests that abdominal US can be helpful in detecting pheochromocytomas [12]. Given both ionizing radiation and contrast dye are teratogenic to the fetus, both CT and angiography are contraindicated in pregnancy. While metaiodobenzylguanidine (MIBG) is selectively taken up by adrenergic tissues, MIBG scans are similarly contraindicated in pregnancy (Table 2) [2, 6].

26.5   Treatment

Total eradication of an offending adrenal mass involves surgical resection. However, depending on the stage of pregnancy and the type of tumor, medical management may be more appropriate therapy … at least initially. While most functioning adrenal tumors

should be removed sooner rather than later, adding a fetus to the equation alters "best management". Surgical resection in the first trimester is controversial because of the increased risk of fetal morbidity and mortality. Surgical intervention in the third trimester carries a high risk of spontaneous delivery, and adrenalectomy during this late stage is usually deferred until delivery or postpartum. The safest time for adrenal resection is the second trimester: less teratogenicity, less fetal morbidity and mortality, and less likely to induce premature delivery.

As described elsewhere in this text, after the diagnosis of pheochromocytoma has been confirmed and the tumor localized, the first line of therapy is pharmacologic. Alpha-blockade is performed preferably with phenoxybenzamine, as there is no evidence that this drug is teratogenic to the fetus. If symptoms continue and are not well controlled with this alpha-blocker, then a beta-blocker may be added, but this is controversial during pregnancy. Propranolol is commonly used but can cause intrauterine growth retardation (IUGR) (Table 2); therefore, its use should be very temporary (<72 h) or fetal monitoring must occur frequently.

Operative resection is the only curative treatment for pheochromocytoma. However, urgent surgical intervention must be weighed against the potential morbidity and/or mortality of the fetus and mother versus the risk of medically managing blood pressure through delivery. In early pregnancy, before 24 weeks' gestation, adrenalectomy carries more risk: 44% risk of fetal demise. A 22% risk of fetal death occurs if resection is performed after 24 weeks [6]. Despite these statistics an operation may need to be performed within the first 24 weeks if the mother and fetus are deteriorating or in an attempt to protect both from labile blood pressures. Delaying operation on the other hand creates an increased risk of stroke, myocardial infarction, or hemorrhage into the tumor [10]. If surgical delay is chosen, then it is best to treat the patient med-

Table 2. Contraindications in pregnancy

Imaging study	Complications
Computerized tomography	Teratogenic to fetus
Metaiodobenzylguanidine	Teratogenic to fetus
Medications	Complications
Spironolactone	Feminizing affect on male fetuses
ACE inhibitor (angiotensin-converting enzyme)	Oligohydramnios and neonatal renal failure
Propranolol (beta-blockers)	Intrauterine growth retardation (IUGR)

ically until the fetus is viable and ready for cesarean section. Vaginal birth and concomitant adrenalectomy is contraindicated because of the 31% risk of maternal mortality for such a practice; unfortunately a 19% risk of maternal mortality is associated with a planned C-section [6]. Detection of the pheochromocytoma during the third trimester is cause to postpone operation until a pre-planned C-section delivery of a mature fetus can occur [12]. In the interim medical management is usually sufficient.

Although timing of intervention is difficult for pheochromocytomas, such is not the case for cortisol-producing tumors. Resection should be performed immediately, as early as 12 weeks' gestation, due to the proven detrimental affects of extreme hypercortisolemia on the fetus. According to a report of 60 women with 69 pregnancies, fetuses growing in the presence of cortisol-producing tumors are at an increased risk to be delivered stillborn (12%), or prematurely (52%), spontaneously abort (12%), or are born with IUGR (25%) [15]. While it is better for the fetus to have the mother receive surgical treatment, at least one study (*n*=43) suggests there are significant risks associated with adrenalectomy: premature birth (47%), IUGR (35%), neonatal death (12%), and perinatal death (12%) [3]. Additional studies find that if the patient delays operation until after the delivery, the risk is great for: premature birth (72%), IUGR (26%), neonatal death (7%), stillbirth (12%), and perinatal death (19%) [10].

Medical treatment remains controversial as to its effectiveness in the case of Cushing's syndrome. Prebtani et al. [13] suggest that in the first trimester medical therapy should be used and operation can wait until the second semester. In the third trimester medical therapy is advised until fetal development is complete. Part of the dispute is due to the limited number of reported cases and data. If the tumor is discovered in the third trimester, there are three published cases where ketoconazole was successfully used despite its known teratogenic association and its ability to cause transplacental passage and reduction of fetal steroid production [13]. Lo has suggested the usage of metyrapone to treat the hypercortisolism. Metyrapone is an inhibitor of 11-beta-hydroxylase and leads to a reduction of cortisol levels. This treatment could be used to stabilize patients prior to operation or as an alternative for poor surgical candidates. While metyrapone has the potential to cross the placenta and affect fetal adrenal steroid synthesis, there have been no identifiable adverse effects reported [9]. Prior to elective operation, hypertension and diabetes should be controlled as well.

With primary aldosteronism in pregnancy, surgical intervention is preferred but medical management is a viable option. Hypokalemia must be corrected immediately because of its detrimental affect on fetal energy supply resulting in IUGR [4]. Operation, if selected, should be performed in the early second trimester. After resection, potassium levels and hypertension immediately improve. If the adenoma is detected in the third trimester, medical management is suggested, using potassium supplementation and anti-hypertensives, such as methyldopa, beta-blockers, calcium channel blockers, or hydralazine. Spironolactone and angiotensin converting enzyme (ACE) inhibitors are contraindicated in pregnancy. Spironolactone has feminizing affects on male fetuses. ACE inhibitors cause oligohydramnios and neonatal renal failure.

26.6   Operative Strategy

The rarity of these tumors is such that most of the literature on adrenal tumors during pregnancy focuses on the removal of pheochromocytomas. A pheochromocytoma may be removed by open or laparoscopic techniques without interfering with the gravid uterus, but the risk of spontaneous abortion is increased with laparotomy [2]. Regardless of the technique, the patient must be carefully positioned. Facilitating exposure for the surgeon is paramount, but keeping the gravid uterus off the inferior vena cava (IVC) to maintain venous return to the heart is important. Left lateral decubitus positioning for a right adrenalectomy (Fig. 10) and use of the reverse Trendelenburg

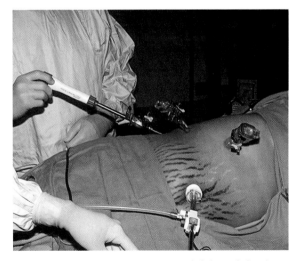

Fig. 10. Preoperative view depicting left lateral decubitus positioning for a right adrenalectomy

position for resecting either gland minimizes IVC compression.

There are laparoscopic considerations to be aware of. The unknown effects of the carbon dioxide (CO_2) pneumoperitoneum on the fetus, possible risk of uterine damage during trocar placement, premature labor due to increased intra-abdominal pressure, and fetal acidosis are all possible harms to the fetus [12]. Given thousands of pregnant women have safely undergone laparoscopic cholecystectomy, laparoscopic adrenalectomy during pregnancy should similarly be safe and efficacious. Two well documented adrenalectomies in pregnant women showed no maternal hypotension, hypoxia, increased end-tidal carbon dioxide, or decreased fetal heart rate during laparoscopic operations [1]. With the use of laparoscopy during pregnancy there is less fetal depression secondary to the decreased use of narcotics, a lower rate of maternal wound complications, diminished postoperative maternal hypoventilation, and more rapid return to a full diet for the mother which decreases nutritional stress on the fetus [12].

If the surgeon decides that adrenalectomy will not occur intrapartum, then tumor removal may occur at delivery or postpartum. This decision depends on the ability to locate the tumor at the time of the C-section. It is suggested that a longer longitudinal incision be made to facilitate easier localization and removal. During an open adrenalectomy, control of excess catecholamine release is maintained via deep anesthesia and adrenergic blocking medications. Magnesium sulfate has been shown to inhibit catecholamine release, block catecholamine receptors directly, and have a direct dilator affect on vessel walls. Once the tumor is removed the mother's symptoms are relieved and postpartum complications are minimal, assuming the patient is well hydrated.

In patients with cortisol-producing tumors, the collective literature suggests the frequency of maternal and fetal complications in patients undergoing adrenalectomy *during* pregnancy is lower than those having adrenalectomy *postpartum* [1]. Nonetheless, debate continues as to whether or not surgical intervention can be postponed until after the delivery. Pricolo et al. [14] found that in a study which included 19 women with 26 pregnancies involving cortisol-producing adrenal adenomas, that fetal and neonatal complications, when adrenalectomy was performed intrapartum, compared favorably (1 in 7, 14%) to operations performed postpartum (12 complications in 19 patients, 63%). Similarly, resection during pregnancy generated fewer maternal complications

(7%) than postpartum adrenalectomy (84%). Early surgical resection to correct hypercortisolism appears safer for both mother and child. The general consensus is that surgical intervention depends on the severity of hypercortisolism and the gestational age of the fetus [13]. If adrenalectomy is postponed until after the delivery, vaginal delivery is preferred over C-section because of the mother's poor tissue healing and potential for wound breakdown [3].

26.7   Summary

Adrenal tumors causing problems during pregnancy are rare. Having such lesions diagnosed before childbirth is extraordinarily uncommon and typically serendipitous. Most *functional* adrenal tumors require surgical resection or medical intervention to prevent IUGR or fetal death. Therefore, when a pregnant woman presents with hypertension without proteinuria and/or without thrombocytopenia (typical for preeclampsia), the physician *must* begin to explore the possibility of pheochromocytoma. Primary hyperaldosteronism and cortisol-producing adenomas are even more difficult to detect, but clinical suspicion with confirmatory laboratory analysis and imaging studies (MRI is best choice) allow physicians the opportunity to intervene earlier. While most patients can undergo delayed resection following childbirth (Fig. 11), surgeons should opt for adrenalectomy in the second trimester for most cortisol-producing tumors and those pheochromocytomas and aldosteronomas that remain refractory to pharmacologic therapy.

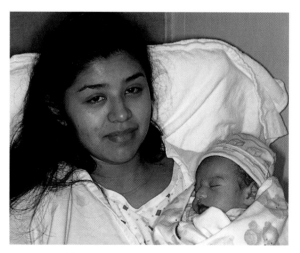

Fig. 11. Healthy mother and child following adrenalectomy at 39 weeks' gestation

References

1. Aishima M, Tanaka M, Haraoka M, Naito S (2000) Retroperitoneal laparoscopic adrenalectomy in a pregnant woman with Cushing's syndrome. J Urol 164:770–771

2. Botchan A, Hauser R, Kupfermine M, Grisaru D, Peyser MR, Lessing JB (1995) Pheochromocytoma in pregnancy: case report and review of the literature. Obstet Gynecol Surv 50:321–327

3. Buescher MA, McClamrock HD, Adashi EY (1992) Cushing syndrome in pregnancy. Obstet Gynecol 79:130–137

4. Fujiyama S, Mori Y, Matsubara H, Okada S, Maruyama K, Masaki H, Yonemoto T, Nagata T, Umeda Y, Matsuda T, Iwasaka T, Inada M (1999) Primary aldosteronism with aldosterone-producing adrenal adenoma in a pregnant woman. Intern Med 38:36–39

5. Harrington JL, Farley DR, van Heerden JA, Ramin KD (1999) Adrenal tumors and pregnancy. World J Surg 23:182–186

6. Keely E (1998) Endocrine causes of hypertension in pregnancy – when to start looking for zebras. Semin Perinatol 22:471–284

8. Linos DA (2000) Management approaches to adrenal incidentalomas (adrenalomas). A view from Athens, Greece. Endocrinol Metab Clin North Am 29:141–157

9. Lo KW, Lau TK (1998) Cushing's syndrome in pregnancy secondary to adrenal adenoma. A case report and literature review. Gynecol Obstet Invest 45:209–212

10. Lyman DJ (2002) Paroxysmal hypertension, pheochromocytoma, and pregnancy. J Am Board Fam Pract 15:153–158

11. Okawa T, Asano K, Hashimoto T, Fujimori K, Yanagida K, Sato A (2002) Diagnosis and management of primary aldosteronism in pregnancy: case report and review of the literature. Am J Perinatol 19:31–36

12. Pace DE, Chiasson PM, Schlachta CM, Mamazza J, Caddeddu MO, Poulin EC (2002) Minimally invasive adrenalectomy for pheochromocytoma during pregnancy. Surg Laparosc Endosc Percutan Tech 12:122–125

13. Prebtani AP, Donat D, Ezzat S (2000) Worrisome striae in pregnancy. Lancet 355:1692

14. Pricolo VE, Monchik JM, Prinz RA, DeJong S, Chadwick DA, Lamberton RP (1990) Management of Cushing's syndrome secondary to adrenal adenoma during pregnancy. Surgery 108:1072–1078

15. Sheeler LR (1994) Cushing's syndrome and pregnancy. Endocrinol Metab Clin North Am 23:619–627

27 Adrenal-Sparing Surgery

Richard A. Hodin, Antonia E. Stephen

CONTENTS

27.1 Introduction

Partial adrenal resection, also known as adrenal-sparing surgery or subtotal adrenalectomy, is the removal of an adrenal tumor with preservation of the normal surrounding adrenal tissue. The aim of a partial adrenal resection is to safely and completely resect the adrenal mass while leaving intact a functional portion of the gland. Partial adrenalectomy was initially described using the standard, open technique [8, 22], whereas recent reports refer to a laparoscopic approach [7, 9, 10, 16, 25]. Laparoscopy lends itself nicely to partial adrenalectomy because of the high level of magnification that allows for a more detailed inspection of the adrenal gland, aiding in the distinction between the tumor mass and the normal adrenal tissue. The focus of this chapter is on laparoscopic partial adrenal resection, with a description of the indications, preoperative evaluation, operative technique, and postoperative follow-up of patients undergoing this procedure. Despite some reported successes with partial adrenalectomy, it is important for the reader to keep in mind that the current standard of care for patients undergoing surgery for an adrenal mass is complete resection (Fig. 1).

27.2 Indications

The two most common disorders for which a partial-adrenal resection may be performed are bilateral pheochromocytoma and unilateral solitary aldosteronoma.

27.3 Bilateral Pheochromocytoma

Both the multiple endocrine neoplasia syndromes and von Hippel Lindau disease predispose to the development of pheochromocytomas of the adrenal medulla. Approximately 50% of patients with MEN 2-A and MEN 2-B will develop pheochromocytomas, and unlike those with non-familial disease, patients with an inherited predisposition are far more likely to develop bilateral tumors [3]. These tumors are thought to slowly develop in the background of adrenal medullary hyperplasia [2]. Patients who develop bilateral pheochromocytomas require bilateral adrenal resection, following which they are left with essentially no functional adrenal cortical tissue and require lifelong steroid replacement with the attendant side effects of steroids and risk of acute adrenal insufficiency. Because these tumors involve only the adrenal medulla, it is an appealing concept to remove only the tumor itself and the adrenal medullary tissue, and leave in place the steroid-producing adrenal cortex. Several cases of partial adrenal resection for patients with familial pheochromocytoma have been described [8, 10, 16, 22]. In those patients with synchronous tumors, the bilateral adrenal resection can be done at one operation. In patients with a familial predisposition to pheochromocytoma who develop a unilateral tumor, a partial adrenal resection should still be considered, as approximately one-third of these patients will go on to develop a pheochromocytoma in the remaining gland [3]. The preoperative evaluation and technique of partial adrenal resection for bilateral pheochromocytoma is discussed later in the chapter.

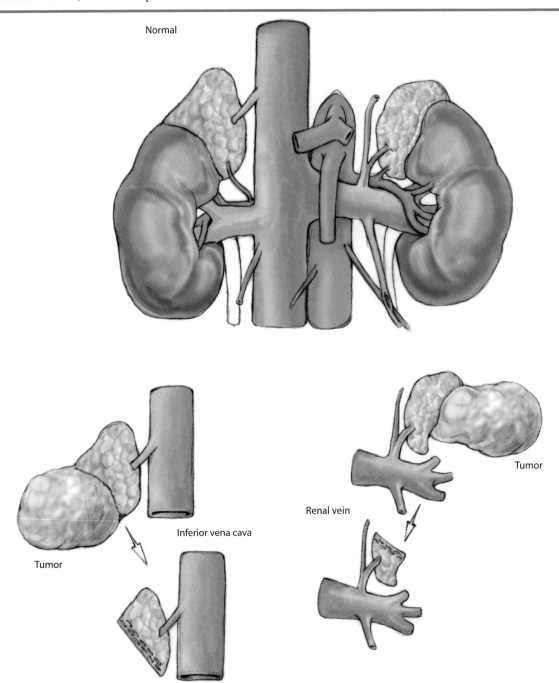

Fig. 1. Illustration of the technique of subtotal adrenalectomy. This was published in one of the earlier case reports describing open partial adrenal resection. In this case, a 48-year-old airline pilot, who was strongly opposed to requiring steroid supplementation, underwent a bilateral partial adrenal resection for pheochromocytoma (*IVC*, inferior vena cava; *RV*, renal vein). (From [22], with permission)

27.4   Solitary Aldosteronomas

Partial adrenalectomy has also been described for patients with solitary cortical tumors, most commonly for aldosterone-producing tumors (Conn syndrome). Unlike patients with bilateral pheochromocytomas, patients with unilateral adrenal tumors are not at risk of steroid dependence following complete resection, provided they have a normal, functioning gland on the other side. However, in the event of a tumor or hemorrhage of the opposite adrenal gland, a partial resection of the aldosteronoma leaves the patient with functional adrenal tissue. Because aldosteronomas are usually small (<2 cm), solitary, and eccentrically located at the margin of the adrenal gland, a limited resection is technically feasible. In addition, these tumors are almost always benign and are unlikely to recur. As such, some authors have suggested that aldosteronomas can be safely enucleated, leaving the remainder of the gland and its blood supply undisturbed [11]. One report of laparoscopic adrenal-sparing surgery in 13 patients with solitary aldosteronomas suggested exclusion criteria for partial resection as a diameter greater than 3 cm, tumors located in a concentric position in the gland, and tumors directly attached to the adrenal vein [9]. Using these criteria maximizes the chance of safe enucleation of the tumor with the preservation of a sufficient amount of well-vascularized adrenal tissue.

27.5   Other Tumors

Partial adrenalectomy has been described for patients with adrenal cortical tumors other than aldosteronoma, including Cushing's adenomas [7, 25]. Once again, commonly used inclusion criteria include a tumor size less than or equal to 3 cm. In one study, if the tumor was located in the central portion of the gland or the spared remnant was expected to be less than 50% of the total adrenal gland, a partial adrenal resection was not performed [7]. Another study identified the ideal size of a tumor appropriate for partial resection as 1.1–2.5 cm, citing both the difficulty in reliably locating a tumor less than 1 cm in diameter within the gland, and the challenge of resecting a tumor greater than 2.5 cm while preserving functional adrenal tissue [25].

In general, a nonfunctional tumor is a rare indication for partial adrenal resection. It may be indicated in selected cases of a benign tumor such as a ganglioneuroma or myelolipoma [7]. However, the usual indication for removal of a nonfunctioning adrenal mass is size greater than 4–5 cm or suspected malignancy, both contraindications to partial resection. The possibility of adrenocortical carcinoma or metastatic cancer of the adrenal gland is an absolute contraindication to partial adrenal resection.

27.6   Preoperative Evaluation

The preoperative evaluation of patients being considered for partial adrenalectomy is of paramount importance. As with all patients undergoing adrenal surgery, a complete hormonal evaluation is performed and localization studies are undertaken to identify the side of the tumor. Once this is done, there are several additional considerations in patients for whom a partial adrenal resection is considered. A thin slice (3–5 mm slice interval) computerized tomographic (CT) scan provides excellent detail of the structure of the adrenal and underlying abnormality. With current technology, CT can detect lesions as small as a few millimeters in diameter [26]. In cases where a partial resection is considered, it is imperative to exclude additional lesions or masses in the adrenal gland. For example, in a patient with a hormonally active tumor on the left side and more than one mass in the left adrenal gland, it is impossible to determine which mass is productive. In that scenario, a complete adrenal resection should be performed [7]. The location of the tumor within the gland can be helpful in planning the surgical approach; in general, anterior, peripherally located tumors are technically easier to resect than those located posteriorly or centrally within the gland. The CT should be done both unenhanced and with intravenous contrast, as it is important to define preoperatively the location of the tumor in relation to the main adrenal vein. In addition, delayed images are necessary to determine the likelihood of malignancy, an important consideration in the work-up of any adrenal mass, and of obvious importance in those considered for a partial resection. In order to minimize the chance of performing a partial resection for a malignancy, Jeschke et al. performed partial adrenal resection only on those patients with an adrenal mass with attenuation of 11 HU or less on the unenhanced images, and 37 HU or less on the delayed-enhanced images [9]. Several references [12, 14] are cited in the aforementioned study as evidence for the reliability of these criteria in distinguishing an adenoma from a carcinoma.

In addition to CT, magnetic resonance imaging (MRI) is commonly utilized in the work-up of pheochromocytomas, which appear bright on T2-weighted

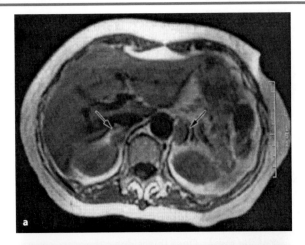

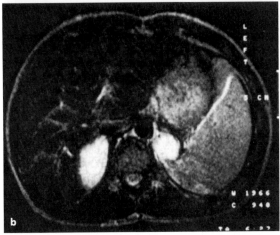

Fig. 2. a Preoperative magnetic resonance image revealing bilateral adrenal masses in an 81-year-old woman with bilateral pheochromocytomas. (From [10], with permission). **b** T2-weighted magnetic resonance image of a young man with bilateral pheochromocytomas. (From [25], with permission). Both of these patients subsequently underwent bilateral partial adrenal resection

images. This can be helpful in identifying patients with MEN-2A or familial disorders who may have bilateral lesions. Preoperative MRI of patients with bilateral pheochromocytomas are shown in Fig. 2 [10,25]. Computed tomography, MRI, and nuclear scintigraphy all play an important role in the postoperative follow-up of these patients, as outlined later in the chapter.

27.7   Technique

The technique of laparoscopic adrenalectomy is well described in Chaps. 31–33. Patient positioning, trocar placement, and exposure of the adrenal gland in adre-

nal-sparing resection are the same as that for complete adrenal resection [18]. Laparoscopy provides a view of the adrenal gland with parenchymal detail not possible in the open approach, such that the tumor tissue is more readily identified. Both the transperitoneal and retroperitoneal approaches are described for partial adrenal resection. As is true in cases where a complete resection is performed, the transperitoneal approach, as popularized by Gagner and many others, is more commonly used [4]. However, it has been suggested that the retroperitoneal approach may better lend itself to partial resections by providing a more detailed view of the adrenal and more precise differentiation between normal and abnormal tissue [25].

Intraoperatively, it is imperative to distinguish the normal adrenal tissue from the tumor itself, and to rule out additional lesions in the gland that may not have been apparent on preoperative studies. Intraoperative ultrasound can be used to examine the entire adrenal gland and hence localize the tumor and define its relation to adrenal vessels and surrounding structures. Intraoperative ultrasound has been described for both partial and complete adrenal resection [5, 7, 10, 16]. Once the adrenal gland is exposed, the intraoperative ultrasound probe is inserted through one of the 10-mm ports and the adrenal gland identified cephalad to the kidney. The tumor is visualized within the substance of the adrenal gland and, depending on the type, may appear hyper- or hypoechoic in relation to the normal adrenal tissue [21]. The extent of resection needed and the size of a potential adrenal remnant can be accurately assessed. Synchronous lesions prohibiting a partial resection are identified. Following tumor resection, intraoperative ultrasound is used to inspect the gland to ensure a complete resection. Due to the small size of many adrenal lesions, and what can be a subtle distinction between normal and abnormal tissue, the use of intraoperative ultrasound when performing a partial adrenal resection is strongly recommended. An example of a preoperative and laparoscopic intraoperative ultrasound in a patient with an aldosterone-producing tumor is shown in Fig. 3 [21].

Several different techniques are described for tumor resection in adrenal-sparing surgery. It is generally agreed that manipulation and dissection of the preserved remnant should be avoided as much as possible. Many authors advocate preservation of the adrenal vein and at least one of the arteries to ensure continued blood supply and function of the remaining tissue [1, 7, 19]. In addition, division of the main adrenal vein may cause congestion of the remaining adrenal

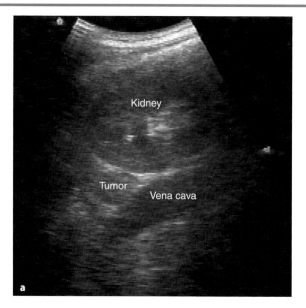

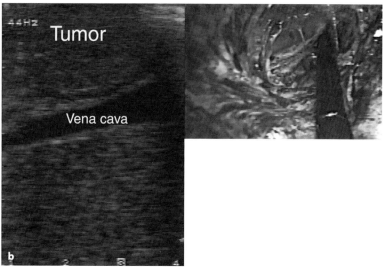

Fig. 3a, b. Ultrasound images of a patient with a right-sided aldosterone-secreting tumor. **a** Percutaneous ultrasound obtained with the patient in the lateral decubitus position demonstrates a 2.6 cm adrenal mass above the superior pole of the right kidney. **b** Intraoperative laparoscopic ultrasound (*left panel*) further localizes the tumor and clearly shows its relationship to the inferior vena cava. *On the right* is a laparoscopic view of the ultrasound probe over the tumor. (From [21], with permission)

tissue and difficulty in obtaining adequate hemostasis [7]. In cases of pheochromocytoma, dissection of the gland while the vein is intact may lead to the release of excessive amounts of catecholamines and hemodynamic instability. This risk can be minimized with pre- and intraoperative pharmacologic management along with gentle handling of the tumor [9, 15]. Some authors contend that preservation of the main adrenal vein is unnecessary since adequate venous drainage will occur through collateral pathways. Kaouk et al., in a case report of bilateral partial adrenal resection for pheochromocytoma, describe dividing the left main adrenal vein and preserving the right. There was no additional bleeding noted from the left side, and there were minimal hemodynamic fluctuations as a result of leaving the right vein intact [10]. In a study of 22 patients who underwent laparoscopic partial adrenalectomy, the decision of whether or not to divide the main adrenal vein depended on the individual case, taking into account the location, size, and type of tumor. In that report, the adrenal vein was preserved in half of the cases (Table 1) [25].

Table 1. A summary of the series published by Walz et al. Between 1994 and 1997, 22 patients underwent unilateral subtotal laparoscopic partial adrenal resection using the retroperitoneal approach. Division of the main adrenal vein was decided on an individual case basis, depending on the relationship of the vein to the adrenal tumor. Details of patient follow-up are included [25]

No.	Age / sex	Diagnosis	Site	Tumor size (cm)	Preservation of main vein	Adrenal part preserved*	Follow-up months	Follow-up comment
1	42 F	Conn adenoma	L	1.5	no		31	Normokalemia, normotensive without medication
2	44 M	Non-functioning tumor (expected metastasis)	L	3	no		29	Alive after pneumonectomy for cancer
3	44 M	Non-functioning tumor	R	4.5	no		27	-
4	34 M	Pheochromocytoma	R	6	no		26	Normotensive without medication, catecholamines normal
5	10 F	Adrenal cyst	L	1.5	yes		25	-
6	45 F	Conn adenoma	L	2	yes		23	Normokalemia, normotensive without medication
7	44 F	Conn adenoma	L	2.5	yes		18	Normokalemia, normotensive without medication
8	34 M	Pheochromocytoma	L	3	no		17	MEN IIa: catecholamines normal; basal cortisol serum level normal, substitution with 10 mg cortisol / day orally
9	38 F	Conn adenoma	R	2	yes		14	Normokalemia, normotensive without medication
10	58 F	Conn adenoma	L	2	yes		13	Normokalemia, normotensive without medication
11	37 F	Conn adenoma	R	1.5	no		11	Normokalemia, normotensive without medication
12	36 F	Conn adenoma	L	1	no		10	Normokalemia, normotensive without medication
13	68 F	Conn adenoma	L	2	yes		10	Normokalemia, normotensive with reduced dosage of antihypertensive agents
14	49 F	Pheochromocytoma	R	4	no		8	Men IIa: contralateral adrenalectomy 1987; catecholamines normal; basal cortisol serum level normal, no substitution necessary
15	57 M	Conn adenoma	R	1	no		7	Normokalemia, normotensive with reduced dosage of antihypertensive agents
16	34 F	Pheochromocytoma	L	2	no		7	Normotensive without medication, catecholamines normal
17	30 F	Cushing adenoma	L	3	no		4	Requires cortisol-substitution
18	70 F	Cushing adenoma	L	2	yes		2	Requires cortisol-substitution
19	42 M	Conn adenoma	L	2	yes		2	Normokalemia, normotensive without medication
20	30 F	Cushing adenoma	R	2.5	yes		2	Requires cortisol-substitution
21	27 F	Cushing adenoma	L	2.5	yes		1	Requires cortisol-substitution
22	57 F	Conn adenoma	R	1.5	yes		1	Normokalemia, normotensive without medication

MEN: multiple endocrine neoplasia.
Dark area: preserved part.

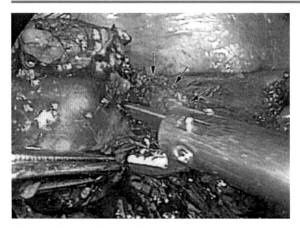

Fig. 4. Technique of partial left adrenalectomy using the harmonic scalpel. This patient had bilateral pheochromocytomas, and underwent bilateral laparoscopic partial resections. The tumor is shown *on the left side* of the picture, while the *arrows* indicate the preserved adrenal remnant. (From [10], with permission)

It should be emphasized that the tissue surrounding the gland must be adequately mobilized and the margins well exposed prior to beginning a partial resection [9]. In doing so, it should be kept in mind that excessive manipulation and dissection of the normal adrenal tissue can disrupt the blood supply and compromise its long-term function. A number of different instruments and techniques can be used for the tumor excision. One author describes outlining the edges of resection with the bipolar electrocautery in order to demarcate the resection margin and minimize bleeding from the surface of the gland [9]. Following cauterization of the surface, the tumor is resected with endoscissors. A fine endoscopic instrument with electrocautery, such as endoscissors, allows for precise dissection along a plane

between normal tissue and tumor. Alternatively, the harmonic scalpel can be used for resection, and may provide better hemostasis (Fig. 4) [10, 25]. Neither the endoscissors nor the harmonic scalpel will provide adequate hemostasis for the main adrenal vein, which requires suture ligatures, clips, or a vascular stapler. In general, electrocautery or the harmonic scalpel is adequate for most of the small vessels, with only the main vein requiring a ligature or clip.

The vascular stapler can also be used for the resection itself, to divide the tissue between the tumor and normal adrenal [7]. This may be most appropriate in cases of small, peripherally located lesions, and will generally achieve excellent hemostasis. Some argue, however, that the relatively large size of the endoscopic staplers do not allow for adequate precision in separating normal from abnormal tissue in a gland as small as the adrenal and may risk sacrificing more normal adrenal parenchyma than necessary [9, 10]. In addition, authors who advocate the use of a stapler for resection warn that in patients with familial pheochromocytoma and adrenal medullary hyperplasia, the tissue may be too thick to safely accommodate division with a vascular stapler. Imai et al. published a report of five patients who underwent laparoscopic partial adrenalectomy using the vascular stapler. All had solitary tumors that were either aldosterone or weakly cortisol producing. Patient data and tumor size are shown in Table 2, and drawings depicting the tumor location within the adrenal are illustrated in Fig. 5. All tumors were peripherally located, such that it was technically feasible to perform the partial resection using the stapler [7].

An alternative method of resection has been described by Walther et al. After the laparoscopic ultra-

Table 2. A summary of the five patients who underwent laparoscopic partial adrenal resection as published by Imai et al. These patient data emphasize that partial adrenal resection can be performed safely with a complete tumor resection [7]

Case	Disease	Age	Sex	Side	Operating time (min)	Blood loss[a]	Tumor size[b] (mm)	Margin[c] (mm)
1	APA[d]	40	M	R	210	Minimal	20	5
2	APA[d]	50	F	R	132	Minimal	7	5
3	APA[d]	56	M	L	120	Minimal	23	10
4	WFA[e]	70	F	L	105	Minimal	26	9
5	WFA[e]	76	M	R	145	Minimal	20	5

[a] Estimated blood loss very little in all cases.
[b] Maximal diameter of tumor.
[c] Length between tumor margin and cutting edge.
[d] Aldosterone producing adenoma.
[e] Weak functioning adrenocortical adenoma.

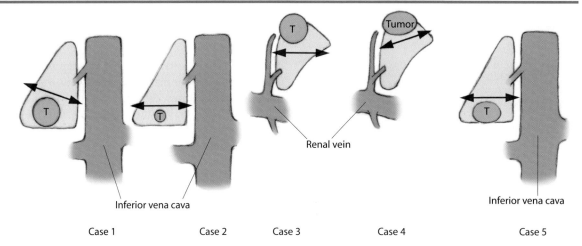

Fig. 5. Location of the adrenal tumor and the line of resection in five patients who underwent laparoscopic partial adrenal resection for aldosterone or cortisol secreting tumors. In these cases, the resection was performed using the vascular stapler (*T*, tumor; *IVC*, inferior vena cava; *C*, adrenal central vein). (From [7], with permission)

sound is used to identify tumor and normal tissue, suture ligatures are placed through the adrenal gland adjacent to the tumor. These sutures separate the tumor from a thin rim of normal, cortical tissue, and the endoscopic scissors are used to excise the tumor. The previously placed sutures provide hemostasis, and additional sutures are placed as needed. These authors found that the harmonic scalpel produced similar results with regards to hemostasis [24].

Since a partial resection is carried through the well-vascularized substance of the adrenal gland instead of the relatively avascular plane between the adrenal and the kidney, a major concern is possible postoperative bleeding from the raw surface of the gland. It is generally agreed that the pressure of the pneumoperitoneum reduces bleeding from the remaining adrenal parenchyma intraoperatively. In order to reduce the incidence of postoperative bleeding, several authors advocate the use of fibrin glue or Surgicel to seal over the resection margin prior to releasing the pneumoperitoneum [1,9,19]. It is also a good idea to release the pneumoperitoneum and check for bleeding prior to removal of the trocars.

In general, the resection is carried out with the goal of a 0.5–1.0 cm margin, depending on the tumor type. In cases of an aldosterone-producing adenoma, it is generally agreed that a 2–3 mm resection margin is adequate [9, 11] since these tumors are almost always benign, infrequently recur, and can be reliably diagnosed on preoperative studies. In one study of eight patients undergoing adrenal-sparing surgery for aldosterone-producing tumors, the authors describe simply enucleating the tumor after dissecting around

the margin with electrocauterized endoscissors [11]. This is not recommended for familial pheochromocytoma, which occurs in the setting of diffuse medullary hyperplasia and is far more likely to recur. Since medullary tissue is largely present only in the main portion of the gland, preservation of only the tail of the gland may ensure a more complete resection of adrenal medullary tissue [10].

Table 3 represents a list of recently published reports on laparoscopic partial adrenal resection. All of the studies listed in Table 3 report minimal intraoperative blood loss and no need for postoperative blood transfusion. The operative time did not differ significantly compared with complete adrenal resection. In one study, the authors compare the operative time and blood loss in 22 patients undergoing partial adrenalectomy to 46 patients undergoing complete adrenalectomy during the same time period [25]. The operating time for subtotal resection was, on average, 20 min shorter than that for the complete resections (not a statistically significant difference), and blood loss was minimal in both groups. Hospital stay in patients undergoing partial adrenal resection was similar to that for patients undergoing complete adrenal resection. There are no reports in the literature of major intraoperative or immediate postoperative complications following partial adrenal resection. In the early postoperative period, all patients should undergo appropriate clinical and/or biochemical testing to ensure complete excision of hormonally active tumors; i.e. plasma potassium levels in the case of aldosteronomas.

Table 3. A comprehensive summary of the published literature on laparoscopic partial adrenalectomy with a list of the different techniques used to perform the resection

Author	No. of patients	Indication for surgery	Operative technique	Follow-up
Walz et al. 1998 [25]	22	Solitary aldosteronoma	Electrocautery, harmonic scalpel, clips	Mean 11 months
		Cortisol-producing adenoma Pheochromocytoma Non-functional tumor		
Jeschke et al. 2003 [9]	13	Solitary aldosteronoma	Endoshears, bipolar, fibrin glue	Median 39 months
Kok et al. 2002 [11]	8	Solitary aldosteronoma	Endoscopic scissors with electrocautery, enucleation Vascular stapler in one patient	Mean 25 months
Al-Sobhi et al. 2000 [1]	7	Solitary aldosteronoma	Bipolar, harmonic scalpel, fibrin glue	Median 12 months
Imai et al. 1999 [7]	5	Solitary aldosteronoma Cortisol-producing adenoma	Vascular stapler	3 months
Neumann et al. 1999 [16]	4	Bilateral pheochromocytoma	Not specified	2–24 months
Walther et al. 2000 [24]	3	Pheochromocytoma	Harmonic scalpel and suture ligatures	3 weeks–3 years
Kaouk et al. 2002 [10]	1	Bilateral pheochromocytoma	Harmonic scalpel, clips	3 months
Radmayr et al. 2000 [19]	1	Bilateral pheochromocytoma	Bipolar, harmonic scalpel, fibrin glue	2 months

27.8   Follow-up

The two main issues with regard to long-term follow-up in patients who have undergone partial adrenalectomy are function of the spared adrenal tissue and recurrence of the resected tumor. In patients who have undergone bilateral partial adrenal resection, the patients are followed closely for the possible requirement for steroid supplementation. Measurements of serum cortisol, with or without adrenocorticotrophic hormone stimulation, are routinely done in patients who have had bilateral resections. An adequate serum cortisol level, or an appropriate response to stimulation, indicates function of the preserved tissue.

It is more difficult to reliably assess the function of the preserved adrenal tissue in cases of unilateral partial adrenal resection. CT scans with intravenous contrast obtained during the 6-month postoperative period can assess the blood supply in the adrenal remnant. Perfusion of the remaining tissue indicates viability, but does not directly assess hormonal function. Nuclear scans are a more reliable test of adrenal gland function, since iodocholesterol-labeled agents are tak-

en up by adrenal tissue with intact steroidogenesis pathways and intracellular cholesterol [26]. These tests are often expensive and time-consuming, however, and may not be indicated for routine follow-up.

It is necessary to follow patients for tumor recurrence who have undergone partial adrenal resection. This is true for all such patients, but is of special concern in patients with familial pheochromocytoma and bilateral adrenal medullary hyperplasia. Because laparoscopic adrenal resection was introduced only in the past decade, the follow-up for patients who have had laparoscopic partial adrenal resection is not long enough to draw valid conclusions. It is helpful, however, to review the literature and follow-up for patients who had open partial adrenal resections, as many were operated on over a decade ago. In a report by Lee et al. from MD Anderson, 14 patients underwent open bilateral cortical-sparing adrenalectomy for familial pheochromocytoma [13]. The patients were followed for a median of approximately 11 years. Thirteen of the 14 patients did not require steroid supplementation and had normal postoperative plasma cortisol concentrations. Three patients had recurrent pheochromocytoma at 10, 14, and 27 years. Neumann et al. published their results of open partial adrenal resection for pheochromocytoma, and report a recurrence 6 years postoperatively. Irvin et al. reported three patients in whom a bilateral resection was performed, and two patients recurred, at 4 and 7 years, one dying from a stroke prior to re-exploration (Irvin et al. 1983, personal communication). This review of the open literature supports the conclusion that although partial resection may be successful in preserving adrenal function in patients with bilateral pheochromocytomas, there is a significant risk of tumor recurrence in these patients, often many years following surgery.

27.9   Literature Summary

There are several published series and case reports in the literature on laparoscopic partial adrenalectomy. The largest series includes 22 patients who underwent subtotal adrenalectomy by the retroperitoneal approach [25]. A summary of this study is shown in Table 1. There were no major complications and all of the patients with hormone secreting tumors were biochemically cured. There were two patients with MEN-IIa who had previously undergone a total adrenalectomy on the contralateral side. One of these patients is off steroids while the other requires low-dose steroid supplementation. The remainder of the patients underwent unilateral adrenal resection with an intact adrenal on the other side. The authors conclude that in selected cases, subtotal adrenalectomy is a safe procedure that can maintain adrenal function of the preserved cortex. It is important to note that there is only one patient with bilateral resections in whom preserved cortex is evident, and also that the follow-up time is relatively short (mean 11 months, range 1–31 months). Jeschke et al. performed partial adrenalectomy in 13 patients with solitary aldosterone-producing adenomas. There were no intraoperative or postoperative complications, and all tumors were completely resected. Patients had significant improvement in their hypertension, and serum aldosterone levels returned to normal in all patients. The patients were followed up at 3 months with enhanced CT scans, all of which showed good blood supply to the adrenal remnant. There was not, however, a more specific assessment of function of the remaining adrenal tissue. Investigators in Germany and Austria reported their results in four patients who underwent bilateral adrenal-sparing surgery for hereditary pheochromocytoma [16]. After a follow-up that ranged from 2 to 24 months, all patients had normal 24-h urine catecholamine excretion, with a normal cortisol response to ACTH stimulation. Although these results indicate preservation of cortical function and successful tumor resection, the follow-up time is relatively short to draw conclusions with regard to tumor recurrence. Kaouk et al. from the Cleveland Clinic reported a case of an 81-year-old woman with bilateral pheochromocytoma who underwent partial adrenal resection [10]. Because of tumor location, the right main adrenal vein was preserved, and the left divided. There was no major intraoperative hemodynamic instability and the total operative time was 5 h. Three months postoperatively the patient had no evidence of residual or recurrent tumor; however, she did require steroid supplementation. As described in the technique section, Imai et al. report resection of five solitary hormone-producing tumors of the adrenal using the vascular stapler (Table 2, Fig. 4). There was minimal blood loss, no complications, and normal aldosterone levels in those patients with aldosterone-producing tumors. The follow-up period, however, was limited to 3 months, and there is no assessment of adrenal remnant function. A comprehensive summary of recently published cases of laparoscopic partial adrenal resections is listed Table 3.

27.10   Conclusions

The advent of operative laparoscopy has revolutionized adrenal surgery, and with partial resection some surgeons are challenging the limits of adrenal surgery, seeking to investigate new and possibly improved methods of caring for patients with these rare tumors. The published literature on the subject supports the conclusion that partial adrenalectomy is a technically feasible and safe procedure. The normal postoperative hormone values documented in published studies indicate that tumors of an appropriate size and location within the gland can be completely resected while leaving in place residual cortical tissue. Still in question, however, is whether or not the remaining tissue is reliably functional. In the few cases of bilateral subtotal resection, some patients still required steroid supplementation during the follow-up period of the study. Another major consideration is tumor recurrence, especially in patients with familial pheochromocytoma and adrenal medullary hyperplasia. Although the goal of a subtotal resection in cases of pheochromocytoma is to remove the entire adrenal medulla while preserving only the adrenal cortex, preservation of the cortex may leave behind enough adrenal medullary tissue to risk a future recurrence. In summary, partial or subtotal adrenal resection is a safe procedure, which may be considered in certain select cases where preservation of adrenal tissue is paramount to the well-being of the patient. Documentation of preserved adrenal function and published studies of long-term follow-up will need to be done, however, to justify partial adrenalectomy as a routine procedure for adrenal tumors.

References

1. Al-Sobhi S, Peschel R, Bartsch G, Gasser R, Finkenstedt G, Janetschek G (2000) Partial laparoscopic adrenalectomy for aldosterone-producing adenoma: short and long-term results. J Endourology 14:497–499

2. Carney JA, Sizemore GW, Tyce GM (1975) Bilateral adrenal medullary hyperplasia in multiple endocrine neoplasia, type 2: the precursor of bilateral pheochromocytoma. Mayo Clin Proc 50:3–10

3. Evans DB, Lee JE, Merrel RC, et al. (1994) Adrenal medullary disease in multiple endocrine neoplasia type 2: Appropriate management. Endocrinol Metab Clin North Am 23:167

4. Gagner M, Lacroix A, Bolte E (1992) Laparoscopic adrenalectomy in Cushing's syndrome and pheochromocytoma. N Engl J Med 327:1033

5. Heniford BT, Iannitti DA, Hale J, Gagner M (1997) The role of intraoperative ultrasonography during laparoscopic adrenalectomy. Surgery 122:1068–73

6. Reference deleted

7. Imai T, Tanake Y, Kikumori T, Ohiwa M, Matsuura N, Mase T, Funahashi H (1999) Laparoscopic partial adrenalectomy. Surg Endosc 13:343–345

8. Irvin GL 3rd, Fishman LM, Sher JA (1983) Familial pheochromocytoma. Surgery 94:938–40

9. Jeschke K, Janetschek G, Peschel R, Schellander L, Bartsch G, Henning K (2003) Laparoscopic partial adrenalectomy in patients with aldosterone-producing adenomas: indications, techniques, and results. Urology 61:69–72

10. Kaouk JH, Matin S, Bravo EL, Gill IS (2002) Laparoscopic bilateral partial adrenalectomy for pheochromocytoma. Urology 60:1100–1103

11. Kok KYY, Yapp SKS (2002) Laparoscopic adrenal-sparing surgery for primary hyperaldosteronism due to aldosterone-producing adenoma. Surg Endosc 16:108–111

12. Korobkin M, Brodeur FJ, Francis IR, et al. (1998) CT time-attenuation washout curves of adrenal adenomas and nonadenomas. AJR Am J Roentgenol 170:747–52

13. Lee JE, Curley SA, Gagel RF, Evans DB, Hickey RC (1996) Cortical-sparing adrenalectomy for patients with bilateral pheochromocytoma. Surgery 120:1064–70

14. Lee MJ, Hahn PF, Papanicolaou N, et al. (1991) Benign and malignant adrenal masses: CT distinction with attenuation coefficients, size, and observer analysis. Radiology 179:415–8

15. Neumann HP, Bender BU, Reincke M, Eggstein S, Laubenberger J, Kirste G (1999) Adrenal-sparing surgery for phaeochromocytoma. Br J Surg 86:94–7

16. Neumann HP, Reincke M, Bender BU, et al. (1999) Preserved adrenocortical function after laparoscopic bilateral adrenal sparing surgery for hereditary pheochromocytoma. J Clin Endocrinol Metab 84:2608–10

17. O'Riordain DS, O'Brien T, Crotty TB, et al. (1995) Multiple endocrine neoplasia type 2B: More than an endocrine disorder. Surgery 118:936

18. Quinn TM, Rubino F, Gagner M (2002) Laparoscopic adrenalectomy, chap 27. In: ACS Surgery: Principles and Practice. American College of Surgeons, Chicago

19. Radmayr C, Neumann H, Bartsch G, Elsner R, Janetschek G (2000) Laparoscopic partial adrenalectomy for bilateral pheochromocytomas in a boy with von Hippel-Lindau disease. Eur Urol 38:344–8

20. Raue F, Frank-Raue K, Grauer A (1994) Multiple endocrine neoplasia type 2: Clinical features and screening. Endocrinol Metab Clin North Am 23:137

21. Siperstein A, Berber E (2002) Laparoscopic ultrasonography of the adrenal glands. In: Gagner M, Inabnet WB (eds) Minimally invasive endocrine surgery. Lippincott Williams & Wilkins, Philadelphia, pp 175–183

22. van Heerden JA, Sizemore GW, Carney JA, Brennan MD, Sheps SG (1985) Bilateral subtotal adrenal resection for bilateral pheochromocytomas in multiple endocrine neoplasia, type IIa: a case report. Surgery 98:363–6

23. Reference deleted

24. Walther MM, Keiser HR, Choyke PL, Rayford W, Lyne JC, Linehan WM (1999) Management of hereditary pheochromocytoma in von Hippel-Lindau kindreds with partial adrenalectomy. J Urol 161:395–8

25. Walz MK, Peitgen K, Saller B et al. (1998) Subtotal adrenalectomy by the posterior retroperitoneoscopic approach. World J Surg 22:621–6

26. Zielke A, Rothmund M (1997) Adrenal imaging procedures. In: Clark OH, Duh QY (eds) Textbook of endocrine surgery. WB Saunders, Philadelphia, pp 466–474

28 Anesthesia for Adrenal Surgery

Stavros G. Memtsoudis, Cephas Swamidoss, Maria Psoma

CONTENTS

28.1 Introduction

The successful diagnosis and treatment of patients with adrenal tumors requires a well orchestrated multidisciplinary approach. This chapter emphasizes the perioperative anesthetic concerns associated with adrenal resections. While not meant to be all-inclusive, it highlights important factors in anesthetic decision-making. The surgeon's appreciation of anesthesia-related concerns can facilitate the patient's evaluation and avoid delays in assessment. The goals of the anesthesiologist include: (1) gathering information about the patient's adrenal disease and general health status, (2) identification of specific problems associated with the patient's condition, (3) institution of interventions that will minimize perioperative risks and (4) development of a concise anesthetic and perioperative plan tailored to the patient's individual needs.

In general, anesthesia for non-functional adrenal tumors follows the principles for general abdominal surgical cases. Functional tumors, though, require special considerations and are discussed.

28.2 Pheochromocytoma

Preoperative Evaluation and Considerations ▶ Approximately 50% of pheochromocytoma related deaths in the hospital occur during induction of anesthesia or during surgery for other causes [1], underlining the important role the anesthesiologist assumes in the treatment of this disease. The patient's clinical presentation is usually related to massive release of catecholamines originating from chromaffin tissue. The typical symptom complex (headache, tachycardia and diaphoresis) is secondary to the secretion of catecholamines, which results in paroxysmal or sustained hypertension, tachydysrrhythmias and ectopic electrocardiographic (ECG) patterns [2, 3]. About 30% of patients with pheochromocytoma will present with left ventricular dysfunction secondary to catecholamine induced cardiomyopathy [4]. Intravascular hypovolemia requiring fluid resuscitation may necessitate insertion of a pulmonary artery catheter to carefully monitor left ventricular filling pressures [5]. Preoperative cardiac workup including an echocardiographic examination may be indicated in addition to the routine preoperative testing. A search for hypertension induced end-organ damage should be included in the assessment. Careful physical examination including fundoscopy may reveal valuable information. Basic central nervous system (CNS) and renal function can be assessed through a precise history and basic laboratory testing. An extremely nervous and tremulous patient, with muscle weakness and weight loss, may often be encountered and may require sedative therapy.

Glucose levels may be elevated as a result of increased sympathetic discharge [6]. Concomitant alpha-adrenergic blockade for hemodynamic treatment (see below) can prove beneficial because it supports endogenous insulin secretion. Exogenous insulin therapy may be necessary. A blood count may reveal polycythemia reflecting hemoconcentration, indicating the need for fluid resuscitation. Its adequacy can be monitored by a decrease in the hematocrit of 5% [6]. Rarely, pheochromocytomas are associated with medullary thyroid cancer as part of the multiple endocrine neoplasm (MEN) 2 syndrome. In these cases a careful airway examination to rule out tracheal involvement and displacement is indicated.

Further testing and examination should be directed by the patient's history and physical examination.

Preoperative Therapy ▶ Preoperative sympatholytic therapy with alpha- and beta-adrenoreceptor blockers and fluid resuscitation remains the standard of care for the patient with pheochromocytoma. Phenoxybenzamine has been in use for over 50 years [7] and has proven to be safe and cost-effective [8]. While its covalent, non-competitive binding to alpha-1-adrenoreceptors results in the intended sympatholytic effect, its non-selectivity results in potential problems that need to be addressed by the anesthesiologist. Blockade of presynaptic alpha-2-adrenoreceptors leads to an interruption of the feedback loop regulating the release of norepinephrine in presynaptic nerve endings. This disinhibition can lead to detrimental effects in the heart such as tachycardia. Beta-adrenergic blockade may become necessary [2, 4], but requires caution in patients with myocardial depression. The irreversibility of the blockade, secondary to alkylation of the receptor by the drug, makes the synthesis of new receptors the rate limiting step for its reversal [9]. This may lead to prolonged hypotension in the immediate postoperative period. In addition, CNS effects, primarily somnolence in patients receiving phenoxybenzamine, have been described [4]. This observation may be secondary to its clonidine-like effect on alpha-2-adrenoreceptors and may require the anesthesiologist to adjust anesthetic drug dosing.

The selective, competitive alpha-1-adrenoreceptor blocker doxazosin has the advantages of reversible binding at the receptor, not crossing the blood brain barrier, and obviating the drug-induced need for concomitant beta-blockade in the preoperative period [2, 10]. Other drugs in current use include prazosin, terazosin and metyrosine. The latter interferes with the synthesis of catecholamines and has proven an valuable adjunct to antiadrenergic blockade [11]. Continuation of alpha-1-adrenoreceptor blocker therapy until the day of surgery is recommended [6].

In addition to the use of beta-1-blockers to counteract the presynaptic effects of phenoxybenzamine, these drugs may be utilized to prevent epinephrine secreting tumor-induced tachycardia [2]. It is strongly recommended that beta-blockade should be instituted only after alpha-blockade, to prevent cardiac failure secondary to drug induced myocardial depression in the setting of increased afterload [6].

Anesthetic Management ▶ The most commonly employed anesthetic technique for the resection of pheochromocytoma is general endotracheal anesthesia with or without neuraxial blockade via an epidural catheter [2]. The main goal of the anesthetic management is to anticipate and treat surges of sympathetic discharge. Despite preoperative adrenergic blockade, labile intraoperative hemodynamics are common [12]. The anesthesiologist's familiarity with the procedure and cooperation with the surgeon is important to identify and anticipate phases of increased stimulation. Intubation, positioning, incision and surgical manipulation of the tumor are only a few points during the procedure that warrant increased vigilance [13]. Availability of fast acting antihypertensives and the avoidance of drugs that stimulate the sympathetic autonomic system are necessary.

Preoperative medication can be useful to treat the anxious patient, thus reducing the level of sympathetic output. Benzodiazepines like midazolam seem a likely choice and can be titrated to effect without major impact on hemodynamics. If opioids are used, synthetic derivatives, such as fentanyl and sufentanil, should be favored over morphine, which can release histamine and stimulate catecholamine release [6]. Under adequate sedation and local anesthesia, invasive hemodynamic monitoring with a peripheral arterial line should be established prior to induction of anesthesia. If central venous and pulmonary pressure monitoring is deemed necessary as per the patient's cardiovascular status, the placement pre-induction has to be balanced against the hazards of potential adverse hemodynamic derangements. In the hands of the experienced practitioner this procedure can be performed safely at this time. The same is true for the potential insertion of an epidural catheter [2, 13].

Induction of anesthesia is achieved by intravenous injection of propofol, etomidate or barbiturates in combination with synthetic opioids. Ketamine should not be used, due to its ability to stimulate the sympathetic nervous system and cause hypertension and tachycardia. Once loss of consciousness has been induced, anesthesia can be deepened by ventilation of the patient's lungs with an inhalational agent. While virtually all anesthetic gases have been successfully used in the past, halothane and desflurane should be used with caution. Halothane has the potential to sensitize the myocardium to catecholamine and increase the risk for arrhythmias. Desflurane, although quickly titratable, can stimulate the sympathetic nervous system, especially when concentrations are being increased rapidly [6, 14]. Iso- and sevoflurane are common choices.

Paralysis to facilitate endotracheal intubation and ventilation can be achieved with a variety of drugs, such as *cis*-atracurim and vecuronium, both of which are virtually devoid of histamine releasing effects and are hemodynamically inactive. Pancuronium, which has sympathetic properties, and atracurium and mivacurium, which are associated with histamine release, should be used judiciously. Although probably not clinically significant, the choice of succinylcholine for rapid sequence induction may theoretically lead to hypertension due to tumor compression by abdominal muscle contraction or histamine release [6]. In this setting, rocuronium should be considered as an alternative.

Placement of an endotracheal tube should only be performed in the setting of adequate levels of anesthesia. The use of intravenous boluses of esmolol, lidocaine or additional opioids just prior to intubation may help to blunt the reflexive sympathetic discharge associated with laryngoscopy [6].

Maintenance ▸ Following induction, anesthesia is usually maintained by administration of a volatile anesthetic with or without the addition of nitrous oxide. Opioids are supplemented as needed. If an epidural catheter is in place it may be dosed with local anesthetics, opioids or a combination, thereby decreasing systemic requirements for pain medication. Local anesthetics may be useful in the control of hypertension. Opioids administered alone may have the advantage that they do not cause the degree of sympathectomy seen with local anesthetics and, therefore, will not aggravate potential hypotension after the pheochromocytoma is resected.

Hypertensive episodes during the procedure should be anticipated and can be treated with the combination of: (1) changes in the concentration of the volatile agent used and (2) infusions of intravenous drugs with rapid onset and short half-life. Commonly, nitroprusside, phentolamine, trimetaphan, nitroglycerine or nicardipine are used, the choice being dependent on the anesthesiologist's familiarity and comfort with the drug [13]. Intravenous magnesium infusions have also been used successfully [2]. If difficulties in controlling blood pressure are persistent, cessation of manipulation by the surgeon should be requested.

Although preoperative adrenergic blockade may have been satisfactory, additional administration of direct adrenoreceptor blocking drugs is often indicated intraoperatively. Labetalol and esmolol lend themselves to intraoperative use, because of their relatively short action [15]. Careful titration of beta-blockers is necessary to prevent cardiac pump failure in patients with catechol-induced cardiomyopathies. Transesophageal echocardiography may be indicated in this select patient population [16]. In addition to the hemodynamic monitoring, electrolyte and glucose monitoring should be available. Hyperglycemia preoperatively may be followed by hypoglycemia after isolation of the tumor [17]. The ability to treat either abnormality should be readily available.

Conclusion of Surgery and Postoperative Considerations ▸ The use of short acting drugs is especially advantageous in light of frequently encountered hypotension after resection of the tumor. Lightening of anesthetic depth, intravenous fluid administration and use of vasopressors, such as phenylephrine, are often necessary and are guided by invasive monitoring. In contrast, many other patients remain hypertensive and require continuation of sympatholytic therapy. In the otherwise healthy individual and in the absence of complications, extubation is usually performed at the conclusion of surgery. Electrolyte and glucose monitoring should be continued until values have stabilized.

28.3   Conn's Syndrome

Preoperative Evaluation and Considerations ▸ Primary hyperaldosteronism results from the uninhibited secretion of aldosterone from either hyperplastic adrenal glands, mineralocorticoid-secreting adenomas or, rarely, cancers. Clinical sequelae are hypokalemia, hypomagnesemia, alkalosis, weakness, paresthesias, tetany, nephropathy induced polyuria and refractory hypertension [3, 6, 18, 19]. Fluid retention secondary to sodium absorption by the kidneys may result in an extracellular volume increase of up to 30% [18], thus contributing to the possibility of congestive heart failure in these patients. Other mechanisms have been proposed by which aldosterone may be involved directly in the propagation of cardiac dysfunction [20]. Electrolyte abnormality induced arrhythmias are additional concerns [18]. Inverted T-waves and U-waves may be visible on the ECG [3]. If surgery is planned and myocardial compromise is suspected, a thorough cardiac workup is indicated. Invasive monitoring with a pulmonary artery catheter or transesophageal echocardiography may be indicated during the procedure. A potentially increased sensitivity to neuromuscular blockade should be considered in the patient with muscle weakness [18]. Respiratory muscle weakness may lead to decreased pulmonary reserve and cough reflexes.

The anesthesiologist should be aware that chronic hypokalemia by itself can lead to cardiomyopathy with fibrosis, nephropathy, depression of baroreceptor activity and antagonistic effect on insulin secretion [18]. Careful consideration when administering drugs and anesthetics that can further impact these systems is warranted.

The occasional presentation of primary hyperaldosteronism with pheochromocytoma or acromegaly should alert the anesthesiologist to the possibility of unexpected phases of paroxysmal hypertension or a difficult airway [21]. The presence of concomitant osteoporosis warrants special care during positioning of the patient.

Preoperative Treatment ▶ The goals of preoperative management are: (1) control of hypertension, (2) optimization of cardiac function, (3) restoration of the intravascular fluid status and (4) correction of acid-base and electrolyte abnormalities.

The aldosterone antagonist spironolactone has been recommended for the treatment of hyperaldosteronism. One to 2 weeks of treatment may be necessary for the onset of effects [14, 22]. Spironolactone may also be helpful in those patients receiving prolonged treatment with ACE inhibitors for hypertension and heart failure. Increased aldosterone levels ("aldosterone escape") have been found in this patient population [18]. Overall, an individually tailored combination of antihypertensives and diuretics is indicated. Of interest, it has been suggested that intraoperative hemodynamics may be more stable when electrolytes and hypertension are controlled with preoperative spironolactone therapy when compared to other antihypertensive drugs.

In addition to hypertension, hypokalemia-related problems are responsible for most other complications in this population. Hypokalemia should be corrected preoperatively, realizing that completely normal values may not be achievable. The total body deficit may be as high as 400 mEq, requiring at least 24 h for repletion to avoid cardiac toxicity [14]. Potassium depletion may be higher in patients with a high sodium intake [18]. Potassium repletion may be difficult without con-

comitant repletion of magnesium stores. Development of tonic muscle contractures has been reported to occur secondary to potassium repletion in Caucasians with Conn's syndrome [23]. Hypovolemia from excessive use of diuretics should be corrected.

Anesthetic Management ▶ General endotracheal anesthesia is most commonly used for patients with Conn's syndrome. Epidural use of local anesthetics requires definitive intravascular volume repletion preoperatively in order to avoid sympathectomy-induced hypotension.

Preoperative Medication ▶ Administration of benzodiazepines may be indicated in the anxious, hypertensive patient. Preoperative opioids, which depress the respiratory drive, should be administered with caution and with monitoring in the patient with pulmonary muscle weakness. If bilateral adrenal resection or manipulation is planned, a stress dose of cortisol should be considered preoperatively and continued for 24 h [6].

Induction ▶ Induction agents should be chosen according to the patient's hemodynamic status. Intravenous barbiturates and opioids should be titrated carefully. Previously hypertensive patients may become profoundly hypotensive if hypovolemia is inadequately corrected. Depressed hypokalemia-induced baroreceptor function may contribute to this problem. The necessity for insertion of invasive hemodynamic monitoring prior to induction is dependent on the patient's cardiovascular status. Etomidate is characterized by the absence of hemodynamic effects, but can suppress adrenal function even after a single dose [24]. Although the clinical significance is not clear, this fact should be kept in mind in the patient in whom postoperative hypocortisolism is expected.

Excessive hyperventilation after loss of consciousness may lead to aggravation of hypokalemia and should be avoided [6]. When choosing a paralytic agent the increased sensitivity of patients with Conn's syndrome should be kept in mind. Hypokalemia and alkalosis can potentially lead to a prolonged effect of non-depolarizing neuromuscular blockers [18]. Thus, drugs of shorter action like vecuronium and *cis*-atracurium should be favored over ones with a longer half-life like pancuronium. Careful monitoring of neuromuscular blockade with a twitch monitor may be helpful in the further titration of drugs.

Maintenance ▸ Inhaled anesthetic agents, with or without the addition of nitrous oxide or intravenous anesthetics, are acceptable. Sevoflurane and enflurane, which are burdened with potential nephrotoxicity, should probably be avoided in the patient with nephropathy [6]. The myocardial depressive effects of halothane should be kept in mind when treating patients with cardiomyopathy.

The intraoperative use of an epidural catheter should include careful consideration of its hemodynamic consequences. Intravascular volume assessment, a preoperative problem in this patient population, may become even more difficult in the setting of positive pressure ventilation, vasodilatory effects of anesthetics and intraoperative fluid losses. Intravascular monitoring may become necessary at this point [6]. Glucose and electrolyte levels should be checked frequently.

Conclusion of Surgery and Postoperative Considerations ▸ Neuromuscular block reversal and assessment of patient strength should precede extubation, especially if preoperative weakness is encountered. A sustained head lift or a strong hand grip for a minimum of 5 s can be considered sufficient. Tidal volumes should be observed to ensure adequate ventilatory effort. If an epidural catheter is in place, it should be dosed to allow for lung excursions not inhibited by pain, thereby avoiding systemic opioids. Careful observation of electrolytes should continue, since potassium deficiency may be observed as long as a week after surgery [25]. Temporary or permanent mineralocorticoid or glucocorticoid therapy may become necessary, depending on the extent of the resection. Hypertension may persist into the postoperative period and pharmacologic treatment should continue [18].

28.4 Cushing's Syndrome from an Adrenal Source

Preoperative Evaluation and Considerations ▸ Surgery for Cushing's syndrome carries the highest perioperative mortality risk among the indications for adrenalectomy discussed in this chapter [14, 26]. Adrenalectomy for hypercortisolism requires the anesthesiologist's full understanding of all aspects of the clinical complex associated with Cushing's syndrome. The inappropriate secretion of cortisol can lead to weight gain, hypertension, diabetes, myopathy, renal calculi, osteoporosis and psychologic changes often requiring pharmacotherapy [3, 6].

There are many anesthetic considerations. The patient's typical physique (i.e. obesity concentrated centrally with facial fat thickening [6]) presents the anesthesiologist with the potential of a difficult airway. A thorough evaluation with a back-up plan for emergency surgical airway access (tracheostomy) must be devised should conventional modes of intubation fail. The presence of obstructive sleep apnea should be considered and integrated in the perioperative plan [27]. Additional considerations related to obesity involve multiple organ systems. Decreased chest wall compliance and functional residual capacity in the presence of increased oxygen consumption results in a severely reduced pulmonary reserve. Increased carbon dioxide production requires increased minute ventilation to maintain normocarbia and further contributes to the likelihood of perioperative pulmonary complications [28]. Pulmonary function testing and a chest X-ray may be indicated preoperatively to rule out any additional and reversible compromise. Steroid myopathy involving ventilatory muscle may further aggravate pulmonary function. If chronic hypoxemia is present, polycythemia may develop and increase the risk for thromboembolic events.

Cardiovascular aberrations include hypertension, cardiac dysfunction secondary to chronically increased blood volume and cardiac output. Pulmonary hypertension may develop in the presence of obstructive sleep apnea. Sudden death is a known complication of morbid obesity and thorough preoperative cardiac work-up is strongly suggested [28]. Obesity and chronic exposure to high levels of steroids and glucose can damage the vasculature and make it difficult to obtain vascular access.

Glucose intolerance is common and should be treated perioperatively. Liver function may be affected and implications for drug metabolism should be kept in mind. Liver function testing should be considered.

Increases in weight should be differentiated from the loss of muscle mass. Myopathy and resulting muscle weakness should lead to a careful titration of neuromuscular blocking agents. Intravenous drugs should be dosed according to ideal rather than actual body weight and titrated to effect.

Abnormalities involving the intestinal tract include increased intra-abdominal pressure, intragastric fluid and increased probability of the existence of a hiatal hernia, all of which put this patient population into a high risk category for pulmonary aspiration [28].

Steroid-induced osteoporosis warrants caution during positioning for surgery.

Hypokalemia and fluid retention are common features of Cushing's syndrome [14].

Preoperative treatment options for hypercortisolism secondary to adrenal etiology are limited and focus on optimizing the patient's intravascular fluid status, electrolyte balance and glucose levels. Spironolactone may be used to treat aldosterone-induced hypervolemia and potassium wasting. Inhibitors of steroid production such as metyrapone and mitotane have limited use. Hypertension should be controlled with pharmacotherapy as needed [14].

Anesthetic Management ▷ General anesthesia, with or without epidural anesthesia, is used for the patient with Cushing's syndrome and management is tailored towards problems related to obesity. Epidurally delivered analgesia should be used whenever possible during the postoperative course in order to minimize systemically administered respiratory depressant opioids. This allows for early breathing exercises and helps to decrease the chance of pulmonary complications arising from atelectasis and hypoventilation. In light of both the difficulties in identifying landmarks and the potential vertebral collapse secondary to osteoporosis in the obese patient with Cushing's disease, an epidural catheter should be inserted preoperatively in the sitting position and should be tested for satisfactory function [28].

Preoperative medication should be kept to a minimum to avoid compromise of the patient's respiratory status. If preoperative medication is deemed necessary, careful monitoring, especially for the patient with sleep apnea, is indicated. Intramuscular injections should be avoided because of the chance of erroneous injections into fatty tissue. Aspiration precautions should include strict adherence to fasting guidelines, administration of non-particulate antacids by mouth, and use of prokinetic drugs and intravenous antacids. A combination of H2-receptor blockers, metoclopramide and sodium citrate can be given [28]. Hydrocortisone replacement therapy may be necessary and should be started at the time of resection of the tumor [14]. Chronic suppression of the contralateral adrenal gland or resection of both glands can lead to acute hypocortisolism.

Induction ▷ The combination of a potentially difficult airway and the increased chance of pulmonary aspiration may warrant an awake fiberoptic intubating technique with the patient in the sitting position [28]. A well informed patient will usually understand this safety maneuver. The procedure can be performed using the nasal approach under mild sedation and after anesthetizing the nasal and oropharyngeal cavities. Intranasal phenylephrine spray may reduce the risk of bleeding while intravenous glycopyrrolate may improve visibility by reducing secretions. Surgical backup for emergency tracheostomy should be available. If the patient's airway allows for standard intubation with a laryngoscope, a rapid sequence induction with cricoid pressure becomes mandatory. Pre-oxygenation is ever more important due to the decreased functional residual capacity that predisposes the obese patient to faster hypoxemia than their non-obese counterpart [29]. Initial administration of neuromuscular blockers should be reduced and effects monitored in light of the common occurrence of myopathy and hypokalemia. Cardiovascular monitoring pre-induction is dictated by the patient's cardiovascular status.

Maintenance ▷ After induction of anesthesia and confirmation of endotracheal tube placement a nasogastric tube should be placed and intragastric contents suctioned. A combination of epidural local anesthetics with a volatile inhalational anesthetic is acceptable for maintenance of anesthesia. When dosing the epidural, the dose should be reduced by up to 25% compared with a patient of normal weight. This phenomenon reflects a decreased volume of the epidural space secondary to higher intra-abdominal pressures leading to a larger space occupation by engorged vessels [30]. It should be kept in mind that lipid soluble drugs may be stored in fatty tissue and undergo prolonged clearance when administered repeatedly or for a prolonged time. In this context, an inhalational anesthetic agent with relatively low lipid solubility such as desflurane or sevoflurane may be preferred to isoflurane and halothane. Nitrous oxide should be avoided in patients with pulmonary hypertension as aggravation of symptoms can result from its use. Its potential to distend the bowel in the setting of already difficult surgical exposure makes it an unlikely choice. Intravenous drugs with short half-lives and low lipid solubility should be chosen. The use of propofol or barbiturates may lead to a prolonged time for awakening [31].

Ventilation may prove problematic and the use of large tidal volumes and positive end-expiratory pressure with acceptance of high peak airway pressures may become necessary. The laparoscopic approach with increased intra-abdominal pressures is of particular concern and necessitates complete cooperation between the surgeon and anesthesiologist. A reverse Trendelenburg position, if feasible, may be helpful in alleviating difficulties. Careful monitoring of the intravascular fluid status, serum glucose and electrolytes perioperatively is indicated.

Conclusion of Surgery and Postoperative Considerations ▶

Neuromuscular blockade should be reversed and the patient should be fully awake and following commands before extubation of the trachea can be considered. The upright sitting position and dosing of the epidural catheter can facilitate improved breathing dynamics. The patient with sleep apnea may be electively transferred intubated to an intensive care setting to allow for careful monitoring of arterial blood gases and clearance of residual anesthesia. Extubation should be performed in the presence of a physician skilled in airway management. Satisfactory levels of analgesia can be achieved with epidural use of local anesthetics. Opioids, even when used neuraxially, can cause respiratory depression in the susceptible patient with sleep apnea [32]. Supplementation with nonsteroidal analgesics may be beneficial.

Steroid replacement therapy becomes necessary, especially after bilateral adrenalectomy. Cardiovascular instability can occur secondary to adrenal insufficiency. Monitoring of electrolytes and glucose levels needs to be continued until stable levels have been achieved.

28.5   Addison's Disease

Hypocortisolism per se is not an indication for adrenal gland resection and will be mentioned only briefly. Nevertheless, destruction of the adrenal cortex by cancer, granuloma or hemorrhage may rarely require adrenalectomy. Management of anesthesia follows many of the aforementioned principles and does not involve any special considerations other than cortisol replacement and therapy. With the exception of etomidate, which can depress remaining adrenal function, all other anesthetic drugs may be used without special consideration, unless concomitant diseases need to be considered [6]. The involved clinicians should be familiar with signs and symptoms of hypocortisolism and be ready to treat the problems arising from it.

28.6   Monitoring

The monitoring for adrenalectomy procedures varies with the pathology and general health status of the individual patient and has been discussed, in part, above.

ECG, blood pressure and pulse oxymetry monitoring should be employed on a standard basis. An arterial line should be placed pre-induction in patients with pheochromocytomas in order to be able to assess and treat the cardiovascular response to induction and intraoperative stimulation. Postoperative surveillance should be continued. The respiratory management of the patient with Cushing's disease and sleep apnea may be facilitated by the knowledge of a pre-induction arterial blood gas. Frequent arterial blood gas analysis may be facilitated by the presence of an arterial line. In all other cases, the insertion of invasive hemodynamic monitoring, including central venous and pulmonary artery catheters, should be considered according to the patient's cardiopulmonary status and the need for invasive volume monitoring. Transesophageal echocardiography may be indicated in selected patients. Urine output monitoring with a Foley catheter may assist in the assessment of intravascular fluid status. Warming devices should be employed and patient temperature monitored. Hypothermia may delay awakening, reversal of neuromuscular blockade and may increase bleeding. A twitch monitor is useful, especially in patients with preoperative muscular weakness. Continuous end-tidal CO_2 monitoring should be used and may reveal valuable information during laparoscopic procedures and in patients with compromised lung function. Electrolyte and glucose monitoring is advised in patients with functional adrenal tumors.

28.7   Adrenalectomy Related Perioperative Complications

Adrenalectomies have become relatively safe procedures over the last few decades. Advances in anesthetic monitoring and surgical technique have contributed to this safety. Nevertheless the perioperative physician should be familiar not only with possible problems arising from the patient's specific pathology, but also with problems related to the procedure itself.

The rate of pneumothoraces approaches 20% [3, 14] and a high level of suspicion should prevail. Intraoperative evaluation can often prevent surprises and emergent intervention in the recovery room. Signs in the intubated patient are related to the size of the pneumothorax and can include increased peak airway pressures as well as hypoxemia. The extubated patient may complain of chest pain and difficulty breathing. Insertion on a chest tube may be necessary.

Estimated blood loss is usually below 300 ml [2], but hemorrhage after difficult resection should be expected. Retroperitoneal bleeding may not become obvious until late if one relies on drainage output as an indicator of hemorrhage. Hemodynamic depression may be secondary to inadequate fluid resuscitation, bleeding and hypocortisolism, especially after bilateral procedures. Cardiogenic causes should be in the differential diagnosis, in view of the high incidence of cardiomyopathies in this patient population. Respiratory complications warrant vigilance especially in the obese patient with Cushing's disease. Complications related to laparoscopy are discussed separately.

28.8   Pain Management

The visual analogue pain score varies by surgical technique and lies between 6–9 with the open approach [3]. Diaphragmatic function is depressed after upper abdominal surgery and contributes to the development of atelectasis [33, 34]. Pain management can improve respiratory function and contribute to the prevention of pulmonary complications secondary to splinting [33]. Successful analgesia can help the patient with early ambulation and thus may decrease the chance of thromboembolic events. The risk of adverse cardiac events may be reduced as well [35].

The epidural technique has the advantage that it can be used intra- and postoperatively. The major advantage of an epidural catheter for pain management is the relatively low dose of opioids needed in comparison to the systemic dose that would be necessary for satisfactory analgesia. In our experience, epidural patient-controlled analgesia with a continuous baseline rate provides good pain relief and high patient satisfaction. The combination of a low concentration of local anesthetic such as bupivacaine 0.08% with or without the addition of an opioid has a high success rate. At this concentration of local anesthetic, sympathectomy and hypotension, as well as involvement of motoneurons, are negligible. The most commonly encountered problems are pruritus, nausea and breakthrough pain. The first two are related to the use of opioids and can be treated with antihistamines, antiemetics or low dose infusion of naloxone. If complaints persist, the opioid can be removed from the infusion.

Contraindications are an uncooperative patient and the inability to treat complications from inadvertent intrathecal or intravascular migration. Coagulopathies preclude the instrumentation of the epidural space due to the risk of epidural hematoma formation and neurologic complications thereof. The use of low dose heparin or NSAIDS at the time of epidural catheter insertion is controversial [33]. In experienced hands, the small risk of neurologic deficits from epidural catheter placement should be significantly lower than that of pulmonary embolism in this patient population. Heparinization should probably be withheld for some time if a bloody tap is encountered during placement. If removal of the catheter is planned, the last dose of prophylactic unfractionated heparin should not be given within 6–12 h. Neurologic assessment and inspection of the catheter site for signs of infection and bleeding should be routinely employed.

Complications include postdural puncture headache and intrathecal or intravascular injection. Aspiration at frequent intervals can help exclude the latter two. Care should be taken to adjust dosing for obese patients as discussed earlier.

If an epidural catheter is not available, the intravenous administration of opioids and NSAIDS can be considered. Morphine or hydromorphone are commonly delivered via patient-controlled analgesia with good result. Although respiratory depression may be a concern, the use of patient controlled analgesia is considered to be safe, and the incidence of respiratory depression has been reported to be between 0.31% and 0.7%. Old age, hypovolemia and the use of a continuous infusion may be risk factors [33]. Skilled staff should be available to monitor and treat respiratory depression.

NSAIDS such as Ketorolac may decrease the overall requirements for opioids. Caution in patients with renal dysfunction, peptic ulcer disease and its antiplatelet action must be considered when using these drugs.

28.9   Anesthetic Implication of Laparoscopic Surgery for Adrenalectomy

The laparoscopic approach for adrenalectomy has become a successful and safe alternative to open surgical removal over the last decade [36, 37]. The advantages are faster postoperative recovery, earlier ambulation, shorter hospital stays and less pain [38, 39]. Special concerns are raised when using this technique for the resection of pheochromocytomas. The compression of the tumor by the pneumoperitoneum has been associated with increased secretion of catecholamines and intraoperative hemodynamic changes [40, 41].

This problem though can be managed safely in the hands of a vigilant anesthesiologist and pheochromocytoma resection can be successfully performed with this approach [38, 41]. Catecholamine release by direct manipulation may actually occur less during laparoscopy [38].

General endotracheal anesthesia with or without the adjunct use of an epidural is usually favored for laparoscopic adrenalectomy. The proximity of the surgical field to the diaphragm and the addition of a pneumoperitoneum is usually not well tolerated from a respiratory point in the spontaneously breathing patient. Anesthesia can be maintained with inhalational agents or be conducted as a total intravenous technique (TIVA). It has been suggested that inhalational agents may be more appropriate for functioning adrenal adenomas while TIVA may have benefits in non-functioning tumors [42].

Regardless of the technique, both anesthesiologists and surgeons should be familiar with the physiologic changes and complications associated with a pneumoperitoneum.

Respiratory changes include a decrease in compliance and functional residual capacity and an increase in peak airway pressures [43]. All are secondary to the elevation of the diaphragm. The insufflation of CO_2 results in systemic absorption and is related to the level of intra-abdominal pressure [44]. The combination with impaired ventilation leads to CO_2 retention, necessitating hyperventilation by increasing the respiratory rate in order to maintain normocapnia. Patients with chronic obstructive pulmonary disease (COPD) may be particularly challenging to treat.

Hemodynamic changes include a reduction in cardiac output that is partially attributed to decreased venous return [45, 46]. Preoperative intravenous volume administration may help alleviate this problem. The increased peripheral vascular resistance seen with the institution of a pneumoperitoneum may be deleterious for patients with limited cardiac reserve [47]. Decreases in renal perfusion and venous stasis in the lower extremities should be kept in mind. Avoidance of nephrotoxins and deep venous thrombosis prophylaxis should be considered.

Complications from pneumoperitoneum include subcutaneous emphysema, as well as pneumothorax and pneumomediastinum. Endobronchial intubation from cephalad movement of the carina may occur. Gas embolism secondary to intravascular or intraorgan gas injection is a feared complication. The severity of clinical sequelae are related to the volume and rate of gas entry [48]. The formation of an air-lock in the right ventricular outflow tract constitutes the worst scenario and can lead to cardiovascular collapse and paradoxic gas emboli. Diagnosis and treatment are similar to those of air embolism. Cessation of gas insufflation, head-down and right-side-up position to displace the air, hyperventilation with pure oxygen and aspiration of gas through a multi-orifice central venous catheter are recommended. Cardiopulmonary resuscitation with vasopressors may become necessary. Rapid absorption of CO_2 is of benefit but this complication can nevertheless be fatal [45].

Vagal tone can increase during insufflation secondary to activation of peritoneal stretch receptors and bradycardia or asystole may result. Release of the pneumoperitoneum and atropine administration may be required [45].

In conclusion, the laparoscopic technique for adrenal surgery is safe and offers advantages over the open approach. Complications are rare, but mandate the close cooperation of anesthesiologists and surgeons for successful management and outcome.

References

1. Sutton MG, Sheps SG, Lie JT (1981) Prevalence of clinically unusual pheochromocytoma: Review of a 50-year autopsy series. Mayo Clin Proc 56:354–60
2. Prys-Roberts C (2000) Pheochromocytoma – recent progress in its management. Br J Anaesth 85:44–57
3. Weigel RJ, Oberhelman HA, Steven K (1999) Endocrine surgery –adrenalectomy. In: Jaffe RA, Samuels SI (eds) Anesthesiologist's manual of surgical procedures, 2nd edn. Lippincott Williams and Wilkins, Philadelphia, PA, pp 481–484
4. Hull CJ (1986) Pheochromocytoma: diagnosis, pre-operative preparation, and anesthetic management. Br J Anaesth 58:1453–68
5. Mihm PG (1983) Pulmonary artery pressure monitoring in patients with pheochromocytoma. Anesth Analg 62:1129–33
6. Stoelting RK, Dierdorf SF (2002) Endocrine disease – adrenal gland dysfunction. In: Stoelting RK, Diedorf SF (eds) Anesthesia and co-existing disease, 4th edn. Churchill Livingstone, Philadelphia, pp 425–434
7. Iseri LT, Henderson HW, Derr JW (1951) The use of adrenolytic drug, regitine, in pheochromocytoma. Am Heart J 42:129–36
8. Witteles RM, Kaplan EL, Roizen MF (2000) Safe and cost effective preoperative preparation of patients with pheochromocytoma. Anesth Analg 91:302–4
9. Hamilton CA, Dalrymple H, Reid JL (1982) Recovery in vivo and in vitro of α1-adrenoreceptor responses and radioligand binding after phenoxybenzamine. J Cardiovasc Pharmacol 4 (Suppl I):S125–8

10. Babamoto KS, Hirokawa WT (1992) Doxazosin: a new α1-adrenegic antagonist. Clin Pharm 11:415–27

11. Steinsapir J, Carr AA, Prisant LM, Bransome ED Jr (1997) Metyrosine and pheochromocytoma. Arch Intern Med 158:901–6

12. Kinney MAO, Warner ME, van Heerden JA, Harlocker TT, Young WF Jr, Schroeder DR, Maxson PM, Warner MA (2000) Preanesthetic risks and outcomes of pheochromocytoma and paraganglioma resection. Anesth Analg 91:1118–23

13. Bogdonoff DL (2002) Pheochromocytoma: Specialist cases that all must be prepared to treat? J Cardiothor Vasc Anesth 16:267–9

14. Roizen MF (2000) Anesthetic complications of concurrent diseases. In: Miller RD (ed) Anesthesia, 5th edn. Churchill Livingstone, Philadelphia, PA, pp 903–1015

15. Nicholas E, Deutschman CS, Allo M, Rock P (1988) Use of esmolol in the intraoperative management of pheochromocytoma. Anesth Analg 67:1114–7

16. Ryan T, Timoney A, Cunningham AJ (1993) Use of transesophageal echocardiography to manage beta-adrenoreceptor block and assess left ventricular function in a patient with pheochromocytoma. Br J Anaesth 70:101–3

17. Levin H, Heefetz M (1990) Phaeochromocytoma and severe protracted postoperative hypoglycemia. Can J Anaesth 37:477–8

18. Winship SM, Winstanley JHR, Hunter JM (1999) Anaesthesia for Conn's syndrome. Anaesthesia 54:564–74

19. Danforth DN, Orlando MM, Bartter FC, Javadpour N (1977) Renal changes in primary aldosteronism. J Urol 117:140–4

20. Zannad F (1995) Aldosterone and heart failure. Eur Heart J 16:98–102

21. Seidman PA, Kofke WA, Policare R, Young M (2000) Anaesthetic complications of acromegaly. Br J Anaesth 84:179–82

22. Weinberger MH, Grim CE, Hollifield JW, Ken DC, Ganguly A, Kramer NJ, Yune HY, Wellman H, Donohue JP (1979) Primary hyperaldesteronism: diagnosis, localization and treatment. Ann Intern Med 90:386–95

23. Gangat Y, Triner L, Baer L, Puchener P (1976) Primary aldosteronism with uncommon complications. Anesthesiology 45:542–4

24. Wagner RL, White PF, Kan PB, Rosenthal MH, Feldman D (1984) Inhibition of adrenal steroidogenesis by the anesthetic etomidate. N Engl J Med 310:1415–21

25. Celen O, O'Brien MJ, Melby JC, Beazley RM (1996) Factors influencing outcome of surgery for primary aldosteronism. Arch Surg 131:646–50

26. Welbourn RB (1985) Survival and cause of death after adrenalectomy for Cushing's disease. Surgery 97:16–20

27. Hiremath AS, Hillman DR, James AL, Noffsinger WJ, Platt PR, Singer SL (1998) Relation between difficult tracheal intubation and sleep apnea. Br J Anaesth 80:606–11

28. Vierra MA, Howard KH (1999) Operations for morbid obesity. In: Jaffe RA, Samuels SI (eds) Anesthesiologist's manual of surgical procedures, 2nd edn. Lippincott, Williams and Wilkins, Philadelphia, PA, pp 352–6

29. Berthoud MC, Peacock JE, Reilly CS (1991) Effectiveness of preoxygenation in morbidly obese patients. Br J Anaesth 67:464–6

30. Stoelting RK, Dierdorf SF (2002) Nutritional diseases and inborn errors of metabolism – obesity. In: Stoelting RK, Diedorf SF (eds) Anesthesia and co-existing disease, 4th edn. Churchill Livingstone, Philadelphia, pp 441–51

31. Juvin P, Vadam C, Malek L, Dupont H, Marmuse JP, Desmonts JM (2000) Postoperative recovery after desflurane, propofol, or isoflurane anesthesia among morbidly obese patients: a prospective, randomized study. Anesth Analg 91:714–9

32. Boushra NN (1996) Anaesthetic management of patients with sleep apnoea syndrome. Can J Anaesth 43:599–616

33. Ready B (2000) Acute perioperative pain. In: Miller RD (ed) Anesthesia, 5th edn. Churchill Livingstone, Philadelphia, PA, pp 2323–2350

34. Ford GT, Whitelaw WA, Rosenthal TW (1987) Diaphragm function after upper abdominal surgery in humans. Am Rev Respir Dis 127:431–6

35. Beattie WS, Buckley DN, Forrest JB (1993) Epidural morphine reduces the risk of postoperative myocardial ischemia in patients with cardiac risk factors. Can J Anaesth 40:532–41

36. Gagner M, Lacroix A, Bolte E (1992) Laparoscopic adrenalectomy for Cushing's syndrome and pheochromocytoma. N Engl J Med 327:1033

37. Jacobs JK, Goldstein RE, Geer RS (1997) Laparoscopic adrenalectomy: A new standard of care. Ann Surg 225:495–502

38. Sprung J, O'Hara JF Jr, Gill IS, Abdelmalak B, Sarnaik A, Bravo EL (2000) Anesthetic aspects of laparoscopic and open adrenalectomy for pheochromocytoma. Urology 55:339–343

39. Duh QJ, Siperstein AE, Lark OH, Schecter WP, Horn JK, Harrison MR, Hunt TK, Way LW (1996) Laparoscopic adrenalectomy. Comparison of the lateral and posterior approaches. Arch Surg 131:870–876

40. Joris JL, Chiche JD, Canivet JL, Jaquet NJ, Legros JJ, Lamy ML (1998) Hemodynamic changes induced by laparoscopy and their endocrine correlates: effects of clonidine. J Am Coll Cardiol 32:1389–96

41. Joris JL, Hamoir EE, Harstein GR, Meurisse MR, Hubert BM, Charlier CJ, Lamy ML (1999) Hemodynamic changes and catecholamine release during laparoscopic adrenalectomy for pheochromocytoma. Anesth Analg 88:16–21

42. Darvas K, Pinkola K, Borsodi M, Tarjanyi M, Winternitz T, Horanyi J (2000) General anesthesia for laparoscopic adrenalectomy. Med Sci Monit 6:560–63

43. Bardoczky GI, Engelman E, Levarlet M, Simon P (1993) Ventilatory effects of pneumoperitoneum monitored with continuous spirometry. Anaesthesia 48:309–11

44. Lister DR, Rudston-Brown B, Warriner CB, McEwen J, Chan M, Walley KR (1994) Carbon dioxide absorption is not linearly related to intraperitoneal carbon dioxide insufflation pressure in pigs. Anesthesiology 80:129–36

45. Joris JL (2000) Anesthesia for laparoscopic surgery. In: Miller RD (ed) Anesthesia, 5th edn. Churchill Livingstone, Philadelphia, PA, pp 2003–24

46. Sharma KC, Brandtstetter RD, Brensilver JM, Jung LD (1996) Cardiopulmonary physiology and pathophysiology as a consequence of laparoscopic surgery. Chest 110:810–5

47. Harris SN, Ballantyne GH, Luther MA, Perrino AC Jr (1996) Alterations of cardiovascular performance during laparoscopic colectomy: A combined hemodynamic and echocardiographic analysis. Anesth Analg 83:482–7

48. Mazoit JX, Umbrain V, Romain M, Samii K, d'Hollander A (1996) Effects of carbon dioxide embolism with nitrous oxide in the inspired gas in piglets. Br J Anaesth 76:428–34

29 Open Left Anterior Adrenalectomy

Dimitrios A. Linos

CONTENTS

29.1   Positions/Incisions (Fig. 1)

The patient lies in the supine position. The preferred incision for open anterior left adrenalectomy is as for right adrenalectomy an extended left subcostal incision. The midline incision may be used if the patient has a narrow costal angle or in the rare case of multiple adrenal paragangliomas/pheochromocytomas.

29.1.1   Approaches to the Left Adrenal Gland

The left adrenal gland can be approached via four different routes:
1. Through the gastrocolic ligament
2. Through the lienorenal ligament
3. Through the transverse mesocolon
4. Through the lesser omentum

The best approach is through the gastrocolic ligament into the lesser sac.

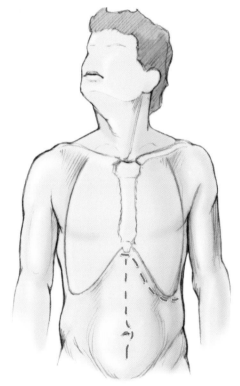

Fig. 1

29.2   Step I: Entering the Lesser Sac/Exposure of the Pancreas (Fig. 2)

The lesser sac is entered through the gastrocolic ligament. Gentle traction with two hands on the transverse colon and countertraction of the greater omentum will demonstrate the avascular plane that can be easily incised by diathermy. The lesser sac needs to be widely opened so that the anterior surface of the pancreas is well visualized. Occasionally if exposure is inadequate the splenic flexure of the colon can be mobilized. Adhesions from the posterior wall of the stomach to the pancreas are cauterized.

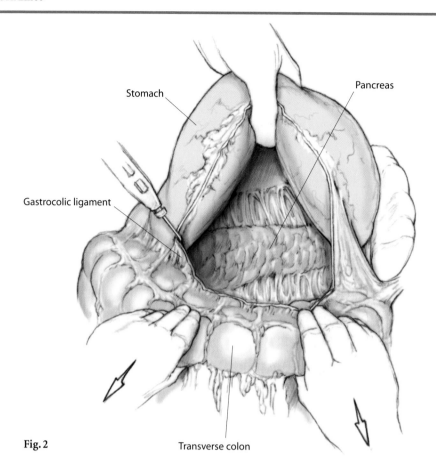

Stomach

Pancreas

Gastrocolic ligament

Fig. 2

Transverse colon

29.3   Step II: Mobilization of the Inferior Border of the Pancreas (Fig. 3)

The peritoneum along the inferior border of the pancreas is incised using cautery. The incision continues all the way from the body to the tail of the pancreas.

29.4   Step III: Exposure of the Adrenal; Ligation of the Left Adrenal Vein; Mobilization of the Left Adrenal Tumor (Fig. 4)

The left adrenal is exposed by lifting the inferior surface of the pancreas upwards. Gerota's fascia is opened and the upper pole of the kidney is retracted inferiorly. With blunt dissection the left renal vein is seen. Following this large vein 3–4 cm from the kidney's hilum a smaller, good size though long vertical vein will appear that leads into the adrenal tumor. This is the left adrenal vein. With a right angle clamp it is dissected and securely divided and ligated. When the tumor is large or highly vascular more large veins can be encountered requiring similar ligation while protecting the integrity of the left renal vein. Once the two to three large veins are ligated the remaining adrenal tumors can be easily mobilized. The smooth collaboration between the surgeon, who exposes each encountered small vessel with a long right-angle instrument ("disecteur"), and his first assistant, who coagulates them using his long "bovie", is the secret of the bloodless removal of the adrenal gland and tumor in toto.

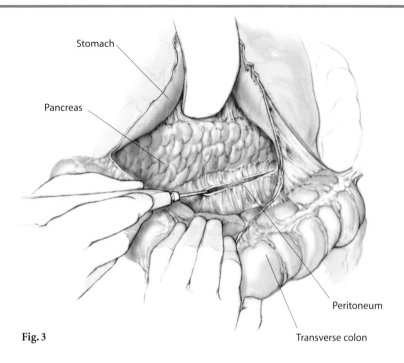

Stomach

Pancreas

Peritoneum

Transverse colon

Fig. 3

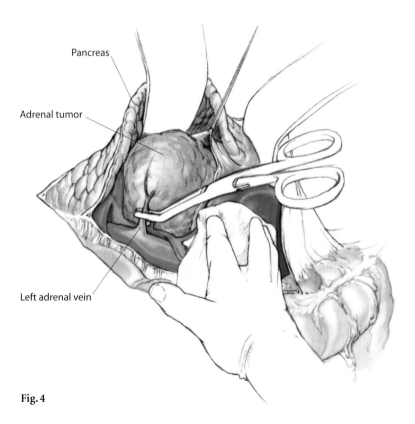

Pancreas

Adrenal tumor

Left adrenal vein

Fig. 4

30 Open Right Anterior Adrenalectomy

Dimitrios A. Linos

CONTENTS

30.1 Positions/Incisions (Fig. 1)

The position of the patient is supine. A pillow between his right flank and lower chest turns the torso about 20° to the left. Hyperextension of the operating table will allow more working space in the subcostal and lateral area. The preferred incision is an extended (both laterally and medially) generous right subcostal incision.

The alternative incision is an upper vertical midline incision with adequate infraumbilical extension especially in patients with narrow costal angle. This type of incision may also facilitate exploration of extra-adrenal pheochromocytomas/paragangliomas. Rarely, especially in very large adrenal carcinomas, a thoracoabdominal incision may be necessary for better exposure and control.

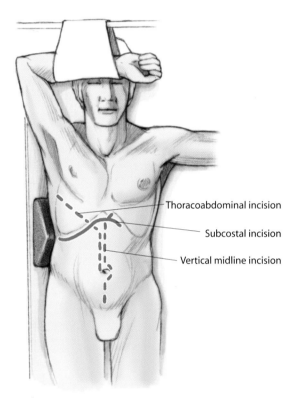

Thoracoabdominal incision

Subcostal incision

Vertical midline incision

Fig. 1

30.2   Step I: Kocher Maneuver (Fig. 2)

After initial hand evaluation of the abdomen is done to assess possible unknown preoperatively pathology, the hepatic flexure of the colon is mobilized inferiorly and the right lobe of the liver is retracted upwards. The aim in the first step is to expose and mobilize the second portion of the duodenum (Kocher maneuver). Scissors or monopolar diathermy is used to divide the lateral attachments of the duodenal loop.

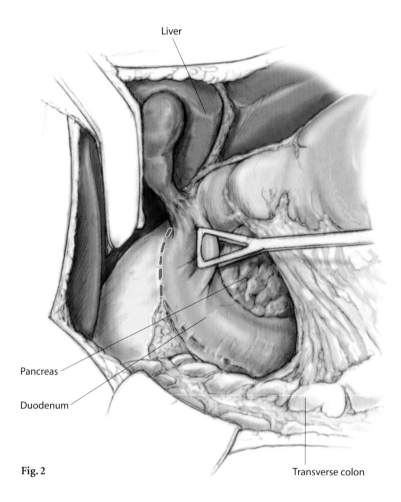

Fig. 2

30.3   Step II: Exposure of the IVC (Fig. 3)

The next and very important step is to expose the inferior vena cava from behind the duodenal loop to as high as possible. This exposure will lead to the adrenal tumor that is usually located higher than initially expected. On the other hand, this (at least 8–10 cm) exposure of the IVC will allow vascular control of the dangerous excessive bleeding that may occur inadvertently during the removal of the tumor, especially while trying to divide the right adrenal vein.

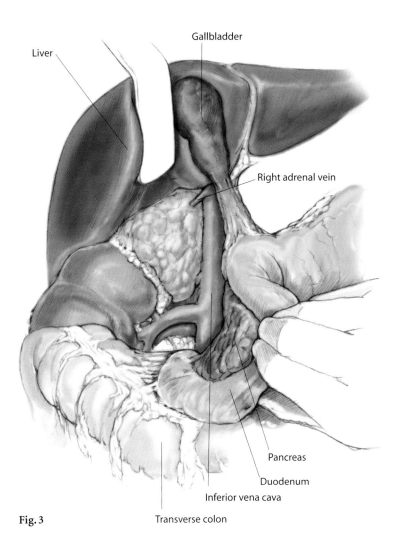

Fig. 3

30.4   Step III: Exposure of the Tumor/Initial Mobilization (Fig. 4)

With the inferior vena cava safely exposed, the left hand of the operating surgeon pulls the upper pole of the right kidney downwards to better expose the adrenal tumor. Gerota's fascia is widely opened and the tumor is clearly seen. A vein retractor is necessary to retract the IVC medially in order to expose the inner border of the adrenal tumor, which usually continues behind the IVC.

Mobilization of the tumor starts by freeing its medial attachments along the inferior vena cava, starting from the lower end and moving upwards toward the main "dangerous" right adrenal vein. Rather small arteries and veins will be encountered that can be cauterized and occasionally ligated depending on their size.

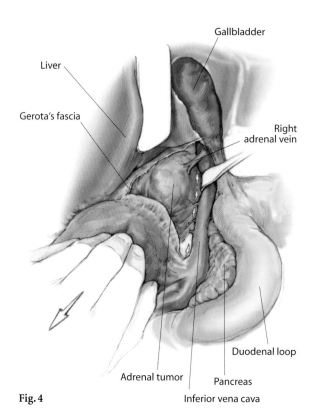

Fig. 4

30.5   Step IV: Identification and Control of Right Adrenal Vein (Fig. 5)

The main right adrenal vein is wide and short, draining directly into the inferior vena cava usually coming from the most superior and medial "corner" of the adrenal. A good and bloodless exposure of the area is necessary; the tip of a suction keeps the field dry to allow dissection of the main adrenal vein, allowing the placement of two clips on the caval site and one on the gland site. Fine long scissors or a knife blade can be used to safely divide the vein. In case of inadvertent avulsion or slippage of the caval clips serious hemorrhage can start. A Satinsky vascular clamp should immediately be placed along the previously exposed IVC for bleeding control and vascular repair.

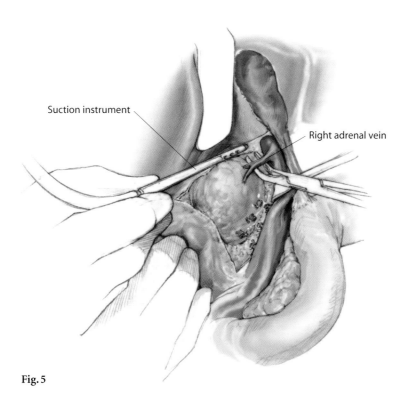

Suction instrument

Right adrenal vein

Fig. 5

30.6   Step V: Mobilization of the Tumor
(Fig. 6)

With the right main adrenal vein clipped and divided, the rest of the mobilization can be more easily and quickly done using monopolar diathermy and occasional ligation or clipping of larger vessels. The mobilization starts from the superior edge of the adrenal tumor that can be more easily seen with continuous downwards retraction of the right kidney. Special at-

tention is required during this phase because occasionally a large accessory subhepatic adrenal vein draining into the right hepatic vein can be encountered, requiring early recognition and safe division. The mobilization continues from the superior aspect of the tumor laterally along the essentially avascular plane requiring cautery use only. At the same time the posterior aspect of the tumor is mobilized from its loose connection to the diaphragm.

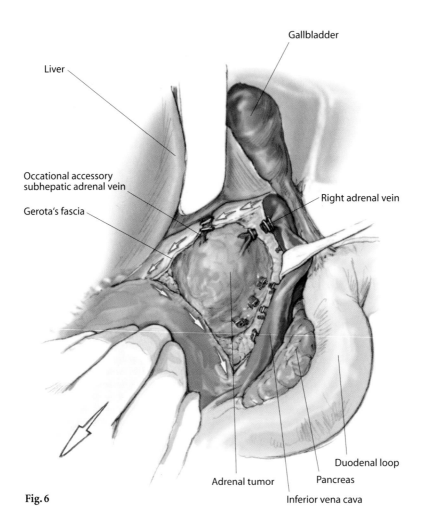

Fig. 6

31 Open Posterior Adrenalectomy

Dimitrios A. Linos

31.1   Position

The patient is turned to the prone position after intubation. Pillows or blankets are placed underneath the chest and pelvis allowing the peritoneal organs to fall away from the retroperitoneum. The table is flexed into the jackknife position to eliminate lumbar lordosis. The knees are flexed and the lower legs supported with soft pillows.

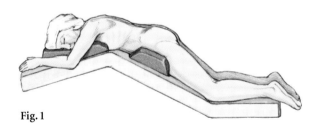

Fig. 1

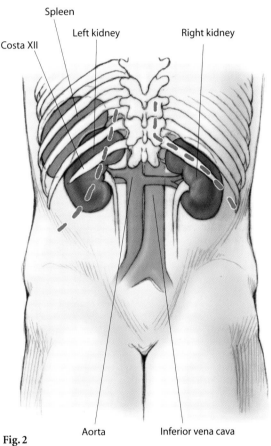

Fig. 2

31.2   Incisions

The classical Young curvilinear incision extending from the 10th rib (4–5 cm from the midvertebral line) to the iliac crest (8–10 cm from the midvertebral line) is usually used. Nevertheless, since the adrenal gland lies beneath the origin of the 12th rib from the vertebral body, a single straight incision over the 12th rib with a small vertical upward extension, if needed, is adequate in most cases.

31.3   Step I: Resection of the 12th Rib

The first step of the posterior approach is resection of the 12th rib (or the 11th rib in the rare case that the 12th is rudimentary). To get there the latissimus dorsi and the lumbodorsal fascia are cut with diathermy and the sacrospinalis muscle is retracted medially. Using the diathermy and the periosteal elevator the rib is removed subperiosteally all the way up to its junction with the vertebral body. Care is taken to avoid injuring the underlying pleura and the subcostal nerve.

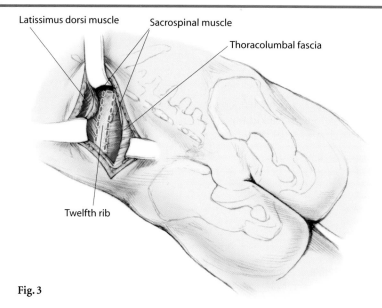

Latissimus dorsi muscle   Sacrospinal muscle

Thoracolumbal fascia

Twelfth rib

Fig. 3

31.4   Step II: Reflection of the Pleura

The second step is to reflect upward the pleura that lie immediately beneath the resected rib. This is done carefully with blunt or sharp dissection, but occasionally holes are made in the pleura. They should be recognized and repaired at this point. The underlying pleura diaphragm can be either divided using diathermy or retracted upward to expose the underlying adrenal and upper pole of the kidney.

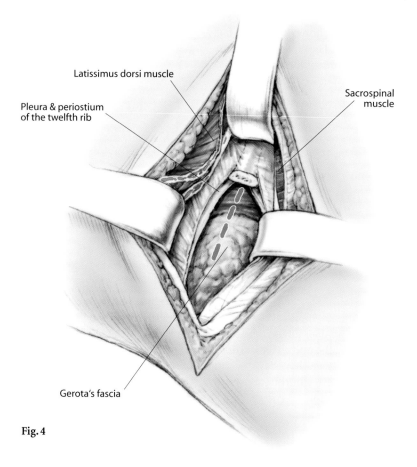

Latissimus dorsi muscle

Sacrospinal muscle

Pleura & periostium of the twelfth rib

Gerota's fascia

Fig. 4

31.5 Step III: Recognition of the Left Adrenal

Gerota's fascia is incised and the posterior surface of the kidney is visualized. Downward retraction is necessary to better expose the adrenal. On the left side it is found medial to the upper pole of the kidney. The left adrenal vein is recognised coming off the left renal vein. As with all adrenal approaches the remaining veins and arteries are usually small requiring cauterization and rarely ligation. The adrenal tumor along with the healthy adrenal tissue, intact, should be mobilized from the surrounding tissues, leaving last its connections with the kidney, which act as retractors until then.

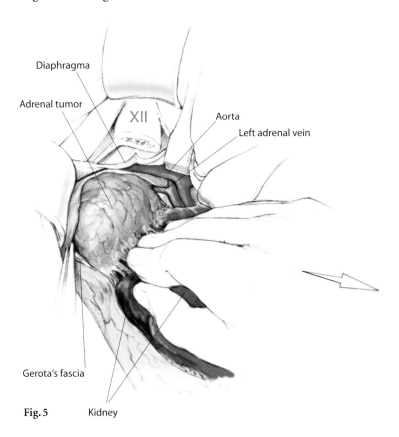

Fig. 5

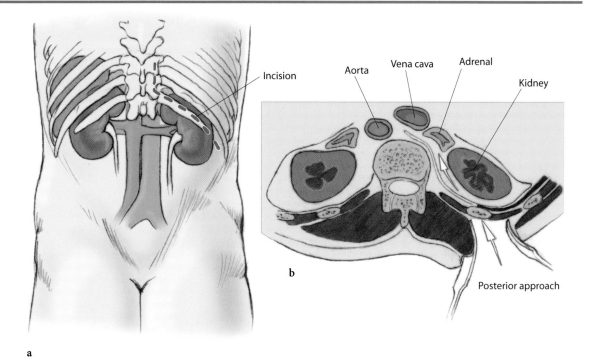

a

Incision

Aorta   Vena cava   Adrenal

Kidney

b

Posterior approach

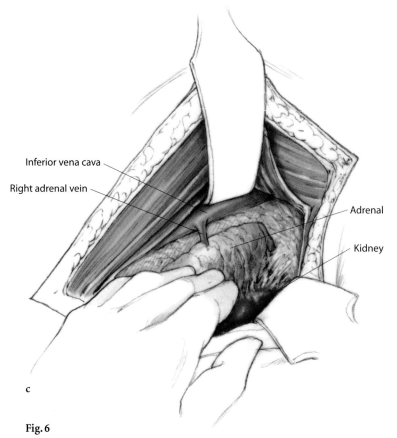

Inferior vena cava

Right adrenal vein

Adrenal

Kidney

c

Fig. 6

31.6   Step IV: Recognition of the Right Adrenal

Be careful when making the initial incision remembering that the right adrenal in the prone position lies on the "left" side of the patient (**a**). The advantage of the posterior approach is the almost immediate reach of the adrenal following the resection of the 12th rib (**b**). The recognition and careful preparation before ligation of the short right adrenal vein as it comes off the inferior vena cava is of paramount importance for the safe and smooth progress of the adrenalectomy (**c**).

32 Right Anterior Laparoscopic Adrenalectomy

Dimitrios A. Linos

CONTENTS

32.1 Position of Patient

The correct position for right laparoscopic adrenalectomy is supine with slight elevation (20° to 30°) of the right side by positioning of appropriate sheets or pillows. Slight overextension of the operating table may also be useful to arc the torso further and provide more working space. The monitor is positioned in the familiar position for laparoscopic cholecystectomy for the surgeon and the operating team is similarly positioned.

The only additional precautions are: (a) placement of a urinary catheter since the operation may last longer than expected and (b) the availability of a tray with all the necessary instruments (including a Satinsky curved clamp) for an immediate open approach should a major complication occurs during surgery, especially with an inferior vena cava injury.

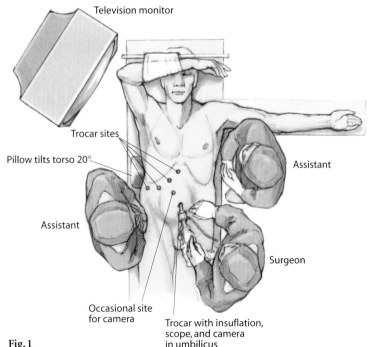

Fig. 1

32.2   Position of the Trocars

The initial camera trocar is placed in the umbilicus, as in laparoscopic cholecystectomy, for easier access and delivery of the adrenal tumor. We always use the open Hassan technique, which is faster and safer than the Veress needle technique. Occasionally when we deal with a very obese patient we can place the initial camera trocar closer to the subcostal area in the middle and below the remaining working trocars and avoid the umbilical site. For large adrenal tumors it is more helpful to use an additional trocar for the camera at a later stage of the procedure and still start with the umbilical incision, which can be extended at the end of the procedure to allow a larger tumor to be extracted.

There are four additional trocars that are placed in a straight line, 1–2 cm below the subcostal margin starting medially from the subxiphoid, a 10–12 mm trocar that will accommodate the liver retractor and finish as far lateral as possible with a 5-mm trocar for the first assistant's grasper. Between these trocars, two additional 10-mm trocars are placed to accommodate the operating surgeon's equipment and the second "helping instrument" of the first assistant, which is usually the suction-irrigation tip.

32.3   Step I

The first step is to retract the liver with the gallbladder upwards. The retroperitoneum is incised in order to further retract the liver and reach as high as possible. The retractor (preferably cloth covered to avoid liver injury) will be held upwards during the whole procedure by the second assistant.

Two landmarks are identified: the kidney laterally and the inferior vena cava (IVC) medially.

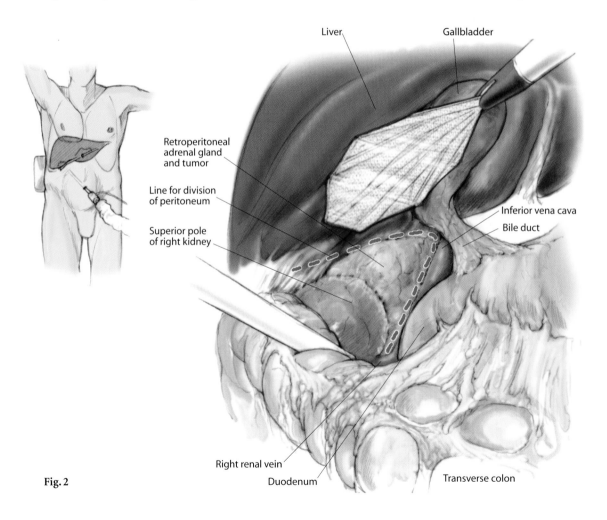

Fig. 2

32.4   Recognition of the Adrenal Gland

Once the posterior liver edge is pushed upwards and the retroperitoneum incised, the surgeon should recognize the yellow color of the normal adrenal tissue and the adrenal tumor. Again the upper pole of the right kidney must be seen and felt and the IVC clearly seen. The right adrenal vein cannot be seen at this point; its recognition and division should be left for later on. In contrast to left laparoscopic adrenalectomy, where the adrenal vein can be seen and divided at the earliest stages, the right adrenal vein lies too high, and it is not wise to go for it first.

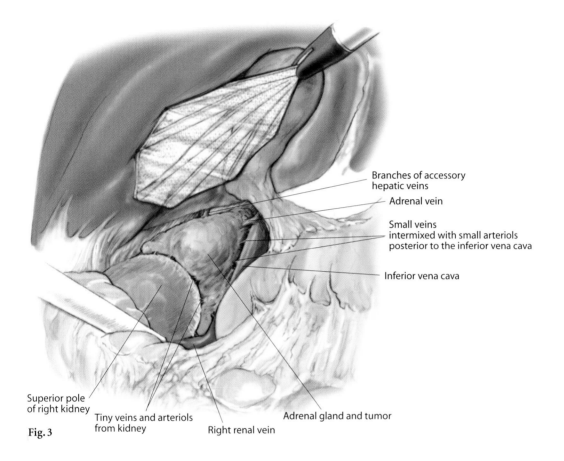

Branches of accessory hepatic veins

Adrenal vein

Small veins intermixed with small arteriols posterior to the inferior vena cava

Inferior vena cava

Adrenal gland and tumor

Right renal vein

Tiny veins and arteriols from kidney

Superior pole of right kidney

Fig. 3

32.5   Mobilization of the Adrenal Tumor

The plan to mobilize the right adrenal tumor has two steps. The first step is the "easy" one; it starts from the inferior edge of the adrenal, continues with the lateral one (detaching the adrenal from the upper pole of the kidney) moving upward and along the liver edge. During these efforts, posterior mobilization is also done since there are no vessels between the diaphragm and the adrenal gland. The second step is the more difficult one and includes mobilization and detachment of the right adrenal gland from the inferior vena cava. This steps ends with the division of the right adrenal vein.

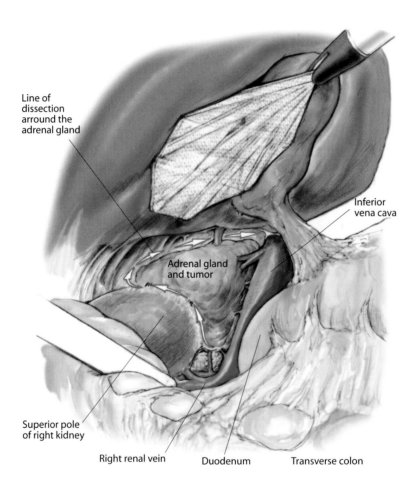

Fig. 4

Line of dissection arround the adrenal gland

Inferior vena cava

Adrenal gland and tumor

Superior pole of right kidney

Right renal vein

Duodenum

Transverse colon

32.6   Division of the Adrenal Vessels

The adrenal arteries and veins (with the exception of the main right adrenal vein) are very small and easily dealt with the use of cautery. There is usually no need to use endoclips. The newer forms of energy such as Ultracision (Ethicon Endosurgery Inc.) and Ligasure (Valley Laboratory) are no better than the cheaper cautery attached to the common dissector. One should be patient and careful to skeletonize every small vessel and then cauterize it in order to avoid unnecessary bleeding.

The first assistant has the main role of exposing these vessels by pushing apart the tissues in between the vessels. In this figure the assistant applies traction-countertraction between the upper pole of the kidney and the adrenal using a grasper instrument and the tip of the suction-irrigation instrument. The suction-irrigation instrument is a very useful instrument because it keeps the space we work in open and clean from smoke and blood at all times.

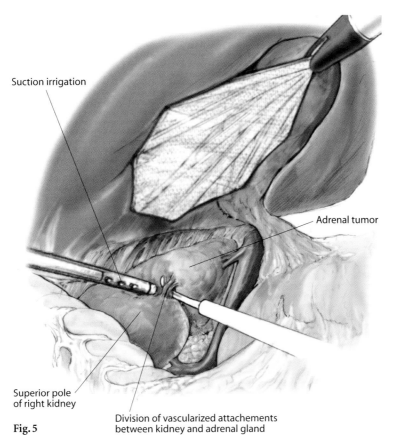

Suction irrigation

Adrenal tumor

Superior pole
of right kidney

Division of vascularized attachements
between kidney and adrenal gland

Fig. 5

32.7   Exposure and Ligation of the Right Adrenal Vein

The fear of the surgeon during right adrenalectomy remains unsuccessful ligation of the right adrenal vein. The laparoscopic approach allows a better view thus a better exposure and safer ligation of this short and wide branch of the inferior vein cava. The usual laparoscopic dissecting instrument should clearly expose the adrenal vein as it enters and usually divides in the upper pole of the adrenal. The space is limited but adequate to place at least two clips on the side of the inferior vena cava and one on the adrenal side. The small scissor dividing the adrenal vein gives the already mobilized adrenal its freedom (and breath to the operating surgeon). One should be careful that occasionally there might be more than one adrenal vein originating from the IVC or even from the hepatic veins.

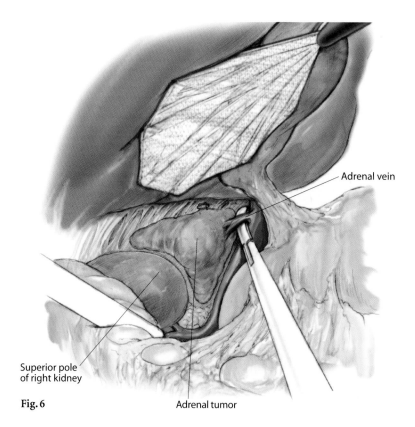

Adrenal vein

Superior pole of right kidney

Fig. 6   Adrenal tumor

32.8   Removal of the Tumor

After the right adrenal vein is safely divided we can then rotate the adrenal tumor all ways in order to cauterize its last attachments to the surrounding tissues. Soon the whole adrenal gland with its tumor is hanging free at the end of our grasper. The tumor is grasped by the right adrenal vein remnant trying to avoid rupture of the adrenal capsule. We want to inspect the borders of the adrenal gland and remove any yellow pieces left behind. The Endobag can easily accommodate adrenal tumors as large as 15 cm in diameter. The Endobag is removed from the umbilical site that occasionally has to be extended. After irrigation to confirm that no bleeders are present a drain is left that usually comes out the next day.

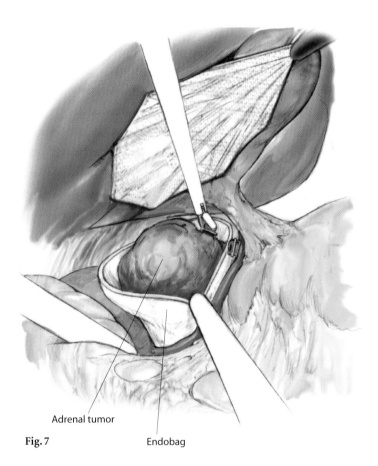

Adrenal tumor

Fig. 7   Endobag

33 Left Anterior Laparoscopic Adrenalectomy

Dimitrios A. Linos

CONTENTS

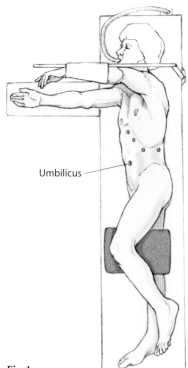

Umbilicus

Fig. 1

33.1 Position of the Patient

The patient is positioned in the lateral right decubitus position. A pillow is placed under the flank and the table is angled to increase the space between the costal margin and iliac crest. The surgeon stands on the right of the table with the monitor across behind the head of the patient. The assistant stands opposite to the patient.

33.2 Placement of Trocars

The first trocar for the camera is placed in the umbilicus using the open technique. In the case of an obese patient a separate camera trocar is placed below and underneath the trocars for the instruments. These four additional trocars are placed along a subcortal line. The first one is placed in the midline to accommodate the endoretractor. The remaining three are placed at 5-cm intervals with the last outer one as laterally as possible. All trocars are 10–12 mm diameter in order to accommodate all the necessary instruments expect the very lateral one, which can be a 5-mm one.

33.3 Step I: Mobilization of the Left Colonic Flexure/Exposure of the Upper Pole of the Left Kidney and Pancreas

The left colonic flexure and descending colon are mobilized inferiorly and medially in order to expose the underlying upper pole of the left kidney. The tip of the surgeon's working instrument could "sense" the hard surface of the kidney behind the Gerota's fascia and the overlying retroperitoneal fat.

Further division of the gastrocolic ligament and mobilization of the transverse colon downward allows exposure of the pancreas. The use of new forms of energy such as Ligasure (Valley Laboratory) and Ultracision (Ethicon Endosurgery, Inc.) may expedite this and subsequent steps.

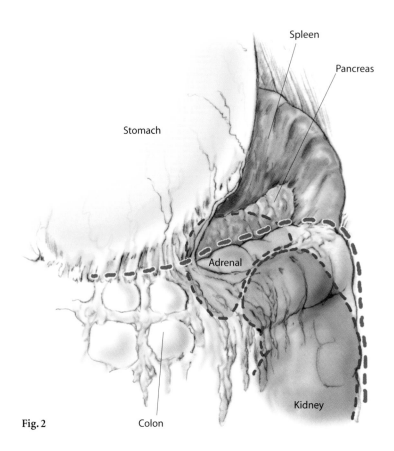

Fig. 2

33.4 Step II: Mobilization of the Inferior Border of the Pancreas Along with the Lower Pole of the Spleen; Exposure of the Left Adrenal Tumor

The retroperitoneum along the inferior border of the pancreas is opened with diathermy. The attachment of the lower pole of the spleen to the upper pole of the kidneys is divided. The main purpose is the upward mobilization of the inferior surface of the pancreas along with the spleen. The characteristic yellow color of the adrenal tumor will now start appearing behind Gerota's fascia. The laparoscopic retractor is now inserted to keep the pancreas away from the adrenal.

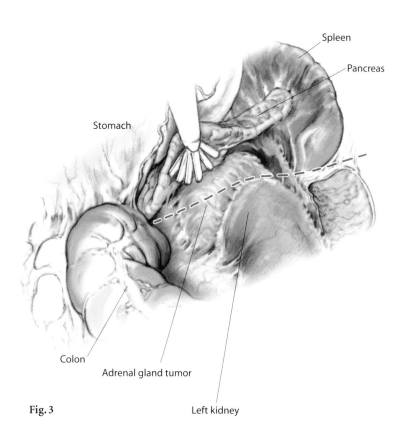

Spleen

Pancreas

Stomach

Colon

Adrenal gland tumor

Left kidney

Fig. 3

33.5   Step III: Mobilization of the Adrenal Tumor

1. We start the mobilization of the tumor from its inner border in the essentially avascular space between the pancreas (that is retracted and protected by the endoretractor) and the adrenal. We continue deep along this plan mobilizing most of the posterior surface of the tumor.
2. We then move along the superior surface that again is essentially without major vessels requiring separate clip ligation.
3. We continue mobilizing the external border of the tumor from the inner surface of the superior pole of the kidney. There are few vessels requiring careful hemostasis to keep the vision clear.

4. The most "difficult" part of this mobilization comes on the inferior border of the adrenal tumor especially recognizing and dividing the left adrenal vein that comes off the left renal vein 2–3 cm from the hilum of the kidney. The pulsating left renal artery needs also to be recognized and protected.

Most left adrenal arteries and veins are small and only the left main adrenal vein (and occasionally another medial accessory vein coming from the inferior phrenic) needs clip ligation. Monopolar diathermy and/or other sources of energy (Ultracision, Ligasure) provide safe and fast hemostasis.

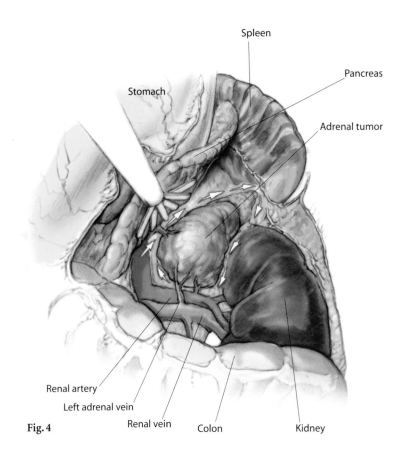

Fig. 4

Labels: Spleen, Pancreas, Adrenal tumor, Stomach, Renal artery, Left adrenal vein, Renal vein, Colon, Kidney

33.6   Step IV: Removal of the Tumor/ Drainage

The tumor is grasped by the left adrenal vein remnant or surrounding non-adrenal tissue, trying to avoid rupture of its capsule. It is positioned in the Endobag, which is retracted through the initial umbilical port. The umbilicus has the advantage that we can easily extend the incision to accommodate large tumors with minimal esthetic cost. A drain is positioned for 24 h.

34 Laparoscopic Lateral Transabdominal Adrenalectomy

Sanziana Roman, Robert Udelsman

34.1   Background

Early successful laparoscopic adrenalectomy was reported in 1992 by Gagner et al. [2, 3]. Since then, the efficacy, safety and advantages of this approach as compared to open techniques have been proven in several retrospective studies [4, 5, 7, 8]. Investigators have shown decreased hospital stays, increased patient comfort and faster return to normal bowel function and physical activity. It is clear that laparoscopic adrenalectomy can be performed safely in skilled hands for benign adrenal tumors less than 8–10 cm and small, isolated metastases to the adrenal gland. Most endocrine surgeons agree that malignant primary tumors of the adrenal gland are still considered a contraindication for the laparoscopic approach.

Various anatomical laparoscopic approaches have been performed, including lateral transabdominal, supine transabdominal, and retroperitoneal approaches. The majority of surgeons have adopted the lateral transperitoneal approach for laparoscopic adrenalectomy. This chapter reviews the principles of laparoscopic adrenal surgery, including anatomic considerations and the technical aspects for both right and left laparoscopic adrenalectomy.

34.2   Anatomic Considerations

The adrenal glands are retroperitoneal organs located along the superomedial aspect of both kidneys, embedded in Gerota's fascia and surrounded by retroperitoneal fat. The glands have a fibrous capsule and a chromate yellow hue due to the high lipid content of the cortex. The fibrous capsule should be kept intact throughout the dissection, thus avoiding cell spillage and possible implantation.

The adrenal glands weigh 4–7 g in the normal adult. The right adrenal gland is more pyramidal in shape, lying under the right hepatic triangular ligament, lateral and somewhat beneath the vena cava and superomedial to the right kidney. The left adrenal gland is more flattened, bounded superiorly by the posterior omental bursa, stomach and the superior pole of the spleen, medially by the periaortic tissue, and inferiorly by the tail of the pancreas and the splenic vessels. Both adrenal glands rest posteriorly on the respective crus of the diaphragm.

They are highly vascular structures, deriving their arterial blood supply from a rich plexus of branches from the inferior phrenic arteries, aorta and renal arteries. Most commonly, they have a single central vein, but multiple veins can be found. The right adrenal vein is typically short, 0.3–1 cm long, draining directly into the vena cava. The left adrenal vein is usually 2–3 cm long, draining from the inferomedial aspect of the adrenal gland into the superior aspect of the left renal vein. The inferior phrenic vein may join the left adrenal vein before its entry into the renal vein (Fig. 1).

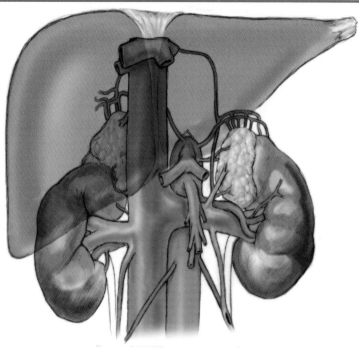

Fig. 1. Normal adrenal anatomy

34.3 Indications for Laparoscopic Adrenalectomy

Laparoscopic adrenalectomy is indicated for virtually all benign functional adrenal tumors as well as nonfunctional tumors that require extirpation due to tumor size, growth, or imaging characteristics. The indications for 100 consecutive laparoscopic adrenalectomies as reported by a single surgeon are seen in Fig. 2 [10].

34.4 Technique of Laparoscopic Transabdominal Lateral Adrenalectomy

The technique for both right and left laparoscopic adrenalectomy follows the principles of open adrena-

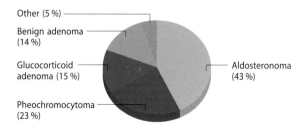

Other (5%)
Benign adenoma (14%)
Glucocorticoid adenoma (15%)
Pheochromocytoma (23%)
Aldosteronoma (43%)

Fig. 2. Indications for surgery in 100 consecutive laparoscopic adrenalectomies [10]

lectomy. The dissection is carried out in an extracapsular manner. Grasping the adrenal gland with laparoscopic instruments should be minimized, if possible, in order to avoid fracture of the gland, spillage of tumor cells and possible implantation. If the gland has been fractured significantly, the surgery may need to be converted to an open adrenalectomy. Grasping the periadrenal fat or gently pushing and elevating the gland results in adequate exposure. Control of the blood supply may be obtained by electrocoagulation, ultrasonic dissector, or endoscopic clips. The gland should be removed intact in an impermeable endoscopic device, so that the specimen may be examined pathologically in its entirety.

34.4.1 Patient Positioning

A well-padded beanbag may used under the patient on the operating table. After general anesthesia is induced and all necessary monitoring is accomplished, a urinary drainage catheter and an orogastric tube are placed. It is essential that the stomach be decompressed, especially on the left side. The patient is placed in the lateral decubitus position, right side up for a right adrenalectomy, or left side up for a left adrenalectomy. The table is flexed, the patient's lower leg is bent, while the upper leg is kept straight,

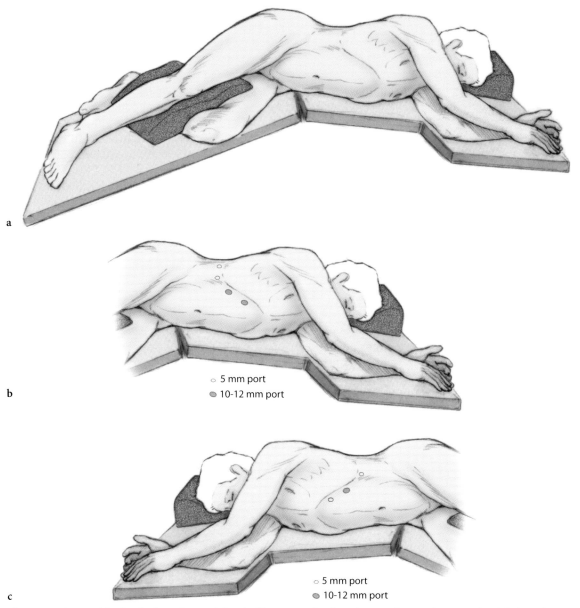

Fig. 3. a Patient positioning for lateral transabdominal laparoscopic adrenalectomy. **b** Port placement for right lateral transabdominal laparoscopic adrenalectomy. **c** Port placement of left lateral transabdominal laparoscopic adrenalectomy

and the kidney rest of the table is elevated. All pressure points must be carefully padded to prevent neurovascular injury. These maneuvers will maximize the space between the costal margin and the iliac crest (Fig. 3a). This positioning will also allow gravity retraction of adjacent organs and excellent exposure to the retroperitoneum. It will not permit access to the contralateral adrenal. For a concomitant bilateral adrenalectomy, the patient will need to be repositioned at the conclusion of the first adrenalectomy.

The video monitors are positioned on each side of the patient's head. The surgeon stands on the ventral side of the patient. The assistant and/or camera operator can stay on the same side or opposite side of the surgeon, according to exposure necessity [1, 8].

34.4.2   Laparoscopic Right Adrenalectomy

The port sites are demonstrated in Fig. 3b. Most commonly, four ports are utilized. In exceptional cases, additional ports may be inserted. Pneumoperitoneum is achieved through the site of the first port, which is located lateral to the rectus muscle in the anterior axillary line along the costal margin. Alternatively, this port may be placed midway between the umbilicus and the right costal margin. A Veress needle may be used to achieve pneumoperitoneum to 12–15 torr. In some cases, particularly patients with pheochromocytoma or chronic obstructive pulmonary disease, the pneumoperitoneum is poorly tolerated. In these cases, one can accomplish the operation laparoscopically using decreased insufflation pressures. A 10 mm port is placed and a 30 degree side-viewing telescope is utilized to visualize the insertion of the remaining ports. Two 5 mm ports are placed along the costal margin toward the flank. An additional port is placed medially to the first port for a liver retractor. This may be either a 5 mm or a 12 mm port, given the available liver retractors. A 5 mm 30 degree side-viewing telescope may also be available. This may be used in the 5 mm ports at various points in the case for optimization of visualization and angle of dissection.

It is important to mobilize the right lobe of the liver by detaching the right triangular ligament from its lateral and inferior attachments using the ultrasonic dissector or electrocautery (Fig. 4). This permits visualization of the retrohepatic vena cava and the entire adrenal gland. Care should be taken in dissecting over the vena cava as small communicating veins between the cava and the liver may bleed profusely if not controlled. Mobilization of the right lobe will also allow retraction and elevation of the liver, thus avoiding injury to the liver parenchyma.

The adrenal gland is easily identified once the liver is mobilized. The dissection is then carried out laterally and superiorly. Small arterial branches can be divided with the cautery or ultrasonic dissector. The right adrenal vein is located usually medially and posteriorly, draining into the vena cava. Once the vein is gently dissected, it should be doubly clipped and transected (Fig. 5). Wide adrenal veins may need to be sequentially clipped or ligated. Slipped clips or sutures from the proximal stump bleed briskly and control may be difficult. Undue traction on the adrenal vein may tear the vena cava. Direct gentle caval compression may be attempted with an endoscopic Kittner dissector to minimize blood loss. If vascular control cannot be obtained en-

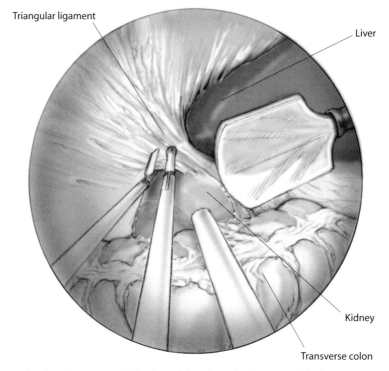

Fig. 4. Right laparoscopic adrenalectomy: mobilization of the triangular ligament of the liver

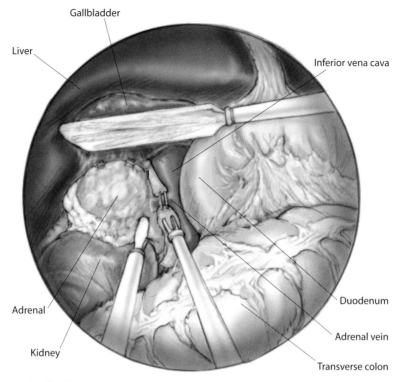

Fig. 5. Right adrenal vein clipping

doscopically, the operation may need to be converted to an open procedure.

Accessory veins may be clipped or cauterized. The adrenal gland may extend beneath the vena cava. Gentle blunt medial traction of the cava and lateral dissection of the gland releases the medial side of the adrenal. Inferiorly, the gland is dissected away from the superior pole of the kidney. The inferior adrenal pole may extend close to the renal vein.

The dissection is kept close to the adrenal capsule to avoid injury to hepatic veins superiorly, vena cava medially and the renal vein or accessory polar arteries inferiorly and posteriorly.

The gland is then extracted via an endoscopic pouch through one of the 10–12 mm port sites. If the tumor is large, the port site may need to be slightly enlarged. Morsellation of the gland is not recommended, as it compromises pathological examination.

34.4.3 Laparoscopic Left Adrenalectomy

The patient is positioned in the left side up lateral decubitus position as described above. Three trocars are usually employed (Fig. 3c). Pneumoperitoneum is achieved through the first 10 mm port site located along the left costal margin, lateral to the rectus muscle. An additional 5 mm port is placed superiorly along the costal margin and a third port, either 5 mm or 10 mm, is placed in the axillary line. Care should be taken in inserting this port as the splenic flexure of the colon may be adherent to the flank area. Occasionally, this will need to be mobilized prior to insertion of the third port. The 10 mm or 5 mm 30 degree telescope is employed via the flank port site, while the dissectors and grasper are used in the medial ports.

Using the grasper and either the coagulation scissors or the ultrasonic dissector, the colon is displaced inferiorly and the spleen is mobilized medially by incising the splenorenal ligament. An edge of ligament should be left on the spleen for grasping purposes, thus avoiding manipulation injury to the spleen. The dissection of the ligament is carried up to the diaphragm to the level of the gastric cardia. This allows full medial rotation of the spleen and utilizes gravity for exposure. Great care should be exercised to avoid injury to either the diaphragm or the stomach, especially when using the ultrasonic dissector.

With the spleen retracted medially, the pancreatic tail is gently dissected off the retroperitoneum. The posteriorly located splenic vessels will be in view as the pancreas is mobilized medially.

Occasionally it is difficult to locate the left adrenal gland in the retroperitoneal fat. This is often the case in patients with Cushing's syndrome. In such cases, the intraoperative laparoscopic ultrasound can be utilized though the 10 mm port.

The anterior surface of the adrenal gland can be bluntly dissected free from the tail of the pancreas. This dissection is carried out to the medial edge of the adrenal gland, where the arterial supply is encountered. Branches off the aorta, left phrenic artery and renal artery can be taken close to the adrenal capsule with the cautery or ultrasonic dissector. The branches should be clearly visualized and dissected prior to cautery. Utilizing the ultrasonic dissector is preferred to endoclips, thus avoiding clip clutter.

The lateral and superior aspect of the adrenal gland is then dissected free from retroperitoneal fat using the ultrasonic dissector. Inferiorly, the adrenal gland is gently dissected off the superior pole of the kidney. The renal capsule should not be injured in order to avoid bleeding.

The adrenal vein is found in the inferomedial aspect of the gland draining in an oblique direction into the renal vein. The adrenal vein is bluntly dissected and double endoscopic clips are applied. It is important to note that the inferior phrenic vein may join the adrenal vein prior to its entry into the renal vein (Fig. 6). It is extremely important to avoid injury to the left renal vein.

In operations for pheochromocytoma, the vein is preferably taken early in the dissection, thus avoiding systemic catecholamine release with the surgical gland manipulation. Prior to clipping of the adrenal vein, the anesthesiologist should be made aware, in order to prepare for the hemodynamic effects of reduced circulating catecholamines.

Utilizing a 5 mm 30 degree angled telescope in various ports has the advantage of visualizing the adrenal from different views, which may facilitate the dissection.

Once the adrenal gland is free, it is removed in an endoscopic pouch through the 10 mm port site. Hemostasis is assured by releasing some of the pneumoperitoneal pressure in order to prevent small venous compressive effect. All port sites larger than 5 mm are closed in layers with fascial approximation and skin closure. A closed suction drain is rarely employed.

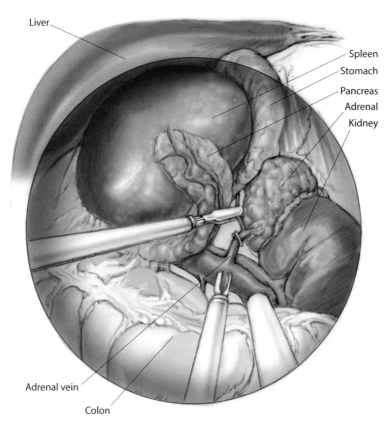

Fig. 6. Left adrenal vein clipping

34.5 Complications

34.5.1 Short-Term Complications

Most complications of laparoscopic adrenalectomy are shared with the open techniques. Potential complications from insertion of the Veress needle include bowel perforation, liver injury and splenic injury. The liver may be injured with the liver retractor during a right adrenalectomy. Gentle retraction and adequate release of the right triangular ligament minimizes this risk. Small capsular tears usually do not necessitate treatment, as they are self-limited. The spleen may also be injured by retraction with the grasper. Leaving a layer of the phrenolienal ligament on the splenic capsule affords a grasping area and avoids direct manipulation of the splenic capsule. Small capsular tears also tend to be self-limited. Good visualization of the operative field is important in dissection; therefore placing the patient in the lateral decubitus position and slight reverse Trendelenburg will keep irrigation fluid and blood out of the operative field. Meticulous dissection in a clear operative field is key to avoiding significant bleeding from the adrenal veins, vena cava and the renal vein. Major hemorrhage should prompt open conversion.

Injury to the pancreas, colon or duodenum can be avoided by careful dissection and manipulation.

34.5.2 Long-Term Complications

Adrenal capsular tear and cell spillage has been reported, with subsequent implantation of tumor cells along the paracolic gutters and the retroperitoneum [6]. Adrenal cell spillage should be avoided by careful manipulation of the gland during dissection and removal.

In patients with Cushing's syndrome positional skeletal fractures can be experienced. These patients may also develop pneumonias. Patients who undergo bilateral adrenalectomy and/or those with Cushing's syndrome will develop adrenal insufficiency postoperatively unless replaced with glucocorticoids. The addisonian crisis may present with abdominal pain, nausea, vomiting, fever, malaise, weakness and leukocytosis. Cardiovascular collapse with hypotension and shock may develop rapidly, if the crisis is not recognized and treated promptly with parenteral glucocorticoids.

Patients with pheochromocytoma may develop postoperative hypotension and rebound hyperinsulinism.

Patients who undergo resection of an aldosteronoma are at risk for postoperative mineralocorticoid insufficiency, manifested by hyperkalemia.

34.6 Postoperative Care

Patients who undergo unilateral or bilateral adrenalectomy for Cushing's syndrome should be given exogenous glucocorticoids and an appropriate taper should be scheduled. Once the patient can take oral medications, a maintenance dose of hydrocortisone or equivalent of 12–15 mg/m^2 is administered daily. The steroid therapy should continue until normal function of the hypothalamic-pituitary-adrenal axis has been achieved. Patients who undergo bilateral adrenalectomies also require mineralocorticoid replacement with fludrocortisone acetate 100 µg per day [9].

Usually, patients will only necessitate parenteral narcotics for 24 h, and be switched to oral pain medication thereafter. Clear liquids may be started within 24 h and have diet advancement as tolerated. Most patients will be discharged within 24–48 h postoperatively with no physical restrictions. Most patients return to work within 10–15 days.

Patients with pheochromocytoma should have urinary catecholamines measured within 6 months postoperatively and then annually.

References

1. Brunt ML (2000) Laparoscopic adrenalectomy, chap 34. In: Eubanks WS, Swanstrom LL et al. (eds) Mastery of endoscopic and laparoscopic surgery. Lippincott Williams and Wilkins, Philadelphia
2. Gagner M, Lacroix A, Bolte E (1992) Laparoscopic adrenalectomy in Cushing's syndrome and pheochromocytoma. N Engl J Med 327:1033
3. Gagner M, Lacroix A, Prinz RA, Bolte E, Albala D, Potvin C, Hamet P, Kuchel O, Querin S, Pomp A (1993) Early experience with laparoscopic approach for adrenalectomy. Surgery 114:1120–4; discussion 1124–5
4. Linos DA, Stylopoulos N, Boukis M, Souvatzoglou A, Raptis S, Papadimitriou J (1997) Anterior, posterior, or laparoscopic approach for the management of adrenal diseases? Am J Surg 173:120–5
5. Prinz RA (1995) A comparison of laparoscopic and open adrenalectomies. Arch Surg 130:489–494
6. Terachi T, Yoshida O, Matsuda T, et al. (2000) Complications of laparoscopic and retroperitoneoscopic adrenalectomies in 370 cases in Japan: a multi-institutional study. Biomed Pharmacother 54 Suppl 1:211s–214s

7. Thompson GB, Grant GS, van Heerden JA, et al. (1997) Laparoscopic versus open posterior adrenalectomy: a case controlled study in 100 patients. Surgery 122:1132–1136

8. Udelsman R (2000) Adrenal. In: Norton JA, Bollinger RR et al. (eds) Surgery: basic science and clinical evidence, chap 40. Springer-Verlag, New York

9. Udelsman R, Ramp J, Gallucci WT, et al. (1986) Adaptation during surgical stress: a reevaluation of the role of glucocorticoids. J Clin Invest 77:1377–1378

10. Zeh H, Udelsman R (2003) One hundred laparoscopic adrenalectomies: a single surgeon's experience. Ann Surg Oncol (in press)

35 Posterior Retroperitoneoscopic Adrenalectomy

Martin K. Walz

CONTENTS

35.1   Introduction

The posterior retroperitoneoscopic approach to the adrenal glands is based on the combination of the classical open posterior route and the technique of minimally invasive surgery. By doing so the advantages of both methods are integrated: the direct approach and limited access minimizing operative trauma. In 1993 and 1994 the technique of posterior retroperitoneoscopic adrenalectomy was independently developed at different locations. Early descriptions were published from Turkey, United States of America, Italy, and Germany [5, 7, 8, 13]. Further studies demonstrated operative feasibility [15] and – compared with the laparoscopic approach – shorter operative times and less blood loss [1]. Currently, the posterior retroperitoneoscopic access has become one of the standard approaches for adrenalectomy. In this chapter we present the surgical technique, results, and our experience based on more than 350 retroperitoneoscopic adrenalectomies.

35.2   Surgical Technique

35.2.1   Preparation

Posterior retroperitoneoscopic adrenalectomy is performed under general anesthesia with laryngeal intubation and assisted ventilation. In addition, a nasogastric tube is placed routinely. In patients with a pheochromocytoma, previous cardiac diseases or severe arterial hypertension, a central venous catheter and an arterial line are inserted. Swan-Ganz catheters and urinary catheters are not used routinely. Patients with pheochromocytomas are pretreated with high-dosage phenoxybenzamine up to a final level of 2–3 mg/kg body weight [19]; patients with hyperaldosteronism receive spironolactone 3–4 weeks prior to operation. Intraoperatively, intravenous antibiotics (i.e. 2 g cefazolin) are given.

35.2.2   Positioning

The procedure is performed with the patient in the prone, half-jackknife position (Fig. 1). Ideal placement is essential to create sufficient space between the ribs and the iliac crest: the hip joints and the knees are bent (75–90°) and fixed in this position. The patient is positioned without lordosis on mattresses allowing inclination ("sagging") of the abdomen. The lateral abdominal wall is placed in a vertical line with the table allowing free movement of all instruments.

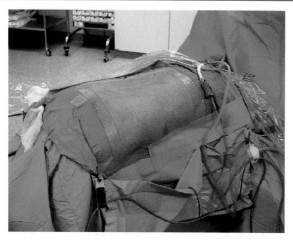

Fig. 1. Positioning of the patient in posterior retroperitoneo-scopic adrenalectomy. Hip joints and knees are bended

35.2.3   Placement of Trocars

Initially, a 1.5 cm transverse incision just below the tip of the 12th rib is made. The retroperitoneal space is reached by blunt and sharp dissection of the abdominal wall. A small cavity is prepared with a finger for digitally guided insertion of two 5 mm trocars about 5 cm lateral and medial to the initial incision site with particular attention to the subcostal nerve. Thus, safe trocar placement is possible without visual control. The medial 5 mm trocar is inserted at an angle of about 45°, allowing a direct view of the adrenal region and avoiding bending of the camera. The lateral 5 mm trocar is placed exactly lateral and below the 11th rib. A blunt trocar with an inflatable balloon and an adjustable sleeve is introduced into the initial incision site and sealed by balloon inflation. The capnoretro-peritoneum is created by maintaining a CO_2 pressure of 20–25 mmHg. Retroperitoneoscopy is performed with a 5 mm 30 degree endoscope that is initially introduced via the middle trocar and later positioned via the medial trocar near the spine (Fig. 2a, b). The initial view shows the fascia of Gerota, which must be opened by dissection (Fig. 3a, b).

35.2.4   Preparation of the Adrenal Gland

After creation of the retroperitoneal space underneath the diaphragm by displacing the fatty tissue inferiorly, the upper pole of the kidney is seen. By doing so the area of the adrenal gland is visualized. The kidney is retracted downwards by one of the instruments from the middle or lateral trocar. Sometimes it is necessary

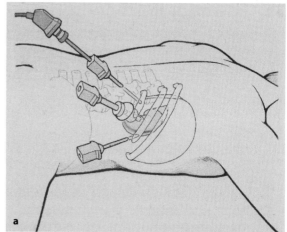

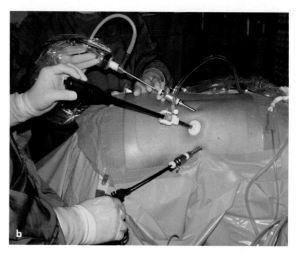

Fig. 2a, b. Positioning of the trocars for posterior retroperitoneoscopic adrenalectomy. (**a** Modified from [16])

to place a fourth trocar below the first line of ports in order to pull the kidney down by a separate retractor.

Mobilization of the adrenal gland begins medially and caudally between the diaphragm and the adrenal gland. In this area, on the right, the gland arteries cross the vena cava posteriorly. These vessels are separated by electrocoagulation or clip application. Clips are useful, especially in well-vascularized pheochromocytomas. By lifting up the adrenal gland the caval vein is demonstrated posteriorly in its retroperitoneal-cranial segment (Fig. 4). The vena cava is clearly visualized by the clearing of any fibro-fatty tissue. During this phase the renal vein and artery must not be identified. Sometimes, an upper pole artery of the kidney crosses the caval vein. The short suprarenal vein becomes clearly visible running posterolaterally usually close to the diaphragm. This key vessel is meticulously prepared for a length of 1 cm and dissected between

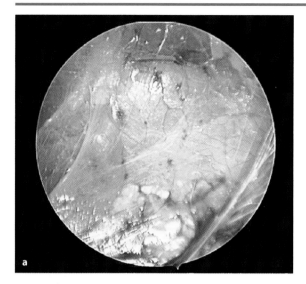

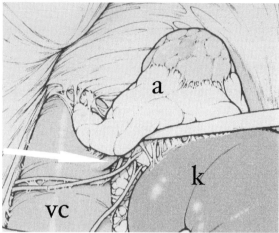

Fig. 4. Right-sided posterior retroperitoneoscopic adrenalectomy. View after creation of the retroperitoneal space (*vc*, vena cava; *a*, adrenal gland with tumor; *k*, upper pole of the right kidney; *arrow*, adrenal vein). (Modified from [16])

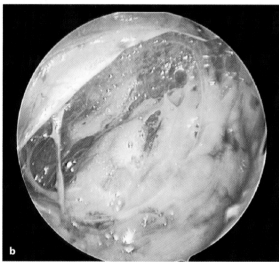

Fig. 3. a Initial view on Gerota's fascia. **b** After dissection the perirenal and periadrenal fatty tissue becomes visible

structures. The harmonic scalpel is also practical but creates relatively dense fog in the small retroperitoneal working space (300–400 ml).

35.2.5 Partial Adrenalectomy

If a partial adrenalectomy is planned, the margin of the neoplasia has to be precisely identified. Therefore, it may be necessary to resect a portion of the surrounding fatty tissue. Additionally, retroperitoneoscopic ultrasonography utilizing a 10 mm flexible 10 MHz probe is utilized. After clear identification, the tumor is resected with a margin of 0.5–1.0 cm of normal tissue. These resections are regularly performed by electrocoagulation with or without clip application [17]. Preservation of the adrenal vessels depends on the individual situation and is not related to cortical function [4, 19].

clips (Fig. 5a, b). Mobilization of the right adrenal gland is completed by lateral and cranial dissection where further small vessels can be found.

For a left-sided retroperitoneoscopic adrenalectomy, the adrenal gland vein must be prepared in the space between the adrenal gland and the diaphragmatic branch medial to the upper pole of the kidney (Fig. 6). After dissection of the main vein (Fig. 7a, b), preparation of the adrenal gland is continued medially, laterally, and cranially. All manipulations of the adrenal gland are performed carefully using blunt palpation probes to prevent injury to gland tissue. For the whole dissection the monopolar electrocautery probe is used allowing a precise preparation of all essential

35.2.6 Final Steps

Extraction of the adrenal tissue is performed through the middle incision with a retrieval bag system (e.g., Endocatch, Tyco Norwalk, CT, USA). Depending on the tumor size the incision site occasionally has to be enlarged. Skin and fascia closure are performed after the optional retroperitoneal drain insertion with reabsorbable materials. On the day of the operation bed rest is abandoned and complete oral intake is allowed.

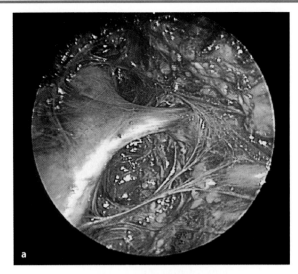

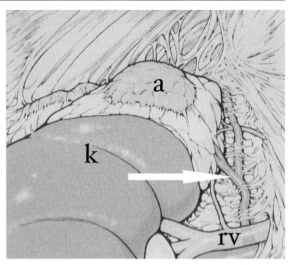

Fig. 6. Left-sided posterior retroperitoneoscopic adrenalectomy. View after creation of the retroperitoneal space (*rv*, renal vessels; *a*, adrenal gland; *k*, left kidney; *arrow*, adrenal vein joining the diaphragmatic vein). (Modified from [16])

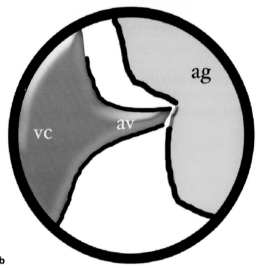

Fig. 5a, b. Right-sided retroperitoneoscopic adrenalectomy (*vc*, vena cava; *av*, adrenal vein; *ag*, adrenal gland)

35.3   Indications and Contraindications
(Table 1)

The posterior retroperitoneoscopic approach to the adrenal glands is indicated in adrenal tumors up to 6–7 cm in diameter, and in those patients with adrenal hyperplasia. Tumors less than 4 cm in size, and patients with little retroperitoneal fatty tissue, are ideal candidates for this procedure.

Due to the limited working space and the increased risk of malignancy, tumors larger than 6–7 cm should not be operated via the posterior retroperitoneoscopic access. This also applies to tumors infiltrating neighboring organs or structures especially in patients with adrenal metastases. Another contraindication is a short distance (less than 3–4 cm) between the ribs and the iliac crest in the prone position, i.e. in patients with severe osteoporosis or after spine fractures. In these patients placement of trocars is impossible. In extremely obese patients (body mass index 45) the abdomen causes severe compression of the retroperitoneum. In such situations even a gas pressure of 30 mmHg does not create a sufficient and safe retroperitoneal space.

35.4   Tips and Tricks

35.4.1   Retroperitoneal Space

A basic aspect of posterior retroperitoneoscopic adrenalectomy is the increased gas pressure with levels between 20 and 25 mmHg. This allows the creation of a sufficient space in the retroperitoneum without any relevant hemodynamic changes [6] even in obese patients. Additionally, an initial balloon dissection – as described in the early publications [14] – can be avoided.

35.4.2   Misplacement of Trocars

In rare instances of misplacement of one of the trocars causing tears of the pleura, the procedure can be con-

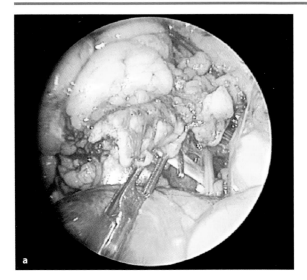

tinued. Sealing of the leakage may be possible by pressure with a blunt tip trocar with a balloon. Additionally, a pleural drain should be inserted until the end of the operation. We have encountered this complication four times and have always succeeded in completing the operation endoscopically. A "leakage" of the peritoneum may occur during right or left posterior adrenalectomies. On the right the posterior part of the right lobe of the liver becomes visible, on the left the spleen or the posterior wall of the stomach can be seen. If this happens, the retroperitoneoscopic procedure can be continued and completed, as significant compression of the retroperitoneum does not occur.

35.4.3 Hemorrhage

The major potential complication is bleeding. By the posterior retroperitoneoscopic approach the risk of arterial bleeding is minimal, as the main renal arteries and the aorta are usually not seen. Clips can control lesions of small arteries, i.e. of the adrenal gland or the upper pole of the kidney. Venous bleeding may occur from suprarenal veins or from the caval vein, but due to the high CO_2 pressure relevant blood loss does not occur. We have seen very few significant hemorrhages from these vessels and a complete control could always be achieved by clip application or temporary compression. Variations in the anatomy of the suprarenal veins are a special problem. They are not found on the left side, but on the right side we encountered such anomalies in about 10% of patients [18]. Especially, conjunctions of adrenal veins with posterior hepatic veins may complicate dissection. Another advantage of the posterior retroperitoneoscopic adrenalectomy is the small space in which the

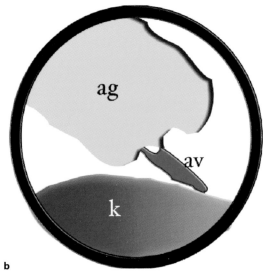

Fig. 7a, b. Left-sided posterior retroperitoneoscopic adrenalectomy (*k*, upper pole of left kidney; *av*, clipped adrenal vein; *ag*, adrenal gland)

Table 1. Indications and contraindications of posterior retroperitoneoscopic adrenalectomy

Indications	Primary functioning tumors (size ≤6–7 cm) i.e.	Pheochromocytoma Conn's adenoma Cushing's adenoma
	Primary non-functioning tumors (size ≥3 cm and ≤6–7 cm) Metastases (≤4 cm and without infiltration of surrounding structures except fatty tissue) Nodular or non-nodular hyperplasia with hypercortisolism	
Contra-indications	Primary adrenal functioning or non-functioning tumors (size >6–7 cm)	Laparotomy or laparoscopic approach
	Malignant tumors (except small metastases) Extreme obesity No distance between ribs and iliac crest	Laparotomy Lateral laparoscopic approach possible Lateral laparoscopic approach possible

whole procedure is performed, limiting the potential maximum blood loss.

35.4.4 Retroperitoneal Fatty Tissue

In patients with large amounts of fatty tissue in the retroperitoneum all surgical procedures for adrenalectomy become extremely difficult. In these patients, typically with Cushing's syndrome or Cushing's disease, the benefit of an endoscopically performed procedure is high especially by avoiding large abdominal incisions. The trick in endoscopic adrenalectomy is to resect the fatty tissue around the upper pole of the kidney and the adrenal gland. Sometimes, this can be performed simply by suctioning of the typically soft and friable fatty tissue. Thereby, the essential anatomic structures and landmarks can be identified within a few minutes.

35.5 Results

35.5.1 Perioperative Results

Studies of posterior retroperitoneoscopic adrenalectomy demonstrate both the feasibility and the safety of this approach (Table 2). The conversion rate to open surgery is about 5% and decreases with growing experience [15, 18]. Operative time ranges between 100 and 200 min; blood loss is minimal. Due to the direct access, we can achieve operative times of less than 30 min

in ideal patients with minimal retroperitoneal fatty tissue and small tumors. Up to now, no perioperative death has occurred after posterior retroperitoneoscopic adrenalectomy. This approach has also been used in recurrent adrenal tumors especially after transperitoneal open operations and in retroperitoneal paragangliomas [19, 20].

Hemodynamic studies show a significant increase of cardiac output, stroke volume, mean arterial pressure, and mean pulmonary arterial pressure following retroperitoneal insufflation in the prone position. Heart rate, systemic vascular resistance, and pulmonary vascular resistance do not change, however, making it a safe procedure in patients with cardiac risk factors [6]. Intraoperatively, absorption of CO_2 by the retroperitoneal tissue without relevant alterations of arterial blood gas analysis has been demonstrated [11]. Further studies show stable pulmonary function in patients undergoing this approach both pre- and postoperatively [9].

35.5.2 Postoperative Results

Long-term results following posterior retroperitoneoscopic adrenalectomy confirm biochemical cure in functioning adrenal tumors even after partial adrenalectomy [12, 17, 18]. Local or locoregional recurrences have not been published. We have noted temporary weakness of the subcostal nerve in about 11% of patients leading to relaxation or hypoesthesia of the abdominal wall [18].

Table 2. Studies of posterior retroperitoneoscopic adrenalectomy with more than ten procedures (*n.d.*, no data)

Author	Year	Adrenalectomies (*n*)	Conversions (*n*)	Operative time (min)	Blood loss (ml)	Remarks
Mercan [8]	1995	11	0	150	n.d.	
Duh [5]	1996	14	0	202	n.d.	Comparison with transperitoneal approach
Walz [14]	1996	30	5	124	40	Five partial adrenalectomies
Baba [1]	1997	13	1	142	32	Comparison with transperitoneal and retroperitoneal-lateral approach
Sasagawa [9]	1998	15	0	162	12	Only partial adrenalectomies
Baba [2]	1999	26	1	144	44	Six procedures: "solo surgery"
Balogh [3]	2000	14	2	128	100	
Walz [18]	2001	142	7	101	54	39 partial adrenalectomies
Sasagawa [12]	2003	47	1	198	41	Only partial adrenalectomies

35.6   Summary

The posterior retroperitoneoscopic approach to the adrenal glands combines the advantages of the posterior open approach and minimal access surgery. This allows for a direct and safe procedure with short operative times and a low complication rate. The approach is not useful for adrenal tumors larger than 6–7 cm in diameter.

References

1. Baba S, Miyajima A, Uchida A, Asanuma H, Miyakawa A, Murai M (1997) A posterior lumbar approach for retroperitoneoscopic adrenalectomy: assessment of surgical efficacy. Urology 50:19–24
2. Baba S, Ito K, Yanaihara H, Nagata H, Murai M, Iwamura M (1999) Retroperitoneoscopic adrenalectomy by a lumbodorsal approach: clinical experience with solo surgery. World J Urol 17:54–58
3. Balogh A, Varga L, Julesz J, Lazar G Jr, Walz MK (2000) [Minimally invasive adrenalectomy with posterior retroperitoneoscopy.] Orv Hetil 141:845–848
4. Brauckhoff M, Thanh PN, Gimm O, Bar A, Brauckhoff K, Dralle H (2003) Functional results after endoscopic subtotal cortical-sparing adrenalectomy. Surg Today 33:342–348
5. Duh QY, Siperstein AE, Clark OH, Schecter WP, Horn JK, Harrison MR, Hunt TK, Way LW (1996) Laparoscopic adrenalectomy. Comparison of the lateral and posterior approaches. Arch Surg 131:870–875
6. Giebler RM, Walz MK, Peitgen K, Scherer RU (1996) Hemodynamic changes after retroperitoneal CO_2 insufflation for posterior retroperitoneoscopic adrenalectomy. Anesth Analg 82:827–831
7. Mandressi A, Buizza C, Antonelli D (1993) Retro-extraperitoneal laparoscopic approach to excise retroperitoneal organs: kidney and adrenal gland. Minim Invasive Ther 2:213–220
8. Mercan S, Seven R, Ozarmagan S, Tezelman S (1995) Endoscopic retroperitoneal adrenalectomy. Surgery 118:1071–1075
9. Sasagawa I, Suzuki H, Izumi T, Tateno T, Shoji N, Kubota Y, Nakada T (1998) Pulmonary function after posterior retroperitoneoscopic surgery. Int Urol Nephrol 30:695–698
10. Sasagawa I, Suzuki H, Tateno T, Izumi T, Shoji N, Nakada T (1998) Retroperitoneoscopic partial adrenalectomy using an endoscopic stapling device in patients with adrenal tumor. Urol Int 61:101–103
11. Sasagawa I, Suzuki H, Izumi T, Shoji N, Nakada T, Takaoka S, Miura Y, Hoshi H, Amagasa S, Horikawa H (1999) Influence of carbon dioxide on respiratory function during posterior retroperitoneoscopic adrenalectomy in prone position. Eur Urol 36:413–417
12. Sasagawa I, Suzuki Y, Itoh K, Izumi T, Miura M, Suzuki H, Tomita Y (2003) Posterior retroperitoneoscopic partial adrenalectomy: clinical experience in 47 procedures. Eur Urol 43:381–385
13. Walz MK, Peitgen K, Krause U, Eigler F-W (1995) Die dorsale retroperitoneoskopische Adrenalektomie – eine neue operative Methode. Zentralbl Chir 120:53–58
14. Walz MK, Peitgen K, Hoermann R, Giebler RM, Mann K, Eigler FW (1996) Posterior retroperitoneoscopy as a new minimally invasive approach for adrenalectomy: results of 30 adrenalectomies in 27 patients. World J Surg 20:769–774
15. Walz MK, Peitgen K, Hoermann R, Giebler RM, Mann K, Eigler FW (1996) Posterior retroperitoneoscopy as a new minimally invasive approach for adrenalectomy: results of 30 adrenalectomies in 27 patients. World J Surg 20:769–774
16. Walz MK (1998) Minimal-invasive Nebennierenchirurgie. Chirurg 69:613–620
17. Walz MK, Peitgen K, Saller B, Giebler RM, Lederbogen S, Nimtz K, Mann K, Eigler FW (1998) Subtotal adrenalectomy by the posterior retroperitoneoscopic approach. World J Surg 22:621–626
18. Walz MK, Peitgen K, Walz MV, Hoermann R, Saller B, Giebler RM, Jockenhövel F, Philipp T, Broelsch CE, Eigler FW, Mann K (2001) Posterior retroperitoneoscopic adrenalectomy: lessons learned within five years. World J Surg 25:728–734
19. Walz MK, Peitgen K, Neumann HP, Janssen OE, Philipp T, Mann K (2002) Endoscopic treatment of solitary, bilateral, multiple, and recurrent pheochromocytomas and paragangliomas. World J Surg 26:1005–1012
20. Walz MK, Neumann HPH, Peitgen K, Petersenn S, Janssen OE, Mann K (2003) Endoscopic treatment of recurrent and extraadrenal pheochromocytomas. Eur Surg 35:93–96

36 Laparoscopic Partial Adrenalectomy

Geoffrey B. Thompson

Cortical-sparing adrenalectomy can be performed in an open or laparoscopic fashion. Small pheochromocytomas can be approached in an open fashion by either a dorsal lumbotomy or an open anterior approach. In patients with VHL lacking extensive intraabdominal adhesions, in those not requiring concomitant major pancreatic and renal procedures, and in patients with small unilateral or bilateral pheochromocytomas, the adrenal glands can be approached laparoscopically. Our preferred method is through a lateral transperitoneal approach. The principles for cortical-sparing surgery are the same as for open and laparoscopic techniques. The adrenal gland is exposed but not mobilized. In open cases, careful palpation is performed along with intraoperative ultrasonography to identify the location of the tumor. In laparoscopic cases, more emphasis is placed on visual inspection and *laparoscopic ultrasonography*, although subtle differences in texture of the gland can be noted with laparoscopic instrumentation. Once the location of the tumor is identified, only that part of the gland is mobilized. This is performed carefully with clips, electrocautery, and harmonic scalpel. Only arterial tributaries to the involved segment(s) (aortic, renal, or phrenic) are divided. If the main adrenal vein is in this region, it too is divided. Provided the remainder of the gland is left in situ, without mobilization, there are sufficient emissary veins running with the remaining arterial tributaries to maintain adequate venous drainage. When an adequate amount of gland has been mobilized, it can be separated from the segments to be spared by means of a stapling device or harmonic scalpel. Once the specimen is removed, it must be examined by the surgeon and pathologist to ensure an adequate margin around the pheochromocytoma (Figs. 1–5).

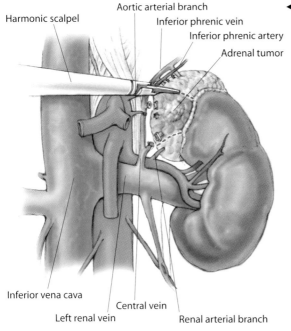

Harmonic scalpel
Aortic arterial branch
Inferior phrenic vein
Inferior phrenic artery
Adrenal tumor
Inferior vena cava
Central vein
Left renal vein
Renal arterial branch

◀ **Fig. 1.** Cortical-sparing left adrenalectomy (CSA) with central resection. Central vein and aortic branches have been divided. No mobilization is performed of remaining upper and lower poles to protect emissary veins and arterial branches (inferior phrenic and renal). Transection is performed laparoscopically using a harmonic scalpel

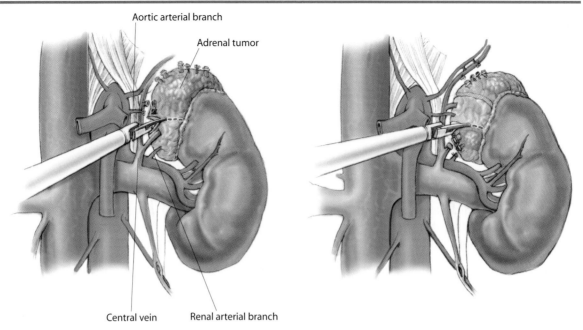

Fig. 2. CSA (*left*) with resection of superior pole tumor. Only inferior phrenic branches are divided

Fig. 3. Upper and lower pole tumors resected. Midportion of gland preserved on aortic arterial branch and emissary veins

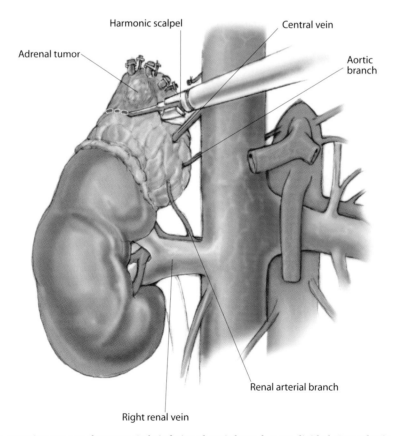

Fig. 4. Right CSA resecting upper pole tumor. Only inferior phrenic branches are divided. Central vein is preserved

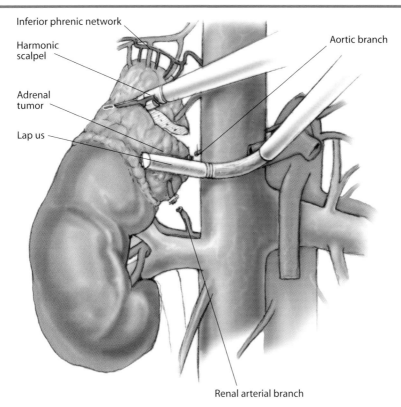

Inferior phrenic network

Harmonic
scalpel

Adrenal
tumor

Lap us

Aortic branch

Renal arterial branch

Fig. 5. Lower pole is resected by dividing aortic and renal arterial branches with their emissary veins. Central vein is preserved.
The intraoperative ultrasound rules out other intraparenchymal nodularity

37 Virtual Reality and Robotic Technologies in Adrenal Surgery

Jacques Marescaux, Francesco Rubino, Luc Soler

CONTENTS

37.1 Introduction

Despite the introduction of laparoscopy, which has revolutionized the practice and concepts of adrenal surgery, several issues still need to be addressed. For instance, in many cases, current diagnostic tools do not allow the accurate prediction of the risk of malignancy in pheochromocytomas; in addition, adrenocortical carcinoma is very rarely diagnosed at an early and potentially curable stage. These limitations become even more important in the era of laparoscopic adrenalectomy since adrenal cancer is considered an absolute contraindication for a laparoscopic approach due to the risk of dissemination. Although recent reports suggest that fears about the oncologic inadequacy of laparoscopic adrenalectomy might be unjustified [1], there is no question that operating an adrenal cancer laparoscopically is much more challenging than operating on a small benign lesion. The surgeon would ideally like to know about the presence of a cancer prior to operation. Furthermore, even the most experienced surgeon would agree that vena caval invasion contraindicates a laparoscopic approach. Unfortunately, this prediction is not possible in all patients.

The management of adrenal incidentalomas is also controversial. Incidentalomas have a frequency of about 1.3% of all patients undergoing abdominal computerized tomographic examinations; this incidence rises to 8% in necropsy series. The incidence of adrenocortical carcinoma, however, is extremely rare at about 1/800,000. Larger adrenal lesions are associated with increased risk of cancer, and incidentalomas larger than 6 cm should be removed; there is general consensus that tumors smaller than 3 cm do not represent an indication for surgery, whether the operation is performed laparoscopically or not. However, there is a tendency to consider the decreased invasiveness of laparoscopic surgery as an argument to broaden surgical indications for smaller sized incidentalomas. Miccoli et al. [2] documented an increase in the number of patients referred for adrenalectomy after the introduction of laparoscopic adrenalectomy, and, in particular more patients were referred who had adrenal metastases and incidentalomas.

Is it justifiable to operate on patients with/and for smaller incidentalomas? Proponents of this strategy argue that this may be the only way to "pick up" adrenal cancers at an earlier stage, and that the minimally invasive removal of an adrenal mass may be preferable to lifelong follow-up, where the likelihood of malignancy is assessed by size on CT scanning, a somewhat arbitrary approach. Furthermore, different size criteria have in fact been used when determining surgical indications in different centers. Importantly, some reports suggest that the cross-sectional anatomy represented by 2-dimensional CT studies may be inaccurate and therefore result in an inadequate estimation of the actual adrenal size and surgical indications which may be inappropriate for the individual patient [3–5]. Thus, better criteria for establishing when incidentalomas should be removed are highly desirable.

There are, in addition, technical issues about adrenal surgery for consideration. Since the initial report by Gagner in 1992 [6], laparoscopic adrenalectomy has rapidly become the surgical procedure of choice for the treatment of benign adrenal lesions. However, laparoscopic adrenalectomy can at times be challenging. This is the case in obese patients, where even tumoral glands may be very difficult to identify. Previous surgery on the kidney, pancreas, or spleen may render the transperitoneal approach challenging especially for surgeons with limited laparoscopic experience. In general, the advent of minimally invasive techniques has further emphasized the importance and potential danger to patients of the learning curve in surgery, creating a need for alternative training models and improvement in surgical education to enhance patient safety.

The introduction of new technologies may possibly help surgeons address and hopefully solve many of the issues mentioned.

In recent years, computer-based image acquisition modalities have matured to the point that they are now capable of accurate 3D reconstructions of an organ system or body region. The advantages of these virtual reality (VR) systems consist in the creation of a virtual environment where complex structures are represented in a fully 3-dimensional manner, which gives the surgeon the ability to interact with the image as if it truly exists, understanding the anatomy of a structure, the features of a lesion, performing tasks and manipulations, as well as navigation within the lumen of blood vessels.

37.2   Current Clinical Applications of Virtual Reality in General Surgery

By using dedicated computer software, virtual reality 3D reconstructions are obtained by the processing of the digital data of current 2D imaging modalities, usually CT scan or MRI acquisitions. Applications of virtual reality have thus far been used mainly for preoperative diagnostic evaluations, which included virtual gastroscopy, bronchoscopy and colonoscopy as well as virtual reconstruction of liver tumors prior to resection.

At the European Institute of Telesurgery we have developed an institutional software program for 3-D virtual cholangioscopy, based on cholangioMRI (MRCP) data acquisition. The software reconstructs the anatomy of the biliary system, including the gallbladder, the common bile duct as well as the intrahepatic biliary branches; this enables virtual navigation and transparency of all structures as well as the automated detection of stones. In a clinical study [7] we found that the 3D virtual cholangiography had sensitivity and specificity rates higher than standard MRCP,

and provided a detailed preoperative reconstruction of the biliary anatomy.

The development of systems for 3D reconstruction of liver anatomy and hepatic lesions has been shown to improve tumor localization ability. Lamade' and coworkers [8] have reported a clinical study showing that the ability to adequately assign a tumoral lesion to a liver segment was significantly increased by 3D reconstruction when compared with 2D computed tomographic scans. Computer engineers of the "Virtual Surgery Team" at our Institute have developed a fully automated software program that, from CT scan images, provides, in less than 5 min, an automated 3D reconstruction of anatomical and pathological structures of the liver as well as invisible functional information such as portal vein labeling and anatomical segment delineation according to the Couinaud definition. In our experience, clinical application and correlation of this method in more than 40 patients showed that automated delineation of anatomical

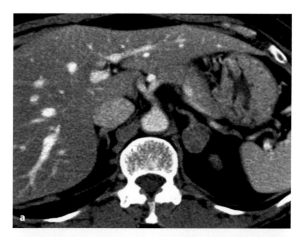

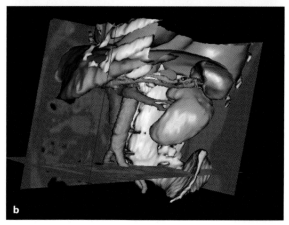

Fig. 1. a CT scan demonstrating a 3-cm left adrenal mass; **b** its VR reconstruction

structures was sufficiently accurate and even more sensitive and specific than manual delineation performed by a radiologist.

37.3 Possible Applications of VR in Adrenal Surgery

37.3.1 The EITS VR Software

We have applied a 3D VR software program developed at our Institution for reconstruction of the adrenal glands in five patients presenting with adrenal lesions. From spiral CT contrasted images with 2 mm slices, using a Unix SGI octane 2 computer station with a R12000 processor at 400 MHz and 1 Gb of RAM, our VR software automatically detected, delineated and reconstructed most intra-abdominal organs. The adrenal glands were automatically reconstructed and tu-

mors were hand delineated (Fig. 1). This preliminary clinical experience demonstrated the feasibility of using VR systems for 3D reconstruction of the adrenal glands and its lesions, and suggested a number of possible interesting applications.

37.3.1.1 Diagnostics

The interest in VR for the diagnosis of adrenal lesions is due to the fact that it has the unique advantage of automatically reconstructing the gland and facilitating the delineation of the lesion in the gland. In newer versions of the software we should also be able to achieve automatic delineation of lesions as well. The differentiation between the structure of the normal gland and pathological lesions can be enhanced with high contrast by combining the use of thresholding, mathematical morphology and colors. Furthermore, more

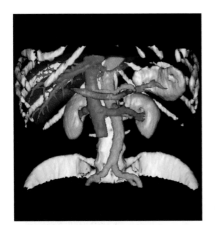
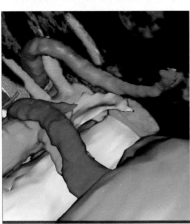
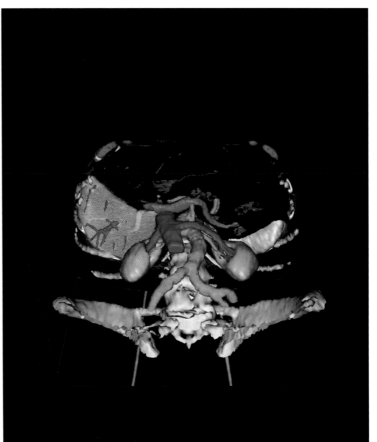

Fig. 2. Although best viewed on a computer monitor screen, these still pictures show how we create a virtual environment where complex structures are represented in a fully three-dimensional way. The surgeon has the ability to interact with the image, and understand the anatomy of a structure, the features of a lesion and the relationship with different organs and vessels

than conventional imaging, the 3D reconstruction helps understanding the reciprocal relationship between the gland, the lesion and adjacent organs. This is also facilitated by the unique ability of VR to allow visualization of structures from virtually any angle of view, as opposed to the flat image obtained with a CT scan or an MRI scan (Fig. 2).

Another important feature of this virtual reality adrenal reconstruction is that it allows "navigation" within the lumen of vessels (Fig. 3), with the obvious implication for the preoperative investigation of venous thrombosis or tumoral invasion in the inferior vena cava or renal veins. Furthermore, simultaneous reconstruction of other organs such as the liver allows evaluation of patients with plurimetastatic diseases, facilitating the monitoring of the response to chemotherapy (Fig. 4).

Moreover, VR allows for precise and measurable evaluation of the volume of an adrenal lesion, which might be better than simply using diameter size as a parameter to evaluate the potential malignancy of a tumor and the surgical indications in patients with incidentalomas. We are currently trying to investigate the accuracy of VR in assessing the size and volume of adrenal glands and lesions in comparison to conventional imaging methods. Further investigation will be needed to understand the significance of volume in predicting the nature of a lesion.

37.3.1.2   Education and Training

To date, surgical residents' education has been highly dependent upon the patients that actually present to

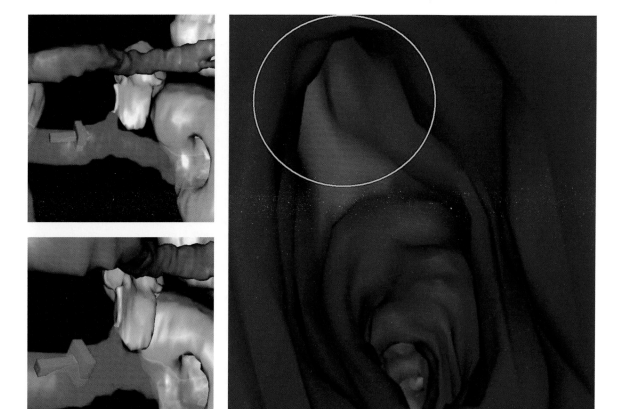

Fig. 3. VR allows the use of virtual transparency of organs and vessels and, importantly, the intraluminal navigation in hollow organs or vessels. The pictures show the VR reconstruction of one of our patients with a left adrenal lesion (in *green*). The image *on the right* shows the inside view of the left renal vein, with the *yellow circle* indicating the origin of the main adrenal vein. This navigation allows the detection of eventual stenosis for thrombosis or tumoral invasion. The *left image* shows a red cursor indicating the real-time position inside the lumen

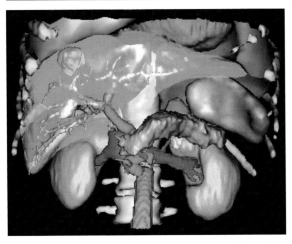

Fig. 4. Three-dimensional VR reconstruction of a patient presenting with metastatic lesions involving the liver and the left adrenal. The virtual transparency of the liver shows the inner portal vessels. Metastatic lesions are colored in *green* and easily recognized from the normal parenchyma

simulators. The trainees can practice, for instance, laparoscopic adrenalectomy to achieve a higher degree of proficiency before performing the procedure clinically.

The ability to objectively assess technical skills and performance by tracking hand motion and the economy of the trainee's movements with the computer has important implications. Digital representation of the human form allows the incorporation of anatomical, functional and pathological data, so that next generations of virtual reality systems and simulators could be used as part of a certification processes.

In total, all the opportunities afforded by VR and simulation may improve the level of surgical education and result in a better quality of performance in clinical adrenal surgery.

37.3.1.3 Preoperative Planning

We have used our software to simulate the first steps of a laparoscopic adrenalectomy in our patients. VR reconstructions can indeed be used to perform a "virtual laparoscopy" (Fig. 5) to help in planning a correct trocar and instrument positioning, calculating the ideal distance between trocars according to the patient's specific body habitus and internal anatomy (Fig. 6).

Unlike neurosurgery and orthopedic surgery where firm bony reference frames are available, in adrenal surgery virtual operation planning, on the basis of 3D reconstruction of soft tissues, has to overcome the obstacles of the inherent mobility and flexibility of the abdominal organs, especially when simulating a transperitoneal laparoscopic approach. As a result, current virtual reality systems have not yet achieved the necessary level of perfection to be used for a reliable simulation. In the near future, however, it is likely that the technical issues will be solved and better surgical simulators will become available. The 3D reconstruction of the patient's specific anatomical structures and lesions, as well as anomalies, can certainly help surgeons better comprehend and plan the proposed procedure for each patient, as well as anticipate possible dangers and identify the optimal plane for dissection or resection.

A further application of VR is the preoperative simulation and planning of robotic assisted surgery. Combining virtual laparoscopy with a virtual Zeus robotic system we experimented with the possibility of simulating the surgical gestures required for a specific procedure in a given patient with the system able to process this information and anticipate possible con-

the service during their period of rotation, with consequent risk of lack of exposure to important types of surgical procedures. Adrenal surgery is not common practice in every hospital and training center. There may be residents that very rarely have the opportunity to participate in a laparoscopic adrenalectomy. Virtual reality and surgical simulators can provide the opportunity to expose each resident to a wider surgical experience and to make the training more uniform for residents in a single training program or even across many institutions.

Virtual reality images, similar to other digital data, can also be easily transferred real-time to distant locations, for tele-education programs in which education from a distant expert can be transmitted to those of the local faculty. An example of this was provided by Silverstein et al. [9], who used a teleimmersive virtual reality environment for simultaneously teaching liver segments and portal vein anatomy to senior surgical residents at two different locations. These authors reported effective acquisition of the new knowledge with no difference between those residents who were with the instructor and those at the remote location as shown by a 24-question examination test administered prior to and after the anatomy workshop.

Extremely important for education and training in adrenal surgery is the ability of VR to provide a safe training environment where errors can be made without consequences to a patient ("learning curve") and where the learning process is based upon learning the cause of failure. This is the basic concept of surgical

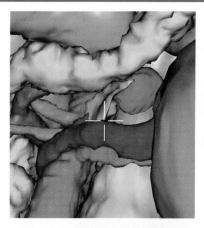
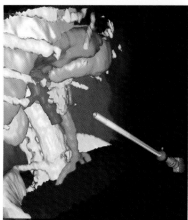
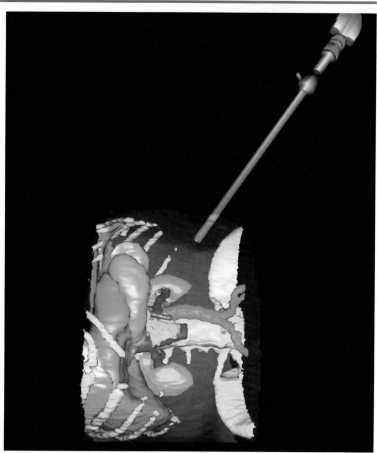

Fig. 5. The concept of virtual laparoscopy. The patient's abdominal organs as well as the skin are reconstructed from a CT scan. The virtual laparoscope is inserted and the internal view is shown just as it would be when using a regular laparoscope in the same patient. Virtual laparoscopy could be used to replace laparoscopic diagnostic explorations or to perform surgical planning

flict between robotic arms and therefore being helpful in planning ideal robotic arm positioning for a smoother operation. This can apply to robotic assisted adrenalectomy as well as to other procedures.

37.3.1.4   The Concept of 4D and the Interest of VR in Patients with Adrenal Incidentalomas

Follow-up of adrenal lesions using medical imaging is limited to a subjective mental reconstruction. VR can be used for assessment of the evolution in time of the volume and morphology of tumors. At our Institute the images of 3D reconstruction of one patient with adrenal and liver metastasis undergoing chemotherapy and one patient with an adrenal incidentaloma were evaluated over time. The virtual images obtained by serial follow-up CT scans were processed by the software and superimposed resulting in a precise and

measurable evaluation of the volume of the lesion and its evolution over time. This is the concept of 4D VR, that is, 3D in time. The main difficulty encountered at the present time lies in the difference in position of the patient and the organ. New global positioning systems and magnetic sensor tools are currently in the developmental stage to overcome this major drawback. However, 4D imaging for the assessment of the evolution of adrenal tumors is a promising novel tool and concept that represents a major step forward for the objective follow-up of tumor growth, with important implications for the management of adrenal incidentalomas as well as for evaluating the therapeutic response in cancer patients. We are now in the process of performing clinical investigations to verify the reliability and significance of this concept in adrenal surgery. It is likely that it may rapidly become a valuable option for the follow-up of incidental adrenal lesions.

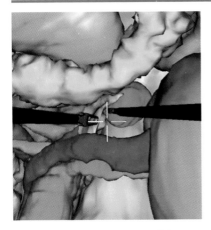
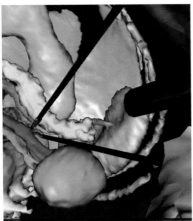
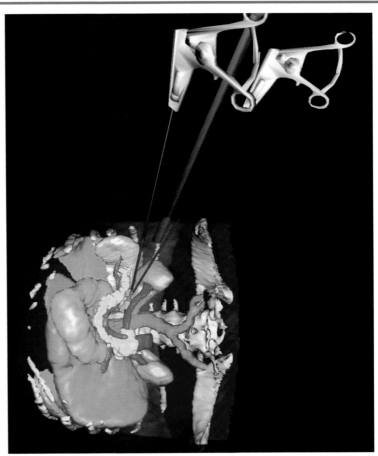

Fig. 6. Planning of trocar positioning in a patient undergoing VR reconstruction. The software allows placement of our virtual patient in the lateral decubitus position. A virtual laparoscope and instruments are placed in the desired position. The smaller windows *on the left* show the inside view and allow planning of the ideal angulation between our dissecting instruments and anticipate possible conflicts. Once the best suitable position has been chosen, the software can calculate the distance, in centimeters, from the ribs as well as between the trocars. This is a preliminary step in the performance of a simulated laparoscopic adrenalectomy

37.4   Robotic Adrenal Surgery

The introduction of robotic systems in surgery was welcomed as an opportunity to improve surgical performance. Indeed, due to their intrinsic characteristics, and the ability to merge together a telemanipulator system with computer interfaces, surgical robots allow tremor filtering, motion downscaling and improved endurance [10, 11]. With these tenets, there have been claims that robotic assisted surgery may, in fact, be better than conventional laparoscopy. However, after being tested in virtually every type of general surgery, robotic systems failed to maintain, at least so far, their promises of making surgery easier for the surgeon and better for the patient. For instance, at the 2003 SAGES Meeting, the data of two multicenter prospective randomized studies performed in the USA were presented [12, 13]. The studies compared robotic assisted cholecystectomy and Nissen fundoplication to the respective procedures performed by conventional laparoscopy. In both operations, the robotic assisted operations were performed with significantly longer operative time than in conventional laparoscopy; however, complications, blood loss and functional outcomes were similar between robotic and conventional laparoscopic surgery. These and other reports are consistent in showing that robotic assisted procedures are as safe and effective as standard laparoscopic procedures but that longer operative times and no significant clinical benefits can be expected from the use of robotic assistance in general abdominal surgery.

Case reports and small case-series about robotic assisted adrenalectomy have been reported [14–16] or presented in several international surgical meetings. One may argue that since adrenalectomy is simply a resective procedure with no anastomosis or extensive suturing or other difficult tasks involved, there is little need, if any, for robotic enhancement of dexterity in laparoscopic adrenalectomy. However, enhancement of dexterity is not the only advantage of robotics.

Our group has shown that robotic assistance can be used for performing surgical operations remotely, even across transatlantic distances [17, 18]. This application of robotics has interest not only for reaching patients located distantly but also to make expert assistance available for surgeons in virtually any location. This may be very helpful when young surgeons perform an operation early in their learning curve, or, for instance, to help endocrine surgeons who have little laparoscopic experience implementing laparoscopic adrenalectomy in their routine practice.

A further advantage of VR simulations is that, in the near future, the digital data of the best simulated procedure could be recorded and replayed by a robot automatically and at a distance. Combining VR with advanced robotics could guide the surgeons through technically challenging procedures and avoid injury to vital structures. The idea of automated surgery is fascinating, but several issues and limitations of current technology need yet to be overcome.

To make dreams come true there is a lot of work to do.

37.5   Conclusions

Virtual reality has great potential to help in several aspects of adrenal surgery, including education and training, preoperative diagnostics, preoperative planning, and intra- and postoperative applications. Furthermore, the possibilities afforded by robotic systems, integrated with virtual and augmented reality capabilities, may further improve surgical technique and possibly blunt the learning curve and reduce the operative risks associated with the early phase of education in new technology.

References

1. Kebebew E, Siperstein AE, Clark OH, Duh QY (2002) Results of laparoscopic adrenalectomy for suspected and unsuspected malignant adrenal neoplasms. Arch Surg 137:948–51
2. Miccoli P, Raffaelli M, Berti P, Materazzi G, Massi M, Bernini G (2002) Adrenal surgery before and after the introduction of laparoscopic adrenalectomy. Br J Surg 89: 779–82
3. Lau H, Lo CY, Lam KY (1999) Surgical implications of underestimation of adrenal tumour size by computed tomography. Br J Surg 86:385–7
4. Linos DA, Stylopoulos N (1997) How accurate is computed tomography in predicting the real size of adrenal tumors? A retrospective study. Arch Surg 132:740–3
5. Barnett CC, Varma DG, El-Naggar AK, et al. (2000) Limitations of size as a criterion in the evaluation of adrenal tumors. Surgery 128:973–82
6. Gagner M, Lacroix A, Bolte E (1992) Laparoscopic adrenalectomy in Cushing's syndrome and pheochromocytoma. N Engl J Med 327:1033
7. Simone M, Mutter D, Rubino F, Dutson E, Roy C, Soler L, Marescaux J (2004) Three dimensional virtual cholangioscopy: a reliable tool for the diagnosis of common bile duct stones. Ann Surg 240(1):82–8
8. Lamade W, Glombitza G, Fischer L, Chiu P, Cardenas CE Sr, Thorn M, Meinzer HP, Grenacher L, Bauer H, Lehnert T, Herfarth C (2000) The impact of 3-dimensional reconstructions on operation planning in liver surgery. Arch Surg 135:1256–1261
9. Silverstein JC, Dech F, Edison M, Jurek P, Helton WS, Espat NJ (2002) Virtual reality: immersive hepatic surgery educational environment. Surgery 132:274–7
10. Garcia-Ruiz A, Gagner M, Miller JH, Steiner CP, Hahn JF (1998) Manual vs robotically assisted laparoscopic surgery in the performance of basic manipulation and suturing tasks. Arch Surg 133:957–961
11. Reichenspurner H, Boehm D, Reichart B (1999) Minimally invasive mitral valve surgery using three-dimensional video and robotic assistance. Semin Thorac Cardiovasc Surg 11:235–240
12. White P, Carbajal-Ramos A, Gracia C, Nunez-Gonzales E, Bailey R, Broderick T, DeMaria E, Hollands C, Soper N (2003) A prospective randomised study of the Zeus robotic surgical system for laparoscopic anti-reflux surgery. Proceedings of the SAGES 2003 Meeting, Los Angeles, CA, March 12-15. S027; 81
13. White P, Carbajal-Ramos A, Gracia C, Nunez-Gonzales E, Bailey R, Broderick T, DeMaria E, Hollands C, Soper N (2003) A prospective randomised study of the Zeus robotic surgical system for laparoscopic cholecystectomy. Proceedings of the SAGES 2003 Meeting, Los Angeles, CA, March 12-15. S061, 89
14. Brunaud L, Bresler L, Ayav A, Tretou S, Cormier L, Klein M, Boissel P (2003) Advantages of using robotic Da Vinci((R)) system for unilateral adrenalectomy: early results. Ann Chir 128:530–5 (French)

15. Desai MM, Gill IS, Kaouk JH, Matin SF, Sung GT, Bravo EL (2002) Robotic-assisted laparoscopic adrenalectomy. Urology 60:1104–7

16. Young JA, Chapman WH 3rd, Kim VB, Albrecht RJ, Ng PC, Nifong LW, Chitwood WR Jr (2002) Robotic-assisted adrenalectomy for adrenal incidentaloma: case and review of the technique. Surg Laparosc Endosc Percutan Tech 12:126–30

17. Marescaux J, Leroy J, Gagner M, Rubino F, Mutter D, Vix M, Butner SE, Smith MK (2001) Transatlantic robot-assisted telesurgery. Nature 413:379–80

18. Marescaux J, Leroy J, Rubino F, Smith M, Vix M, Simone M, Mutter D (2002) Transcontinental robot-assisted remote telesurgery: feasibility and potential applications. Ann Surg 235:487–92

Subject Index